ULTRASONOGRAPHY
in OBSTETRICS and GYNECOLOGY

PETER W. CALLEN, M.D. Associate Professor
Departments of Radiology,
Obstetrics and Gynecology and Reproductive Sciences,
University of California School of Medicine
San Francisco, California

W. B. SAUNDERS COMPANY Philadelphia   London   Toronto
Mexico City   Rio de Janeiro   Sydney   Tokyo

W. B. Saunders Company: West Washington Square
Philadelphia, PA 19105

1 St. Anne's Road
Eastbourne, East Sussex BN 21 3UN, England

1 Goldthorne Avenue
Toronto, Ontario M8Z 5T9, Canada

Cedro 512
Mexico 4, D.F. Mexico

Rua Coronel Cabrita, 8
Sao Cristovao Caixa Postal 21176
Rio de Janeiro, Brazil

9 Waltham Street
Artarmon, N.S.W. 2064, Australia

Ichibancho, Central Bldg., 22-1 Ichibancho
Chiyoda-Ku, Tokyo 102, Japan

Library of Congress Cataloging in Publication Data

Callen, Peter W.
   Ultrasonography in obstetrics and gynecology.

   1. Ultrasonics in obstetrics. 2. Generative organs, Female—Diseases—Diagnosis. 3. Diagnosis, Ultrasonic.
I. Title. [DNLM: 1. Ultrasonics—Diagnostic use.
2. Genital diseases, Female—Diagnosis. 3. Obstetrics.
4. Fetal monitoring. WQ 100 U47]
RG527.5.U48C34   1982   618   82-42616
ISBN 0-7216-2331-X

Ultrasonography in Obstetrics and Gynecology   ISBN 0-7216-2331-X

© 1983 by W. B. Saunders Company. Copyright under the Uniform Copyright Convention. Simultaneously published in Canada. All rights reserved. This book is protected by copyright. No part of it may be reproduced, stored in a retrieval system, or transmitted in any form or by any means, electronic, mechanical, photocopying, recording, or otherwise, without written permission from the publisher. Made in the United States of America. Press of W. B. Saunders Company. Library of Congress catalog card number 82-42616.

Last digit is the print number: 9   8   7   6   5   4   3   2

To Melanie and Brooke

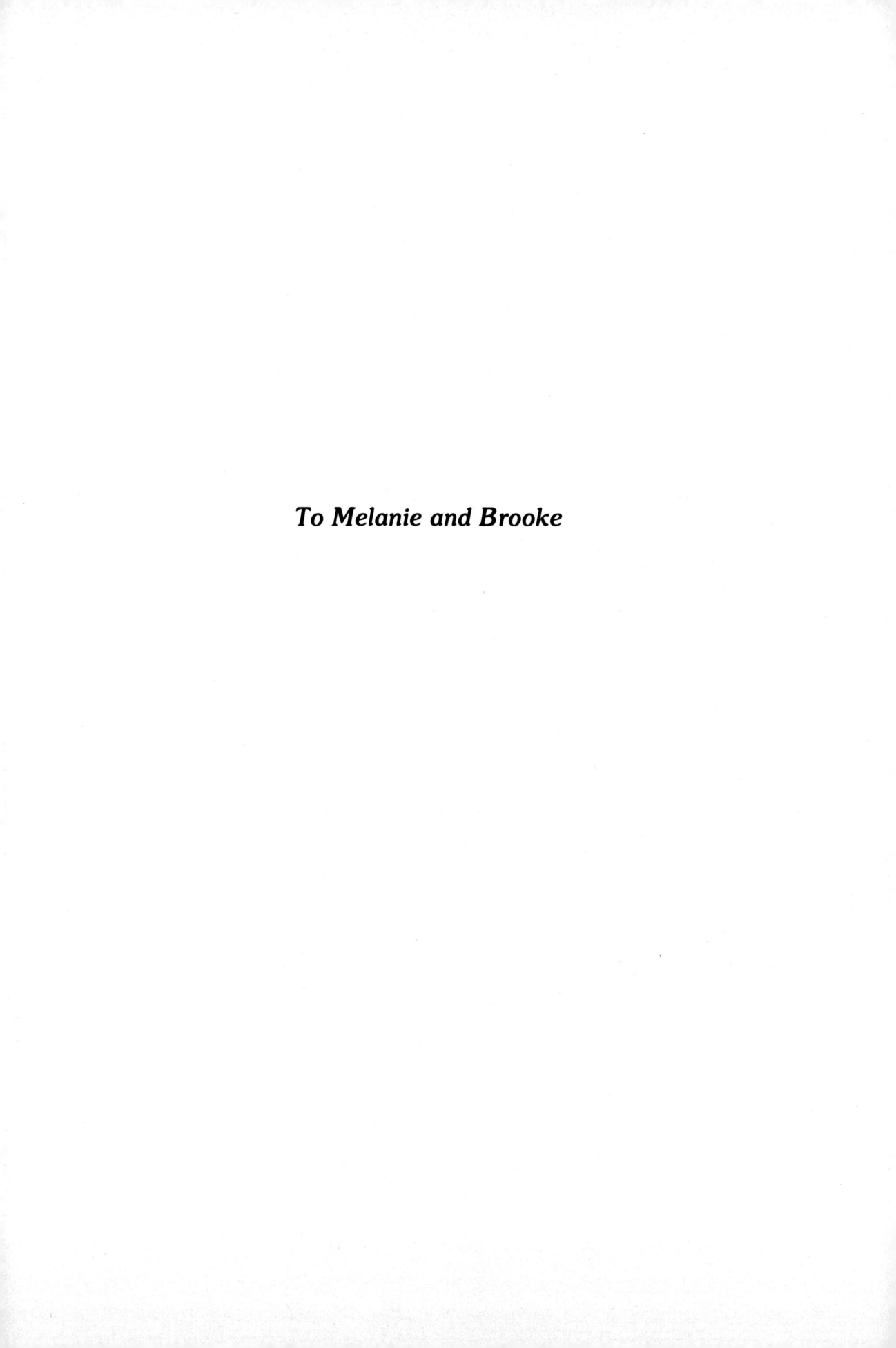

Preface

The field of ultrasonography has undergone dramatic change since its introduction into the arena of medical diagnosis over 20 years ago. Nowhere are the remarkable advances more evident than in the application of diagnostic ultrasound to the obstetric and gynecologic patient. At its inception ultrasound was limited to the most basic descriptions and measurements of the fetus for the purpose of dating and identifying a cystic mass within the female pelvis. Presently, however, subtle abnormalities of almost of every fetal organ system are being imaged routinely in many ultrasound laboratories, and ultrasound is playing a major role in the in utero treatment of several of these anomalies.

The major advances that have occurred in ultrasound have been technological, particularly with regard to real-time instrumentation. There has, however, also been a dramatic improvement in our understanding of the normal anatomy of both the fetus and nongravid female pelvis as well as a clearer understanding of the pathophysiology of many disease processes.

The idea for this text came in late 1981 when I was asked to edit an issue of the *Radiologic Clinics of North America* on Ultrasonography in Obstetrics and Gynecology. While I wished to cover most areas applicable to the sonographer caring for the obstetric and gynecologic patient, I was limited in both space and readership by the nature of this periodical. While textbooks are available that deal with the subject, I felt the need for an up-to-date, practical, and comprehensive text on obstetric and gynecologic ultrasound. Several of the manuscripts utilized in the *Radiologic Clinics* issue are included here but have been expanded with additional information, illustrations, and line drawings. In addition, 11 completely new chapters have been added to make this a comprehensive text.

No single text can serve as an exhaustive review of the anatomy, physiology, and pathology of a medical specialty. This text is certainly no exception. The authors have, however, included a wealth of both "state of the art" illustrations, line drawings, and explanations of the anatomy and pathophysiology of disease to serve both the neophyte and "seasoned" ultrasonographer who wish to gain more knowledge in the area of obstetric and gynecologic ultrasound. To this end I feel the major original goal of this text has been accomplished.

It is difficult to acknowledge all those who have contributed to the compilation of this text. The individual authors are to be congratulated for their excellent reviews of their subject material, providing exhaustive, timely, and practical presentations of their areas of expertise. Many individuals have contributed indirectly, enhancing my own knowledge of the field of ultrasound. These include the technologists with whom I have worked closely over the years as well as the many residents, fellows, and referring clinicians who have continuously challenged the "accepted facts" of ultrasound, ultimately leading to a clearer understanding of both the normal and abnormal. My close associate and friend Roy Filly has served as an inspiration to me in this field not only on the basis of his diagnostic acumen but because of his good judgment and kindness as well. The support of my family cannot be overstated.

It was a pleasure to work with the W. B. Saunders Company. I am indebted for their support, cooperation, and expedient publication of this text. While there are many unnamed people at Saunders who helped in the preparation of this text, this work would not have been possible without the excellent guidance of its Medical Editor, Linda Belfus. She helped to develop the concept for this text and meticulously guided this work in all of its aspects from beginning to completion. She personally put a great deal of effort into the publication of this text and her personable nature made this publishing experience a pleasant one for me. Lastly, I would like to thank my secretary, Jean Quinn, who worked innumerable hours on this text and without whose assistance this work would not have been possible.

PETER W. CALLEN, M.D.

Contributors

Rochelle Filker Andreotti, M.D.
Resident, Department of Radiology, Jackson Memorial Hospital and University of Miami, Miami, Florida

Lincoln L. Berland, M.D.
Assistant Professor of Radiology, Medical College of Wisconsin; Radiologist, Milwaukee County Medical Complex, Froedtert Memorial Luthern Hospital, Milwaukee, Wisconsin

Jason C. Birnholz, M.D.
Radiologist-in-Chief, Lying-in Division, Brigham-Women's Hospital; Assistant Professor of Radiology, Harvard Medical School, Boston, Massachusetts

James D. Bowie, M.D.
Associate Professor of Radiology, Assistant Professor of Obstetrics and Gynecology, and Chief, Section of Ultrasound, Duke University Medical Center, Durham, North Carolina

Peter W. Callen, M.D.
Associate Professor, Departments of Radiology, Obstetrics and Gynecology and Reproductive Sciences, University of California School of Medicine, San Francisco, California

Russell L. Deter, M.D.
Associate Professor and Director of Obstetrical Ultrasound, Department of Obstetrics and Gynecology, Baylor College of Medicine, Houston, Texas

Michael P. Federle, M.D.
Associate Professor of Radiology, University of California; Chief of Computed Body Tomography, San Francisco General Hospital, San Francisco, California

Roy A. Filly, M.D.
Professor, Departments of Radiology, Obstetrics and Gynecology, and Reproductive Sciences, University of California School of Medicine, San Francisco, California

Charles E. Fiske, M.D.
Assistant Clinical Professor, Department of Radiology, University of California School of Medicine, San Francisco, California

Arthur C. Fleischer, M.D.
Assistant Professor of Radiology and Obstetrics and Gynecology, Vanderbilt University Medical Center, Nashville, Tennessee

W. Dennis Foley, M.D.
Associate Professor of Radiology, Medical College of Wisconsin; Chief, Angiography and Co-Director, Section of Digital Imaging, Milwaukee County Medical Complex, Froedtert Memorial Lutheran Hospital, Milwaukee, Wisconsin

Mitchell S. Golbus, M.D.

Professor, Departments of Obstetrics, Gynecology and Reproductive Sciences and Pediatrics, University of California School of Medicine, San Francisco, California

Peter Grannum, M.D.

Assistant Professor, Director of Medical Studies, Department of Obstetrics and Gynecology, Yale University School of Medicine, New Haven, Connecticut

Barry H. Gross, M.D.

Assistant Professor of Radiology, University of Michigan Medical Center, Ann Arbor, Michigan

Frank P. Hadlock, M.D.

Associate Professor of Radiology, Baylor College of Medicine; Chief of Radiology, Women's Hospital of Texas and Jefferson Davis Hospital, Houston, Texas

Michael R. Harrison, M.D.

Associate Professor of Surgery (Pediatric Surgery), University of California School of Medicine, San Francisco, California

Ronald B. Harrist, Ph.D.

Associate Research Biometrician, University of Texas School of Public Health, Houston, Texas

Richard Hattan, M.D.

Instructor in Ultrasound and Radiology, Division of Diagnostic Ultrasound, Department of Radiology, University of Colorado Health Sciences Center, Denver, Colorado

Sidney C. Henderson, M.D.

Associate Professor of Radiology and Chief of Ultrasound Section, University of Oregon Health Sciences Center, Portland, Oregon

John C. Hobbins, M.D.

Professor, Departments of Obstetrics and Gynecology and Diagnostic Radiology, Yale University School of Medicine; Director of Obstetrics, Yale-New Haven Medical Center, New Haven, Connecticut

A. Everette James, Jr., Sc.M., J.D., M.D.

Professor and Chairman, Department of Radiology and Radiological Sciences, Vanderbilt University Medical Center, Nashville, Tennessee

R. Brooke Jeffrey, M.D.

Assistant Professor of Radiology, University of California; Staff Radiologist, San Francisco General Hospital, San Francisco, California

Howard W. Jones, III, M.D.

Assistant Professor of Obstetrics and Gynecology, Vanderbilt University Medical Center, Nashville, Tennessee

Michael L. Johnson, M.D.

Associate Professor of Radiology and Medicine; Director, Division of Diagnostic Ultrasound, Department of Radiology, University of Colorado Health Sciences Center, Denver, Colorado

John Q. Knochel, M.D.

Assistant Professor of Radiology, Oral Roberts University, City of Faith Medical and Research Center, Tulsa, Oklahoma

Frederick W. Kremkau, Ph.D.

Associate Professor of Diagnostic Radiology, Yale University School of Medicine, New Haven, Connecticut

Alfred B. Kurtz, M.D.

Associate Professor of Diagnostic Radiology and Obstetrics and Gynecology, Jefferson Medical College, Thomas Jefferson University, Philadelphia, Pennsylvania

Faye C. Laing, M.D.

Associate Professor of Radiology, University of California, San Francisco; Chief, Ultrasound Section, San Francisco General Hospital, San Francisco, California

Thomas L. Lawson, M.D.

Professor of Radiology, Medical College of Wisconsin; Co-Director, Section of Digital Imaging, Milwaukee County Medical Complex, Froedtert Memorial Lutheran Hospital, Milwaukee, Wisconsin

Timothy G. Lee, M.D.

Professor of Radiology, University of Utah Medical Center, Salt Lake City, Utah

Clifford S. Levi, M.D.

Assistant Professor of Radiology, University of Manitoba; Radiologist, Section of Diagnostic Ultrasound, Health Sciences Centre, Winnipeg, Canada

Edward A. Lyons, M.D.

Associate Professor of Radiology, University of Manitoba; Director, Section of Diagnostic Ultrasound, Health Sciences Centre, Winnipeg, Manitoba, Canada

Michael G. Melendez, M.D.

Chief of Radiology, Bonner General Hospital, Sandpoint, Idaho

Grant K. Rees, R.T.

Visiting Rotary Scholar and Ultrasound Technologist, University of Colorado School of Medicine, Denver, Colorado (from Invercargill, New Zealand)

Matthew D. Rifkin, M.D.

Assistant Professor of Radiology, Jefferson Medical College, Thomas Jefferson University Hospital, Philadelphia, Pennsylvania

Anne Colston Wentz, M.D.

Professor of Obstetrics and Gynecology, Vanderbilt University School of Medicine, Nashville, Tennessee

Contents

1
Ultrasound in the First Trimester of Pregnancy 1
E. A. Lyons and C. S. Levi

2
Estimating Gestational Age In Utero 21
James D. Bowie and Rochelle Filker Andreotti

3
Normal Fetal Anatomy... 41
Michael L. Johnson, Grant K. Rees, and Richard A. Hattan

4
Fetal Anomalies Involving the Thorax and Abdomen 61
*John Q. Knochel, Timothy G. Lee, Michael G. Melendez,
and Sidney C. Henderson*

5
Ultrasonography of the Normal and Pathologic Fetal Skeleton 81
Roy A. Filly and Mitchell Golbus

6
Ultrasound Evaluation of the Normal and Abnormal Fetal Neural
Axis.. 97
Charles E. Fiske and Roy A. Filly

7
Evaluation of Normal Fetal Growth and Detection of Intrauterine
Growth Retardation... 113
Russell L. Deter, Frank P. Hadlock, and Ronald B. Harrist

8
The Placenta 141
Peter Grannum and John C. Hobbins

9
Fetal Behavior and Condition 159
Jason C. Birnholz

10
The Role of Ultrasound in Prenatal Diagnostic Procedures 169
Mitchell S. Golbus

11
Perinatal Management of the Fetus with a Correctable Defect........ 177
Michael R. Harrison

12
Normal Anatomy of the Female Pelvis............................... 193
Alfred B. Kurtz and Matthew D. Rifkin

13
Ultrasound Evaluation of the Ovary 209
*Arthur C. Fleischer, Anne Colston Wentz, Howard W. Jones, III,
and A. Everette James, Jr.*

14
Ultrasound of the Uterus 227
Barry H. Gross and Peter W. Callen

15
**Ultrasonography in the Detection of Intrauterine Contraceptive
Devices** 249
Barry H. Gross and Peter W. Callen

16
**Ultrasonography in Evaluation of Gestational Trophoblastic
Disease** 259
Peter W. Callen

17
Sonographic Evaluation of Pelvic Infections 271
Lincoln L. Berland, Thomas L. Lawson, and W. Dennis Foley

18
Ultrasound Evaluation of Ectopic Pregnancy 291
Faye C. Laing and R. Brooke Jeffrey

19
Pelvimetry 305
Michael P. Federle

20
Ultrasound Instrumentation: Physical Principles 313
Frederick W. Kremkau

Appendix 325

Index 337

1

Ultrasound in the First Trimester of Pregnancy

E. A. Lyons, M.D.,
and C. S. Levi, M.D.

The first trimester of pregnancy is a dynamic period that spans ovulation, fertilization, implantation, and organogenesis. Ultrasound is the only imaging modality that can accurately assess pregnancy during this critical period. To understand fully the normal and abnormal sonographic findings of the conceptus, we present a brief outline of the embryologic changes that occur during the first trimester. For this discussion, menstrual age is used in keeping with the sonographic and obstetric literature.

Ovulation occurs on approximately day 14 of the menstrual cycle. Fertilization occurs in the distal third of the fallopian tube on day 14 or 15 as the ovum and sperm unite to form a zygote. By day 20, the zygote has formed a blastocyst—a fluid-filled cyst lined with trophoblastic cells, which contains a cluster of cells at one side called an inner cell mass (Fig. 1). The blastocyst burrows into the hyperplastic endometrium at the site of the inner cell mass on about day 20 and implantation begins. Implantation is completed by day 23. The maternal endometrial cells adjacent to the blastocyst become modified to supply nourishment to the blastocyst and are referred to as the decidual reaction.

During the fourth week (menstrual age), there is rapid proliferation and differentiation of the syncytiotrophoblast, forming a primitive uteroplacental circulation. Primary chorionic villi are formed and surrounded by pools of maternal blood. The inner cell mass begins to differentiate, forming an embryonic disc, a small amniotic cavity, and a primary yolk sac (Fig. 2). By the end of the fourth week, the primary yolk sac has regressed and a secondary yolk sac forms. Later, because of differential growth, the yolk sac comes to lie on the placenta sandwiched between the amnion and chorion.

During the fifth week two tubes (the primitive heart) develop from splanchnic mesodermal cells. By the end of the fifth week these tubes begin to pump into a primitive paired vascular system. The neural plate and notochord also form in week five. Somites begin to form which eventually give rise to the musculoskeletal system.

Early in the fifth week, the amniotic cavity is freed from the walls of the chorion. An extraembryonic vascular network forms, which connects through umbilical arteries to the primitive embryonic vascular network.

Weeks six to ten are referred to as the embryonic period when essentially all adult internal and external structures form. The embryo develops from a trilaminar disc (endoderm, mesoderm, and ectoderm) to a tubular body with all organ systems established. The embryonic head is disproportionately large, accounting for half of the crown-rump length.

By the end of week six the blood flow is unidirectional and by the end of the eighth week the heart attains its definitive form. The peripheral vascular system develops slightly later and is completed by the end of the tenth week.

The gastrointestinal system has formed and remains herniated into the umbilical cord at the end of the embryonic period. The rectum separates from the urogenital sinus by the end of the eighth week menstrual age and the anal membrane perforates by the end of the tenth week. External genitalia are still in a sexless state at the end of week ten. Limbs are formed with sepa-

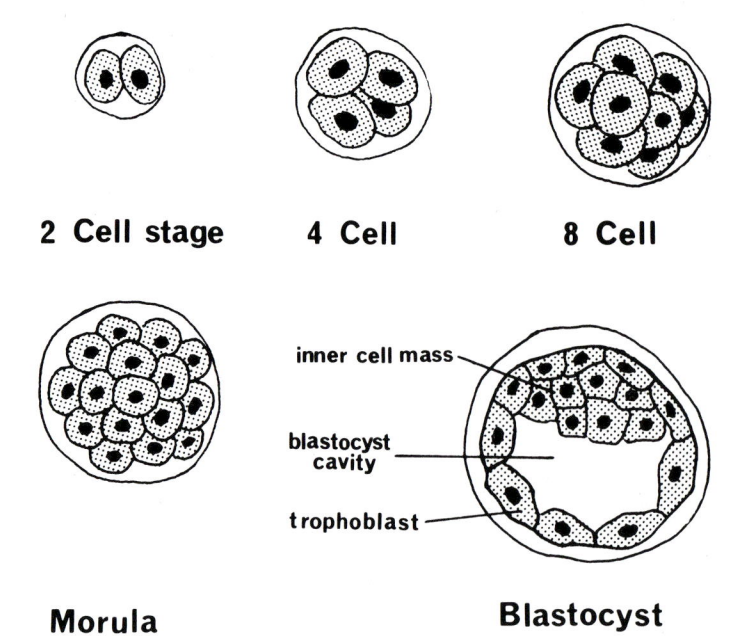

Figure 1. Development of the zygote from a two-cell stage to a blastocyst by five days' gestation.

rate fingers and toes. Nearly all congenital malformations except abnormalities of the external genitalia originate during the embryonic period; the external genitalia do not reach mature fetal form until the end of the fourteenth week.

Early in the fetal period body growth is rapid and head growth is slower, with the crown-rump length doubling between weeks 11 and 14. The intestines return to the fetal abdomen by the end of the twelfth week.

The amnion expands to fill the entire chorionic sac by the end of the tenth week (Fig. 3). At about the same time, the villi in contact with the decidua capsularis begin to degenerate, forming the chorion laeve. The villi are retained in the chorion

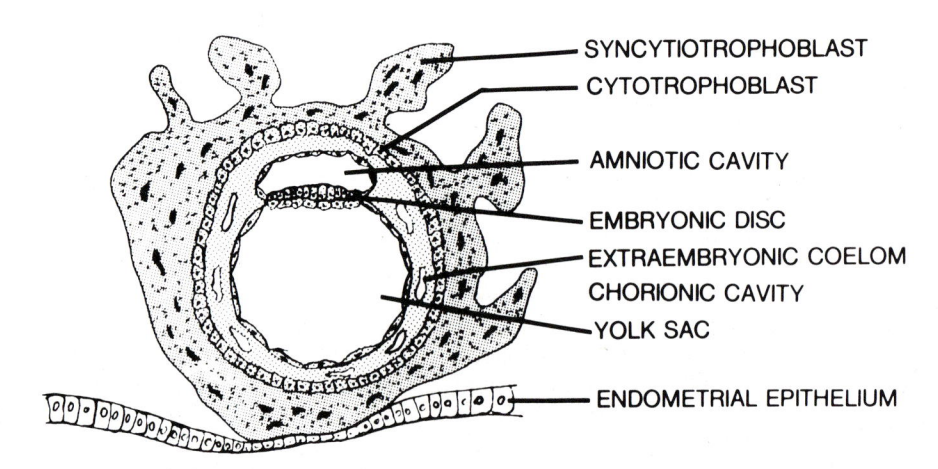

Figure 2. A diagram of the implanted blastocyst 12 days after conception shows formation of the embryonic disc which lies between the primitive yolk sac and the amniotic cavity. Trophoblastic villi are extending into the endometrium.

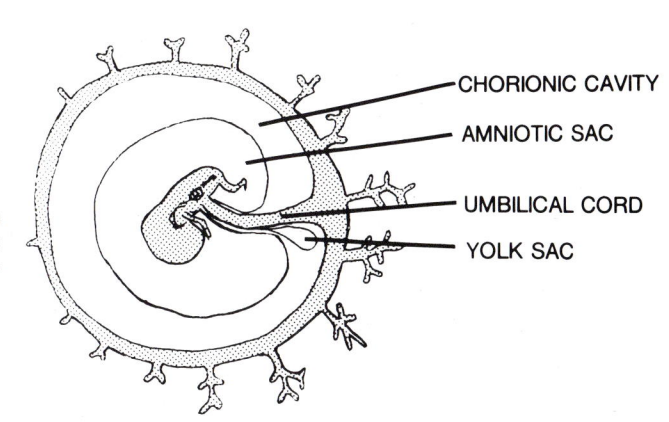

Figure 3. The relationship of the fetus and membranes at the end of the tenth week shows extrusion of the yolk sac by the enlarging amniotic sac.

10 WEEK GESTATION

frondosum, which is in contact with the decidua basalis. The chorion frondosum and decidua basalis form the placenta.

SONOGRAPHIC APPEARANCES AND THE NORMAL FIRST TRIMESTER

Embryonic Sonographic Appearances

Implantation. The earliest that an implanted gestational sac has been identified within the endometrial cavity is at four weeks' menstrual age within days of the expected menstrual period. This is within a few days of the completion of implantation. Only the extraembryonic coelom or chorionic sac is visible because the amniotic cavity is just beginning to form and enlarge. The sacs reported in the literature have been about 8 mm in diameter sonographically, having enlarged rapidly over the preceding seven days. The sac at this point has no internal echoes, since the yolk sac and neural plate are below the resolving power of the equipment (Fig. 4).

The wall of the gestational sac is a combination of cyto- and syncytiotrophoblastic tissue surrounded by decidua. As shown in Figure 5, decidua basalis will lie deep to the sac at the site of implantation, whereas the decidua capsularis surrounds its free surface. If there is no significant fluid or blood within the endometrial cavity, the decidua capsularis and the decidua vera lying on the opposite wall of the endometrium are in opposition and sonographically indistinguishable. In fact, despite the different anatomic layers of decidua, they appear sonographically as a uniform band of sonodensity surrounding the echo-free gestational sac. Until the syncytiotrophoblastic layer rapidly enlarges, giving rise to the chorion frondosum, the exact site of implantation may be impossible to identify.

The exact site of implantation, whether on the anterior or posterior surface of the endometrial cavity, cannot be identified at this early stage. However, it is well known from later sonographic studies that implantation usually occurs in the fundal portion of the uterus, with equal frequency on the anterior or posterior surfaces. Sac implantation has been identified in the cornua, fundus, body of the uterus, the cervical canal, and lower uterine segment. A cornual implantation (Fig. 6) can occur in an otherwise normal uterus or in one with a rudimentary horn from an incomplete duplex uterus. In either instance, continued growth of the gestational sac in a cornual location usually results in cornual rupture with massive hemorrhage and is life-threatening because of the vascularity of this region and its inability to expand adequately.

Low implantation of a gestational sac has been associated with poor outcome, but this is not fully substantiated in the literature. The implantation into the endocervical canal is the exception. This less vascular area cannot support growth of the gestational sac and abortion is inevitable.

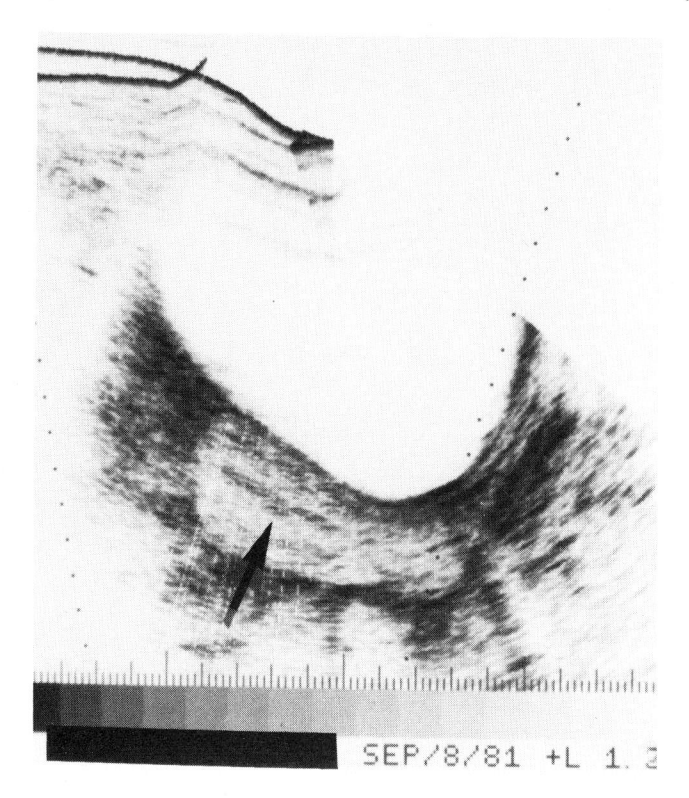

Figure 4. Longitudinal scan of a woman with a pregnancy with a known menstrual age of 4 weeks. The arrow points to a tiny thickening in the endometrial cavity which may be passed off as a variation in normal, but which developed on subsequent studies to a normal gestational sac.

Sac Growth. There is a rapid increase in the volume of the developing gestational sac in the first trimester from 0 to 70 ml at 12 weeks' menstrual age, with a range at 12 weeks of 50 to 120 ml. These estimates were made by Robinson in 1975 and are based on planimetry of serial sections of gestational sacs.

Previous authors (Hellman et al.[3]) have used the volume of the sac or its size to assess gestational age. This technique is not commonly used now because the distended urinary bladder easily compresses the uterine fundus and distorts the gestational sac. Because it has no standard shape allowing rapid volume estimations, exhaustive sectioning and planimetry would have to be carried out on each sac. This would make it an inordinately time-consuming procedure. Because of the biologic variation, the accuracy is ±9 days. Other authors have suggested that the diameter of the sac in centimeters plus three will give an approximation of the menstrual age. Most practitioners become familiar with relative sac sizes from the first appearance of the sac at just over four weeks' menstrual age to the appearance of the fetal pole at seven weeks and will "guesstimate" the menstrual age. At this time of gestation, the menstrual history is usually readily obtainable and reliable and can be used with the size of the sac to estimate age.

The inner cell layer of cytotrophoblast

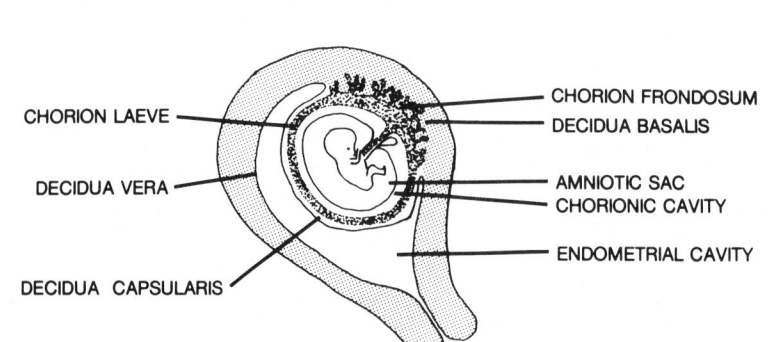

Figure 5. Divisions of the decidua and the chorion in a fetus at 10 weeks' menstrual age.

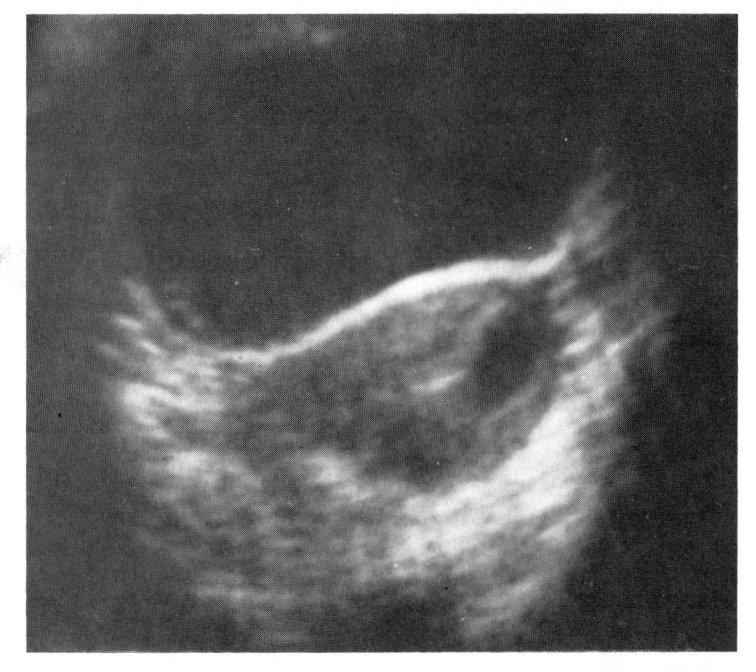

Figure 6. Transverse sonogram through the uterine fundus demonstrates a gestational sac in the left cornua with the central endometrial cavity being obliterated. The pregnancy subsequently aborted.

and outer syncytiotrophoblast rapidly proliferates at four weeks' menstrual age, appearing as a uniformly thick echo-dense ring around the gestational sac. In the fifth and sixth weeks, the syncytiotrophoblast layer invades the hyperplastic endometrium beneath it (the decidua basalis) and appears as a thick echogenic crescent. This is the chorion frondosum or the primitive placenta (Figs. 7 and 8).

On the opposite side of the developing gestational sac, the syncytiotrophoblast degenerates, is thinned out, and forms the chorion laeve.

In 60 per cent of patients between the fifth and eighth week of menstrual age, the endometrial cavity is not sonographically "empty." One may see an echo-free rim surrounding the gestational sac or a triangular area containing low-level echoes (Fig. 8B). This may well represent bleeding caused by implantation; its significance will be discussed later. By its presence, it separates the decidua capsularis from the decidua vera (Fig. 9). One can now appreciate the difference in thickness of the capsularis from the basalis layers. This is thought to represent bleeding from implan-

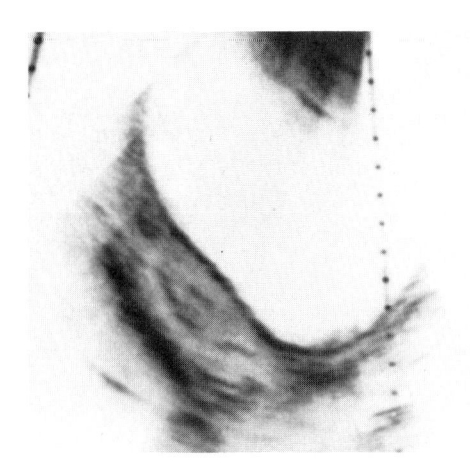

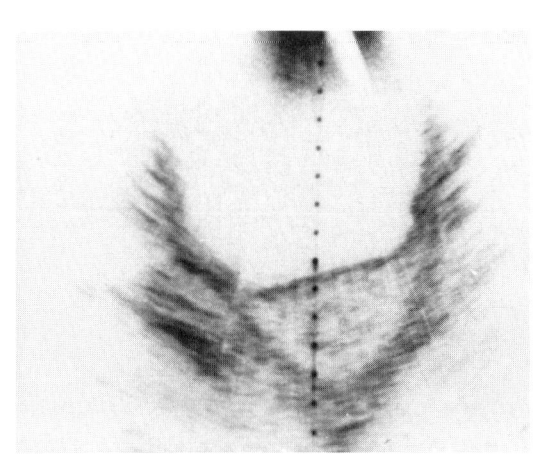

Figure 7. Transverse and longitudinal sonograms of a gestation at 5 weeks, 6 days' menstrual age show a thickening of the endometrial cavity without a well-defined gestational sac.

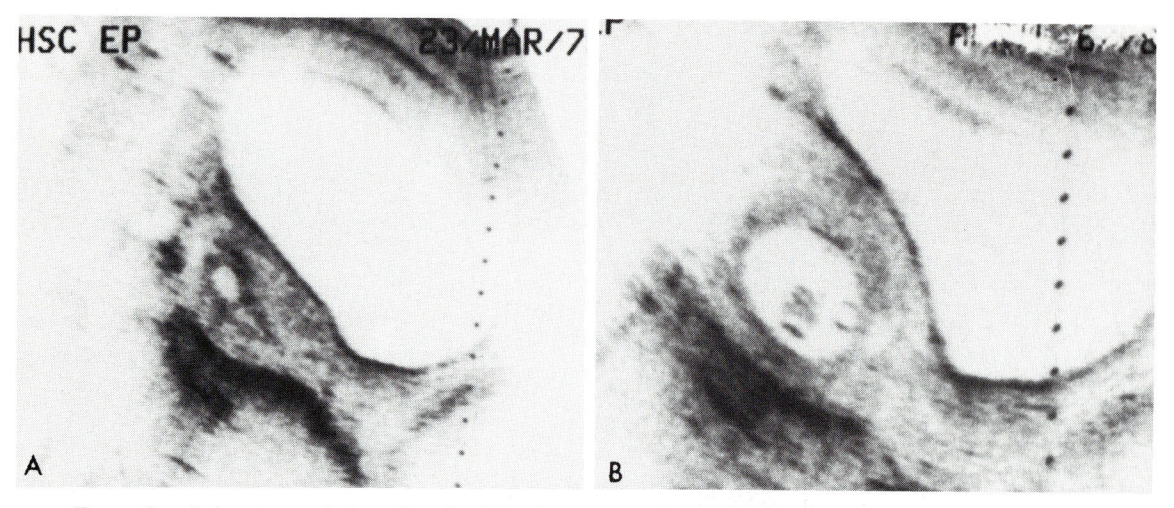

Figure 8. *A*, A gestational sac at 6 weeks, 6 days' menstrual age situated in the uterine fundus. Slight thickening of the trophoblastic reaction anteriorly will be the future site of placental development. *B*, Same patient two weeks later. The site of thickening and placental development can be more readily seen.

tation because on careful examination one can see a slight elevation of the thick chorion frondosum extending partly into the endometrial cavity (Fig. 10).

As the sac enlarges, this space or pseudosac or implantation bleeding disappears and is therefore seen in 50 per cent of patients from eight to 12 weeks and in 20 per cent from 12 to 15 weeks' menstrual age. The shape of the normal gestational sac varies because of compression of the uterine body by the distended bladder caudally and the sacral promontory craniad. An overdistended bladder can almost entirely flatten an otherwise normal sac, making it appear like a decidual cast of an ectopic pregnancy. The sac can be shaped like a dumbbell or be crescentic (Fig. 11). As the bladder volume is reduced, the sac assumes a more normal appearance. It should not take on a crenated appearance, nor should the trophoblastic layer appear abnormally thinned. These findings of anembryonic gestation will be discussed later.

The Fetal Pole. Sonographically, the fetal pole appears at six weeks' menstrual age when embryologically it is 5 mm long. It is otherwise shapeless and lies on the bottom of the gestational sac or adjacent to the placenta (chorion frondosum). By the beginning of the seventh week of menstrual age, it has grown to almost 1 cm, and cardiac activity of the fetus can now be seen. Embryologically, the primitive cardiac tubes now begin spontaneous and rhythmic pulsation. One can also see gross fetal body motions, which may be accentuated as the anterior abdominal wall is tapped smartly,

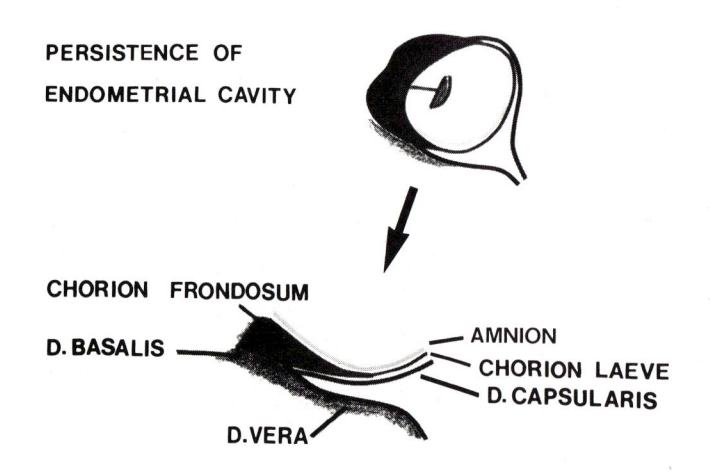

Figure 9. A possible explanation for the pseudosac as a "persistence of the endometrial cavity."

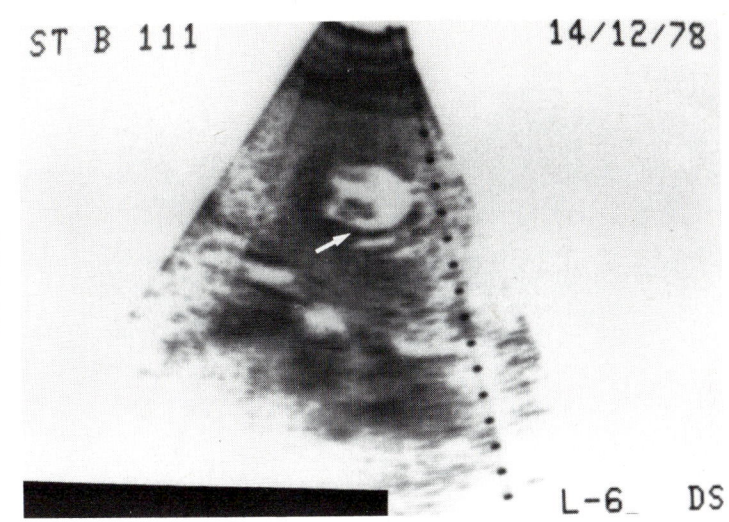

Figure 10. Longitudinal sonogram through a gestational sac showing a tongue of chorion frondosum (*arrow*) extending into the endometrial cavity. The gestation is 7 weeks, 3 days' menstrual age.

sending a shock wave through the gestational sac, bouncing the fetus off of the bottom. One can see a flailing activity as the fetus settles again to the bottom. Cardiac activity of the fetus should be identifiable in 100 per cent of the cases from the seventh week onward.

The fetal pole continues to enlarge and elongate, reaching 5.5 to 6 cm at 12 weeks' menstrual age. The fetal head is approximately the same size as the fetal body and can be identified at approximately 12 weeks' menstrual age. At 12 weeks, the biparietal diameter can be identified and measured.

Measuring the long axis of the fetus or the crown-rump length accurately assesses menstrual age in the first trimester. In 1975 H. P. Robinson, whose studies were confirmed by later workers, established an accuracy of ± 4.7 days in assessing menstrual age.[6] Figure 12 demonstrates the measurement of the long axis of an 11-week fetus lying on the bottom of the amniotic cavity. Care must be taken to obtain the true long axis of the fetus. To this end, a real-time scanner with linear array or sector (as in this case) must be used. The cranial end appears as an enlarged area at one pole of the otherwise shapeless trunk. At this stage, limbs are clearly identified anterior to the trunk (Fig. 13).

Yolk Sac. The primitive yolk sac develops from the inner mass on the side opposite of the amniotic cavity. As the amniotic cavity enlarges, part of the yolk sac is enveloped within the fetus to form part of the primitive gut. The remainder is extruded to lie on the surface of the placenta, near the insertion of the cord between the amniotic and chorionic membranes. The yolk sac can be identified in early fetal life after usually less than eight weeks' men-

Figure 11. Two longitudinal sonograms through different areas of a normal 9 week gestational sac. The image above shows a dumbbell-shaped distortion of this sac due to an overfull bladder. The more normal sac is seen in the lower scan.

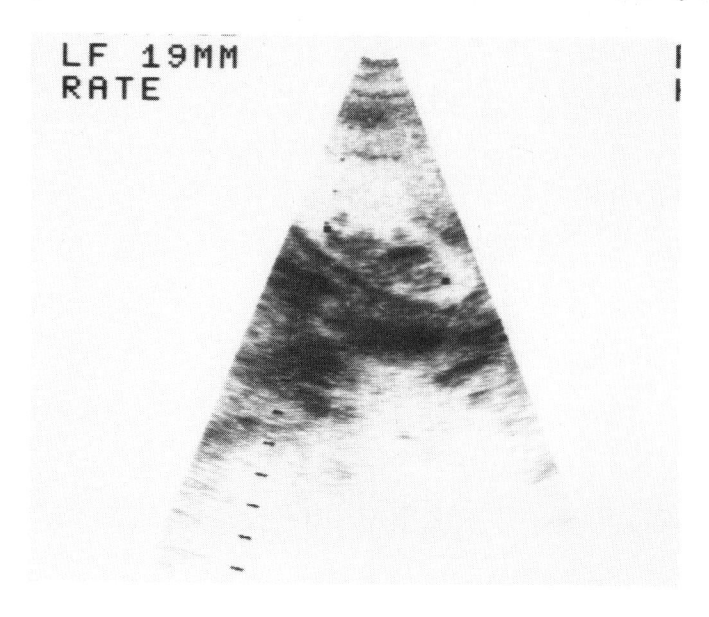

Figure 12. A longitudinal sonogram shows a normal fetus with a crown-rump length of 41 mm, consistent with 11 weeks' menstrual age.

strual age. It is generally a small, rounded, saclike structure measuring less than 1 cm in diameter (Fig. 14). Sonographically, its recognition is unimportant other than to realize its insignificance. Embryologically, however, it is the site of early blood formation and forms the luminal gastrointestinal tract. It should not be present in an anembryonic gestation, since no fetus exists.

Multiple Gestations. Multiple gestations can occur because of the fertilization of several ova but more commonly because of the early and complete division of a fertilized ovum. Division can occur before the blastocyst develops, giving rise to the dichorionic and diamniotic sacs. Division may occur, and more commonly does, after the chorionic sac forms but before the amniotic cavity develops, giving rise to the monochorionic and diamniotic sacs.

Also, commonly, the neural plate divides after the amniotic and chorionic sacs form, with the resultant dichorionic and diamniotic gestations. The different types generally cannot be differentiated sonographically. In the monochorionic, monoamniotic form in which two fetuses are seen to exist within one fluid cavity with no intervening membrane, fetal entanglement fre-

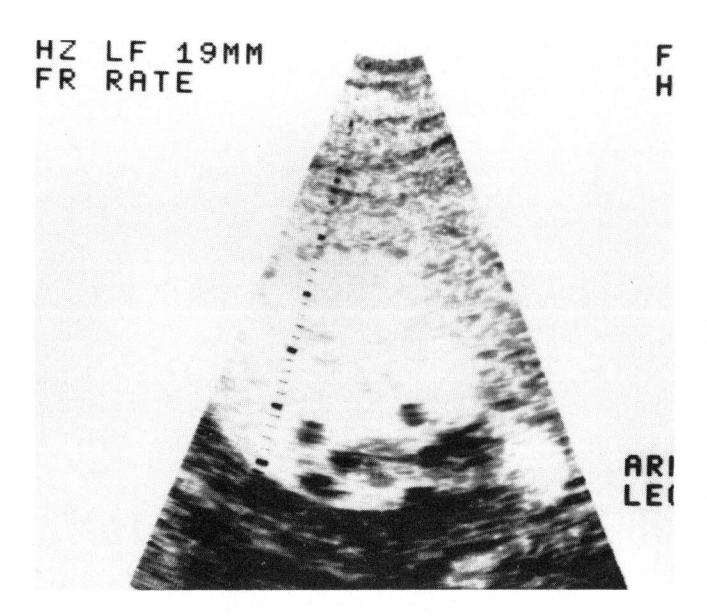

Figure 13. Longitudinal sonogram through the limbs of an 11 week fetus.

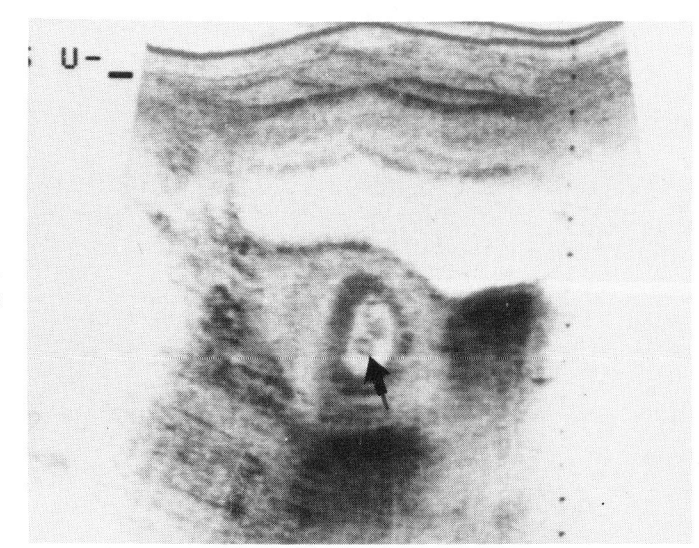

Figure 14. Yolk sac (*arrow*) in a normal gestation at 8 weeks' menstrual age measures 5 mm in diameter.

quently occurs killing one or both offspring. A more common complication is the twin-to-twin transfusion syndrome which results from the interconnection of large fetal vessels in a shared placenta. Figure 15 shows an early normal twin gestation at eight weeks' menstrual age.

An "implantation bleed" should not be mistaken for a second gestational sac. This has previously been called the second sac and has been equated with a blighted ovum that subsequently aborted. If this explanation were accepted, then the incidence of twins could exceed 60 per cent of all first trimester gestations seen in our general ultrasound laboratory. This far exceeds the clinically recognized figure of one in 200 live births.

Triplets, quadruplets, and quintuplets have all been recognized sonographically in the first trimester, and case reports are in the literature. Figure 16 shows quadruplets at nine weeks' menstrual age following Pergonal therapy. One should diagnose a multiple gestation only when multiple gestational sacs and multiple live fetuses are visualized coexistently, so as not to mistake bleeding from implantation for a twin.

In approximately one in 30,000 pregnancies, a multiple gestation will develop with

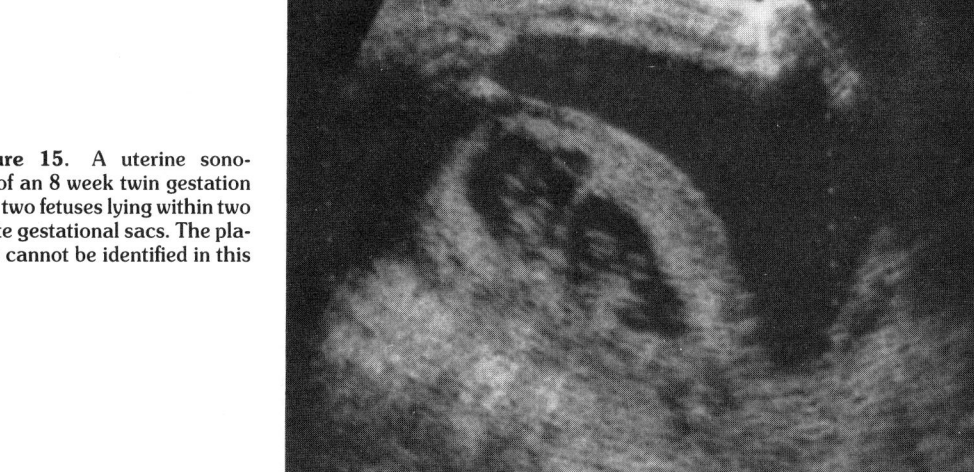

Figure 15. A uterine sonogram of an 8 week twin gestation shows two fetuses lying within two discrete gestational sacs. The placentas cannot be identified in this scan.

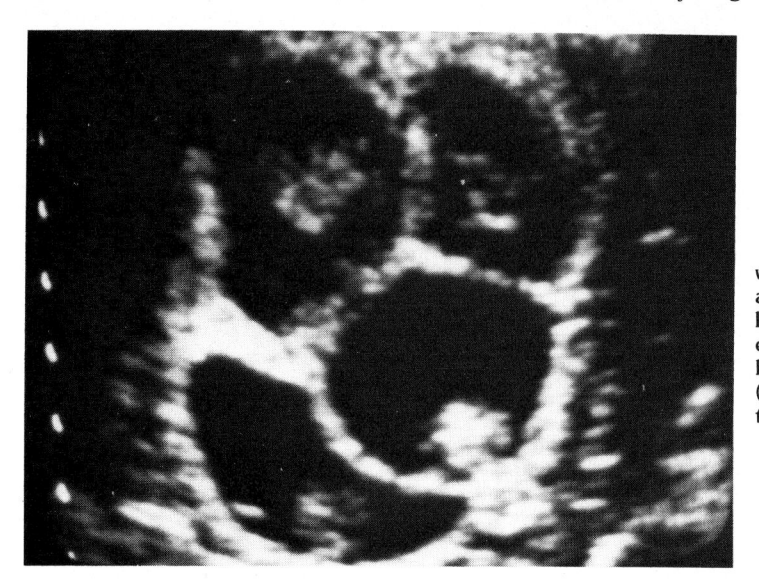

Figure 16. Quadruplets at 9 weeks' menstrual age; all four sacs and fetuses may be seen. This followed Pergonal stimulation and ended at 21 weeks with premature labor and death of all four fetuses. (Courtesy of M. Gillieson, M.D., Ottawa General Hospital.)

one fetus inside the endometrial cavity and the other in an ectopic location. This condition is discussed in a subsequent chapter.

Extraembryonic Structures

Placenta and Membranes. The placenta develops from the hyperplastic invasion of the syncytiotrophoblast of the chorion into the decidua basalis. This thickening is seen usually by the eighth week of menstrual age. The sonographic appearance of the placenta is that of a uniformly echogenic thickening of the gestation sac. The placenta maintains this crescentic shape and its relatively uniform echogenicity throughout the first trimester.

The development of the gestational sac involves the formation and enlargement of the chorionic and the amniotic sacs within the endometrial cavity. The anatomic interrelationships of these three sacs or cavities can give rise to the appearance of intrauterine membranes which are either developmental or acquired. These situations will be discussed as separation of the chorionic and amniotic membranes or their elevation.

Chorioamniotic Separation. The amniotic cavity begins to form 7½ days after fertilization from an accumulation of fluid beneath the superficial layer of cells in the inner cell mass. It enlarges rapidly to surround the fetus and fill the chorionic cavity at about 16 weeks' menstrual age. Prior to 16 weeks, with careful scanning the inner unfused amniotic membrane can be seen sonographically. This appearance we have termed the developmental form of chorioamniotic separation (Fig. 17). Only a small portion of the unfused amniotic sac is visualized. It is very thin, having only five cell layers, one of epithelium and four layers of connective tissue.[1] Figure 18 shows the delicate inner amniotic membrane at 10 weeks.

In a small percentage of cases, the amniotic and chorionic membranes fail to fuse over their entire surface at 16 weeks or separate following initial apposition. This finding, termed acquired chorioamniotic separation, is felt to be of no clinical significance. A recent report by Burrows et al.[2] referred to work by Torpin, who examined a large number of membranes of fetuses affected by the amniotic band syndrome and presented evidence that the chorioamniotic separation was caused by spontaneous or iatrogenic rupture of the amnion with preservation of the chorion. This in turn led to accumulation of amniotic fluid behind or outside the amniotic membrane, resulting in retraction of the amnion in part or in whole up to the base of the umbilical cord where the two membranes are firmly adherent. The type of chorioamniotic separation most commonly seen sonographically is not associated with the amniotic band syndrome reported to cause amputation of digits or even limbs.

Chorioamniotic Elevation. One may see a similar appearance if both the cho-

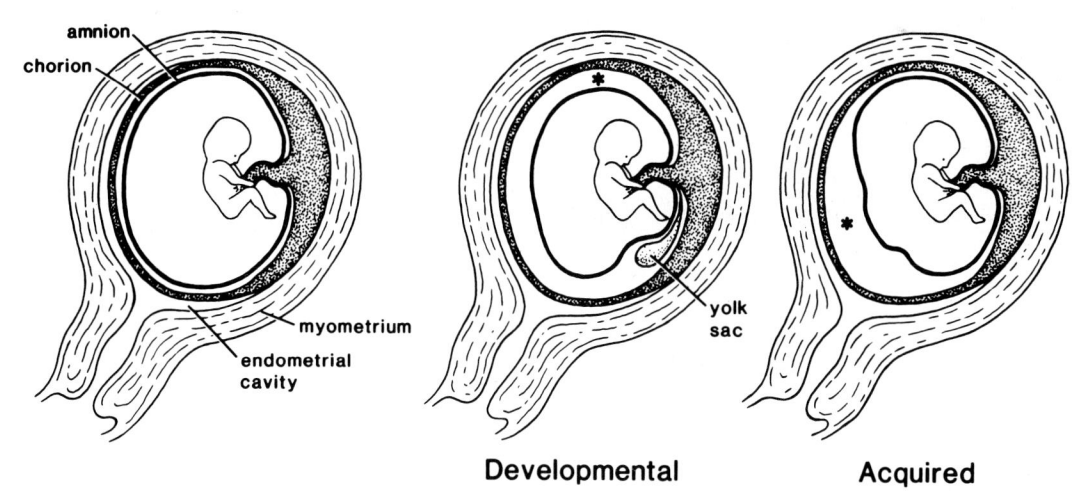

Figure 17. Chorioamniotic separation. The normal (far left) relationship of the amnion, chorion, and endometrial cavity. Prior to complete expansion of the amniotic sac, the amniotic membrane can be identified within the chorionic cavity (*) and lying separately from the chorionic membrane. This is the developmental (middle figure) form of chorioamniotic separation. The acquired form (far right) would presumably occur after the complete expansion of the amniotic sac with subsequent partial collapse and reappearance of the chorionic cavity (*).

rionic and amniotic membranes are elevated by fluid or blood in the endometrial cavity. As mentioned previously, in 60 per cent of first trimester pregnancies between the fifth and eighth weeks of menstrual age, a relatively echo-free, often triangular structure was seen adjacent to an otherwise normal gestational sac and fetus (Fig. 19). There was usually elevation of a "tongue" of chorion frondosum giving rise to the explanation of normal implantation bleeding or an extension of it (see Figs. 9 and 10). If the site of bleeding was adjacent to the internal cervical os, the patient had spotting.

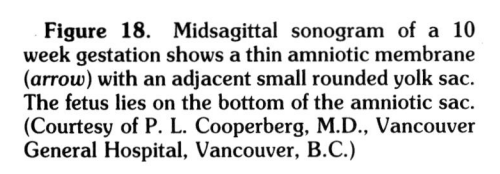

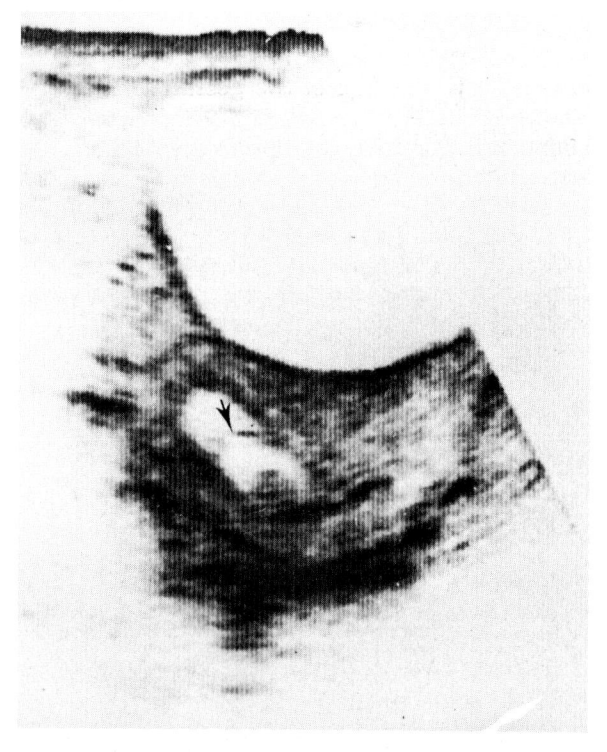

Figure 18. Midsagittal sonogram of a 10 week gestation shows a thin amniotic membrane (*arrow*) with an adjacent small rounded yolk sac. The fetus lies on the bottom of the amniotic sac. (Courtesy of P. L. Cooperberg, M.D., Vancouver General Hospital, Vancouver, B.C.)

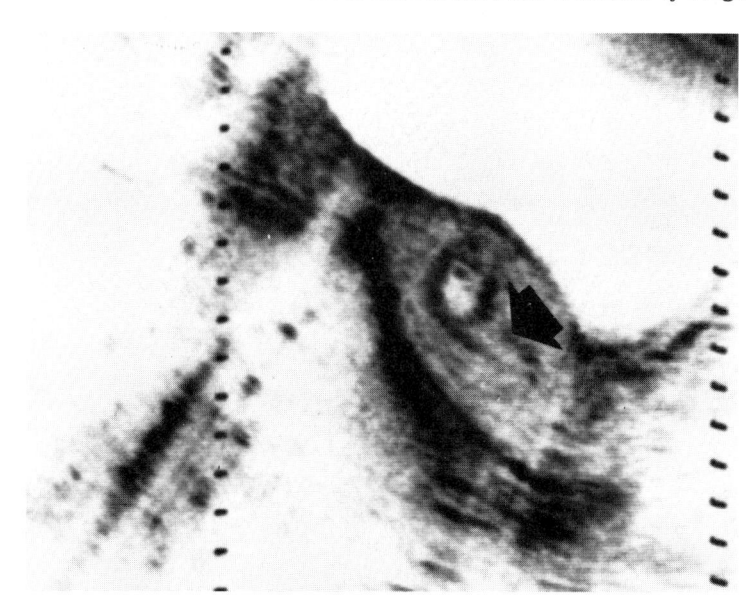

Figure 19. A gestational sac at 5 weeks, 4 days' menstrual age with the sac, uterine fundus, and the triangular and likely blood-filled endometrial cavity below it (*arrow*).

This was not true if it lay away from the os, in the uterine fundus. With only one exception, all of the cases seen went on to a normal full-term delivery of an otherwise healthy infant. In the one exception (Fig. 20), the bleeding was associated with elevation of half of the placenta, and, as one would expect, a follow-up examination three days later showed a complete abortion. Close examination of the triangularly shaped site of bleeding (Fig. 20B) shows a relatively echogenic area arising from the junction of the elevated tongue of tissue, the chorion frondosum, and the decidua basalis, consistent with a blood clot. Peripherally, there was an echo-free zone consistent with unclotted blood. One could readily have predicted, and in fact we did, the outcome in this case.

Extensive chorioamniotic elevation may present the appearance of a sac within a sac (Fig. 21). The inner sac represents the elevated chorioamniotic membranes surrounded by blood in the endometrial cavity. This is an unusual presentation and presumably is associated with a higher incidence of abortion.

In pregnancies between eight and 12 weeks' menstrual age the incidence of implantation bleeding was 50 per cent; this was reduced to 20 per cent in those from 13 to 15 weeks' menstrual age. After 13 weeks' menstrual age the membrane elevation may be either developmental or acquired. In these patients the findings may mimic chorioamniotic separation; however, if the patient is spotting from the vagina, then the fluid collection must lie extrachorionic. Figure 22 shows an extrachorionic fluid collection. The patient had spotting early in pregnancy and then went on to deliver a normal full-term fetus.

Filly (personal communication) has proposed another explanation for implantation bleeding. He suggests that this triangular structure is hyperplastic endometrium with some central fluid or blood. This would be in response to the normally increased levels of circulating estrogen and progesterone in pregnancy. One may not expect to see perigestational sac fluid in every case of a normal intrauterine gestation. It could occur above or below the gestational sac depending on the implantation site and may present as spotting.

The two main arguments in opposition to this explanation are (1) the sonographically evident segmental elevation of a tongue of chorion frondosum, a finding that would favor the implantation bleed and (2) the case shown in Figure 20 of the 50 per cent elevation of the placenta going on to a complete abortion. Hemorrhage would clearly explain all of the findings on the second study at 12 weeks. For the previous week, the study looks identical to most of the other early pregnancies we have labeled implantation bleeding. Most likely there are cases with sonographic findings attributable to implantation bleeding, decidual hyperplasia, or a combination of both. The exact proportion of each and its final explanation are for the most part academic and require further study.

Changes in Uterine Size and Shape. In the nongravid uterus, the anteroposterior diameter of the uterine fundus is approximately 3 to 4 cm whereas the cervix is just less than 3 cm. As early as five weeks' menstrual age the uterine fundus becomes more bulbous whereas the cervix remains essentially unchanged. The uterus enlarges progressively in response to the enlarging gestational sac while its shape is determined by the masses around it: the bladder, the bowel, and the sacral promontory.

Myometrial contractions seen throughout the gestational period appear as rounded masses bulging inward into the endometrial canal or the developing gestational sac. Their echogenicity is identical to that of a normal myometrium. They are a spontaneous event or may be brought on by the massaging action of the ultrasound transducer over the maternal abdomen and pregnant uterus. Myometrial contractions seldom last more than 30 minutes and in early gestation are imperceptible to the patient.

It is important to differentiate myometrial contractions from fibroids, which are much less homogeneous in echo texture, often distort the serosal surface of the uterus, and are persistent throughout the study. The echo texture of these masses may change during pregnancy, beginning relatively echo free with increased vascularity and sometimes degeneration, and becoming more densely echogenic. Small fibroids may be very difficult to identify, especially in the second and third trimesters, and yet clinically may be very tender and painful.

Corpus Luteum Cyst. With the rupture of the echo-free follicular cyst and release of the ovum, the corpus luteum cyst is born. The cyst walls invaginate with the desquamation of granulosa cells and red blood cells. Sonographically the cyst measures less than 2 cm in diameter and contains low level echoes. As the pregnancy is established and the placenta begins to secrete human chorionic gonadotropin, the corpus luteum cyst enlarges to an average of 4 cm in diameter and is maintained until the twelfth week of menstrual age (Fig. 23). On occasion the cyst becomes quite large, even up to 10 cm in diameter. It may also undergo hemorrhagic changes, rupture, and present as an acute abdomen.

FIRST TRIMESTER ABNORMALITIES

Failed Contraception (The Intrauterine Contraceptive Device and Pregnancy). In 2 per cent of women with intrauterine contraceptive devices, the effect is less than adequate and a pregnancy ensues either because the device was improp-

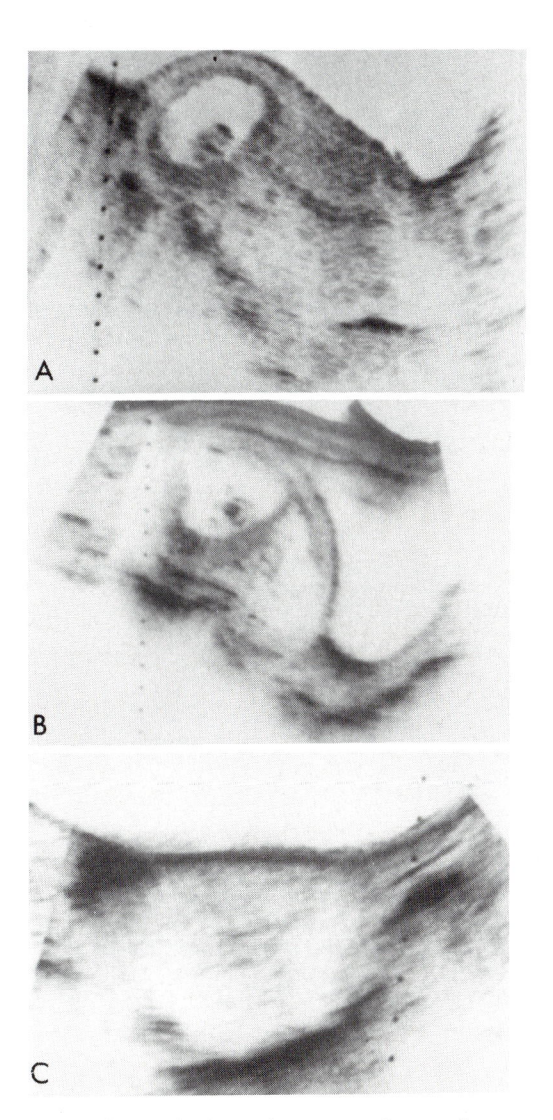

Figure 20. *A*, An 11 week gestational sac with a central placenta previa and below it the triangular pseudosac. *B*, Scan at 12 weeks demonstrates a large triangular hemorrhage with elevation of 50 per cent of the placenta. *C*, A midline scan through the empty uterus.

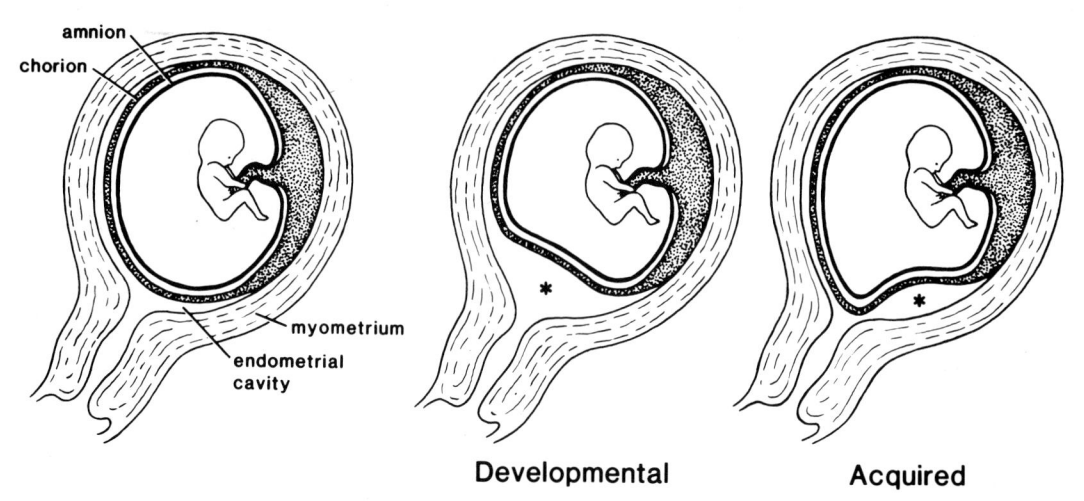

Figure 21. Chorioamniotic elevation. The normal (far left) relationship of the amnion, chorion, and endometrial cavity. Prior to the complete expansion of the chorionic cavity, possibly due to the presence of an implantation bleed, the chorionic and/or amniotic membranes can be identified separately from the decidua vera and the endometrial cavity (*). This is the developmental form of chorioamniotic elevation (middle figure). The acquired form (far right) may occur secondary to marginal sinus rupture with extra-chorionic accumulation of blood.

erly placed into the myometrium or because a properly placed device failed to provide adequate contraception. One can recognize the intrauterine contraceptive device either by its type-specific morphology or by its two parallel, echogenic lines within the endometrial canal. The double line is due to an echo from the anterior and posterior surfaces of the contraceptive device. This is only seen when the transducer beam hits the device perpendicularly, using axial resolution to resolve the anterior and posterior surfaces. It is not seen in the Dalkon shield, which is an unusually thin membrane, but fortunately this product is no longer used. A distal shadow is

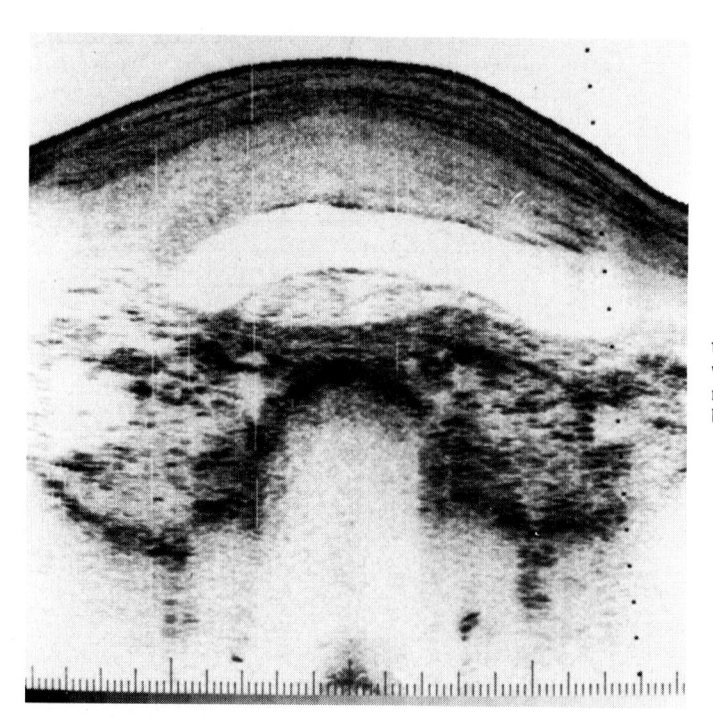

Figure 22. A transverse scan through the uterine fundus shows elevation of the amniotic and chorionic membranes with some low level echoes behind it, likely caused by blood.

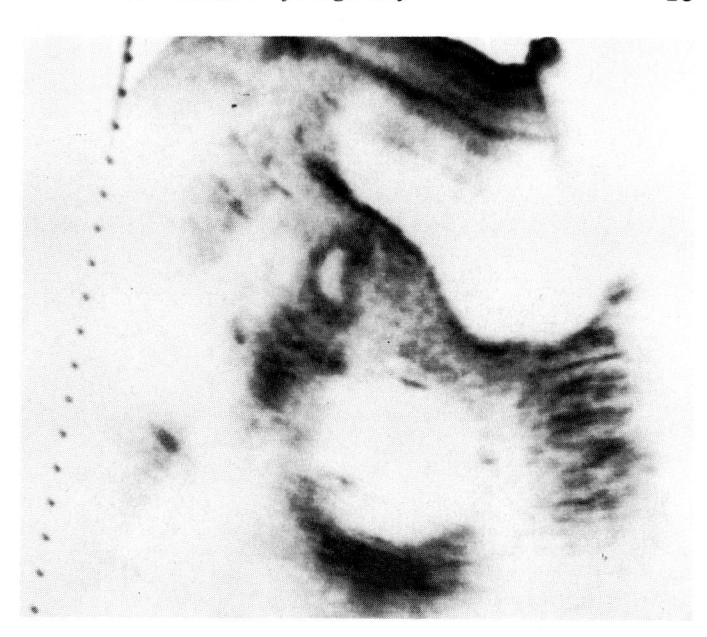

Figure 23. An 8 week pregnancy with part of the gestational sac within the uterine fundus, which is displaced anteriorly by a 5 cm corpus luteum cyst lying in the posterior cul-de-sac.

often seen behind the intrauterine contraceptive device, providing another sonographic clue. The intrauterine contraceptive device may lie within the placental site or away from it. There is no consistent relationship.

If left untouched, at least 40 per cent of pregnancies reaching the second trimester with an intrauterine contraceptive device in place will have serious complications including sepsis, premature rupture of membranes, bleeding, and spontaneous abortion. Gottesfeld recommends the use of real-time ultrasonic visualization; a curette is placed within the cervical canal, and the device is removed. One must use ultrasonic guidance to ensure that the gestational sac is not disrupted during the procedure. In his experience (personal communication), the rate of subsequent abortions after manipulation is less than 5 per cent.

Anembryonic Gestation of Blighted Ovum. The anembryonic gestation is a gestational sac without an embryo. A fertilized ovum develops into the blastocyst, but the inner cell mass and resultant fetal pole never develop. The gestational sac invades the endometrium and acts in part like a normally developing pregnancy. The syncytiotrophoblast invades the endometrium and produces human chorionic gonadotropin, which gives rise to a positive pregnancy test and the enlarged tender breasts and other clinical stigmata of pregnancy. The normal appearances, however, are short-lived. The gestational sac fails to grow and develop normally, and the uterus fails to develop as expected. There is frequently spotting with drops of a brownish fluid representing degenerated blood. The level of circulating human chorionic gonadotropin drops, and the results of the pregnancy test soon become weakly positive or negative. With falling levels of human chorionic gonadotropin, progesterone, and estrogen, the feeling of being pregnant and the associated pelvic fullness and breast tenderness are also lost.

The sonographic findings are rather specific and relate to the size, shape, and thickness of the sac and continuity of the trophoblast. The sac may be smaller than expected for the stated clinical age, appropriate in size, or even slightly large. In serial studies for two weeks, the sac generally does not grow and may in fact get smaller. Of primary importance is that a fetus will never be seen despite a very careful study. The presence of a small fetal pole with no visible motion or heart beat would be a missed abortion and not truly an anembryonic gestation. The difference is semantic only; clinically, the result will be the same. The echogenic trophoblast is usually irregular in thickness with areas in which no trophoblast is seen. This is a very reliable sign seen in almost all cases (Fig. 24). The outline of the sac may have a crenated shape, be angular, or may have the more

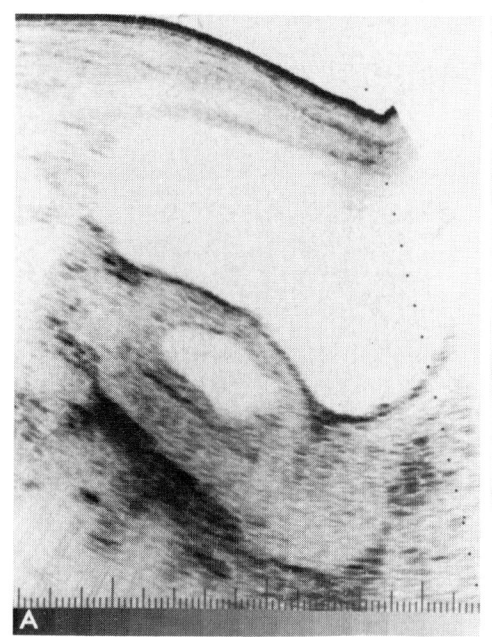

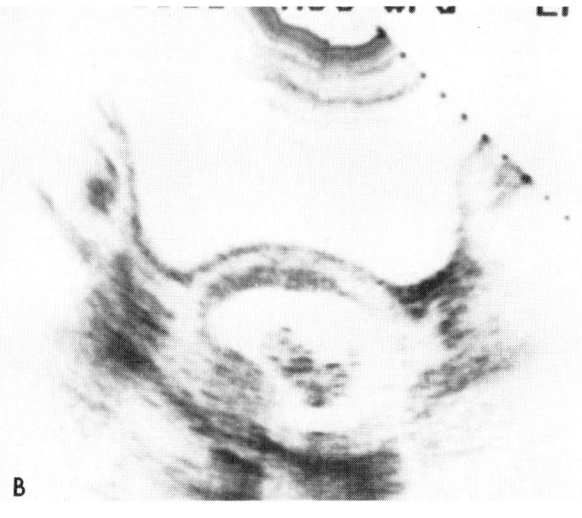

Figure 24. *A*, A midline sonogram of a 10 week gestation showing a blighted ovum with centrally located gestational sac but very poorly echogenic trophoblast peripherally. No fetus was seen. *B*. By comparison a transverse sonogram through the uterine fundus in a 10 week normal gestation demonstrates the normally thickened trophoblast in the right half of the uterus identifying the position of the chorion frondosum.

normal, rounded configuration. The angular irregularities cannot be produced by uterine compression and are presumed to be abnormalities of the primary sac. This is also a reliable sign. Occasionally a fluid-fluid level can be seen within the sac, presumably because of hemorrhage.

The worst-looking sac may still develop normally. It is crucial therefore to always give the fetus the benefit of the doubt. The classic history of a weakly positive or negative pregnancy test, spotting, and loss of that "pregnant feeling" may still be associated with a normally developing fetus. We have occasionally seen such patients in whom the gestational sac was very small, and yet it developed normally. Almost certainly, a patient who has had a blighted ovum and aborted it unknowingly went on to become pregnant again. The ultrasound examination was then done at the beginning of the subsequent normal pregnancy. If one sees a gestational sac smaller than a seven-week sac, one must not diagnose a blighted ovum without a repeat study in one week's time. If, of course, the sac is larger than a sac after eight weeks with no evidence of fetal echoes and a thin, spotty trophoblast, one can diagnose, on one scan alone, an anembryonic pregnancy. The true incidence of blighted ovum is, I feel, unknown and will remain so until someone follows a large series of women in the reproductive years through many menstrual cycles. Only by this method will one identify women whose menstrual periods were a few days late because of hormonal changes and those in whom there was a blighted ovum that aborted spontaneously. The incidence is almost certainly much higher than that reported in the literature.

Trophoblastic Disease. Rarely, and no one knows how often, a blighted ovum undergoes trophoblastic degeneration and becomes a hydatidiform mole. Such a case is shown in Figure 25. This woman went on holiday after the initial sonographic study. She had had amenorrhea for eight weeks and on her return eight weeks later had an enlarged uterus with diffused low-level echoes throughout, indicating a hydatidiform mole. Early moles are usually more echogenic than normal, and such is often the case.

Ectopic Pregnancy. The development of a gestational sac and fetus within the fallopian tube or within the abdominal cavity is tremendously important and will also be discussed in another chapter. The decidual cast seen in some 20 per cent of ectopic pregnancies may resemble sonographically a developing intrauterine gestational sac. With the undistended bladder, the decidual cast should not attain a well-

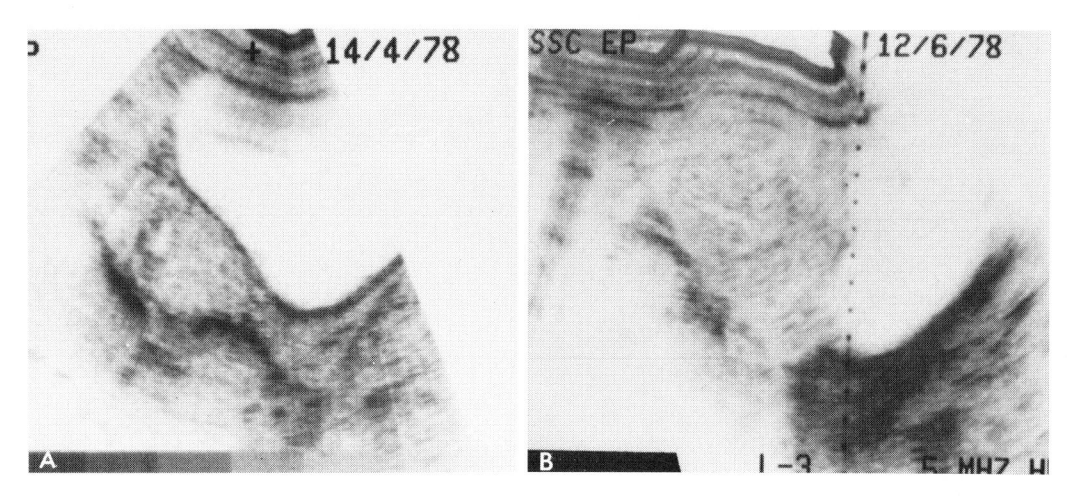

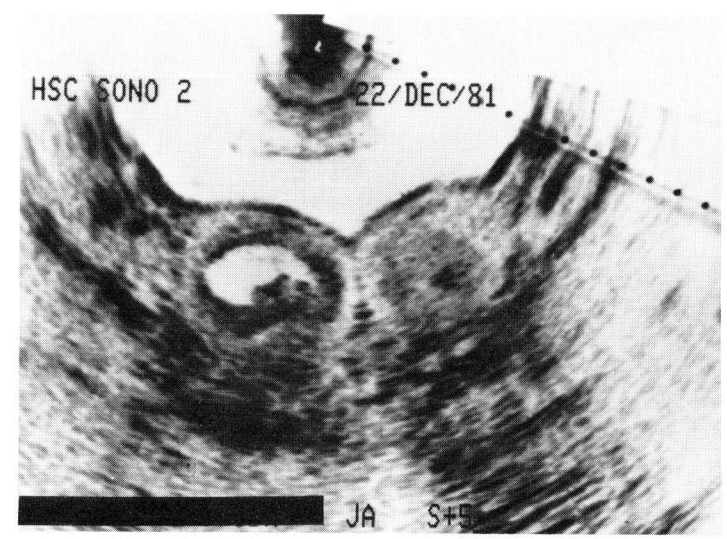

Figure 25. *A*, Longitudinal scan through the uterus shows a very small irregular gestational sac in a woman with amenorrhea of 8 weeks' duration. The changes would be consistent with a blighted ovum. *B*, The uterus is enlarged to the size of a 16 week gestation with no visible gestational sac. The uniformly soft echoes throughout were secondary to a hydatidiform mole.

rounded appearance, whereas the gestational sac will. This is a useful differentiating feature; however, it is still occasionally difficult to diagnose. Finally, in one of 30,000 pregnancies coexistent intrauterine and extrauterine gestation occurs.

Congenital Uterine Anomalies. The most common anomaly visualized sonographically is that of a double uterus with a coexistent pregnancy. The developing gestational sac is usually seen in one horn and often a decidual reaction or cast may be seen in the other (Fig. 26). This is not a common anomaly; however, it is the one most recently recognized sonographically.

A more common anomaly would be a septated uterus, frequently seen on hysterosalpingography. It is, however, unusual to see the septum in the first trimester of pregnancy, and only occasionally is it seen in the second and third trimesters.

Leiomyomata in Pregnancy. As mentioned previously, leiomyomata should be differentiated from normal uterine contractions. In later pregnancy, leiomyomata may be difficult to identify. However, within the first trimester, they are not frequently missed. Their exact location relative to the internal cervical os must be identified to be able to predict and advise

Figure 26. Transverse sonogram through the fundus shows two rounded masses representing the two fundi of a double uterus. The uterus on the right has an 8½ week gestational sac and fetus.

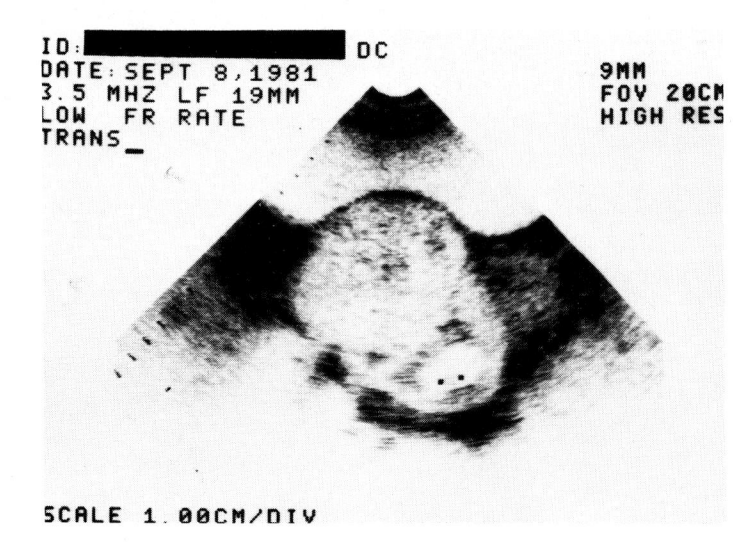

Figure 27. A longitudinal scan through an enlarged uterus with a normal 7 week gestational sac situated in the fundus posteriorly. It is displaced posteriorly by a 7 cm well-defined, solid, nondegenerated fibroid.

obstetric management. A large fibroid in the lower uterine section may well obstruct labor and therefore must be recognized. Fundal fibroids should not present a problem at delivery but are associated with an increased incidence of spontaneous abortion (Fig. 27). In early pregnancy, the position of a fibroid can be misleading if it is displaced by a distended bladder. We had such a case in which the fibroid in a gestation of eight weeks appeared to be in the uterine fundus. Subsequent study at 20 weeks, however, showed it to be in the lower uterine segment. It is clear that in the first study the fibroid was displaced cephalad by the enlarging bladder. The bladder when distended will significantly distort the uterus, displacing it anteroposteriorly, laterally, or even rotating it about the long axis of the uterus.

Fibroids can appear uniformly echolucent initially as seen in this case of a fundal fibroid in a 14 week gestation (Fig. 28). Note the very echolucent and highly attenuating nature of the fibroid with loss of any echoes deep to it.

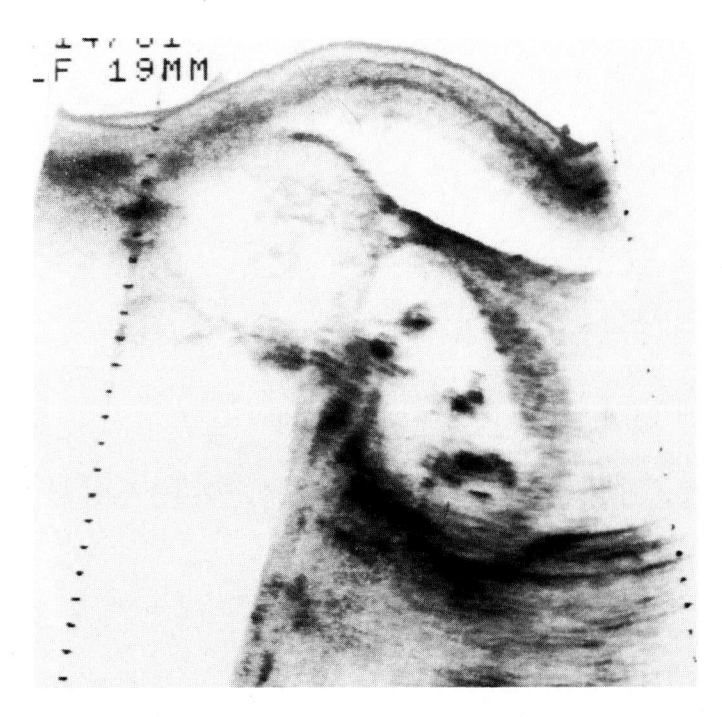

Figure 28. A midline scan shows a 16 week gestation situated in the body of the uterus. The dense echoes in the center of the gestational sac are from fetal limbs. In the uterine fundus there is a 7.5 cm solid mass with marked attenuation of sound posteriorly and an ill-defined back wall. These findings are characteristic of a nondegenerated fundal fibroid.

Fibroids usually distort the serosal surface of the uterus; contractions tend to distort the gestational sac. The contraction has the echogenicity of normal myometrium as opposed to the varying density of the fibroid, which is usually echo poor with marked posterior attenuation (Fig. 28). As the fibroid becomes more vascular and undergoes degeneration, however, its echogenicity increases, and the amount of attenuation decreases.

There are many observations we make sonographically in the first trimester that we can explain quite readily, and yet there are many for which the reason is not yet apparent. For this reason, it is important that one always give the fetus the benefit of doubt and repeat the examination as often as is necessary to assure ourselves of the true diagnosis.

REFERENCES

1. Bourne, C. L.: The microscopic anatomy of the human amnion and chorion. Am. J. Obstet. Gynecol., 79:1070, 1960.
2. Burrows, P. E., Lyons, E. A., Phillips, H. J., et al.: Intrauterine membranes: Sonographic finding and clinical significance. J. Clin. Ultrasound, 10:1, 1982.
3. Hellman, L. M., Kobayashi, M., Fillisti, L., et al.: Growth and development of the human fetus prior to the twentieth week gestation. Am. J. Obstet. Gynecol., 103:789, 1969.
4. Moore, K. L.: The Developing Human. Edition 2. Philadelphia, W. B. Saunders Co., 1977.
5. Robinson, H. P.: Gestation sac volumes as determined by sonar in the first trimester of pregnancy. Br. J. Obstet. Gynecol., 82:100, 1975.
6. Robinson, H. P., and Fleming, J. E. E.: A critical evaluation of sonar crown-rump length measurements. Br. J. Obstet. Gynecol., 82:703, 1975.
7. Sauerbrei, E., Cooperberg, P. L., and Poland, B. J.: Ultrasound demonstration of the normal fetal yolk sac. J. Clin. Ultrasound, 8:217, 1980.

2

Estimating Gestational Age in Utero

*James D. Bowie, M.D.,
and Rochelle Filker Andreotti, M.D.*

Both pregnant women and their doctors estimate gestational age to predict the time of delivery. While knowledge of the gestational age is valuable, we can only roughly estimate the time when labor may begin, since there is some variation, about plus or minus 23 days with a mean of 284 days for 90 per cent of cases,[2] in the duration of pregnancy before the spontaneous onset of labor. A second, perhaps more important reason for estimating gestational age is to estimate organ development or maturity so that prematurity in the newborn can be prevented. Early in pregnancy there is a close but not invariable relationship between the size of the embryo and the stage of organogenesis.[41] Later there is a less well-defined relationship between gestational age and organ function. Neonatal survival is limited primarily by the maturity of the infant's lungs and brain at birth. The absence of lung and brain maturity will lead to significant morbidity and mortality from respiratory distress syndrome and germinal matrix hemorrhage. While the risk for the former is very small after 36 weeks of gestation, and for the latter is reduced after 32 weeks of gestation, individual biologic variation in development may disrupt these relationships. Fetal maturity may often then be assessed directly by biochemical means. Because the normal range for a wide variety of studies performed on the fetus varies with the gestational age, our use of these studies is strictly limited by our estimate of gestational age. Thus the critical first step is to estimate the gestational age within a certain range and at an acceptable confidence level. Finally, in high risk pregnancies estimated gestational ages are important in making decisions about interventions such as the appropriateness of fetal transfusions, the use of betamethasone to accelerate fetal lung maturation, and the timing of diagnostic amniocentesis.

Not everyone uses the same starting point to count gestational age. Fusion of the gametes represents the beginning of the organism, but the complicated process of pregnancy does not begin until implantation of the morula occurs. Since such phenomena are not marked by easily recognized events, the first day of the last normal menstrual period (LNMP) is usually used as the point from which the duration of pregnancy is measured. Obviously this introduces several additional variables which become important in understanding the measures of gestational age we now have available. First, while the time between the LNMP and ovulation is often uniform, there is nevertheless a variation of one or more weeks during which ovulation may occur.[60] This may be even greater in unplanned pregnancies.[7] The rise in basal body temperature is a better indicator of the time of ovulation, which occurs within a narrow range of 36 hours after this event. Fertilization then usually occurs during the next 24 hours while the ovum is viable; implantation follows in about a week. Thus it is apparent that using the LNMP we can only estimate the gestational age to within two to three weeks and, even knowing the time of rise in basal temperature, there may be a two to three day variation in which conception occurs. Because investigators have frequently used LNMP to establish the gestational age when setting a range for some other measure, such as biparietal diameter, then this must introduce a degree of uncertainty which will be included in the final results.

Current methods of estimating gestational age in utero are clinical, biochemical, radiologic, and sonographic. In addition there are a variety of clinical methods for estimating the gestational age for the newborn infant.

Clinical Estimation. The clinical methods for estimating gestational age include the last normal menstrual period (LNMP), basal temperature rise, quickening, first trimester pelvic examinations, measurement of fundal height, and first appreciation of fetal heart beat by means of the fetoscope or Doppler ultrasound. Although these methods have been used for a long time, their accuracy has only recently been investigated. Unfortunately, most of these investigations have relied on the LNMP or time of delivery to establish the gestational age. As a result it is difficult to know the true value of these clinical estimations of gestational age.

Some number of women will not recall when the LNMP occurred. The inability to specify a time for the LNMP has been reported in 20 to 40 per cent of women.[8,19] Perhaps some of the variation in known "dates" is a result of the willingness of the physician to accept a date as accurate. Often there is a bias to recall the first, fifth, or fifteenth day of the month.[67] In some women the LNMP may not be acceptable because of the use of birth control pills, irregular menstrual cycles, or the inability to decide if the menstrual period was normal or not. In yet another group it is thought that the bleeding at the time of implantation which often occurs from three to five weeks after the last normal period is mistaken for the menstrual period.[32] Despite these problems, the first day of the last normal menstrual period remains the most commonly used and probably the best single "clinical" estimator of gestational age. There is evidence that when the patient's recollection of this date is considered reliable, the fetal gestational age is estimated to within three weeks in 90 per cent of cases,[2] but to be 90 per cent certain that a gestational age of 38 weeks has been reached, 42 weeks must elapse.[31]

Other clinical estimators of gestational age have been less thoroughly evaluated but do not appear to be as useful as the LNMP,[2] with perhaps the exception of physical examination of the uterine size in the first trimester. Physical examination during this time is generally considered to be accurate in estimating the gestational age to within a week, although we know of no study done to evaluate the accuracy of this. Also, this measure is known to be misleading if the patient's uterus is abnormal, for example, enlarged by fibroid tumors, congenitally abnormal, or retroflexed, or if the patient is difficult to examine. The measurement of the fundal height of the uterus can be done from the beginning of the second trimester to term. Studies relating this measure to gestational age have shown an accuracy of no more than plus or minus six weeks at the 90 per cent confidence level.[2, 3] Serial measurement of the fundal height as an estimation of fetal growth, however, is a useful clinical tool and may lead to the correct recognition of many abnormalities, such as twins, polyhydramnios, intrauterine growth retardation, and so forth. Fetal heart tones can be detected by Doppler ultrasound at 14 weeks and with a fetoscope at 18 weeks. While these observations often assist in establishing an approximate minimum age, the actual variation in predicting gestational age is greater than fundal height measurement.[2] The maternal appreciation of fetal movement, because of its subjective nature, is not useful in estimating gestational age.

BIOCHEMICAL ESTIMATION

Type II cells of fetal lung alveoli produce active phospholipids collectively called surfactant. Surfactant acts as a detergent to lower the surface tension at air-fluid interfaces within alveoli. This decreases the tendency of the alveolus to collapse at the end of an expiration according to LaPlace's Law: $P = 2T/R$. The respiratory distress syndrome develops when the lung collapses with each expiration because of the high surface tension at air-fluid interfaces. Surfactant is composed of lipids (80 to 90 per cent), protein (10 to 20 per cent), and carbohydrates (1 to 2 per cent). The majority of the lipids are phospholipids. Phosphatidyl choline (lecithin) is the major phospholipid. Important phospholipids in surfactant are dipalmityl lecithin, phosphatidyl inositol (PI), and phosphatidyl glycerol (PG). Dipalmityl lecithin is stored in lamellar bodies which are contained within Type II alveolar cells. The lamellar bodies are released from Type II cells into the alveolar space, and may then be transported in large quantities to the amniotic fluid.[23, 35, 49]

The ratio of lecithin to sphingomyelin (L/S) in amniotic fluid has become a popular method of assessing fetal lung maturity since, in uncomplicated pregnancies, it follows a predictable pattern.[24] Sphingomyelin concentrations change little with gestational age and consequently provide a useful standard for comparison. Lecithin appears in the amniotic fluid at approximately 24 to 26 weeks. Between 31 and 35 weeks there is a gradual rise in lecithin concentration to give a L/S ratio of 2. By 34 to 36 weeks there is an acute rise in lecithin concentration. Gluck and coworkers[25] first showed that the likelihood of respiratory distress syndrome is minimal in a normal gestation when the L/S ratio is 2 or greater.[36] In a recent report of 20 series involving 2170 patients with a mature L/S ratio, 98 per cent of the newborns did not develop respiratory distress syndrome, and less than 2 per cent did develop respiratory distress syndrome. Although the false-positive rate was remarkably small, this was at the expense of a high false-negative rate.[30] Cumulative results from several investigators indicate that in 38 to 46 per cent of the cases in which the L/S ratio was less than 2, the ratio was not predictive of respiratory distress syndrome.[20, 30, 36]

Hallman et al.[28, 29] have recently developed a new technique which may help to identify those neonates who will develop respiratory distress syndrome in the presence of a mature L/S ratio, and a larger group of neonates who do not develop respiratory distress syndrome in the presence of an immature L/S ratio. It was proposed that surfactant containing PI and PG stabilizes alveolar function and surfactant activity. Therefore, alveoli may be more stable at lower volumes when these two phospholipids are present. PI increases with gestational age at rates similar to the L/S ratio up to a value of 2. At approximately 35 to 36 weeks, the PI level decreases. PG first appears at 35 weeks, probably signaling the appearance of mature surfactant. These measurements of PI, PG, and disaturated lecithin may be plotted to obtain a lung profile which permits the clinician to assess the stage of fetal lung development. This test may be especially important in high risk pregnancies in which the L/S ratio is less than 2. In these cases, the L/S ratio may not be predictive since in stressed infants, lung maturity is often accelerated but is not reflected in the L/S ratio. However, PG may be detected earlier than 35 weeks, signaling lung maturity.

In an attempt to eliminate time, effort, and cost in the precise measurement of the L/S ratio, Clements and associates developed the foam stability test, or shake test.[11] The procedure involves mixing amniotic fluid with saline in various proportions and adding this to a similar volume of 95 per cent ethanol. After the mixture is shaken for 15 seconds, the test is positive if adequate surfactant is present to generate stable foam in the presence of ethanol. If the foam persists at the air-liquid interface for 15 minutes, lung maturity may be assumed. The shake test is reported to be a reliable indicator of pulmonary maturity. Thus, a positive test is a valid measure of pulmonary maturity, and the false-positive rate is similar to that of the L/S ratio method. The problems with the shake test are twofold: test results may be altered considerably by contamination with blood or meconium, excessive centrifugation, or exposure to warm room temperature; and false-negative results are common. Comparing the reports of Gluck et al. on the L/S ratio method and Clements et al. on the shake test, an immature L/S ratio is more predictive of respiratory distress syndrome than is an immature shake test.[12, 24]

Investigators have also attempted to assess fetal maturity by using other constituents or properties of amniotic fluid. The most widely cited measurements are amniotic fluid creatinine[22, 64] and Nile blue staining cells.[6] A major drawback of these tests is their inability to assess pulmonary function directly. Fetal organ systems do not mature in parallel, and it is usually the fetal pulmonary system which determines whether the neonate will survive outside the womb. Creatinine in amniotic fluid gradually rises as a pregnancy approaches term, reflecting the increased excretion of creatinine by maturing fetal kidneys. A creatinine level of 2 mg per 100 ml has commonly been used to indicate fetal maturity. Some investigators report confidence in amniotic fluid creatinine as a reliable index of gestational age or fetal weight. However, other investigators have reported that creatinine levels at a given gestational age show wide variation, and are of little value in the determination of fetal maturity.

Amniotic fluid contains desquamated fetal cells of two origins: squamous and sebaceous, which are easily differentiated by staining with Nile blue sulfate. While the squamous cells stain light blue with dark blue nuclei, lipid-containing cells shed from sebaceous glands stain orange to pink in color. Fetal sebaceous glands become functional with increasing gestational age and begin shedding cells late in gestation. Bishop and Corson[6] claimed that the percentage of the "fat cells" in amniotic fluid increases with gestational age. When lipid cells exceeded 20 per cent, a gestational age of over 36 weeks was indicated. Problems involved in the use of the Nile blue sulfate technique include clumping of the fat cells, which makes quantification difficult. A high false-negative rate may also be observed since a low percentage of fat cells does not necessarily indicate prematurity.

RADIOLOGIC AND ULTRASONIC ESTIMATION OF GESTATIONAL AGE

Radiographic estimation of gestational age has been attempted by measuring the size of various fetal structures.[55] The most widely used standard is the appearance of the distal femoral (DFE) or proximal tibial (PTE) ossification center.[61] However, when the gestational age has been established by ultrasonographic determination of crown-rump length (CRL), it is evident that the DFE can often be seen by 32 weeks but sometimes not until 38 weeks while the similar range for the PTE is 33 to 41 weeks. In this same study, 42 per cent of growth-retarded babies had retarded development of epiphyses,[52] confirming evidence from previous studies.[15]

In the last decade or two a great deal has been written or said about the use of ultrasound for the in utero estimation of gestational age. Ultrasound observations can be divided into either quantitative measurements (length, area, volume) or qualitative observations (movement, organ appearance, and so forth). The crown-rump length (CRL), biparietal diameter (BPD), gestational sac (GS) size, and femur length (FL) are the measurements most commonly used. A distinction should be made between measures of size or proportion, for example, head circumference, abdominal circumference, long axis, and measures of age. All dimensional measures are related to both size and age, but some relate more to size and others to age. One way to organize an approach to fetal measures is to first make the best estimation of age that is possible, then determine if size or proportion is appropriate for that age.

The gestational sac is the first structure seen on ultrasound examination in pregnancy. When a single internal diameter of the sac or an average of anteroposterior, transverse, and lateral diameters is used to determine gestational age, the variation for 90 per cent of cases is approximately plus or minus two weeks (Fig. 1, A and B). Volume of the sac as calculated from the sum of cross-sectional areas of parallel scans reduces this range to plus or minus nine days.[53] However, this measure has not been routinely employed because of the need for special instrumentation to measure the sac areas and special care to see that sections are taken at precise intervals. When the embryo cannot be identified, the gestational sac can be used to determine if the pregnancy is advanced enough to expect an embryo to be present. When the embryo is seen, the crown-rump length can be measured (Fig. 1C).

With static scanners, the technique for measuring crown-rump length requires projection of the margins of the embryo onto the patient's skin from a series of parallel images. From this projection the longest axis of the embryo is approximated, and scans are performed until a maximum length is obtained. With real-time scanning the transducer is slowly rotated until a maximum length is found.

The crown-rump length determined by ultrasound examination, when done properly, estimates gestational age between six and 12 weeks with a range of 4.7 days at the 95 per cent confidence level (Table 1).[54] However, this measurement requires considerable skill to do properly, and to know from the actual image that a true maximum was found is difficult. In our experience errors are more common after the twelfth week, and after the fourteenth week we do not measure crown-rump length but use biparietal diameter.

The greatest problem in measurement of crown-rump length early in pregnancy lies

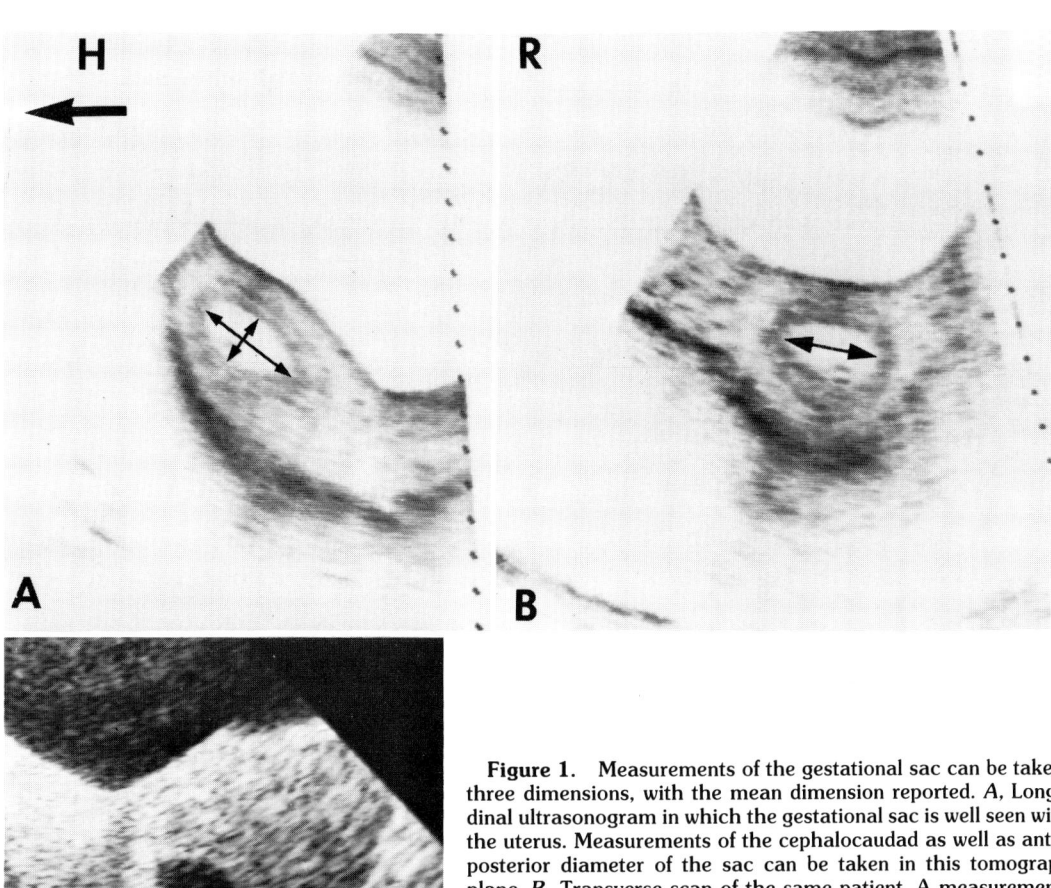

Figure 1. Measurements of the gestational sac can be taken in three dimensions, with the mean dimension reported. A, Longitudinal ultrasonogram in which the gestational sac is well seen within the uterus. Measurements of the cephalocaudad as well as anteroposterior diameter of the sac can be taken in this tomographic plane. B, Transverse scan of the same patient. A measurement of the transverse diameter of the gestational sac completes the third measurement for which an average can be taken. C, Careful scanning of the gestational sac, often with real time equipment, will demonstrate the embryo (*arrow*). The maximum length of this structure is a better measure of gestational age than the sac size.

in knowing whether the maximum length was obtained and measured (Fig. 2). Since the anatomic landmarks are very limited at this time, it is not possible to look at the measured image and know that it represents the optimal one. Good results depend on meticulous application of the appropriate technique, and the skill and dedication of the person doing the scanning. Later in pregnancy, measurement of crown-rump length is affected by flexion and extension movements of the fetus (Fig. 3). Changes in body tone may affect the measurement significantly. After the twelfth week we prefer to confirm our measurements with a measurement of biparietal diameter as well. Measurements of crown-rump length later in pregnancy generally seem to entail less error when the fetus is in a very slightly flexed position, not hyperextended and not fully flexed.

Biparietal Diameter

When setting up this technique in an ultrasound laboratory the important factors are: that the technique duplicates the one used for the standard chart from which the gestational age is determined, that there are adequate criteria for accepting a measurement, and that quality control be done to verify the precision and reproducibility for biparietal diameters in that labora-

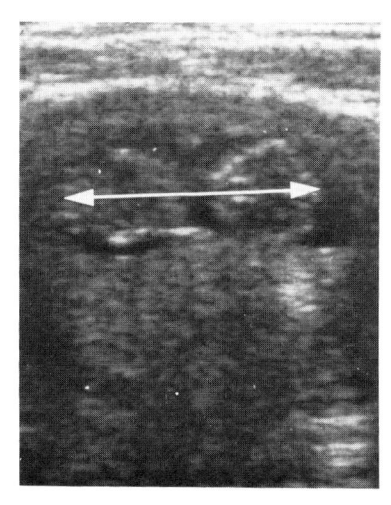

Figure 2. It is important in measuring the crown-rump length to obtain a maximum length. Measurement of the crown-rump length in neutral position can be measured accurately early in gestation. Accurate measurements depend upon obtaining a maximal length (*arrows*).

tory.[9] Two techniques that have been carefully documented are those of Campbell and Sabbagha.[56, 62] These two techniques for static scanners, originally bistable, are equally valid for gray-scale static scanners. Each one begins by identifying the longitudinal axis of the head and after determining the angle of tilt of this axis the scan is rotated to be perpendicular to this line and a series of images are taken until a maximum diameter is obtained. The two important steps are setting the scan plane perpendicular to the appropriate axis and obtaining enough samples. Measurements can be made from an A-mode or the B-mode image. When done properly these give equivalent results. Measurements from B-mode images can be either from a bistable image or a gray scale image and again the results are the same.[62] Finally, measurements from a gray scale, B-mode image can be either from the outer margin of the near

Table 1. *Fetal Crown-Rump Length Against Gestational Age**

CRL (mm)	−2 SD	MEAN WEEKS	+2 SD	CRL (mm)	−2 SD	MEAN WEEKS	+2 SD
7		6.25	7.15	39	10	10.65	11.35
8		6.45	7.3	40	10.1	10.75	11.45
9		6.7	7.55	41	10.2	10.8	11.55
10	6.25	6.9	7.7	42	10.3	10.9	11.65
11	6.5	7.1	7.9	43	10.4	11.05	11.7
12	6.6	7.25	8.1	44	10.45	11.1	11.8
13	6.85	7.45	8.25	45	10.55	11.2	11.9
14	7.00	7.60	8.45	46	10.66	11.3	12
15	7.15	7.75	8.60	47	10.7	11.35	12.05
16	7.3	7.9	8.70	48	10.8	11.45	12.15
17	7.45	8.1	8.9	49	10.9	11.55	12.25
18	7.60	8.2	9.0	50	10.95	11.6	12.3
19	7.75	8.4	9.15	51	11.1	11.7	12.4
20	7.9	8.5	9.3	52	11.15	11.8	12.5
21	8.05	8.6	9.4	53	11.2	11.85	12.55
22	8.15	8.8	9.55	54	11.3	11.95	12.65
23	8.3	8.9	9.65	55	11.4	12.05	12.75
24	8.4	9.05	9.8	56	11.5	12.1	12.8
25	8.55	9.15	9.9	57	11.55	12.2	12.9
26	8.7	9.3	10	58	11.65	12.3	12.95
27	8.8	9.4	10.1	59	11.7	12.35	13.05
28	8.9	9.5	10.25	60	11.8	12.45	13.15
29	9.05	9.65	10.35	61	11.85	12.5	13.2
30	9.15	9.7	10.45	62	11.9	12.6	13.3
31	9.25	9.85	10.55	63	12	12.65	13.4
32	9.35	9.95	10.65	64	12.05	12.75	13.45
33	9.45	10.05	10.75	65	12.1	12.85	13.55
34	9.55	10.15	10.85	66	12.2	12.9	13.6
35	9.6	10.2	10.95	67	12.3	12.95	13.7
36	9.7	10.35	11.05	68	12.35	13.05	13.75
37	9.8	10.4	11.15	69	12.45	13.1	13.8
38	9.9	10.55	11.25	70	12.5	13.15	13.9

* *From* Robinson, H. P., and Fleming, J. E. E.: A critical evaluation of sonar crown-rump length measurements. Br. J. Obstet. Gynecol., *82*:702, 1975, with permission.

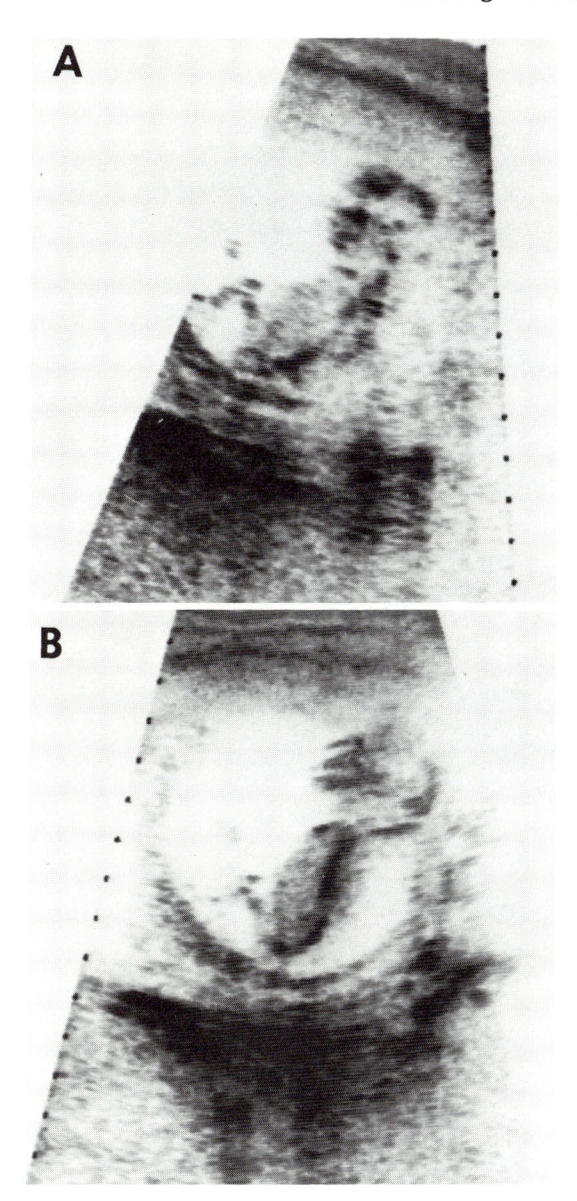

thought to represent samples of the maximum diameter.

With this approach, the most important single criterion is that a midline be present and located in the center between the outer skull echoes.[66] In fact, if this criterion is met and adequate levels are sampled then this criterion alone is sufficient to obtain the maximum biparietal diameter. However, the midline echoes identified must originate in the plane of the interhemispheric cleft. It is possible to find lines in the head which resemble the "midline" but are in fact not in the appropriate interhemispheric plane. To reduce the chance of this error, other criteria are added. These are that the head appear oval and the midline represent a major diameter of the elipse. Other criteria dealing with image quality and occasional anatomic landmarks can be added. These criteria may be classified as "geometric" ones.

Even when the head is oval and the midline is centered, it is possible to obtain "coronal" views, and unless the entire fetal head is scanned carefully the maximum diameter can be missed (Fig. 5). Furthermore, additional determinations such as head circumference and frontal occipital diameters cannot be performed reproducibly unless standard axial views are taken.

A "geometric" approach can be used with real-time systems although the approximations of the angle of tilt of the head are more difficult and the criteria for acceptance must be rigidly applied. It is also possible to use an "anatomic" approach which requires that certain internal structures be

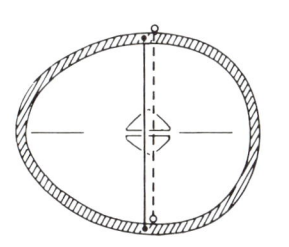

Figure 3. Crown-rump length measurement later in pregnancy. *A,* At this stage of pregnancy it is possible for the fetus to flex. *B,* Same fetus in extended position. Change in position may alter the measurements.

skull line to the inner margin of the far one (O-I) or from the middle of each (M-M), and equivalent results are obtained (Fig. 4).[38] When measuring this diameter it is important to determine that it is perpendicular to the midline, that evidence of midline is seen on either side of the diameter (but not necessarily crossing it), and that it is obtained from an acceptable image. The number used must represent the maximum biparietal diameter. Thus it is appropriate to average measurements only if they are all

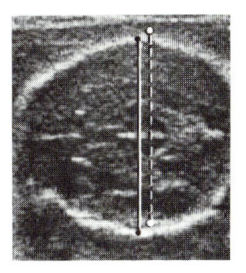

- - - - - - Outer to inner
——— Center to center

Figure 4. Diagram of the points of measurement for obtaining a biparietal diameter. Once an accurate plane of section has been obtained the fetal head may be measured either from the outer margin of the near skull line to the inner margin of the far one or from the center or middle of each skull line.

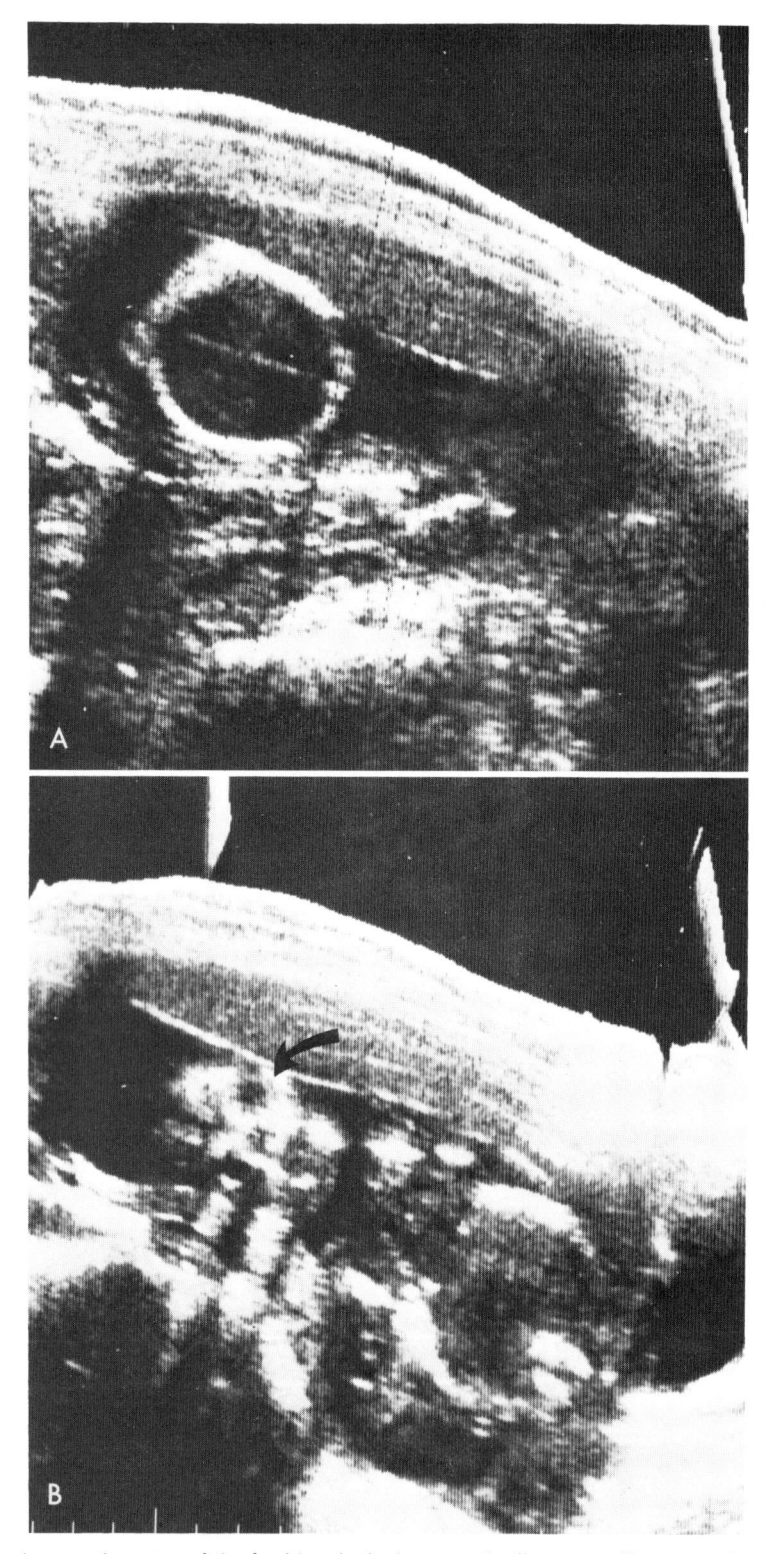

Figure 5. *A*, A coronal section of the fetal head which meets the "geometric" criteria of an oval head with a centered midline. *B*, A section taken parallel to Figure 5A showing the coronal nature of the scan plane. The fetal face (*arrow*) is seen including orbits, maxilla, and mandible.

seen in the brain and several levels are photographed.[33] This serves as a useful check for static scanners and is particularly appropriate for real-time equipment. Images are taken at the base of the brain and progressively higher to the level of the lateral ventricles. This gives some assurance that adequate sampling has occurred.

An anatomic approach requires a knowledge of the appropriate regional fetal anatomy and the ability to visualize the fetus as a three-dimensional structure while the study is being performed (Fig. 6). Our suggestion is that during the initial survey with real-time equipment, the relative position of the fetal spine and head be identified. With this as a guide, the scan plane is positioned so that it is roughly an axial plane of the fetal head. With a rocking motion the head is scanned until the fetal orbits are located. These important landmarks allow an experienced operator to recognize the position of the face relative to the fetal spine and in turn the ultrasound scan plane can be placed in a lateral axial position near the base of the fetal skull. With minor adjustments this scan plane can be positioned parallel to the base of the skull to show the greater wings of the sphenoid bones and the petrous ridges. Using this scan plane as a base, the transducer is moved to obtain a second scan plane parallel and slightly above the first one. This will show the midbrain and basilar artery; often the circle of Willis and middle cerebral arteries can also be visualized. Another plane parallel to this one and slightly higher will show the basal ganglia and thalamus which surround the third ventricle.

Actually several planes can be obtained showing these structures depending on the size of the fetal head and the width of the scan plane. At the upper levels, the septum cavum pellucidum, anterior horns of the lateral ventricles, and quadrigeminal cisterns may be seen. This plane has been chosen by one investigator as the optimal one for the measurement of biparietal diameter.[63] If standard charts based on the maximum biparietal diameter are used, it is either this plane or occasionally one slightly higher as the lateral walls of the lateral ventricles are seen which contain the maximum biparietal diameter (Fig. 7). To complete the axial views of the fetal head, the falx should be visualized, but no measurements should be taken from this level.

Having established a technique and criteria for measuring, each laboratory should have a quality control program. Reproducibility can be checked by performing consecutive studies on the same patient one day apart.[16] The result of the first measurements should not be available during the second study. This is appropriate if one person does all of the studies. Our way of controlling reproducibility is to have each study done twice on every occasion, first by one sonographer then by another, each unaware of the other's results. If the differences in the resultant biparietal diameters are greater than 2 mm, a third examination is done. We check reproducibility continuously because of the number of individuals we are training. For most laboratories, after reproducibility can be shown to be consistently within the 2 mm range, then only periodic quality control is required whenever a new person begins to do the studies, and whenever new equipment is used. Validity is more difficult to establish. We have found actual measurement of newborn heads with calipers to be difficult but this approach has been used. We prefer to select a sample of patients who have normal, average-sized term babies, have well-known last menstrual periods or measured crown-rump lengths, and spontaneously deliver within one week of their expected date. From this group we see if the ultrasound determination of gestational age is within the accepted range. The difficulty that remains to be solved is how to assure that if a measurement is obtained in one laboratory it is equivalent to one done elsewhere.

Interpretation of the Biparietal Diameter. Although it is not clear what degree of variation in biparietal diameter results from racial or socioeconomic differences,[57] maternal disease,[1, 43, 46] or fetal head shape,[26] it is generally agreed that the variation in biparietal diameter measured by ultrasound for a given age of gestation becomes greater as pregnancy progresses. As a result, earlier measurements are more useful than later ones. We believe, now, that the optimal determinations are obtained from 15 to 26 weeks (our own preference is measurement prior to 20

STEPS IN OBTAINING THE BIPARIETAL DIAMETER

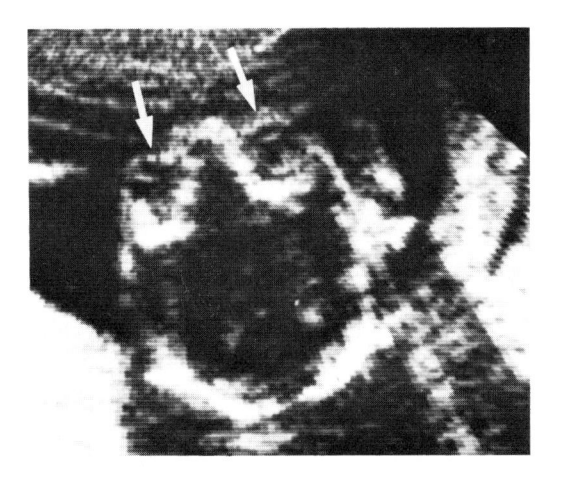

1. Determine the position of the spine as it relates to the head.
2. Obtain an axial scan of the head.
3. Angulate the transducer to image the orbits.

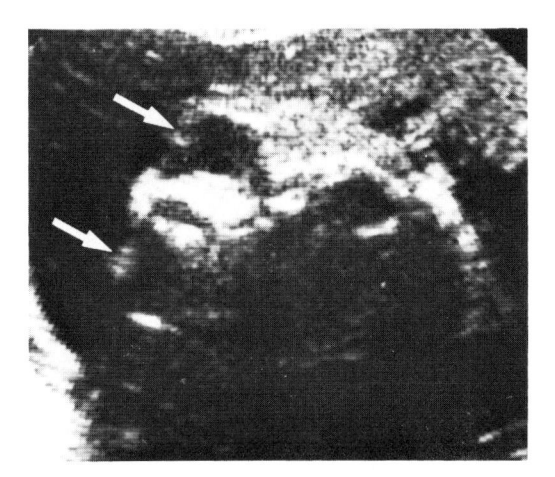

4. Knowing the position of the face relative to the fetal spine, obtain a lateral axial scan near the base of the fetal skull.

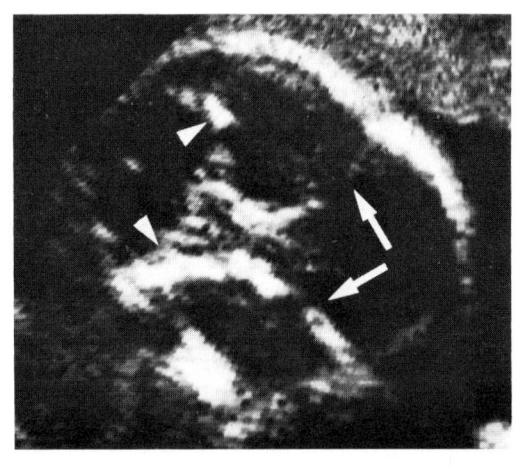

5. Obtain a true axial scan at the base of the skull imaging the "crossed" appearance of the greater wings of the sphenoid (→) and the petrous ridges (▸).

Figure 6. Steps in obtaining a biparietal diameter based upon a knowledge of the fetal anatomy.

Estimating Gestational Age in Utero 31

6. Using the scan plane in (5) as a base obtain a scan plane parallel and above that of the scan imaging the midbrain (→).

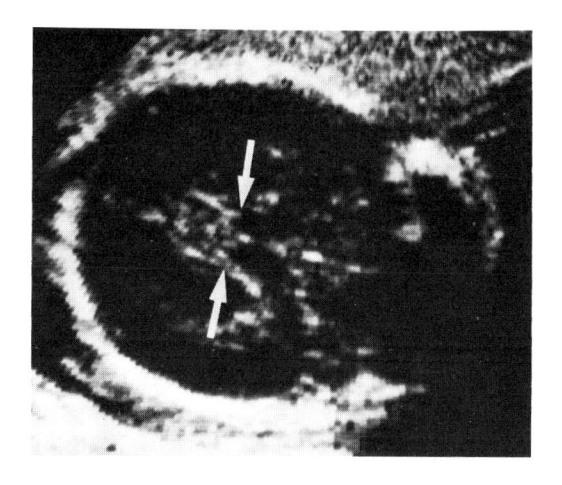

7. If this scan plane demonstrates the orbits, the transducer should be angulated to realign the plane parallel to the skull base.

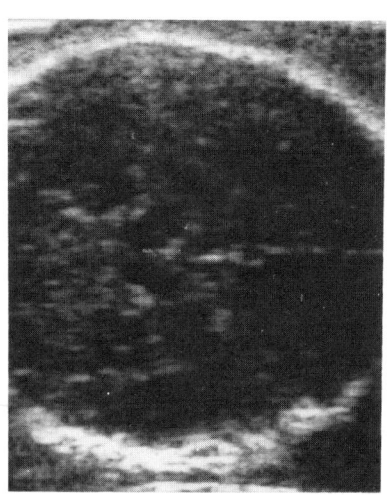

8. The final plane of section at a higher level will pass through the basal ganglia and thalamus (→) which should surround the 3rd ventricle (▸).

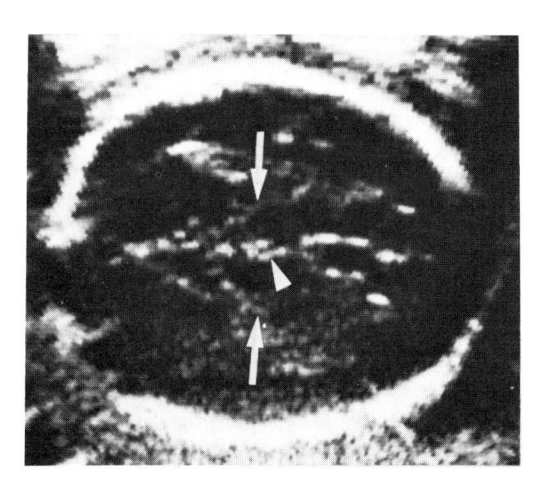

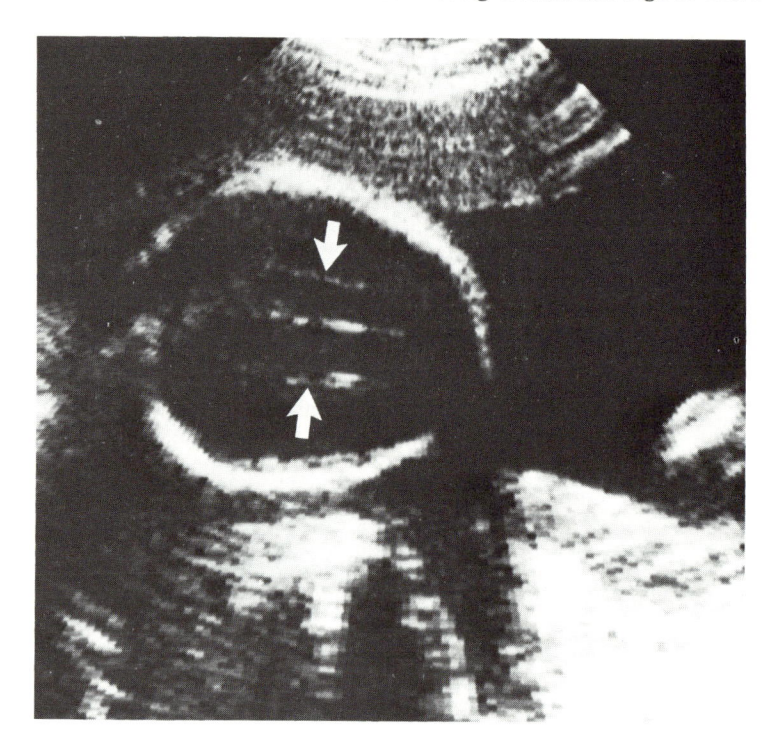

Figure 7. An axial scan at the level of the lateral ventricles which shows the lateral walls of the lateral ventricles (*arrows*).

weeks), that from 27 to 30 weeks there is a progressive increase in variability, and that after 30 weeks satisfactory assignment of gestational age is difficult (Table 2). Greater importance should be given to measurements obtained at earlier times, and generally measurements prior to 26 weeks are thought to be more related to gestational age and afterward more influenced by growth. It is important for each study to give a mean gestational age, an expected range, and the statistical basis for the range (for example, two standard deviations, 95 per cent confidence level, and so forth). This shift of relationship from age to growth is incorporated in a system called growth adjusted sonographic age (GASA).[58] However, until more investigation of this system has occurred, we feel that the average user should not use GASA, particularly since there is increasing evidence that fluctuations in growth rate patterns are a part of normal growth of biparietal diameter,[40] and one underlying assumption of the GASA system is that growth rates rather closely follow a given "percentile" curve.

Some of the variation in measurements of biparietal diameter in the latter part of pregnancy may be accounted for by differences in shapes of fetal heads. Perhaps in some cases there is little change in head shape as pregnancy progresses, but in instances of twins or fetal crowding the head shapes may change and significantly alter measurement of biparietal diameter. For this reason, measurements of head circumference or measures of the ratio of frontal occipital diameter to biparietal diameter have been suggested to monitor head growth later in pregnancy.[27] We begin doing this after 26 weeks.

Establishing a standard image plane based on anatomic landmarks is essential if measurements of head circumference or frontal occipital diameter are to be obtained. It is not entirely clear whether such criteria have been applied to the published charts of circumferences. The level we suggest for measurement is the same as for anatomic biparietal diameter measurement: that is, the high thalamic area which includes anterior horns of lateral ventricles, septum cavum pellucidum, third ventricle, thalamus, and quadrigeminal cisterns. This plan must be sought in a systematic manner as described above, and not just any scan plane with a "box" in the front of midline used. In fact it is easy to obtain an oblique coronal plane to include the septum cavum pellucidum and the third ventricle, and to resemble the standard section but not lie parallel to the base of the skull.

Twins. Because of their relatively small numbers, less is known about the growth patterns of twins than singleton pregnancies. Because it is unclear whether the more rigorous anatomic criteria have been used in the few studies of biparietal diameter in twins, the question of whether the standard charts for singleton pregnancies can be used for twin pregnancies is not answerable. However, it does seem likely that early in pregnancy (prior to 20 weeks), the singleton charts will not differ significantly from those for normal sized twins. As pregnancy progresses there is frequently distortion of head shape in twin pregnancies and our feeling is that accurate measurements of head circumference are absolutely required to compare head sizes of twins and to plot head growth. It has been suggested that a difference of more than 10 per cent in head circumference suggests discordance in twin size.[14] However, we recommend that this information be combined with other measures of fetal size, particularly abdominal circumference, before a diagnosis of discordance be made.

Table 2. *Correlation of Predicted Menstrual Age Based upon Biparietal Diameters*

			BPD Mean Values (mm)			
Menstrual Age (weeks)	Composite Sabbagha and Hughey[1]	Composite Kurtz et al.[2]	Kurtz et al.[2] < 1974	Kurtz et al.[2] > 1974	Hadlock et al.[3] 1982	Shepard and Filly[4] 1982
14	28	27	28	26	27	28
15	32	31	31	29	30	31
16	36	34	35	33	33	34
17	39	38	39	36	37	37
18	42	41	42	40	40	40
19	45	45	46	43	43	43
20	48	48	49	46	46	46
21	51	51	52	50	50	49
22	54	54	55	53	53	52
23	58	57	58	56	56	55
24	61	60	61	59	58	57
25	64	63	64	61	61	60
26	67	66	67	64	64	63
27	70	69	69	67	67	65
28	72	71	72	70	70	68
29	75	74	75	72	72	71
30	78	76	77	75	75	73
31	80	79	79	77	77	76
32	82	81	81	79	79	78
33	85	83	83	82	82	80
34	87	85	85	84	84	83
35	88	87	87	86	86	85
36	90	89	89	88	88	88
37	92	91	91	90	90	90
38	93	92	92	92	91	92
39	94	94	94	94	93	95
40	95	95	95	95	95	97

[1] Sabbagha, R. E., and Hughey, M.: Standardization of sonar cephalometry and gestational age. Obstet. Gynecol., *52*:402, 1978.

[2] Kurtz, A. B., Wapner, R. J., Kurtz, R. J., et al.: Analysis of biparietal diameter as an accurate indicator of gestational age. J. Clin. Ultrasound, *8*:319, 1980.

[3] Hadlock, F. P., Deter, R. L., Harrist, R. B., et al.: Fetal biparietal diameter: A critical re-evaluation of the relation to menstrual age by means of real-time ultrasound. J. Ultrasound Med., *1*:97–104, 1982.

[4] Shepard, M., and Filly, R. A.: A standardized plane for biparietal diameter measurement. J. Ultrasound Med., *1*:145–150, 1982.

Assigning Gestational Age

Assigning gestational age in utero is a complicated task which depends on the use of skill and good judgment. Since this is far from an exact science, we do not offer any fixed rules, although the following guidelines often prove useful. First the ultrasonographer should have some general concept of which parameters are better than others (Table 3). Then generally the best parameter available is used to estimate the gestational age, unless there is some reason to believe that this particular estimator may not be as accurate as usual. For example, a measurement of crown-rump length at 8 weeks would be given priority over the LNMP from memory (with a good history) unless there were special reasons to believe that the crown-rump length was inaccurate. There is little evidence that averaging of data[51] improves the precision of estimations, and we do not suggest that this approach be taken until there is more knowledge about the effects of averaging data from dissimilar sources. When data from several sources agree within a one or two week range, confidence that the estimation is correct is greater than when data are derived from one source only or when different sources give disparate estimations. Perhaps the greatest problem is for the ultrasonographer to estimate the reliability of a clinical parameter; to ignore these parameters is a mistake to be avoided. Serial measurements of biparietal diameter do not improve the precision with which gestational age is known,[44] but may act as information supplementary to other growth parameters such as abdominal circumference.

Recently the length of the fetal femur has been measured in the second trimester (Fig. 8; Table 4). This measure correlated well with gestational age during the period of 14 to 22 weeks with an estimate to within 6.7 days at the 95 per cent confidence level.[45] These data are from a small series and the reliability later in pregnancy is not known. The femoral length may be used as an estimator of gestational age in those cases in which the biparietal diameter cannot be relied upon or obtained because of positions of the fetal head, or abnormalities of the cranium in the second trimester.

A number of simple and complex ultrasound measurements have not been discussed, some perhaps as an oversight, others because we feel they are more closely related to fetal size than to gestational age. These include ultrasonic abdominal diameters or circumferences, chest diameters or areas, somatic size estimations, cranial size data, thigh diameters, and others. In the third trimester these more complex measures may provide answers to some of the questions about fetal size, maturity, and well being.

Table 3. *Clinical Parameters in Estimation of Gestational Age**

PRIORITY FOR ESTIMATING GESTATIONAL AGE	"ESTIMATED" RANGE FOR 95% CASES
1. In vitro fertilization	less than 1 day
2. Ovulation induction	3–4 days
3. Recorded basal body temperature	4–5 days
4. Ultrasound crown-rump length (CRL)	±.7 weeks
5. First trimester physical examination (normal uterus)	±1 week
6. Ultrasound BPD prior to 20 weeks	±1 week
7. Ultrasound gestational sac volume	±1.5 weeks
8. Ultrasound BPD from 20 to 26 weeks	±1.6 weeks
9. LNMP from recorded dates (good history)†	±2–3 weeks
10. Ultrasound BPD 26 to 30 weeks	±2–3 weeks
11. LNMP from memory (good history)	3–4 weeks
12. Ultrasound BPD after 30 weeks	3–4 weeks
13. Fundal height measurement	4–6 weeks
14. LNMP from memory (not good history)	4–6 weeks
15. Fetal heart tones first heard	4–6 weeks
16. Quickening	4–6 weeks

* *Rule* is to always use a more reliable indicator in preference to a less reliable one.

† A "good" history requires knowledge of both LNMP and previous period with regular periods and no use of birth control pills for at least six months prior to the LNMP.

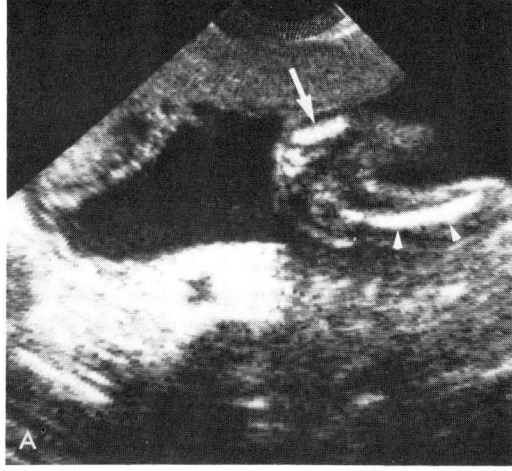

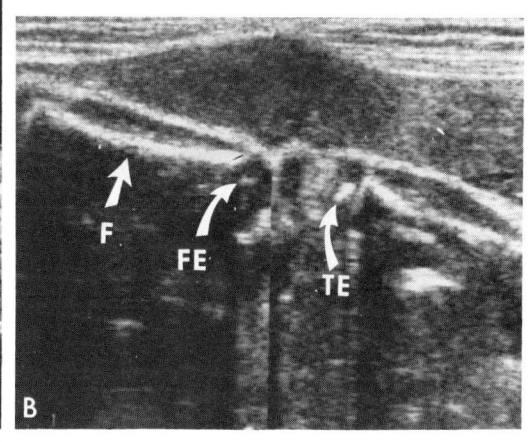

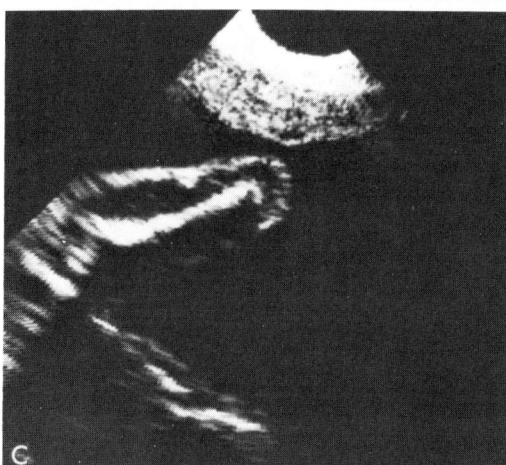

Figure 8. *A,* The femur can be identified by using the iliac bone as a reference point (*arrow*) and rotating the real-time transducer until a femur is seen (*arrowheads*). In this example the optimal length has not been obtained as indicated by tapering of the ends of the bone. *B,* Real-time scan of the entire distal extremity of a fetus. This scan demonstrates the appearance of the femur which is appropriate for measurements. This coronal scan of the femur can be determined by the presence of the femoral head and the position of the bone in the thigh which is closer to the lateral side of the thigh than the medial. This scan which was taken late in gestation demonstrates presence of both the distal femoral epiphysis (FE) and the proximal tibial epiphysis (TE). *C,* A sagittal view of a femur which is indicated by the more center position in the soft tissues.

Other Ultrasound Observations

Qualitative observations of the appearances of fetal organs or identification of certain fetal activities have some potential for establishing age independent of a measurement. These types of observations can be divided into two major categories: those that deal with morphologic changes which are often qualitative and those that deal with dynamic events which are related to fetal movements or activity patterns.

Morphologic changes throughout pregnancy can be observed with ultrasound. Areas which have been studied include: the relative size of the fetal ventricles,[17] the appearance of the choroid plexus,[13] the echogenicity of fetal lungs, the appearance of fetal bowel, the thickness of fetal thigh, the appearance of fetal kidneys, and the appearance of fetal skin. While some observations related to these structures may alone or in combination be used to establish a gestational age, at the time of this writing the evidence is simply too preliminary to be used clinically.

Perhaps a little more is known about some of the dynamic events that can be observed with real-time ultrasound. Fetal movements can be seen with dynamic ultrasound systems. Also, the nature of these measurements change with the duration of pregnancy. Individual limbs can be seen to flex and extend, trunk movements occur, chest wall and diaphragm movements have been described, and bowel peristaltic activity, fetal mouth and tongue movements, and fetal eye movements can be seen.[4] It is probably true that with increasing gestational age, increasingly complex patterns of activity appear,[5] but these are also related to the metabolic state of the fetus and possibly cycles of activity similar to adult wake and sleeping cycles. As a result, although

Table 4. *Comparison of Predicted Femur Lengths at Points in Gestation*

Femur Length (mm)

Menstrual Age (weeks)	Filly et al.[1] 1981	Jeanty et al.[2] 1981†	Hadlock et al.[3] 1982*	Hadlock et al.[3] 1982†
12		09	14	08
13		12	16	11
14	16	16	19	15
15	19	19	21	18
16	22	23	23	21
17	25	26	26	24
18	28	30	28	27
19	32	33	30	30
20	35	36	33	33
21	38	39	35	36
22	41	42	38	39
23	44	45	40	42
24	47	48	42	44
25	50	51	45	47
26	53	54	47	49
27	55	57	49	52
28	57	59	52	54
29	61	62	54	56
30	63	65	57	58
31		67	59	61
32		70	61	63
33		72	64	65
34		74	66	66
35		77	69	68
36		79	71	70
37		81	73	72
38		83	76	73
39		85	78	75
40		87	80	76

*Linear function
†Linear quadratic function

[1] Filly, R. A., Golbus, M. S., Carey, J. C., et al.: Short-limbed dwarfism: Ultrasonographic diagnosis by mensuration of fetal femoral length. Radiology, *138*:653–656, 1981.

[2] Fetal femur length as a predictor of menstrual age: Sonographically measured. Am. J. Roentgenol., *138*:875–878, 1982.

[3] Jeanty, P., Kirkpatrick, C., Dramaix-Wilmet, M., et al.: Ultrasonic evaluation of fetal limb growth. Radiology, *140*:165–168, 1981.

there has been a considerable amount of investigation of these areas, we cannot yet use these data to estimate gestational age in utero. However, some combinations are currently being used with apparent success to estimate fetal well being.

Fetal breathing activity has received considerable attention. Short bursts of four to ten movements have been seen between 20 and 28 weeks of pregnancy. From 28 to 30 weeks longer episodes are observed. Multiple short respiratory efforts with a long period of expiration are found from 30 to 34 weeks followed by a more even ratio of inspiration to expiration from 36 to 39 weeks.[65] Absence of fetal respiratory effort is a poor prognostic sign, although it is difficult to define fetal apnea. Possibly absence of or greater than six seconds between respiratory efforts during a 45 minute observation period after a glucose load is abnormal if the fetus is not depressed by tobacco, alcohol, or drugs.[48]

A combination of observations[39] has been proposed to evaluate fetal well being which includes the evaluation of fetal breathing, fetal movement, fetal tone, estimation of the amount of amniotic fluid, and the nonstress test which measures fetal heart acceleration in response to fetal movement. Clearly there is a great deal more to be learned in the evaluation of fetal gestational age and well being from ultrasound observations.

ESTIMATING GESTATIONAL AGE IN THE NEWBORN INFANT

Once a child is born, a variety of methods are available to estimate gestational age. These are generally based on physical and neurologic criteria.[10] Other methods using biochemical data have been proposed. Our purpose is not to discuss these methods but only to remind the reader that in almost all of these systems, the LNMP was used to establish the validity of the various estimators. As a result the precision with which gestational age is estimated must be expressed as a range which is estimated to be plus or minus 2½ weeks for 90 per cent of cases.[21, 37] Also, physical parameters may be affected by growth retardation and neurologic criteria by illness in the newborn infant.[37, 47] Perhaps these systems are more accurately described as estimations of fetal maturity than of gestational age.

As originally asserted, knowledge of the gestational age can prove very useful in clinical management of the obstetric patient and forms the standard against which many other measures are evaluated for normalcy. Our recommendations for estimating the gestational age are as follows: The first day of the LNMP and first trimester physical examinations are the best clinical ways to estimate gestational age. When these are known, this evidence is sufficient for uncomplicated pregnancies. In other situations it is important to confirm the gestational age by ultrasound measurement of either the crown-rump length or early biparietal diameter. Our own preference is to measure the biparietal diameter prior to 20 weeks, but the range up to 26 weeks is probably acceptable. In all pregnancies in which the LNMP is unknown, early ultrasound confirmation of gestational age should be made.

There will always be a group of patients in whom these goals cannot be achieved. Often this occurs because only in the third trimester is there clinical reason to suspect that the patient's "dates" are incorrect; in other cases the patients may not be seen by a physician until the third trimester. We have no clinically practical solution to this problem. Whenever possible, these problems should be anticipated. When there is no other choice we use the best parameter available as listed in Table 3. It is possible to establish a probability of minimal gestational age for normal pregnancies with a given measurement of biparietal diameter.[59] This estimation should be viewed as a statistical "guess" and greater effort should be spent on estimating fetal size, establishing fetal well being, and looking for direct evidence of intrauterine growth retardation.

REFERENCES

1. Aantaa, K., and Korrs, M.: Growth of the fetal biparietal diameter in different types of pregnancies. Radiology, *137*:167, 1980.
2. Andersen, H. F., Johnson, T. R. B., et al.: Gestational age assessment. Am. J. Obstet. Gynecol., *139*:173, 1981.
3. Beazley, J. M., and Underhill, R. A.: Fallacy of the fundal height. Br. Med. J., *4*:404, 1970.
4. Birnholz, J. C.: The development of human fetal eye movement patterns. Science, *213*:679, 1981.
5. Birnholz, J. C., Stephen, J. C., and Farina, M.: Fetal movement patterns: A possible means of defining neurologic developmental milestones in utero. Am. J. Roentgenol., *130*:537, 1978.
6. Bishop, E. H., and Corson, S.: Estimation of fetal maturity by cytologic examination of the amniotic fluid. Am. J. Obstet. Gynecol., *102*:654, 1968.
7. Boyce, A., Mayaux, M. J., and Schwartz, D.: Classical and "true" gestational post maturity. Am. J. Obstet. Gynecol., *126*:911, 1976.
8. Campbell, S.: The assessment of fetal development by diagnostic ultrasound. Br. Med. J., *2*:730, 1974.
9. Campbell, S.: An improved method of fetal cephalometry by ultrasound. J. Obstet. Gynecol. Br. Commonw., *75*:568, 1968.
10. Casaer, P., and Akiyama, Y.: The estimation of the post menstrual age: A comprehensive review. Dev. Med. Child Neurol., *12*:697, 1970.

11. Clements, J. A., Platzker, A. C. G., Tierney, D. F., et al.: Assessment of the risk of the respiratory distress syndrome by a rapid test for surfactant in amniotic fluid. N. Engl. J. Med., 286:1077, 1972.
12. Clements, J. A., Haustead, R. F., and Johnson, R. P.: Pulmonary surface tension and alveolar stability. J. Appl. Physiol., 16:4444, 1961.
13. Crade, M., Patel, J., and McQuown, D.: Sonographic imaging of the glycogen stage of the fetal choroid plexus. Am. J. Roentgenol., 137:487, 1981.
14. Crane, J. P., Tomich, P. G., et al.: Ultrasonic growth patterns in normal and discordant twins. Obstet. Gynecol., 55:678, 1980.
15. Croll, J., and Grech, P.: Radiological maturity of the small-for-dates fetus. J. Obstet. Gynecol. Brit. Commonw., 77:802, 1970.
16. Davison, J. M., Lund, T., Farr, V., et al.: The limitations of ultrasonic fetal cephalometry. J. Obstet. Gynecol. Brit. Commonw., 80:769, 1973.
17. Denkhaus, H., and Winsberg, F.: Ultrasonic measurement of the fetal ventricular system. Radiology, 131:781, 1979.
18. Depp, R.: Present status of the assessment of fetal maturity. Semin. Perinatol., 4:229, 1980.
19. Dewhurst, D. J., Beazley, J. M., and Campbell, S.: Assessment of fetal maturity and dysmaturity. Am. J. Obstet. Gynecol., 113:14, 1972.
20. Donald, J. R., Freeman, R. K., and Goebelsmann, V.: Clinical experience with amniotic fluid lecithin/sphingomyelin ratios. I. Antenatal prediction of pulmonary maturity. Am. J. Obstet. Gynecol., 115:547, 1973.
21. Dubowitz, L. M. S., Dubowitz, V., and Goldberg, C.: Clinical assessment of gestational age in the newborn infant. J. Pediatr., 77:1, 1970.
22. Foulds, J. W., and Pennock, C. A.: Amniotic fluid creatinine: An unreliable index of fetal maturity. J. Obstet. Gynecol. Br. Commonw., 79:911, 1972.
23. Frosolono, M. F., Charms, B. L., Pawlowski, R., et al.: Isolation, characterization and surface chemistry of a surface-active fraction from dog lung. J. Lipid Res., 11:439, 1970.
24. Gluck, L., and Kulovich, M. V.: Lecithin/sphingomyelin ratios in amniotic fluid in normal and abnormal pregnancy. Am. J. Obstet. Gynecol., 115:539, 1973.
25. Gluck, L., Kulovich, M. V., Vorer, R. C., et al.: Diagnosis of respiratory distress syndrome by amniocentesis. Am. J. Obstet. Gynecol., 109:444, 1971.
26. Hadlock, F. P., Deter, R. L., Carpenter, R. J., et al.: Estimating fetal age: Effect of head shape on BPD. Am. J. Roentgenol., 137:83, 1981.
27. Hadlock, F. P., Deter, R. L., Harrist, R. E., et al: Fetal head circumference. Relation to menstrual age. Am. J. Roentgenol., 138:649, 1982.
28. Hallmann, M., Feldman, B. H., Kirkpatrick, E., et al.: Absence of phosphatidylglycerol in respiratory distress syndrome in the newborn: Study of the minor surfactant phospholipids in newborns. Pediatr. Res., 11:714, 1977.
29. Hallman, M., Kulovich, M. V., Kirkpatrick, E., et al.: Phosphatidylinositol and phosphatidylglycerol in amniotic fluid: Indices of lung maturity. Am. J. Obstet. Gynecol., 125:613, 1976.
30. Harvey, P., Parkinson, C. E., and Campbell, S.: Risk of respiratory distress syndrome. Lancet, 1:42, 1975.
31. Hertz, R. H., Sokol, R. J., et al.: Clinical estimation of gestational age: Rules for avoiding preterm delivery. Am. J. Obstet. Gynecol., 131:395, 1978.
32. Iffy, L., Chatlerton, R. T., and Jakobavito, A.: The "high weight for dates" fetus. Am. J. Obstet. Gynecol., 115:238, 1973.
33. Johnson, M. L., Dunne, M. C., et al.: Evaluation of fetal intracranial anatomy by static and real time ultrasound. J. Clin. Ultrasound, 8:311, 1980.
34. Keniston, R. E., Pernoll, M. L., Buist, S. J., et al.: A prospective evaluation of the lecithin/sphingomyelin ratios and the rapid surfactant test in relation to fetal pulmonary maturity. Am. J. Obstet. Gynecol., 121:324, 1975.
35. King, R. J., and Clements, J. A.: Surface active materials from dog lung. II. Composition and physiologic correlation. Am. J. Physiol., 223:715, 1972.
36. Kulovich, M. V., Hallman, M. D., and Gluck, K. L.: The lung profile. I. Normal pregnancy. Am. J. Obstet. Gynecol., 135:57, 1979.
37. Latis, G. O., Simionato, L., and Ferraris, G.: Clinical assessment of gestational age in the newborn infant. Comparison of two methods. Early Hum. Devel., 5:29, 1980.
38. Lawson, T. L., Alborelli, J. N., et al.: Gray scale measurement of biparietal diameter. J. Clin. Ultrasound, 5:17, 1977.
39. Manning, F. A., Platt, L. P., and Sypus, L.: Antepartum fetal evaluation: Development of a fetal biophysical profile. Am. J. Obstet. Gynecol., 136:787, 1980.
40. Meire, H. B.: Ultrasound assessment of fetal growth patterns. Br. Med. Bull., 37:253, 1981.
41. Moore, G. W., Hutchins, G. M., and O'Rahilly, R.: The estimated age of staged human embryo and early fetuses. Am. J. Obstet. Gynecol., 139:500, 1981.
42. Mukherjie, T. K., Rajegowda, B. K., Glass, L. L., et al.: Amniotic fluid shake test versus lecithin/sphingomyelin ratios in the antenatal prediction of respiratory distress syndrome. Am. J. Obstet. Gynecol., 119:648, 1974.
43. Murato, V., and Martin, C. B.: Growth of the biparietal diameter of the fetal head in diabetic pregnancy. Am. J. Obstet. Gynecol., 115:252, 1973.
44. O'Brien, W. F., Coddington, C. C., and Cefalo, R. C.: Serial ultrasonographic biparietal diameter for prediction of estimated date of confinement. Am. J. Obstet. Gynecol., 138:467, 1980.
45. O'Brien, G. D., Queenan, J. T., and Campbell, S.: Assessment of gestational age in the second trimester by real-time ultrasound measurement of the femur length. Am. J. Obstet. Gynecol., 139:540, 1981.
46. Ogata, E. S., Sabbagha, R. E., Metzger, B. E., et al.: Serial ultrasonography to assess evolving fetal macrosomia. J.A.M.A., 243:2405, 1980.
47. Ounsted, M. K., Chalmers, C. A., and Yudkin, P. L.: Clinical assessment of gestational age at birth: The effects of sex, birth weight, and weight for length of gestation. Early Hum. Devel., 211:73, 1978.
48. Patrick, J., Campbell, K., et al.: A definition of

human fetal apnea and the distribution of fetal apneic intervals during the last ten weeks of pregnancy. Am. J. Obstet. Gynecol., *136*:471, 1980.
49. Pfleger, R. C., and Thomas, H. G.: Beagle dog pulmonary surfactant lipids. Lipid composition of pulmonary tissue, exfoliated lining cells, and surfactant. Arch. Intern. Med., *127*:863, 1971.
50. Pitkin, R. M., and Zwerek, S. J.: Amniotic fluid creatinine. Am. J. Obstet. Gynecol., *98*:1135, 1967.
51. Roberts, C. J., Hibbard, B. M., et al.: Precision in estimating gestational age and its influence on sensitivity of alphafetoprotein screening. Br. Med. J., *1*:981, 1979.
52. Robinson, H. P., Sweet, E. M., and Adam, A. H.: The accuracy of radiological estimates of gestational age using early fetal crown-rump length measurements by ultrasound as a basis for comparison. Br. J. Obstet. Gynecol., *86*:525, 1979.
53. Robinson, H. P.: Gestation sac volume as determined by sonar in the first trimester of pregnancy. Br. J. Obstet. Gynecol., *82*:100, 1975.
54. Robinson, H. P., and Fleming, J. E. E.: A critical evaluation of sonar crown-rump length measurements. Br. J. Obstet. Gynecol., *82*:702, 1975.
55. Russell, J. G. B.: Radiological assessment of fetal maturity. J. Obstet. Gynecol. Brit. Commonw., *76*:208, 1969.
56. Sabbagha, R. E., and Turner, H. J.: Methodology of B-scan sonar cephalometry with electronic calipers and correlations with fetal birth weight. Obstet. Gynecol., *40*:74, 1972.
57. Sabbagha, R. E., et al.: Sonar biparietal diameter: Analysis of percentile growth differences in two normal populations using same methodology. Am. J. Obstet. Gynecol., *126*:479, 1976.
58. Sabbagha, R. E., Hughey, M., and Depp, R.: Growth adjusted sonographic age: A simplified method. Obstet. Gynecol., *51*:383, 1978.
59. Sabbagha, R. E., Turner, H. J., et al.: Sonar BPD and fetal age definition of the relationship. Obstet. Gynecol., *43*:7, 1974.
60. Saito, M., Keijiro, Y., et al.: Time of ovulation and prolonged pregnancy. Am. J. Obstet. Gynecol., *112*:31, 1972.
61. Schreiber, M. H., and Morettin, L. B.: Antepartum prediction of fetal maturity. Radiol. Clin. North Am., *5*:21, 1967.
62. Santos-Ramos, R., Deunhoelter, J. H., and Rersch, J. S.: Sonar fetal cephalometry: Comparison of bistable with gray scale and real time technique. Am. J. Obstet. Gynecol., *136*:805, 1980.
63. Shepard, M., and Filly, R. A.: A standardized plane for biparietal diameter measurement. J. Ultrasound Med., *1*:145–150, 1982.
64. Teohes, L., Ambrose, A., and Ratnam, S. S.: Amniotic fluid creatinine, uric acid and urea as indices of gestational age. Acta Obstet. Gynecol. Scand., *52*:323, 1973.
65. Trudinger, B. J., and Knight, P. C.: Fetal age and patterns of human fetal breathing movements. Am. J. Obstet. Gynecol., *137*:724, 1980.
66. Watmough, D., Crippin, P., et al.: A critical assessment of ultrasonic fetal cephalometry. Br. J. Radiol., *47*:24, 1974.
67. Zador, I. E., Hertz, R. H., et al.: Sources of error in the estimation of fetal gestational age. Am. J. Obstet. Gynecol., *138*:344, 1980.

3

Normal Fetal Anatomy

Michael L. Johnson, M.D., Grant K. Rees, R.T., and Richard A. Hattan, M.D.

During the past few years diagnostic ultrasound has radically changed the care of the obstetric patient. Improvements in instrumentation have made it possible to identify an increasing number of fetal anatomic structures. Better spatial resolution allows definition of small structures such as the fetal renal arteries and diaphragmatic crura, while improvements in contrast resolution, particularly in static articulated arm scanners, have made it possible to recognize subtle differences in fetal soft tissue structures such as the liver, pancreas, and spleen.[2,6,7] With increasing knowledge and awareness of fetal anatomy and anomalies, decisions regarding the timing and mode of delivery are being made that directly affect the health of both the fetus and the mother. The fetus can now be considered a patient in its own right, and neonatology has taken on an entirely new perspective. With recent introduction of intrauterine fetal surgery,[1] certain anomalies can even be treated in utero. Recognition of normal fetal anatomy is important if one is to confidently make a diagnosis of a congenital anomaly.

Visualization of fetal structures is highly dependent on the intrinsic subject contrast of the structure for which one is searching. Thus, highly echogenic structures such as the fetal skeleton are easily recognized, as they are surrounded by relatively echo-poor soft tissue. Fluid-filled, echo-free structures such as the bladder, heart, blood vessels and fluid-filled gut are also easily visualized. Other factors that affect visualization of fetal structures include maternal obesity, fetal position within the uterus, fetal movement, and amount of amniotic fluid.

One important point that cannot be overemphasized is the competency and interest of the ultrasonographer or ultrasonologist performing the scans. Patience and strict attention to detail are important in the proper identification of normal anatomy and detection of anomalies.

TECHNIQUE OF EXAMINATION

An obstetric examination can be divided into two parts. First is the examination of the maternal pelvis, including the adnexa, uterus, placenta, amniotic fluid, number of fetuses, and fetal position. Second is the careful detailed examination of the fetus itself. Before one attempts to identify fetal structures, it is essential to ascertain the lie of the fetus within the uterus. Only after this is done will one know which side of the fetal body, either right or left side, one is observing.

At our institution, serial parasagittal and transverse scans through the uterus are performed at 2 cm intervals. Fetal position is reported as vertex, transverse, oblique, or breech. The position of the fetal spine is indicated. In Figure 1 the fetus is in a vertex presentation with the spine to the maternal right. The fetus is thus lying on his right side and the left side is toward the anterior abdominal wall of the mother. Using real-time equipment this fetal position can be determined very rapidly. Figure 2 further illustrates the various positions within the uterus. In Figure 2A, the fetus is in vertex presentation with its spine on the maternal right; therefore, the fetus is lying on its right side as in Figure 1. The stomach is in the left upper quadrant and the gallbladder on the right side of the abdomen. The other three positions shown in this figure should be carefully evaluated as each is different. By recognizing the internal fetal anatomy, one can determine the fetal lie by visualizing a scan through the

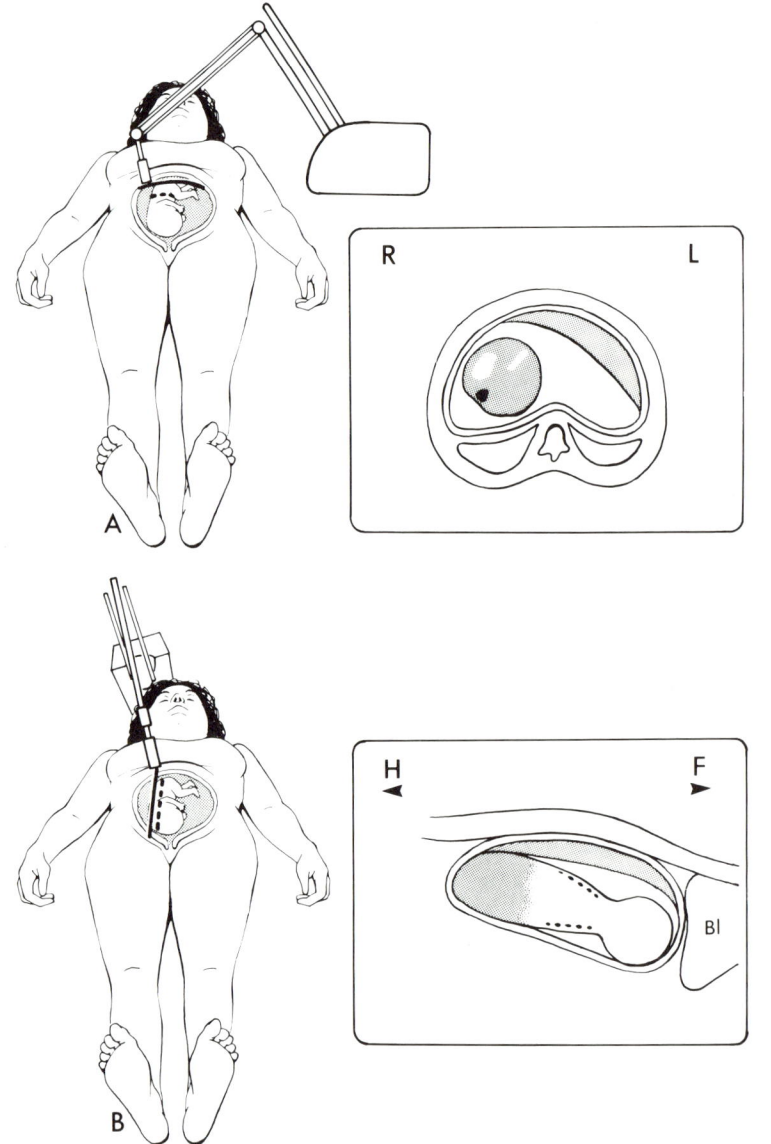

Figure 1. *A*, Diagrammatic illustration of the transverse plane of section of the maternal pelvis. As the fetus is in a vertex presentation, this scan transects the fetal abdomen transversely. *B*, Longitudinal plane of section of the same fetus. These are viewed with the maternal head to the left of the recorded image.

fetal abdomen and knowing the plane of the scan through the mother's abdomen. Once the fetal position is determined, it is possible to orient the scanning arm in the correct plane to image the desired fetal structures. In our experience, static scans with a 5 MHz transducer appear to allow detection of much finer detailed anatomy than does a real-time examination with a 5 MHz transducer. Simple linear and sector scans are used and compound scanning is avoided, as this degrades the image and does not allow visualization of extremely small structures. While many of the illustrations in this chapter were made using a static articulated arm scanner, a combination of static and real-time scanning is often the most ideal method for assessment of the fetus. Real-time scanning is absolutely essential for evaluation of congenital anomalies.

With the exception of the umbilical vein and ductus venosus, most fetal structures, such as the pancreas, gallbladder, and aortic arch, are in the same position within the fetus as in the adult. The only organ slightly displaced in position is the heart, which lies more horizontally in the fetus owing to the large size of the liver. The fetal gallbladder has been noted to lie in the same variety of orientations as the adult gallbladder.

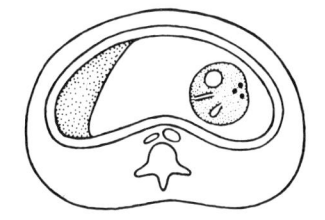

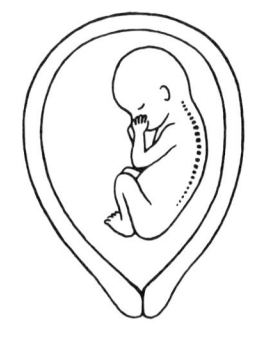

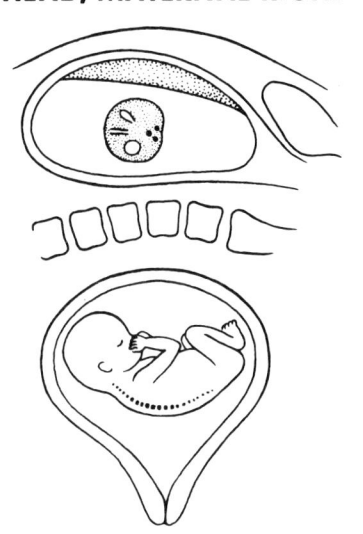

Figure 2. Knowledge of the plane of section across the maternal abdomen (longitudinal or transverse) as well as the position of the fetal spine and left (stomach) and right (gallbladder) sided structures can be used to determine fetal lie and presenting part. *A,* This transverse scan of the maternal pelvis demonstrates the fetal spine on the maternal right with the fetus lying with its right side down (stomach anterior, gallbladder posterior). Remembering that these images are viewed looking up from the patient's feet, the fetus must be in longitudinal lie and cephalic presentation. *B,* When the maternal pelvis is scanned transversely and the fetal spine is on the maternal left with the right side down, the fetus is in a longitudinal lie and breech presentation. *C,* When a longitudinal plane of section demonstrates the fetal body to be transected transversely and the fetal spine is nearest the uterine fundus with the fetal left side down, the fetus is in a transverse lie with the fetal head on the maternal left. *D,* When the longitudinal plane of section demonstrates the fetal body to be transected transversely and the spine is nearest the lower uterine segment with the fetal left side down, the fetus is in a transverse lie with the head on the maternal right. While real-time scanning of the gravid uterus will quickly allow the observer to determine fetal lie and presenting part, this maneuver of identifying specific right and left sided structures within the fetal body forces one to accurately determine fetal position and identify normal and pathologic fetal anatomy.

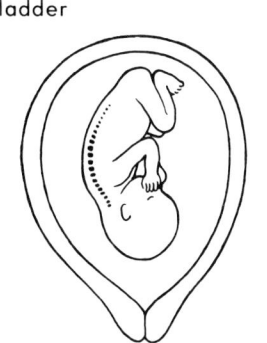

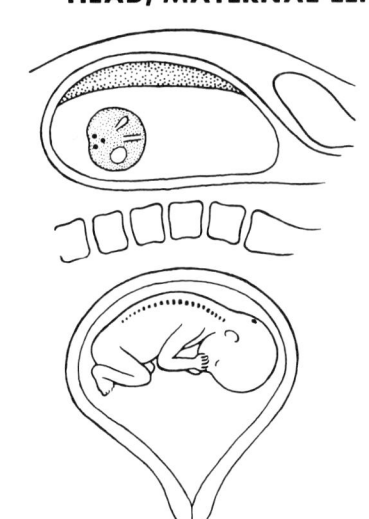

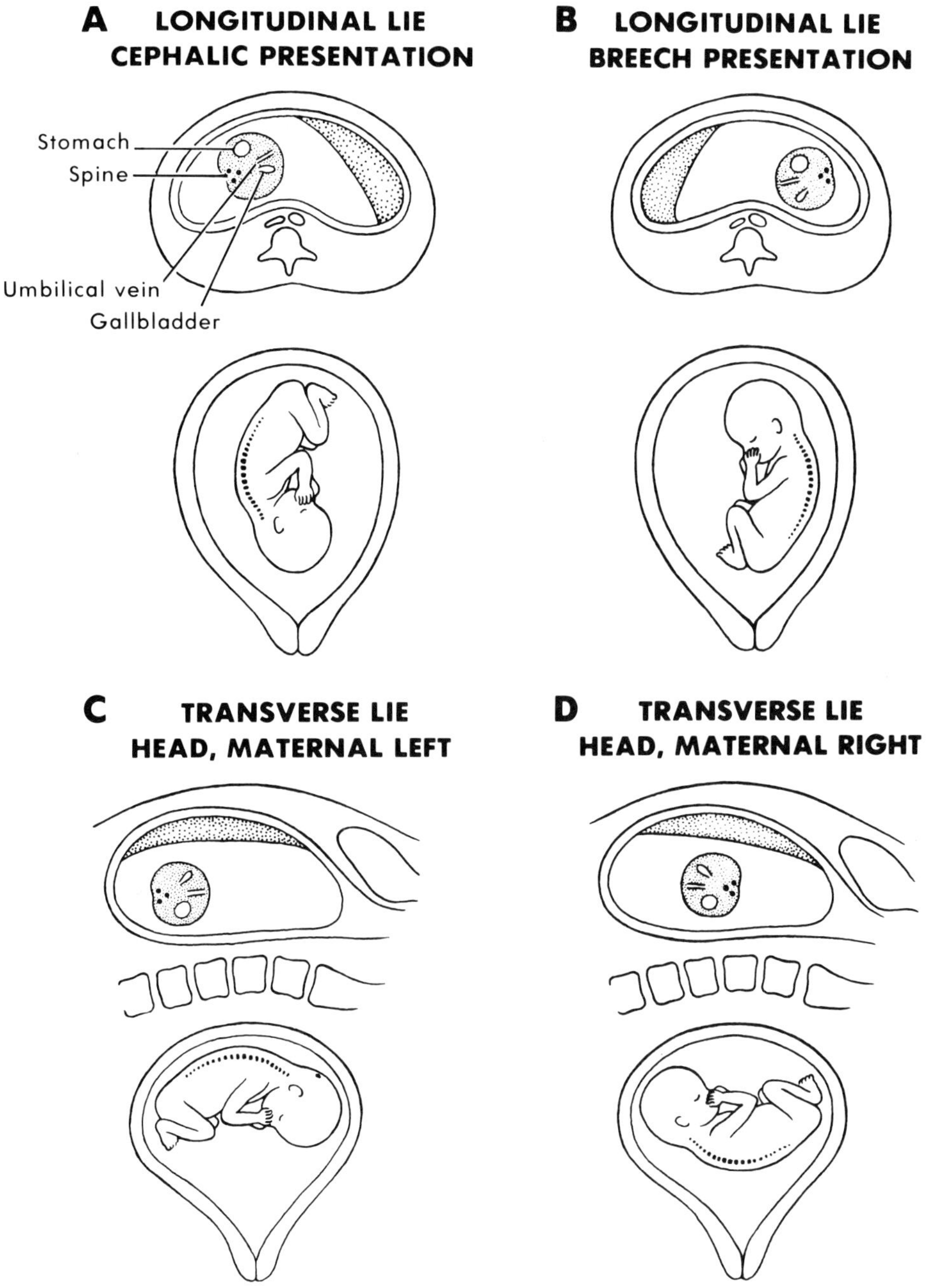

Standard transverse, parasagittal, and coronal scans of the fetus will demonstrate most of the normal anatomy. Examination of the pancreas is aided by the presence of fluid within the fetal stomach and duodenum. Structures that run obliquely in the fetus such as the hepatic veins, ductus venosus, and umbilical vein are best visualized by oblique scans through the fetal abdomen.

EARLY DEVELOPMENT

The earliest age at which embryonic tissue can consistently be seen within the gestational sac is between six and eight postmenstrual weeks. At this stage of development, the embryo is recognized simply as an elliptically shaped mass of tissue without recognizable fetal parts. The maximum length of the fetal head and trunk, or the crown-rump length, is the most reliable estimate of gestational age and is usually obtained between six and 14 weeks (Fig. 3). Real-time ultrasonography greatly facilitates this measurement. Heart activity can be seen as early as six weeks and is recognized as a rapid continuous motion within the fetal pole on real-time examination.

By 10 weeks the embryologic period has ended and the fetal period of development has begun.[11] Thus organs have reached their final anatomic location and structures visualized by ultrasound past this stage will be developing organs that will not change position within the fetus for the remainder of pregnancy. The only exception to this rule is the fact that the yolk sac and fetal bowel within the umbilical cord are present after the end of the embryologic period. The yolk sac can be seen in 50 to 80 per cent of cases between seven and 11 postmenstrual weeks.[10] It appears as a round mass of fluid-filled tissue within the gestational sac that is completely separate from the fetal pole (Fig. 4). This should not be mistaken for a twin gestation or included in the measurement of the crown-rump length.

FETAL CHEST

The most obvious and easily recognized structure within the fetal thorax is the heart. As mentioned previously, fetal heart activity can be seen with real-time scanning as early as six to eight weeks. By 13 weeks' gestation the heart can be recognized as a fluid-filled structure within the fetal thorax, and valve motion can be appreciated by 20 weeks.

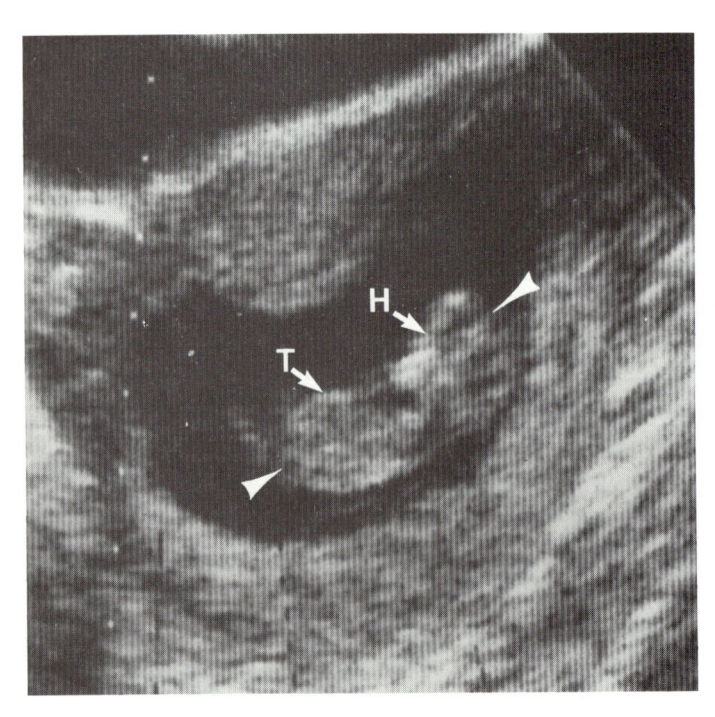

Figure 3. Transverse scan through the uterus demonstrates the long axis of a 10½ week fetus, showing the head (H) and trunk (T). Crown-rump length (CRL) is measured between the arrows and is 3.5 cm. The limbs and cord are not included in the crown-rump length measurement.

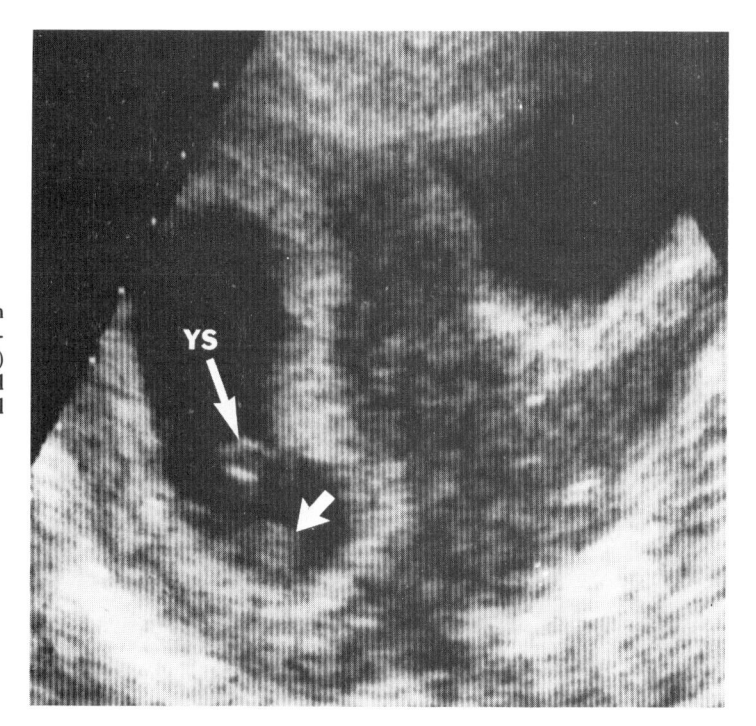

Figure 4. Longitudinal scan through the uterus at 8 weeks' gestation demonstrates the yolk sac (YS) floating above a portion of the fetal pole (*arrow*) within the gestational sac.

When evaluating the fetal heart, one should first determine to which side the heart rests within the thorax. If the position of the heart is abnormal, the cause of the dextroposition should be investigated.

In the second half of pregnancy, detailed analysis of the fetal heart using two-dimensional real-time (Fig. 5) and M-mode studies (Fig. 6) can be performed. When doing fetal echocardiography, one should

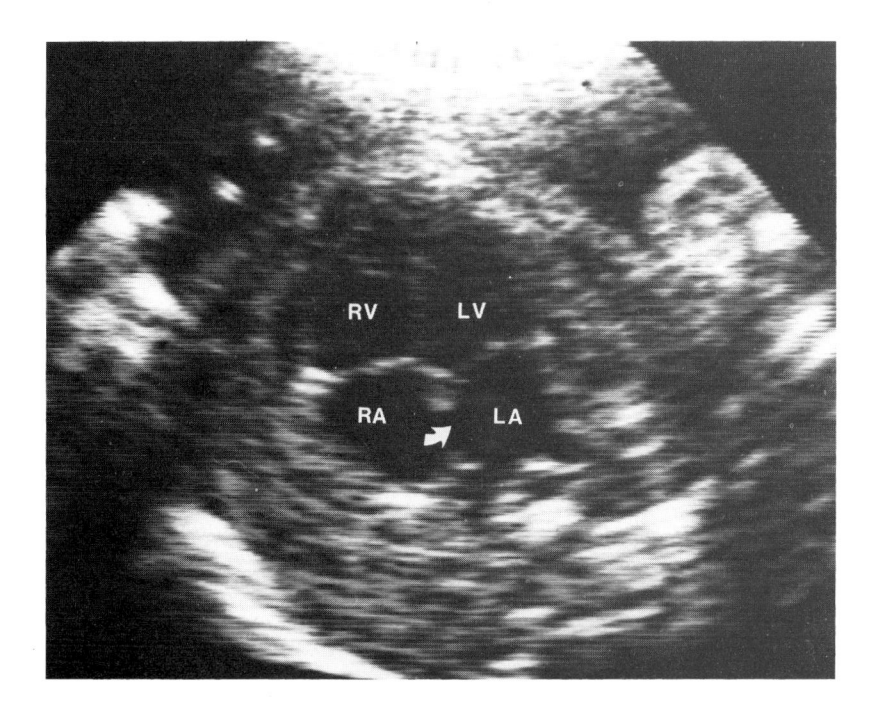

Figure 5. Four-chamber real-time view demonstrates the right atrium (RA), left atrium (LA), right ventricle (RV) and left ventricle (LV). The foramen ovale (*arrow*) is noted between the two atria.

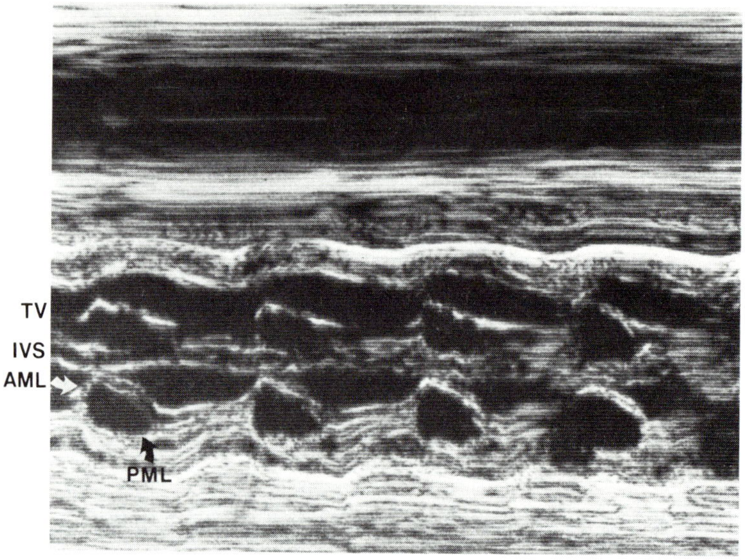

Figure 6. M-mode echocardiogram at the level of the tricuspid and mitral valves. The tricuspid valve (TV) is located anteriorly. Both the anterior (AML) and posterior (PML) leaflets of the mitral valve are seen. The intraventricular septum (IVS) is noted between the two valves.

realize that cardiac anatomy is displayed differently than in the standard pediatric or adult echocardiogram. The most important reason for this difference is the more horizontal orientation of the fetal heart, especially in the second trimester. This horizontal position of the heart is largely due to the relatively large size of the liver, a major hematopoietic organ for the fetus. Because the heart is oriented differently, certain standard echocardiographic scanning planes, such as the apical four-chamber view, are more easily obtained. Other standard planes such as the long axis view of the left ventricle, mitral valve, and aortic valve are more difficult to obtain.

Prenatal and postnatal echocardiography also differ because the fetal lungs are not filled with air and thus provide a good ultrasonic window to view the heart. Thus many more scanning planes are feasible in the fetus than in the postnatal study, in which one is scanning with the lungs inflated with air.

With detailed two-dimensional real-time studies, one can view the inferior vena cava emptying into the right atrium and see the patent foramen ovale and left atrium (see Fig. 5). All four cardiac valves, the aortic root, and both ventricles can be seen in long and short axis. Quantitative cross-sectional measurements for the right ventricle, left ventricle, pulmonary artery, and aortic root in the normal fetus weighing more than 500 gm have been measured.[14] Great vessels can often be recognized exiting the aortic arch (Fig. 7A). On coronal views, the thoracic and abdominal aorta can be demonstrated, and often the aortic bifurcation is seen (Fig. 7B).

The other major organ within the fetal thorax is, of course, the lung. The fetal lung is not fully developed until later in the third trimester, and thus there is very little amniotic fluid within the maturing alveoli. As such, fetal lung has similar echogenicity to other soft tissue structures such as the liver or spleen. With parasagittal scanning, the fetal lung can be recognized above the diaphragm (Fig. 8). At various gestational ages, differences between liver and lung echogenicity can be appreciated and the significance of this is being investigated.[4, 17]

FETAL ABDOMEN

Scans of the fetal abdomen yield useful diagnostic information. The structures that are most often imaged include the fetal stomach, liver, umbilical vein, kidneys, and bladder. Other structures that can also be seen but with less frequency include the fetal adrenal glands, pancreas, spleen, and intra-abdominal vascular anatomy.

The most commonly obtained section through the fetal abdomen is a transverse scan through the stomach and the liver at the level of the intrahepatic portion of the umbilical vein (Fig. 9). This is the most common site for taking fetal trunk measurements. Often only the stomach is well visualized, but occasionally portions of the duodenum may be seen. Behind the fluid-filled stomach, the spleen may be visualized. Fluid-filled loops of nondilated large and small bowel may be seen and are of no clinical significance unless they persist and become dilated. In the term fetus, the loops of bowel may contain meconium and appear quite prominent with solid material within the lumen (Fig. 10).

If the entire length of the intrahepatic umbilical vein is visualized, the scan is not a true transverse projection through the abdomen, but rather an oblique scan.[13] (See Figure 9 on p. 126.) The fetal liver fills the upper abdomen and its vascular structures are often identified (Fig. 11). All figures in this section are oriented as in the standard abdominal scans viewed by computed tomography or ultrasound.

With the exception of three structures, the anatomy of the fetal hepatobiliary system is identical to that of the neonate. The three structures that do differ are the umbilical vein, the portal sinus, and the ductus venosus (Fig. 12). These vessels allow for the unique fetal circulatory system. The fetus receives oxygenated blood from the placenta via the umbilical vein. The um-

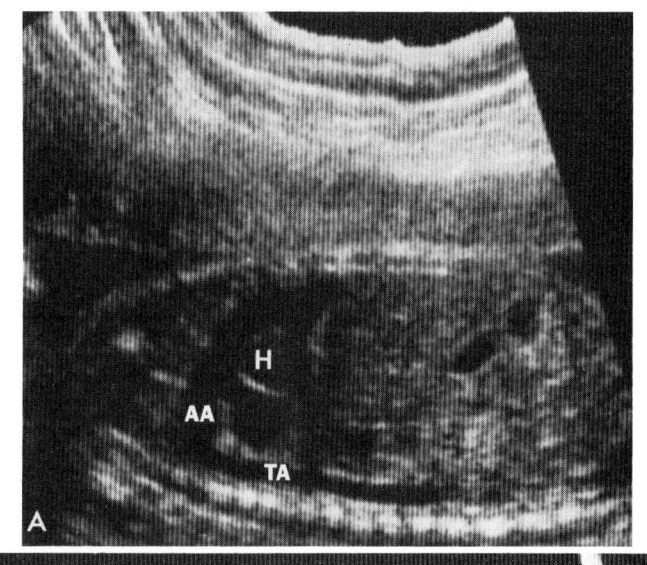

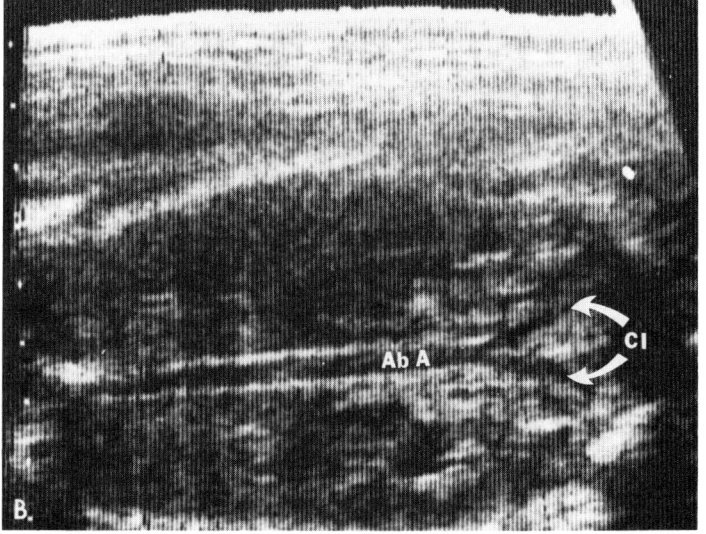

Figure 7. *A*, Parasagittal scan through the chest at 25 weeks' gestation demonstrates the heart (H), aortic arch (AA), and descending thoracic aorta (TA). *B*, Coronal scan at 30 weeks' gestation demonstrates the abdominal aorta (AbA) and the aortic bifurcation with both common iliac arteries (CI).

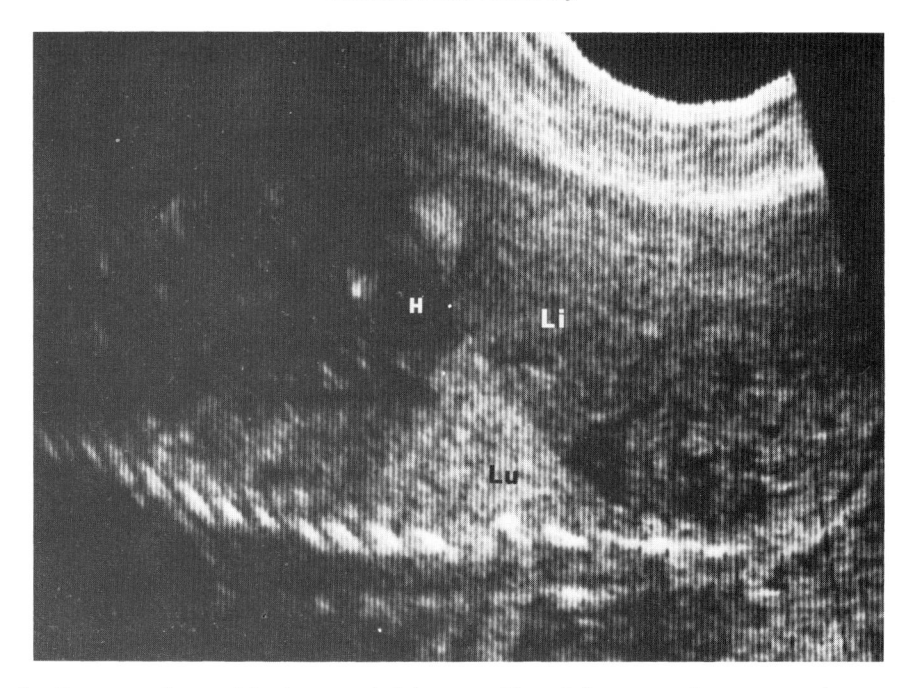

Figure 8. Parasagittal view of the thorax and abdomen at 29 weeks' gestation demonstrates the more echogenic lung (Lu) and liver (Li). The fetal ribs and heart (H) are also seen.

bilical vein, traveling in the umbilical cord, enters the fetus in the midline through the anterior abdominal wall. It then proceeds in a cephalad direction, enters the liver, and continues intrahepatically to terminate at the portal sinus which is the main left portal vein (Fig. 13A). From the portal sinus, the oxygenated blood may flow into the large right portal vein or the smaller ductus venosus. The ductus veno-

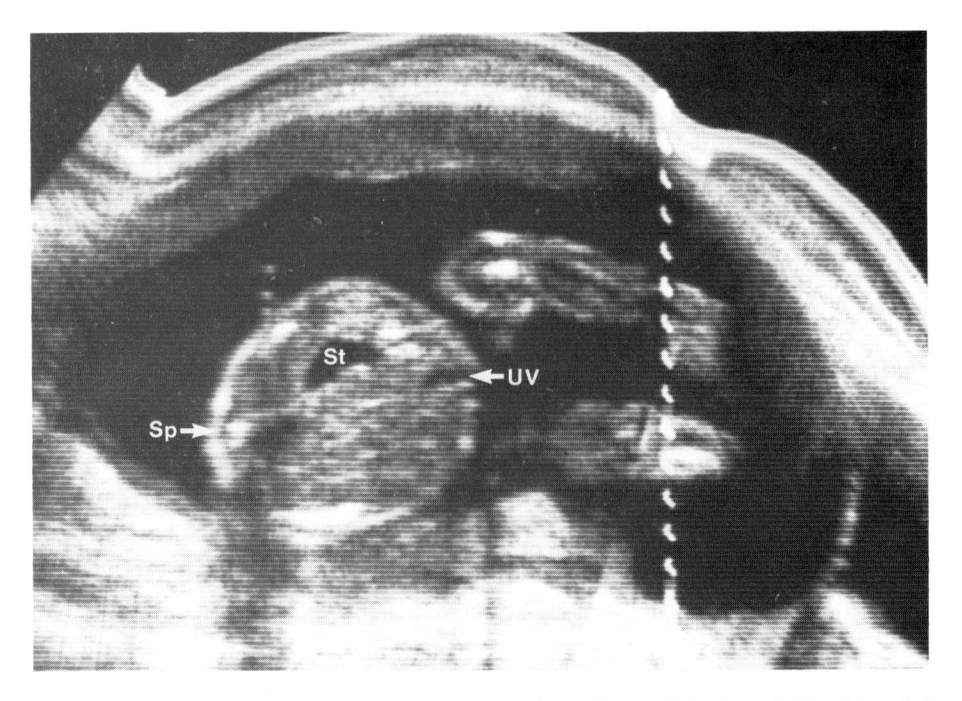

Figure 9. Transverse scan through the fetal abdomen at the level of the umbilical vein (UV) at 31 weeks' gestation. The fetal spine (Sp) and stomach (St) are seen.

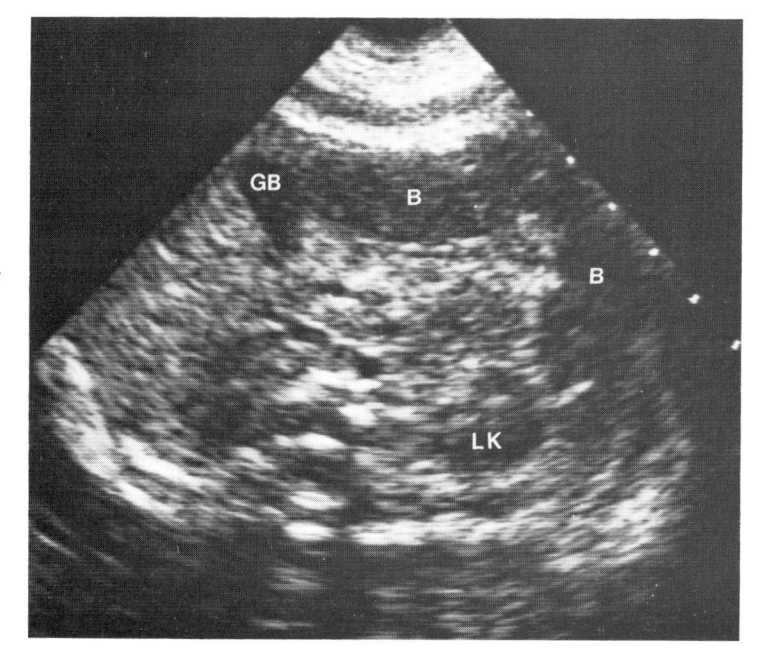

Figure 10. Transverse scan through fetal abdomen at level of gallbladder (GB) and left kidney (LK). The transverse colon and splenic flexure (B) are filled with low level echoes representing meconium.

sus continues in a cephalad direction and enters the inferior vena cava, thereby bypassing the liver parenchyma (Fig. 13B). The blood flow entering the right portal vein flows through the hepatic sinusoids and is drained by the hepatic veins into the inferior vena cava. These vessels are present in both the fetus and neonate but undergo functional changes after birth.

With the cessation of blood flow from the placenta, the umbilical vein and ductus venosus collapse to become the ligamentum teres and ligamentum venosum, respectively. The portal sinus remains patent and becomes the proximal portion of the left portal vein. Blood flow through the ductus venosus is controlled by a sphincter near the umbilical vein. It is thought that this

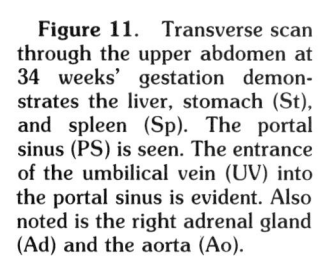

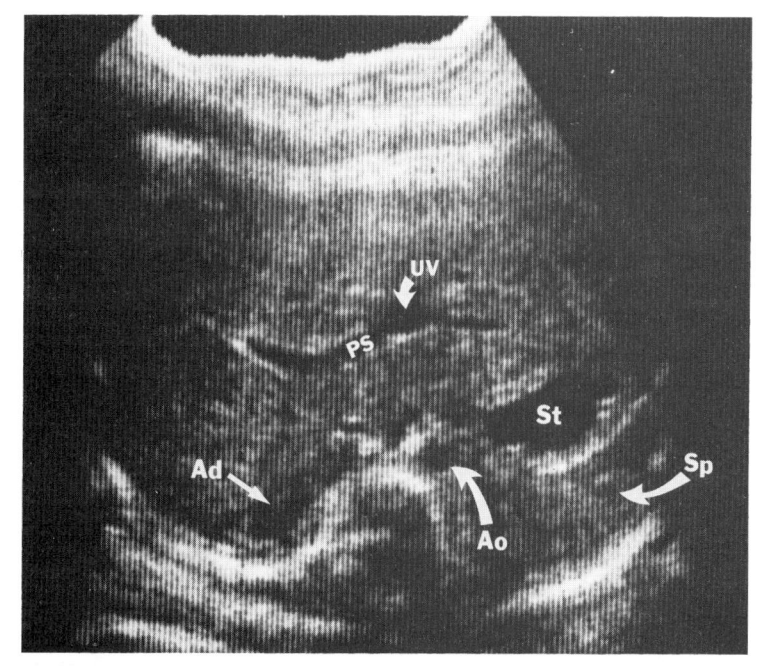

Figure 11. Transverse scan through the upper abdomen at 34 weeks' gestation demonstrates the liver, stomach (St), and spleen (Sp). The portal sinus (PS) is seen. The entrance of the umbilical vein (UV) into the portal sinus is evident. Also noted is the right adrenal gland (Ad) and the aorta (Ao).

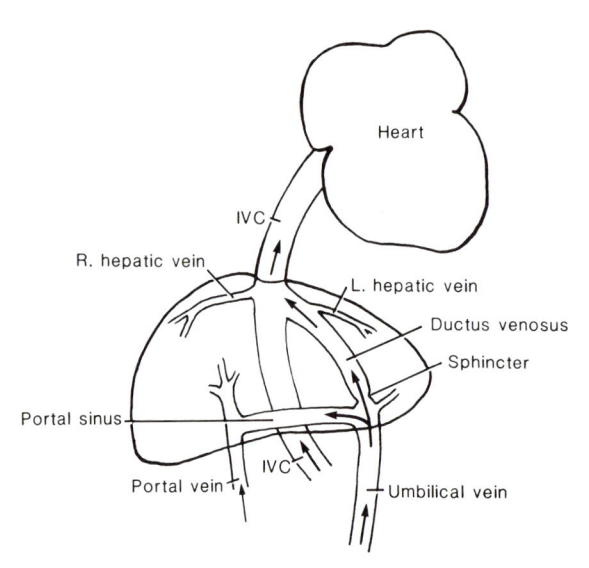

Figure 12. Schematic diagram of the fetal circulatory system demonstrates connections between umbilical vein, portal vein, and inferior vena cava. (Modified from Moore, K. L.: The Developing Human. Clinically Oriented Embryology. Philadelphia, W. B. Saunders Co., 1977.)

sphincter closes as a result of the uterine contractions when the venous return is too high, thus preventing a sudden overload to the heart.[8] The undivided segment of the right portal vein and the division into the anterior and posterior branches of the right portal vein can be seen (Fig. 14).

The hepatic veins can be seen draining the hepatic sinusoids into the distal inferior vena cava or directly into the right atrium. The three hepatic veins are located intersegmentally and course between the four segments of the liver (Fig. 15).

The only portion of the biliary system in the fetus routinely demonstrated is the gallbladder (Fig. 16). The gallbladder lies parallel to the umbilical vein on the right side of the abdomen and may vary in size. Because the long axis of the gallbladder and umbilical vein lie in the same plane, these two structures can often be confused. The umbilical vein should always be located before the gallbladder is identified (see Fig. 13).

The pancreas is more difficult to identify but can be visualized by utilizing the same landmarks as in the adult, such as the superior mesenteric and splenic veins (Fig. 17). The stomach of the fetus can be a useful acoustic window as well as a landmark, as the pancreas lies directly behind the stomach, antrum, and duodenal cap. The fetal pancreas is slightly more echogenic than the liver, but without good landmarks, such as the stomach and mesenteric vessels, it is difficult to appreciate. It can be visualized as a band of echogenic tissue anterior to the great vessels (Fig. 18), without distinct borders.

Identification of the normal kidneys is of great importance in evaluating a fetus because the genitourinary tract is the site of many developmental abnormalities. The kidneys can be identified in the fetus as early as 12 to 14 weeks. The kidneys appear as two relatively sonolucent structures adjacent to the spine on transverse scans (Fig. 19). Closer scrutiny of intrarenal structures will show the echo-poor renal pyramids distributed uniformly throughout the medulla of the kidney (Fig. 20). Renal sinus fat is seen as more echogenic material within the hilus of the kidney. The pelvis of the collecting system is occasionally seen (Fig. 21), and its visualization does not mean obstruction to urine flow. Renal vessels have been seen. Although the kidneys can be seen early in fetal life, they are not reliably found until after 15 postmenstrual weeks. Kidneys of normal fetuses between 15 and 17 weeks are seen less than 50 per cent of the time. In fetuses between 17 and 22 weeks of age, one or both kidneys are seen in 90 per cent of cases.[9]

Assessment of renal size is important because certain abnormalities such as infantile polycystic kidney disease may present with nephromegaly. The ratio of maximum kidney circumference to abdominal circumference is essentially unchanged throughout gestation and measures between 0.27 and 0.30.[5]

Visualization of the fetal bladder is an important step in documenting the pres-

Normal Fetal Anatomy 51

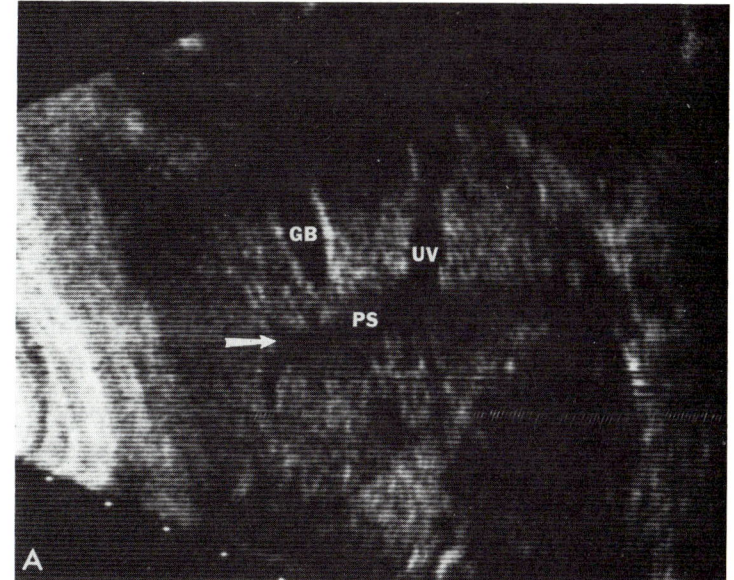

Figure 13. Two oblique transverse sections through the liver at 34 weeks' gestation. *A*, The umbilical vein (UV) is seen entering the portal sinus (PS). The bifurcation of the right portal vein into anterior and posterior segments is seen (*arrow*). The gallbladder (GB) is also seen. *B*, An oblique transverse cut through the same fetus (below) demonstrates the communication of the portal sinus (PS) ductus venosus (DV), and the interior vena cava (IVC) draining into the heart (H). The gallbladder should not be mistaken for the umbilical vein.

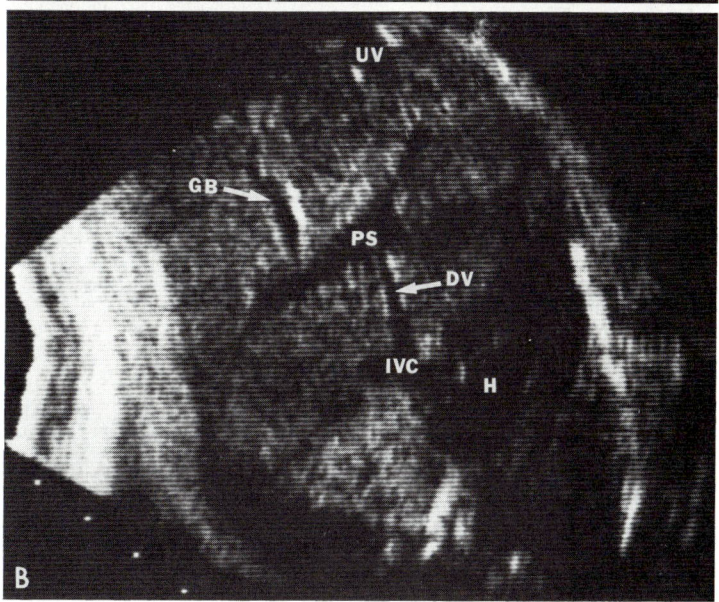

ence of normal renal function. The fetal urinary bladder is noted as a cystic structure present in the pelvis of the fetus (Fig. 22). When the transverse projection is evaluated, the iliac wings are important landmarks. With these structures visualized, one can be confident that the level of the fetal pelvis has been reached. Care must be taken not to confuse amniotic fluid located between the fetal thighs as the fetal bladder. The bladder is a dynamic structure with constant filling and emptying in the normal fetus. Thus, absence of the fetal bladder on a single ultrasound examination does not imply an abnormality. In our department we routinely see the bladder in the majority of fetuses beyond 20 weeks' gestation. In those fetuses in which the bladder is not seen, repeat real-time examinations 30 to 45 minutes later will often demonstrate a normal bladder.

Ultrasonic demonstration of the fetal adrenal gland has been previously reported.[16] Of note is the fact that the adrenal gland in the fetus is relatively large compared with its size in the adult. Approximately 90 per cent of the fetal adrenal gland is cortex, and this tissue quickly involutes after birth

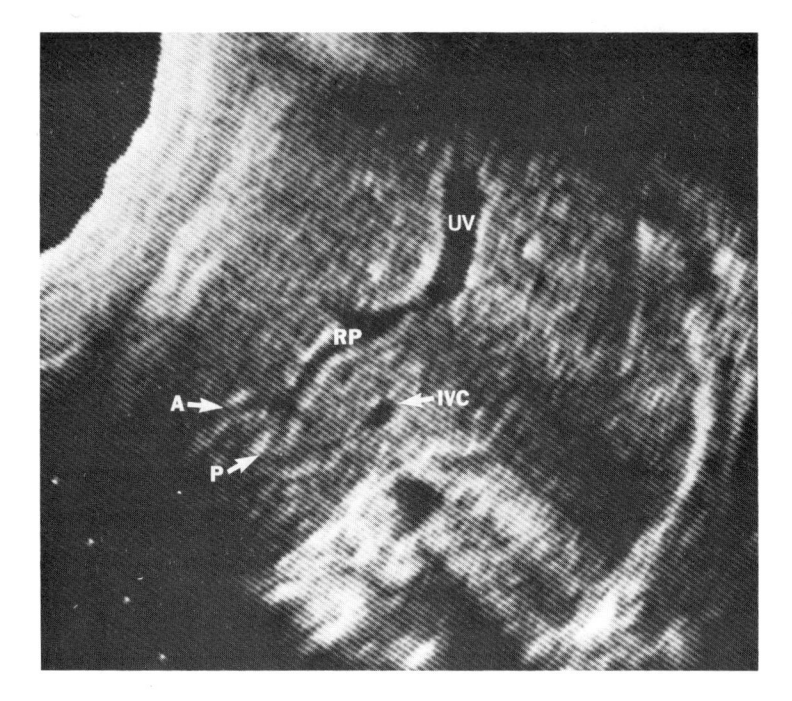

Figure 14. Single pass scan through fetal abdomen demonstrating umbilical vein (UV), right portal vein (RP), and the anterior (A) and posterior (P) branches of the right portal vein. The inferior vena cava (IVC) is seen in cross section.

so that the adrenal assumes a more usual size and triangular shape post partum. The fetal adrenal gland is recognized as an oval mass of echo-poor tissue lying superior to the kidney on the sagittal scan (Fig. 23). On transverse scans the fetal adrenal is seen as a long thin echogenic line of medulla, surrounded on both sides by a thicker sonolucent rim of cortex (Fig. 24). The adrenal gland should be smaller than the normal kidney. Care must be taken to recognize normal renal tissue below the adrenal gland because cases of renal agenesis have been reported in which an adrenal gland in

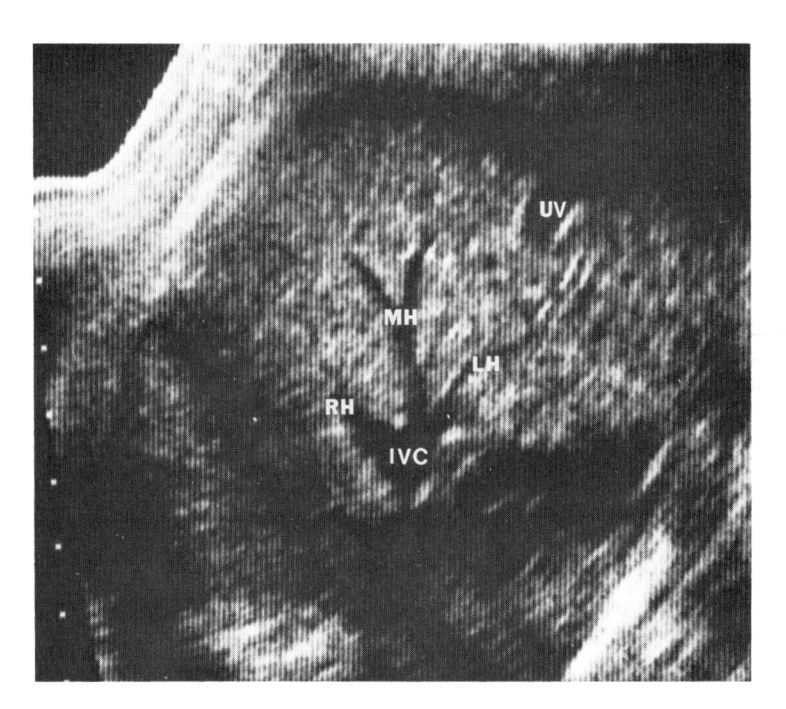

Figure 15. Oblique transverse scan through the upper abdomen at 31 weeks' gestation. The left (LH), middle (MH), and right (RH) hepatic veins are seen separating the four segments of the liver as they drain into the inferior vena cava (IVC). The umbilical vein (UV) is also seen.

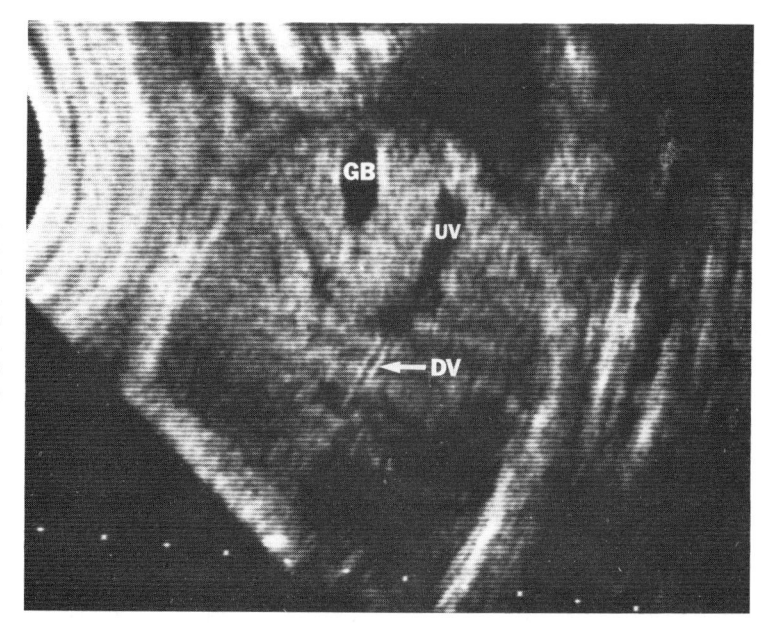

Figure 16. An oblique transverse scan through the abdomen at 31 weeks' gestation demonstrates the length of the umbilical vein (UV). The gallbladder (GB) is noted to the right of the umbilical vein. The ductus venosus (DV) is seen connecting the portal system with the inferior vena cava.

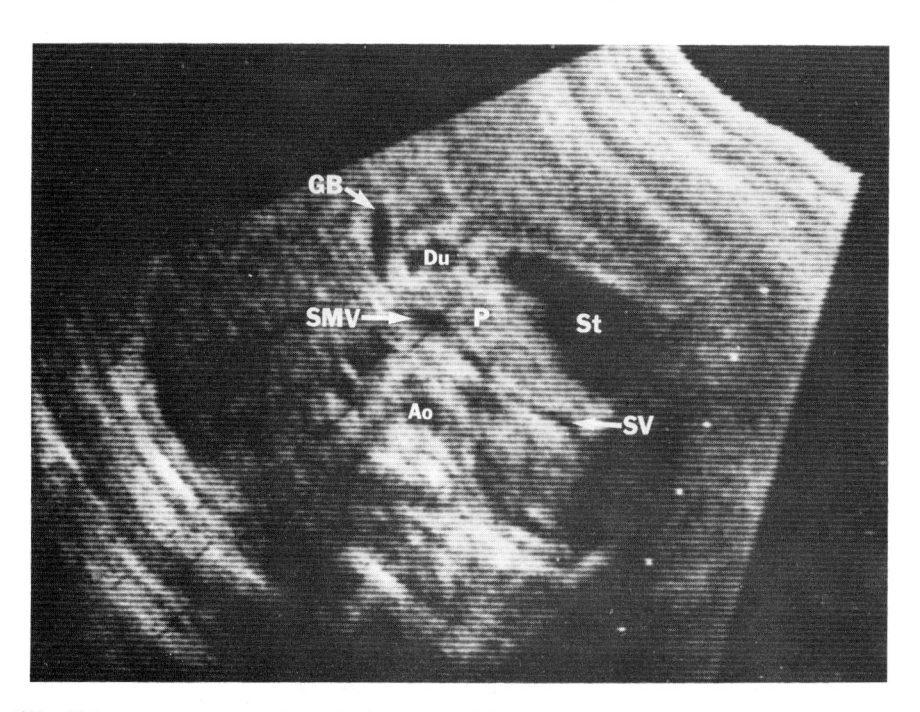

Figure 17. This transverse scan through the upper abdomen at 34 weeks' gestation demonstrates vascular landmarks of the fetal pancreas. The splenic vein (SV) is seen running transversely to join the superior mesenteric vein (SMV). The fetal pancreas (P) is noted anterior to the splenic vein. Also seen are the stomach (St), duodenum (Du), neck of the gallbladder (GB), and the aorta (Ao).

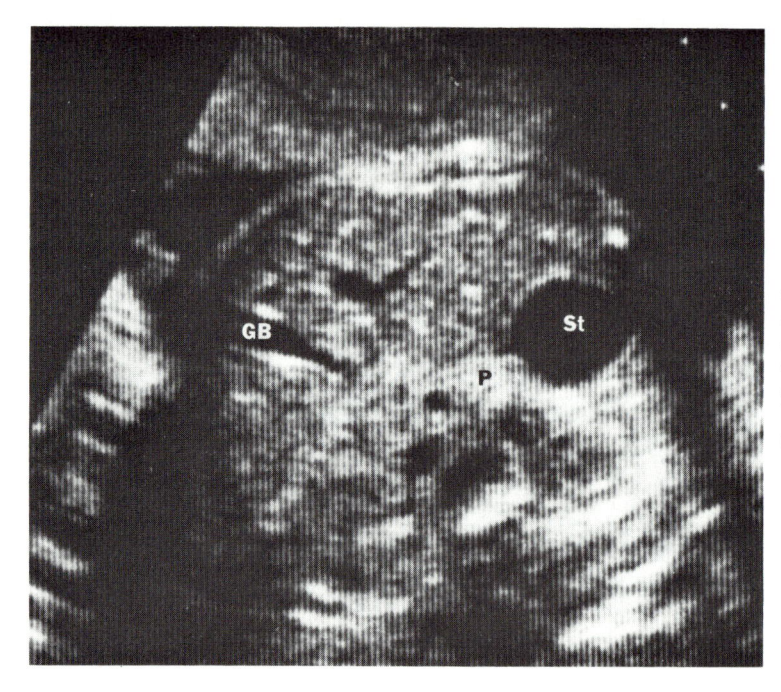

Figure 18. Scan through upper abdomen of a 26 week fetus demonstrating fetal pancreas (P) as a poorly marginated echogenic structure behind the stomach (St) and anterior to the great vessels. The gallbladder (GB) is visualized.

the renal fossa was mistakenly called the kidney.[18] Other examples of fetal adrenals may be seen in Figures 8 and 11.

GENITALIA AND CORD

Fetal genitalia may often be seen, especially with the high resolution real-time examination after 25 weeks' gestation (Fig. 25). In one series, genitalia of 72 of 112 consecutive pregnancies were seen and the sex of the fetus correctly determined in all 72.[15] Approximately equal numbers of female and male infants were present in this series. Mistakes can be made, however, in confusing swollen labia or umbilical cord

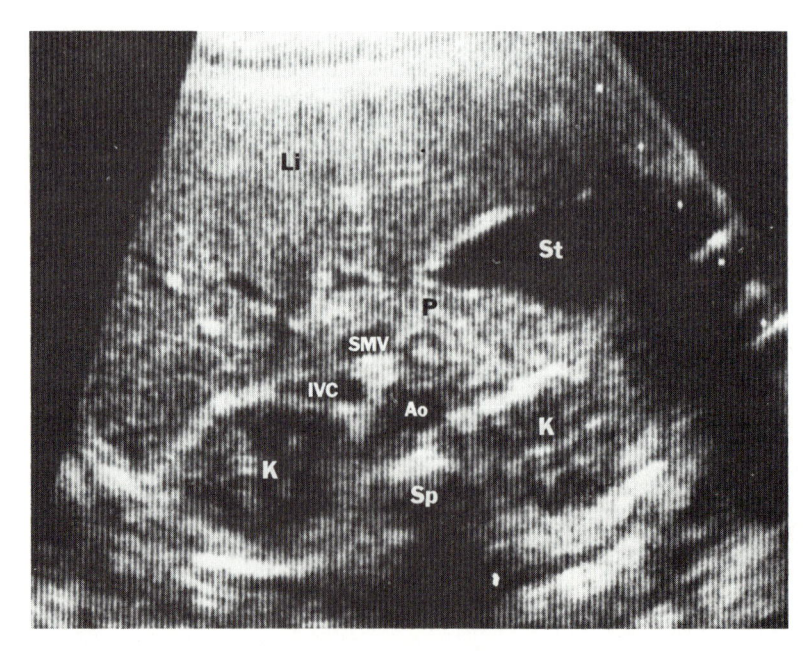

Figure 19. This transverse scan at 34 weeks' gestation demonstrates the echo-poor kidneys (K) on either side of the fetal spine (Sp). Also of note are the liver (Li), pancreas (P), stomach (St), superior mesenteric vein (SMV), inferior vena cava (IVC) and aorta (Ao).

Normal Fetal Anatomy 55

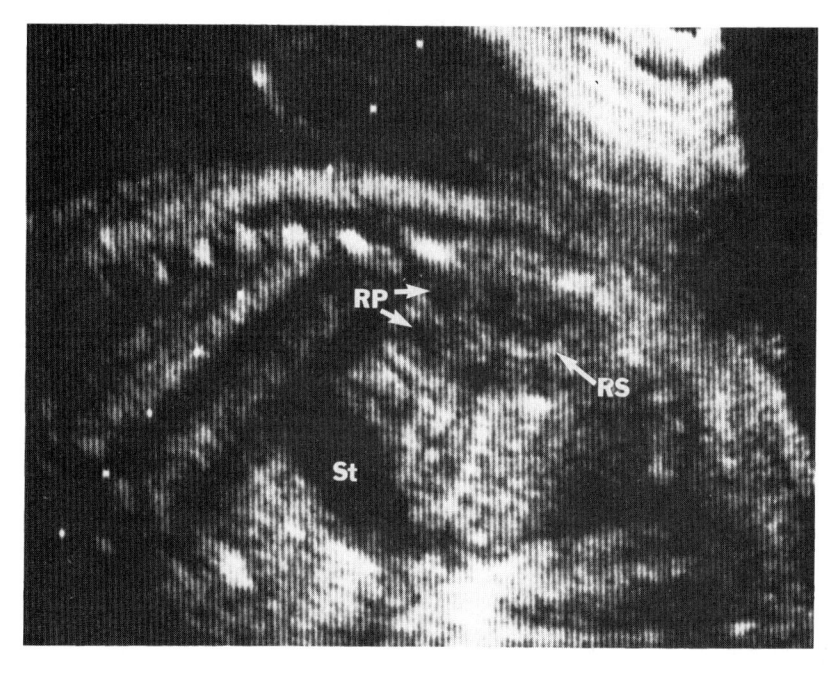

Figure 20. A parasagittal scan through the left kidney at 31 weeks' gestation demonstrates the relatively echo-poor renal pyramids (RP). The echogenic renal sinus (RS) can be seen in the hilus of the kidney. The fetal stomach (St) is also noted.

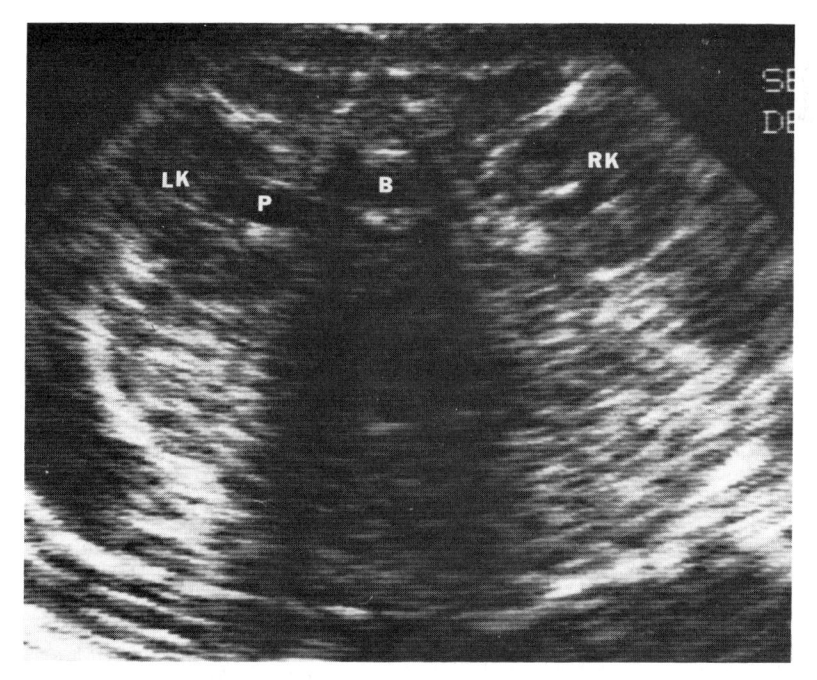

Figure 21. Real-time image through the back of a term fetus demonstrating the left (LK) and right (RK) kidneys. The pelvis (P) is mildly dilated in the left kidney. This was normal at birth. The vertebral body (B) is casting an acoustic shadow.

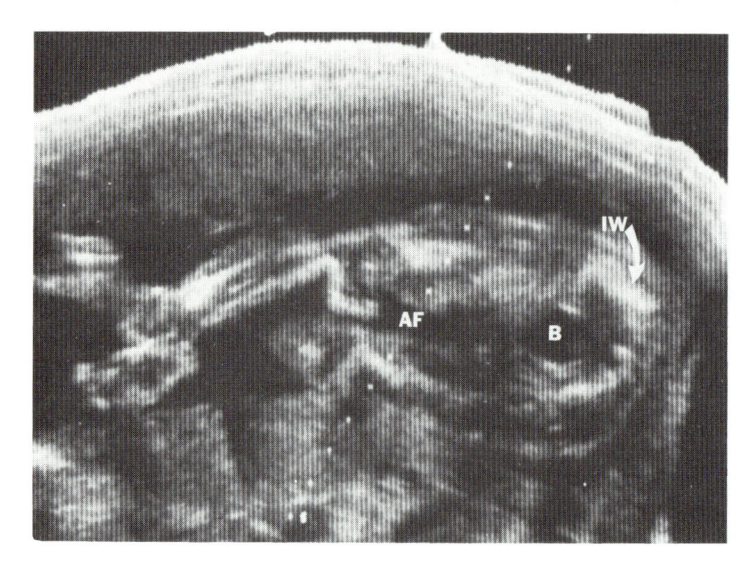

Figure 22. This transverse scan through the fetal pelvis at 26 weeks' gestation demonstrates a filled urinary bladder (B) between the iliac wings (IW). Of note is amniotic fluid (AF) between the fetal thighs.

lying between the legs of a female fetus as male genitalia. We believe that the clinical value of determination of fetal gender by ultrasound is questionable and that an extensive search for genitalia is not warranted.

The umbilical cord is often seen in the second and third trimesters of pregnancy. With the use of real-time examination, pulsations in the cord with a rate equal to the fetal heart rate can be recognized. The cord is best seen when the amount of amniotic fluid is generous. With oligohydramnios, it may be impossible to see the cord, even at term. The normal cord is recognized by two smaller arteries surrounding the larger

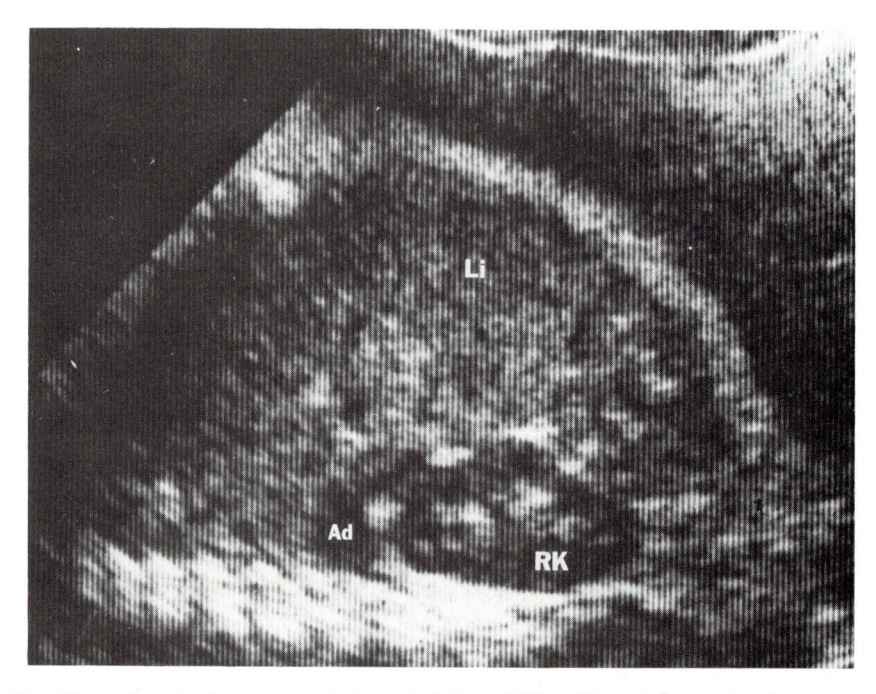

Figure 23. This parasagittal scan through the right kidney (RK) at 33 weeks' gestation demonstrates the echo-poor adrenal gland (Ad) superior to the kidney. Liver (Li) is noted superior and anterior to the kidney and adrenal gland.

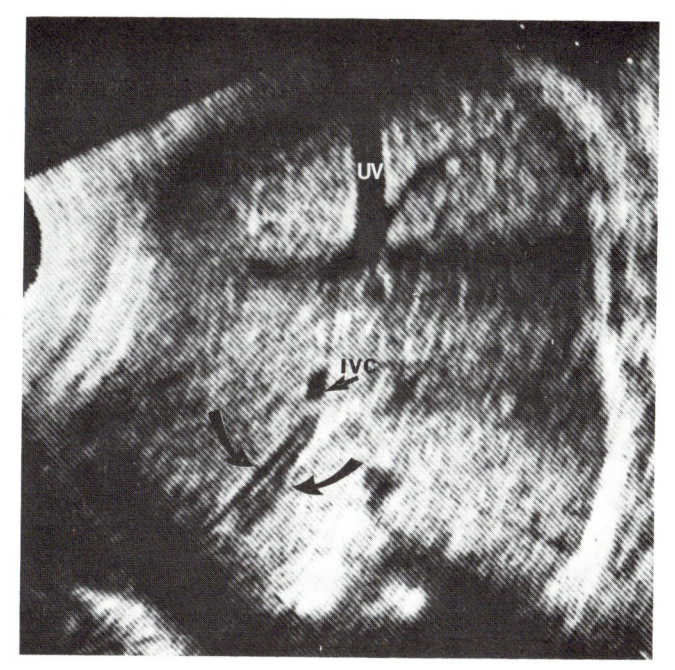

Figure 24. Scan through upper abdomen of fetus demonstrating the right adrenal gland (*curved arrows*). The echogenic medulla is surrounded by the larger sonolucent adrenal cortex. The inferior vena cava (IVC) is just anterior to the adrenal gland and the umbilical vein (UV) is visualized.

umbilical vein (Fig. 26).[12] Arteries can be distributed in any orientation around the vein. The demonstration of a two-vessel cord (that is, artery and vein) is associated with numerous fetal congenital anomalies, including serious cardiovascular and genitourinary abnormalities. The single umbilical artery is also associated with diabetes, twins, and increased neonatal mortality.[3]

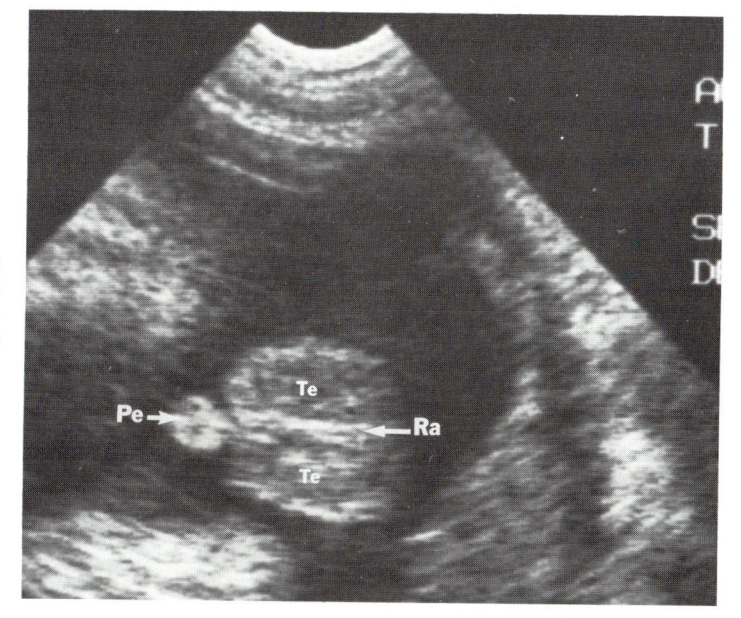

Figure 25. A real-time scan of 36 weeks' gestation demonstrates the penis (Pe) and the scrotum containing the testes (Te). The midline raphe (Ra) is noted between the testicles.

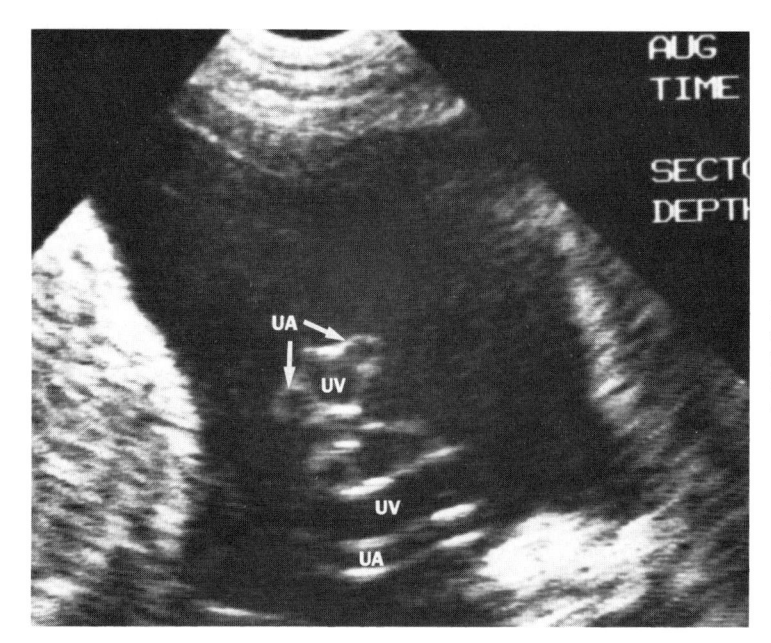

Figure 26. Cross-sectional and longitudinal views of the umbilical cord at 36 weeks' gestation. The two umbilical arteries (UA) and the larger single umbilical vein (UV) are seen.

CONCLUSION

We have attempted to discuss normal fetal anatomic structures that can be imaged with currently available ultrasound equipment. The superb resolution and delineation of fetal anatomy now possible allow consideration of the fetus as a patient, separate and apart from the mother and uterine environment. It is obvious that ultrasound is capable of visualizing a tremendous number of fetal organs. In no way, however, do we intend the reader to assume that we routinely visualize such detailed anatomic structures as the fetal pancreas or spleen. But we do want to emphasize that with care and concern for technical details, many fetal soft tissue structures can be seen. The utility of visualizing the structure of fetal organs has already been demonstrated in the brain, kidney, and several other organs. We believe that the need for visualizing other fetal organs such as the lung, pancreas, and spleen in selected patients will become obvious as more disorders are diagnosed in utero. Ultrasound has assumed an extremely exciting role in perinatal medicine and is presently on the cutting edge in this field.

ACKNOWLEDGMENTS

We would like to thank Ms. Judith Caplan Banjavic for her secretarial assistance, Mr. Kevin Appareti and Mr. Dale Cyr for their technical assistance, and the technologists and student technologists in the Ultrasound Division for their support and care of the patients in our department.

REFERENCES

1. Clewell, W. H., Johnson, M. L., Meier, P. R., et al.: A surgical approach to the treatment of fetal hydrocephalus. N. Engl. J. Med., 306:1320–1325, 1982.
2. Filly, R. A., and Callen, P. W.: Ultrasonographic evaluation of the normal fetal anatomy. In Sanders, R., and James, E. (eds.): Ultrasonography in Obstetrics and Gynecology. New York, Appleton-Century-Crofts, 1980.
3. Froehlich, L., and Fujikura, T.: Follow-up of infants with single umbilical artery. Pediatrics, 52:6–13, 1973.
4. Garrett, W. J., Warren, P. S., Picker, R. H., et al.: Maturation of the fetal lung, liver, and bowel. Abstract presented at American Institute of Ultrasound in Medicine Scientific Meeting, San Francisco, California, August 1981.
5. Grannum, P., Bracken, M., Silverman, R., et al.: Assessment of fetal kidney size in normal gestation by comparison of ratio of kidney circumference to abdominal circumference. Am. J. Obstet. Gynecol., 136:249–254, 1980.
6. Hattan, R. A., Rees, G. K., and Johnson, M. L.: Normal fetal anatomy. Radiol. Clin. North Am., 20:1–14, 1982.
7. Johnson, M. L., Hattan, R. A., and Rees, G. K.: The normal fetus. Semin. Roentgenol., 17:182–189, 1982.
8. Langman, J.: Medical Embryology. Baltimore, Williams and Wilkins, 1969.
9. Lawson, T., Foley, W., Berland, L., et al.: Ultra-

sonic evaluation of the fetal kidney. Radiology, 138:153–156, 1981.
10. Mantoni, M., and Pederson, J.: Ultrasound visualization of the human yolk sac. J. Clin. Ultrasound, 7:459–460, 1979.
11. Moore, K.: The Developing Human. Philadelphia, W. B. Saunders Company 1977.
12. Morin, F., and Winsberg, F.: The ultrasonic appearance of the umbilical cord. J. Clin. Ultrasound, 6:324–326, 1978.
13. Morin, F., and Winsberg, F.: Ultrasonic and radiographic study of the vessels of the fetal liver. J. Clin. Ultrasound, 6:409–411, 1979.
14. Sahn, D., Lange, L., Allen, H., et al.: Quantitative real-time cross-sectional echocardiography in the developing normal human fetus and newborn. Circulation, 62:588–597, 1980.
15. Scholly, T., Sutphen, J., Hitchcock, D., et al.: Sonographic determination of fetal gender. Am. J. Roentgenol., 135:1161–1165, 1980.
16. Silverman, P., Carroll, B., and Moskowitz, P.: Adrenal sonography in renal agenesis and dysplasia. Am. J. Roentgenol., 134:600–602, 1980.
17. Thieme, G., Banjavic, R. A., Johnson, M. L., et al.: Sonographic identification of lung maturation in the fetal lamb. Invest. Radiol, (in press).
18. Toomey, F., Fritzsche, P., Carlsen, E., et al.: Application of aortography and ultrasound in evaluation of renal agenesis. Pediatr. Radiol., 6:168–171, 1977.

4

Fetal Anomalies Involving the Thorax and Abdomen

John Q. Knochel, M.D., Timothy G. Lee, M.D., Michael G. Melendez, M.D., and Sidney C. Henderson, M.D.

The lack of ionizing radiation and absence of any yet proven deleterious effects to the mother or fetus has made ultrasound a unique and powerful tool for evaluating and managing the obstetric patient. Up to this time, ultrasound has been used predominantly to identify placental location, fetal position, fetal number, and fetal gestational size. Now, with improvements in both gray scale ultrasound and real-time ultrasound, the fetus itself has come under increasing scrutiny.[11, 13, 25, 33–36, 55] Alterations in fetal anatomy combined with changes in the placenta or in the amount of amniotic fluid gives the ultrasonographer important clues to underlying fetal abnormalities. Recognition of such fetal abnormalities may drastically alter management, from termination of the pregnancy to in utero interventional procedures.

With the increasing complexity and improvement in perinatal care, the early detection of fetal abnormalities can be crucial to that infant's survival. Anticipation of an abnormal fetus, based on ultrasound findings, provides time to mobilize the specialists required to properly manage the fetus once it is born. This chapter will review sequentially some of those fetal thoracoabdominal abnormalities detectable by ultrasound. Knowledge of normal fetal anatomy is a prerequisite to proper identification of altered fetal structures (see Chapter 3). Interventional procedures and other imaging modalities helpful in the management of fetal abnormalities will also be discussed. It is important to note that in assessing the fetus, one must first ascertain fetal position and then obtain serial transverse and sagittal scans. Only in this way can one establish anatomic relationships and detect subtle deviations from normal.

CERVICAL REGION

A variety of abnormalities can be detected in the fetal cervical region. Differentiation may be made based on whether the mass is cystic or solid, where it is located, and whether or not it is associated with a skull or spinal column defect.[56] Encephaloceles and neural tube defects characterize the latter and are discussed elsewhere. However, because neural tube defects are typically cystic and because associated vertebral column defects may not always be recognized, they should always be considered in any differential of cystic neck masses.

Solid masses include mesenchymal sarcomas, solid teratomas, hemangiomas, and congenital goiter.[2, 30, 64] Cystic masses include cystic hygromas, fetal edema, cystic teratomas, thyroglossal duct cysts, and branchial cleft cysts.[64] While each of these cervical region masses may have certain characteristics that help to distinguish one from another, it should be emphasized that anatomic distinction is not always possible.

Teratomas. Teratomas are congenital tumors, most often benign in infancy and childhood, which are derived from the three embryologic germ layers.[30] They may arise from many locations, but of all sites, the cervical region is the least common. Teratomas may be cystic, solid, or mixed; as such they may be difficult to separate ultrasonically from other lesions. However, shadowing from calcification within the tumor may be seen and may help in making the diagnosis. Teratomas are usually located anteriorly within the neck and there may be associated polyhydramnios (Fig. 1). Respiratory and feeding difficulties are presenting symptoms in many patients and

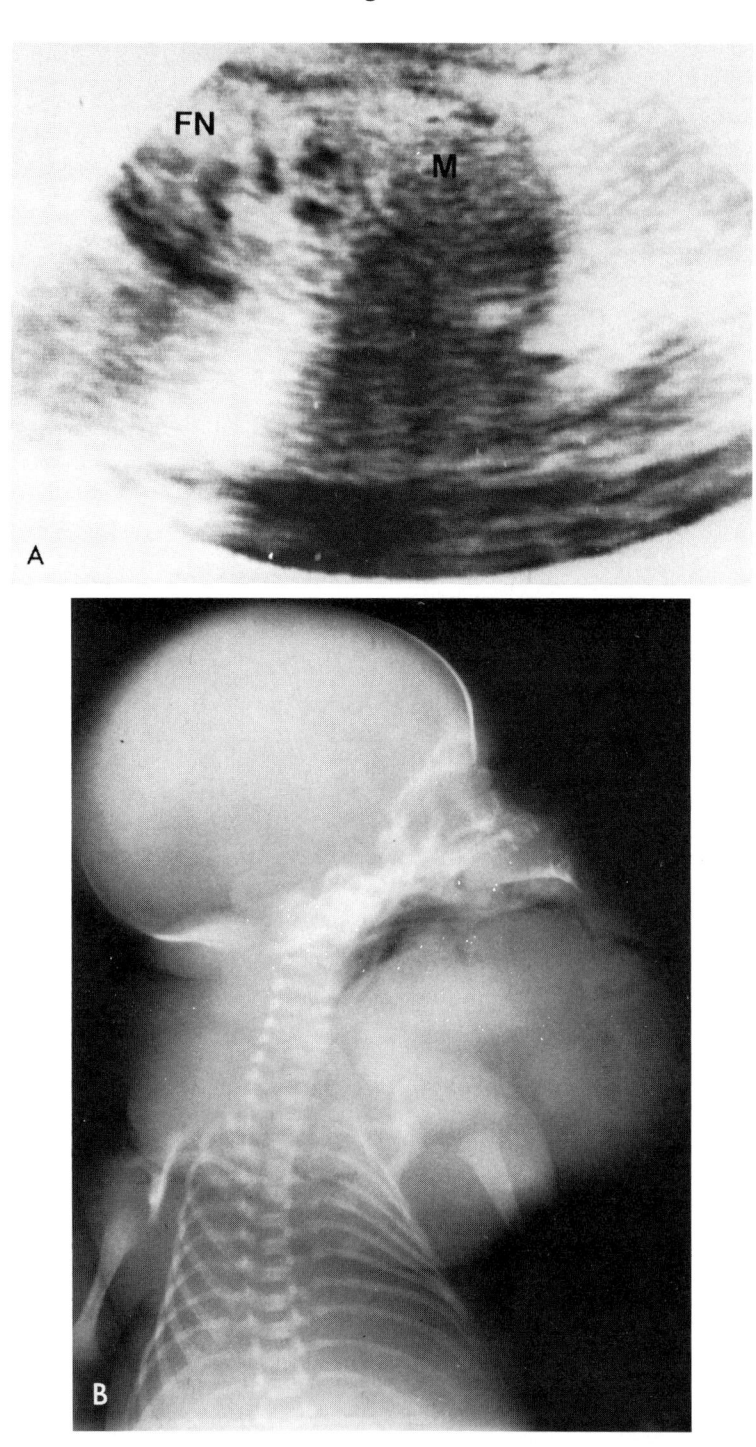

Figure 1. *A*, A sector view of the fetal neck shows an anterior cervical teratoma. Mass (M); fetal neck (FN). *B*, A postpartum lateral radiograph confirms the anterior cervical mass. (Courtesy of Dr. Gayle Williams, Southwest Methodist Hospital, San Antonio, Texas.)

may require immediate surgical intervention.

Edema. A fetus severely hydropic from any cause may have significant amounts of subcutaneous edema. Often there will be associated fetal ascites. The outer margins of the edematous tissue are thick, and a halo effect is evident since the edematous tissue conforms to the outlines of the fetal head and neck. Similarly, the edema may also be seen over the tissues of the fetal thorax and abdomen (Fig. 2).[56]

Cystic Hygroma. Cystic hygromas are benign developmental abnormalities of lymphatic origin. Their ultrasound characteristics are those of a thin-walled multiseptated cystic mass usually located posterior to the fetal head and neck (Fig. 3).[45, 48] Eighty per cent of cystic hygromas occur in the cervical region, but they may also be found in the axilla, groin, or mediastinum. Since 65 per cent of cystic

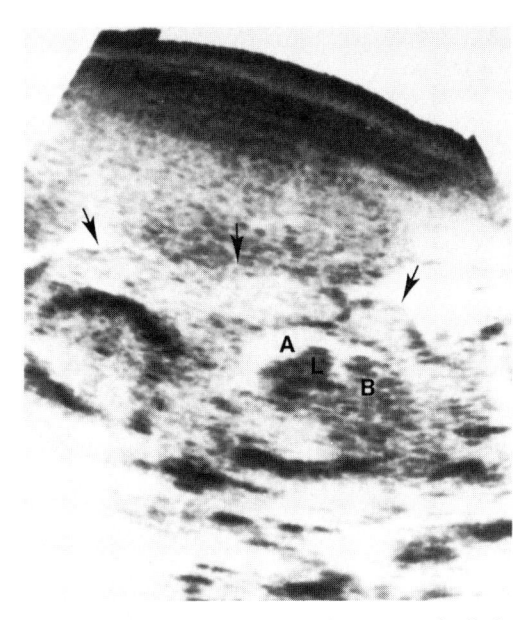

Figure 2. This sagittal scan shows a markedly hydropic fetus. A soft tissue halo (*arrows*) representing edema surrounds the fetus. Ascites (A); liver (L); bowel (B).

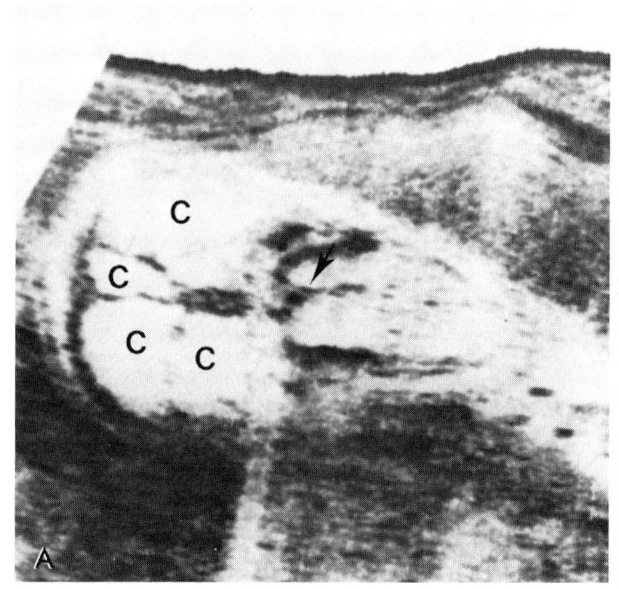

Figure 3. *A*, A posterior multiseptated cystic mass (C) represents a cystic hygroma. Spine (*arrow*). *B*, A large soft tissue mass is seen posterior to the normal cervical vertebra in this lateral radiograph of the same patient with the cystic hygroma.

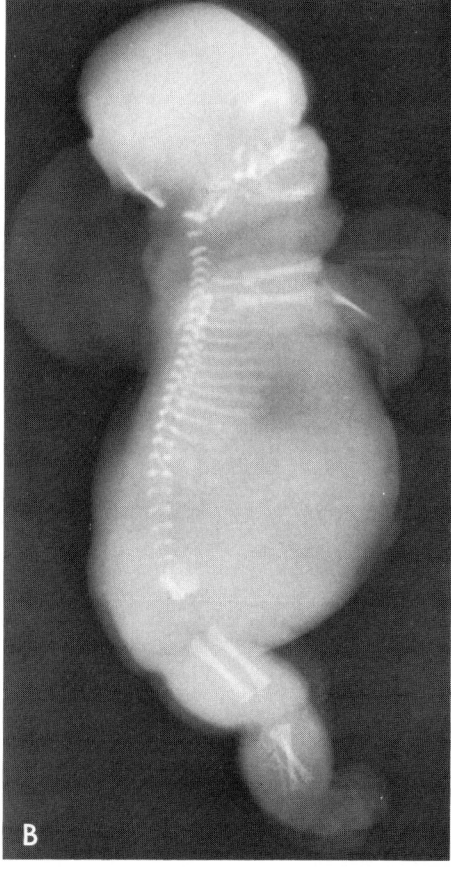

hygromas are apparent at birth,[48] they should be readily detectable antenatally with good ultrasound technique. Large cystic hygromas have been described in association with Turner's syndrome.[39, 47]

Differentiation of cystic hygromas from neural tube defects may be difficult since both can have a similar ultrasound appearance (Fig. 4) as well as elevated levels of alpha-fetoprotein in the amniotic fluid.[39, 47] In those cystic hygromas associated with Turner's syndrome, chromosomal analysis may be helpful. Other ultrasound findings that may be present in cystic hygromas and serve to differentiate them from neural tube defects are fetal ascites, fetal edema, enlarged edematous placenta, and intradermal fluid collections (cystic cutaneous lymphangiectasia).[48] In contradistinction, cervical region masses associated with neural tube defects tend to be localized.

Meningo-Meningomyelocele. Cystic thin-walled neck masses of neural origin are usually localized and may be associated with polyhydramnios. Other differential points are described above. This entity will be discussed elsewhere.

THORAX

Identification of the fetal thorax is made simple by recognition of the characteristic ultrasound pattern of the fetal spine and ribs. Acoustic shadowing from the ribs traversing the more trans-sonic lung tissue establishes the region of the fetal thorax. Extrathoracic masses such as cystic hygro-

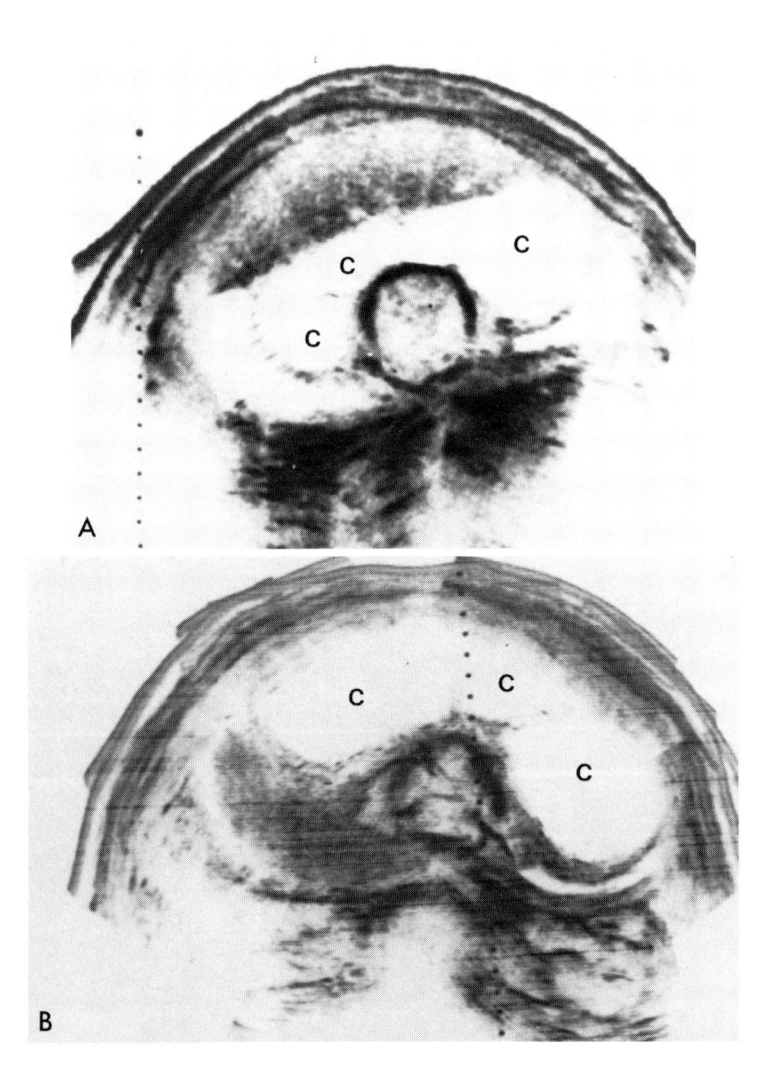

Figure 4. Note the similarity between these two posterior cystic masses (C). *A*, Cystic hygroma. (Courtesy of Dr. Arthur Budge, McKay Dee Hospital, Ogden, Utah.) *B*, Meningomyelocele. (Courtesy of Dr. William J. Little, Medical Arts Building, Kalispell, Montana.)

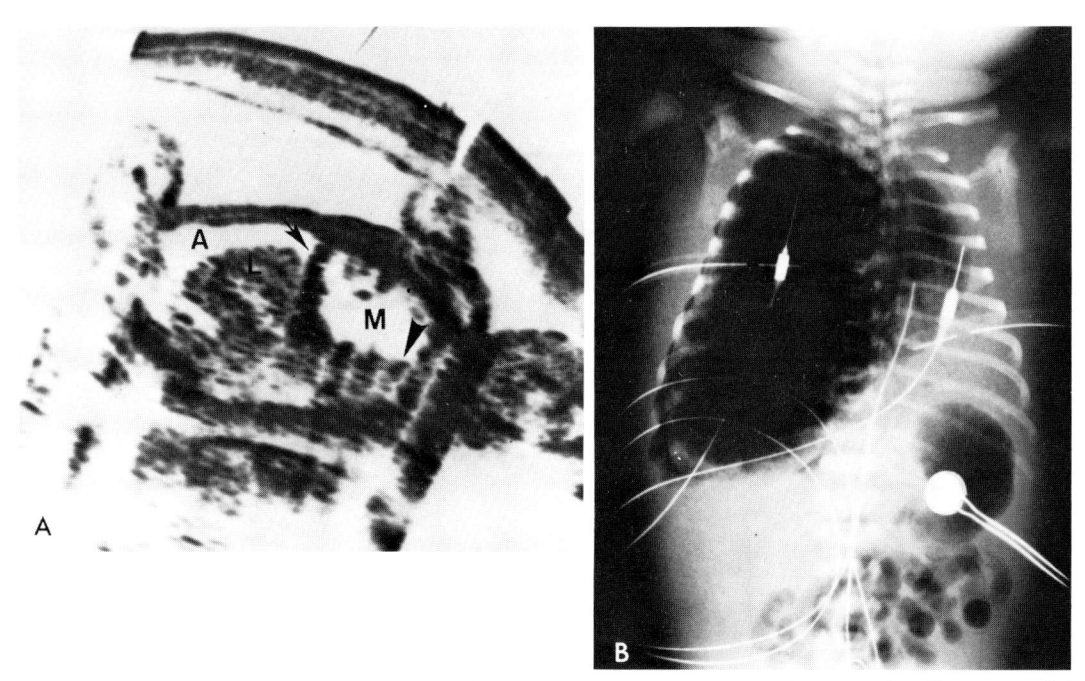

Figure 5. *A*, A cystic mass (M) within the fetal thorax represents a cystic adenomatoid malformation of the lung. Note the inversion of the diaphragm (*arrow*), the compression of the heart and lung (*arrowhead*), and the presence of ascites (A). Liver (L). *B*, Postpartum radiograph confirms the ultrasound findings.

mas and neural tube defects can also be seen in this region. This section will describe fetal intrathoracic abnormalities.

Heart. A left-sided anterior cystic chamber within the thoracic cage represents the fetal heart. Slow scanning with a contact scanner or observation by real-time ultrasound shows the characteristic valve motion of the fetal heart. It is this valve motion that confirms the position of the heart within the thorax and differentiates this structure from other intrathoracic masses. M-mode cardiac scanning can also be performed. Furthermore, fetal heart structures such as the four valves and the intraventricular septum, as well as measurements of the chamber size, have been reported.[25, 63]

Because the cardiac location and intracardiac structures can be defined ultrasonically, a case of an ectopic cordis was diagnosed by showing the heart outside of the fetal chest.[36] Similarly, pericardial effusions can be seen as a halo of anechoic fluid surrounding the fetal heart.[43] Other reports detail such cardiac abnormalities as congenital heart block, single ventricle, and holoacardia.[24, 38, 58]

Other Intrathoracic Abnormalities. The antenatal diagnosis of pleural effusions,[3, 6, 11, 36] diaphragmatic hernia,[25] cystic adenomatoid malformation (Fig. 5),[8, 18] and enteric cyst[25] have been previously reported. In addition, we have encountered a case of mediastinal encephalocele (Fig. 6) and a case of pulmonary sequestration (Fig. 7). The key to the diagnosis of these abnormalities is to define them within the fetal chest above the level of the diaphragm

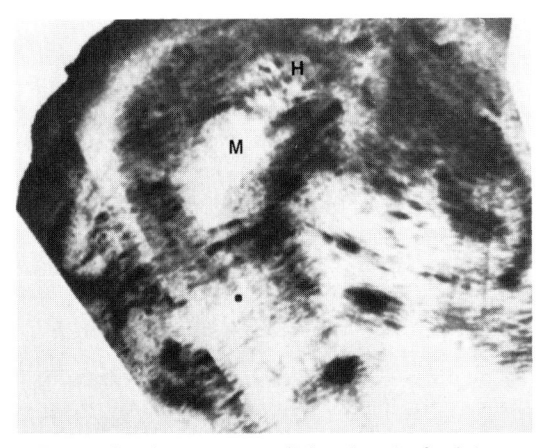

Figure 6. A cystic mass (M) within the fetal thorax displaces the fetal heart (H). This mass can be clearly separated from the heart, which is characterized by the presence of valve motion. This proved to be a mediastinal encephalocele.

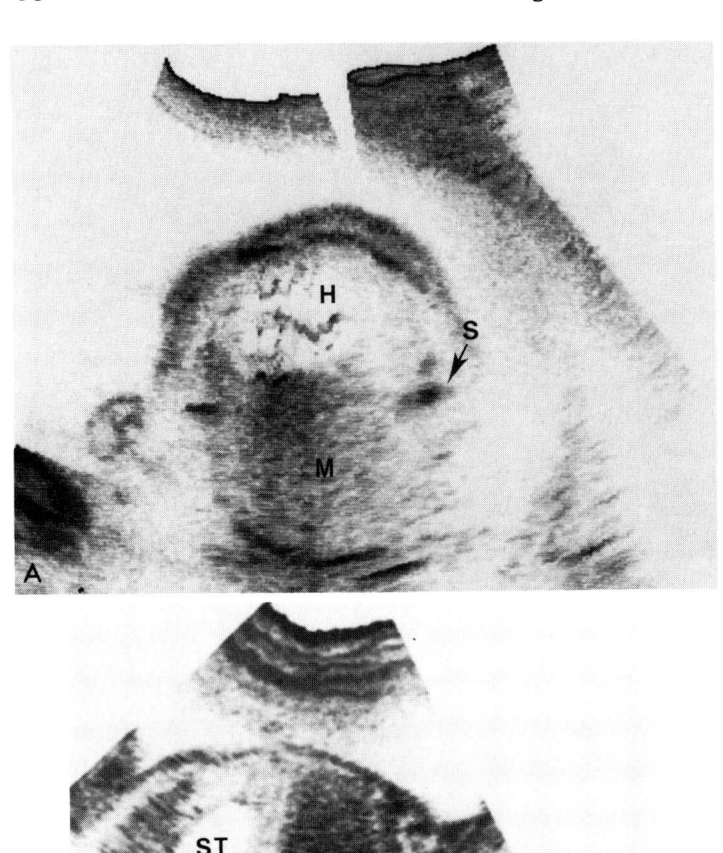

Figure 7. *A*, The solid mass (M), a pulmonary sequestration, displaces the fetal heart (H) to the right. Fetal spine (S). The valve motion of the heart again identifies this structure. *B*, A sagittal view of the fetus shows the intrathoracic solid mass (M) displacing the heart (H) to the right. The left-sided stomach (ST) is below the diaphragm.

Illustration continued on opposite page

and separate them from the fetal heart. Many of these lesions appear cystic, making distinction of one from another difficult. Our case of pulmonary sequestration is unusual in that it was predominantly solid. Regardless of our ability to establish the etiology of these intrathoracic lesions, the consequence to the fetus is similar.

Two effects may occur from elevation of intrathoracic pressure from any of the described intrathoracic abnormalities. First, there may be inversion of the diaphragm with obstruction of venous return and compression of the fetal heart, resulting in heart failure and subsequent edema and development of fetal ascites (Fig. 8). Second, if there is significant mass effect within the fetal thorax, the lungs will not develop properly and the child will be born with underdeveloped lungs (see Fig. 8). Awareness of these impending pulmonary problems can allow for immediate evaluation following birth. In diaphragmatic hernias and cystic adenomatoid malformation

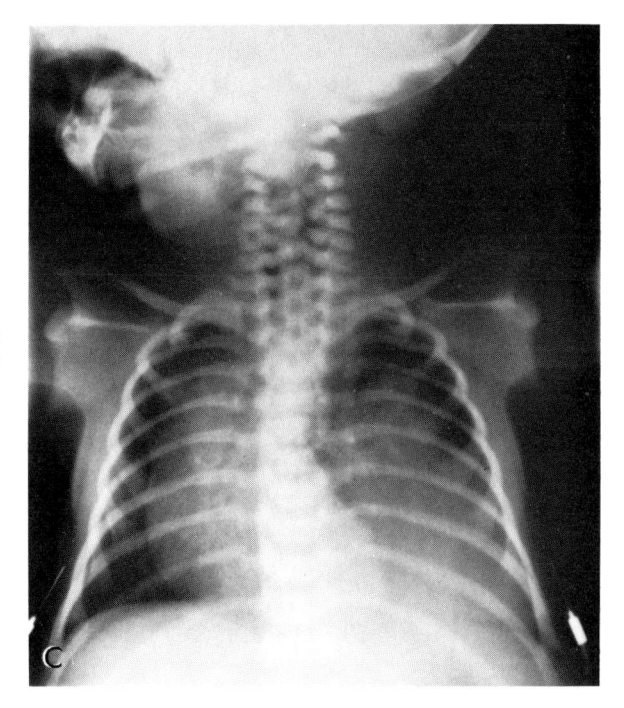

Figure 7. (*Continued*). *C*, A postpartum chest radiograph demonstrates the left chest mass displacing the heart to the right.

of the lung, immediate surgery can be anticipated.[8, 25]

The therapeutic implication of finding thoracic abnormalities by ultrasound is exemplified in the case described in Figure 8. An ultrasound examination was performed in the third trimester of pregnancy. A large fluid collection could be seen in the fetal thorax, displacing the heart and compressing the normal lung. The diaphragm was inverted. Significant vascular compromise was already manifested by a large amount of fetal ascites. At birth the infant was apneic and without a heartbeat. Apgar scores at one minute were 0 - 0. The infant's poor status was thought to be due to the compression effect of the large pleural effusion and associated ascites. Because of the prenatal ultrasound findings, a thoracentesis and paracentesis were immediately performed with removal of 130 and 60 ml of fluid, respectively. The infant improved immediately to an Apgar of 5 and was transferred to the Newborn Intensive Care Unit. Clearly, this infant would not have survived without the prenatal ultrasound diagnosis and the prompt therapeutic procedures that it prompted. In cases in which cardiopulmonary compromise is detected early, the pregnancy can be prolonged by percutaneous needle aspiration of the cystic thoracic mass, thus preserving cardiac function and facilitating development of the fetal lung.

GASTROINTESTINAL TRACT

Esophageal Atresia. Esophageal atresia occurs once in 1500 live births; however, 90 per cent of these cases have a tracheo-esophageal fistula which allows passage of fluid into the fetal stomach.[57] There is, therefore, no polyhydramnios and no abnormality detectable by ultrasound. One review states that in over 5000 obstetric scans, the fetal stomach was identified in all but one.[12] Our experience suggests that the stomach is not identified that often, but that it nevertheless is a commonly seen structure. Certainly, repeated failure to identify the fetal stomach in the presence of polyhydramnios should lead one to consider the possibility of esophageal atresia.

Bowel Obstruction. Just as it is not unusual to see a fluid-filled stomach, so it is not unusual to see fluid-filled bowel within the fetal abdomen. However, prominent fluid-filled loops of bowel with little change in configuration, particularly when

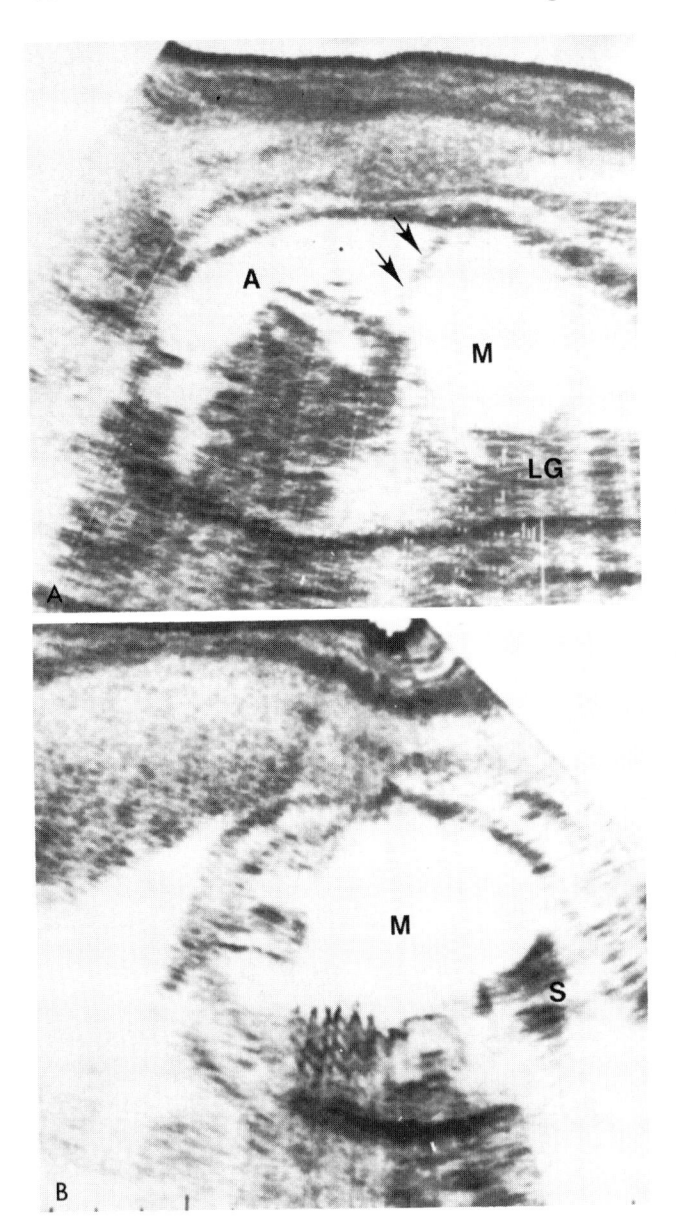

Figure 8. *A*, The diaphragm (*arrows*) is inverted by a large pleural effusion (M). The diaphragm serves as a landmark for identification of the thoracic space. The lung (LG) is compressed. Below the diaphragm there is a large amount of ascites (A) outlining the abdominal viscera. *B*, A cross section of the fetal thorax again shows the mass effect of a large pleural effusion (M) compressing the heart and lung. Wave motion identifies the heart. Spine (S).

Illustration continued on opposite page

seen on repeat scans in the presence of polyhydramnios, should alert the sonographer to the possibility of an obstructed hollow viscus.[10, 35, 65] The most characteristic ultrasound pattern is that seen with duodenal atresia.[4, 37, 41] The so-called double bubble sign so familiar to pediatric radiologists has its counterpart in ultrasound where two fluid-filled structures are seen in the upper portion of the fetal abdomen (Fig. 9). Usually the stomach is the larger of the two and resides in the left upper quadrant. A case of obstruction from an antral web has been described in which there was only a single large fluid collection in the left upper quadrant, representing a dilated fluid-filled stomach.[65] Another report suggests that patients with duodenal atresia may have emesis, in which case fluid-filled structures in the presence of an obstructed system may come and go.[11] Since they are still high in the gastrointestinal

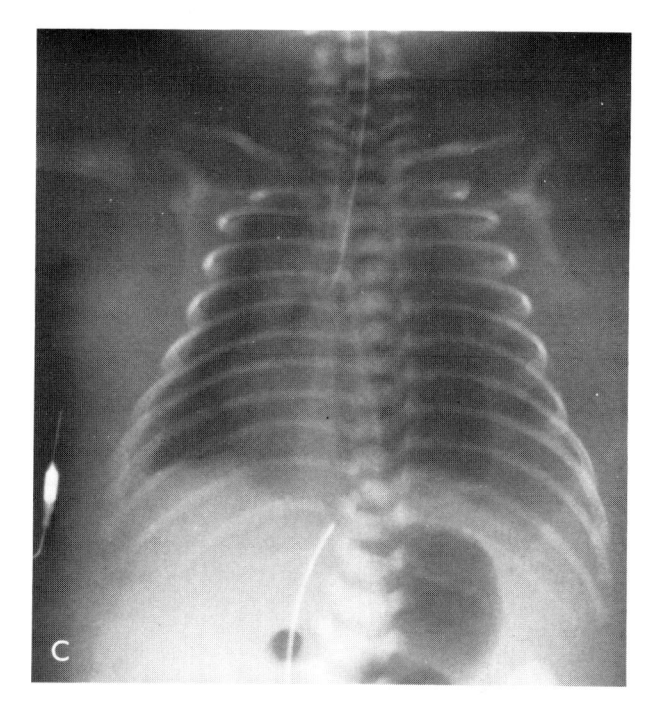

Figure 8. (*Continued*) *C*, In this postpartum chest x-ray film the heart remains displaced to the right. A large pleural effusion still remains following a thoracentesis at the time of birth.

tract, ileal and jejunal atresias may have concomitant polyhydramnios, but more fluid-filled loops of bowel than seen with duodenal atresia (Fig. 10).[15] Anal atresia is associated with fluid-filled loops of bowel that are usually more distal in the gastrointestinal tract and are therefore seen more caudally in the fetal abdomen.[1] This abnormality is usually not associated with polyhydramnios since there is a sufficient length of bowel for resorption of swallowed fluids.[11]

Recognition of these abnormalities is important since it allows for appropriate planning and management at the time of birth. Significant morbidity and mortality can ensue secondary to persistent vomiting, electrolyte imbalance, or aspiration of gastric contents if obstruction of the gastrointestinal tract is not recognized at delivery and there is undue delay in making the diagnosis.[4] Confirmation of the ultrasound findings can be made antenatally by amniography. This is an invasive procedure and generally is not necessary since confirmation can be obtained quickly post partum with insertion of a nasogastric tube and aspiration of gastric contents. If necessary, air can be introduced via the nasogastric tube and its progress followed with an abdominal radiograph. Physical examination and barium studies are useful if the lesion is located more distally.

Other conditions that may lead to obstruction of bowel loops include malrotation syndrome, microcolon, and meconium ileus. The presence of a large thick-walled bladder and hydronephrosis in the presence of polyhydramnios should lead one to suspect the presence of megacystic-microcolon-intestinal hypoperistalsis syndrome.[31, 59] Other cystic structures occurring in the

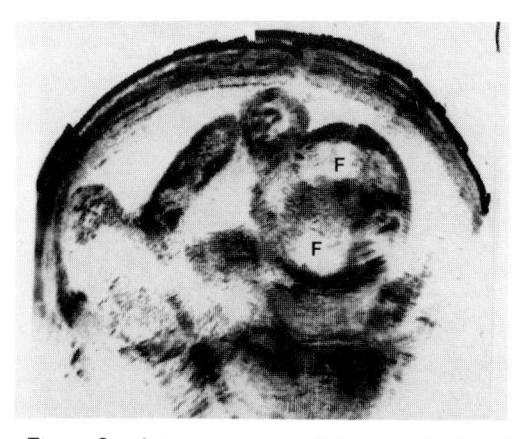

Figure 9. A transverse scan of the upper fetal trunk shows two fluid-containing structures (F) identical to the radiographic "double bubble" of duodenal atresia. Polyhydramnios is present.

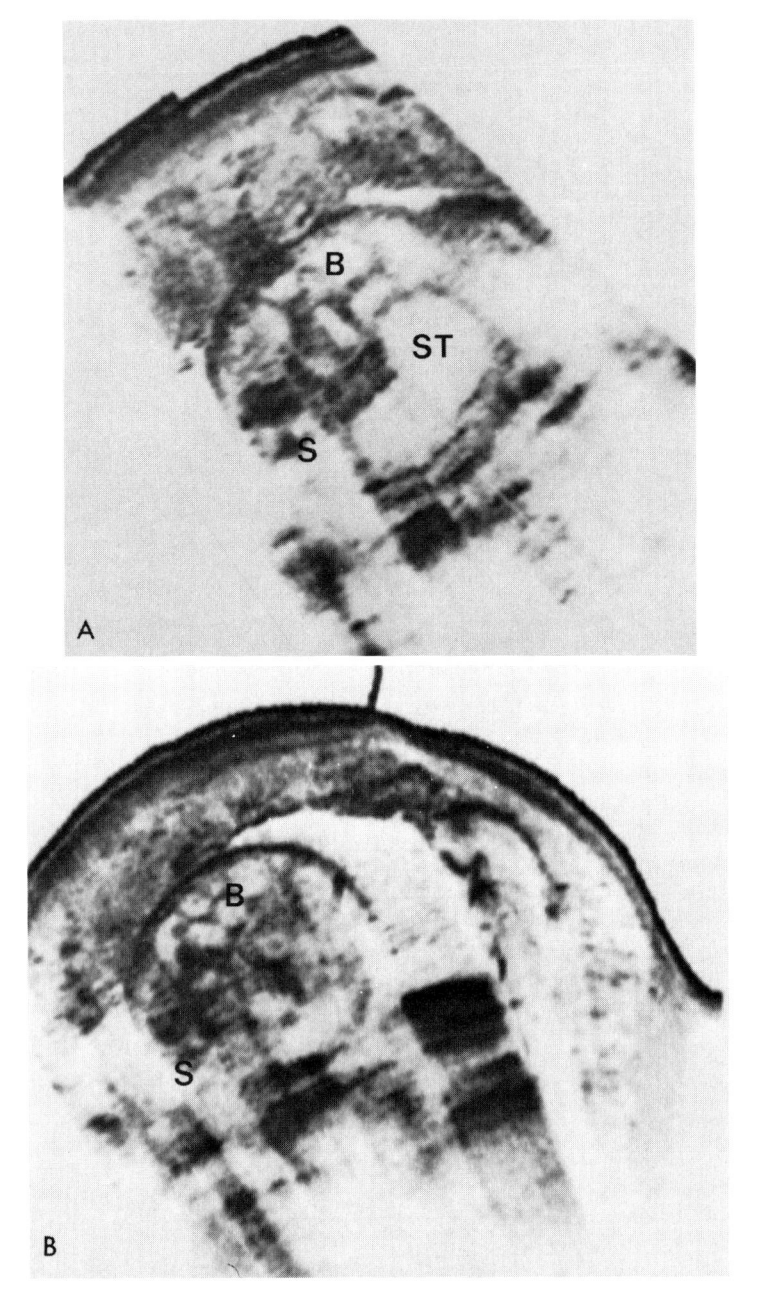

Figure 10. Numerous fluid-filled loops of bowel (B) are seen in the fetus with jejunal atresia. Stomach (ST); fetal spine (S).

fetal abdomen should be considered in the differential diagnosis of bowel obstruction. Examples include choledochal cyst, intestinal duplication, and ovarian cyst.[7,16,34,52] Further, when fetal bowel obstruction is suspected at the time of ultrasound examination, great care must be taken to differentiate bowel loops from cystic disease of the kidney or an obstructed urinary tract. In differentiating these two groups of abnormalities it is well known that gastrointestinal lesions are usually associated with polyhydramnios whereas renal lesions are not. The position of the abnormality within the fetal abdomen may also be a helpful differential feature, with renal lesions generally being paraspinal or posterior in location, while bowel lesions are anterior. An exception to this observation is the fetal bladder, which is an anterior structure. Distinction is not always possible between abnormalities of the bowel and urinary

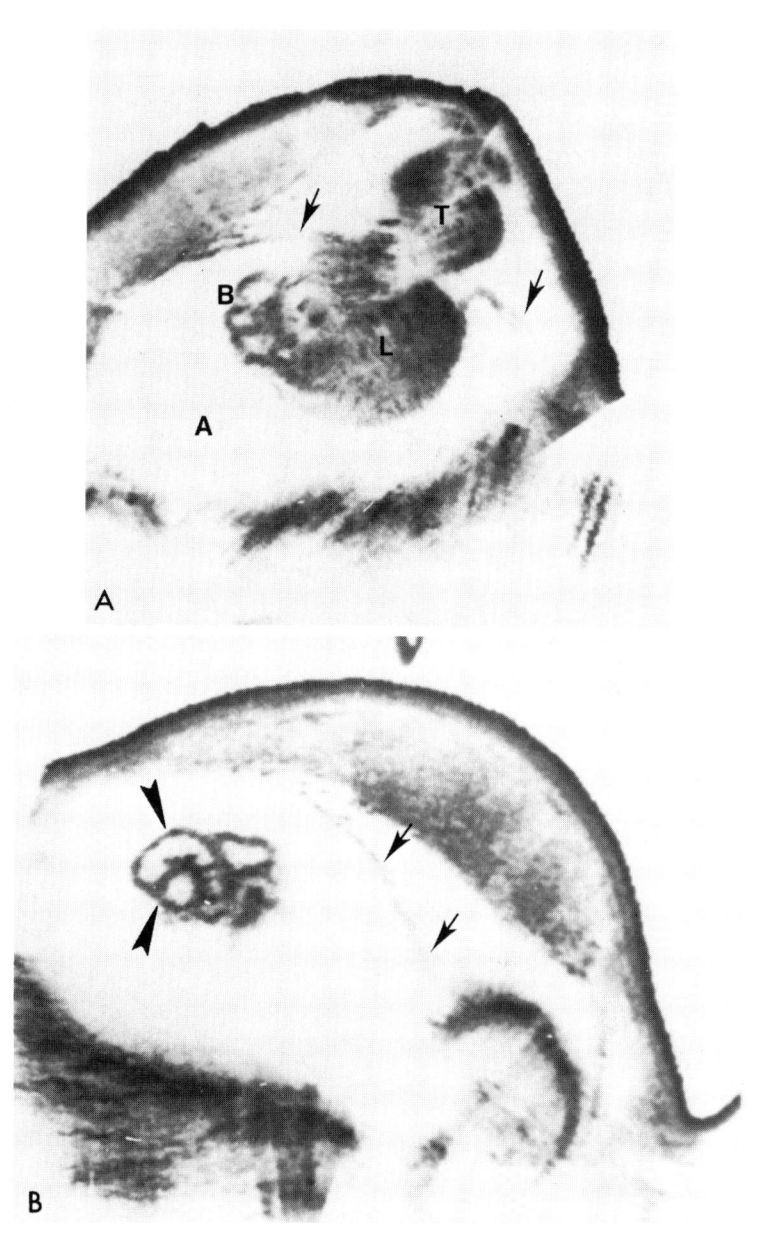

Figure 11. *A,* Extrusion of abdominal viscera results in a small fetal trunk (T). Careful scanning shows the membrane (*arrows*) of the omphalocele displaced away from the viscera by a large amount of ascites (A). Liver (L); bowel (B). *B,* The floating fetal bowel (*arrowheads*) is similarly seen in gastroschisis. However, identification of a covering membrane (*arrows*) qualifies this abnormality as an omphalocele. This was proved at autopsy.

Illustration continued on opposite page

tract based on the above anatomic considerations, especially when each involves gross dilatation of structures.

Anterior Wall Defects. Defects in the fetal anterior abdominal wall consist of umbilical cord hernias, omphaloceles, and gastroschisis. The embryogenesis of each of these entities is described elsewhere.[29] More simply, umbilical cord hernias can be considered similar to omphaloceles, but are smaller in size. Both omphaloceles and gastroschisis represent herniation of abdominal contents. In omphaloceles, the abdominal contents, which include both bowel and liver or spleen, are herniated to the base of the umbilical cord. The omphalocele, therefore, is covered by parietal peritoneum or amniotic membrane.[53, 62] In addition, omphaloceles have a high association with multiple congenital anomalies.[40]

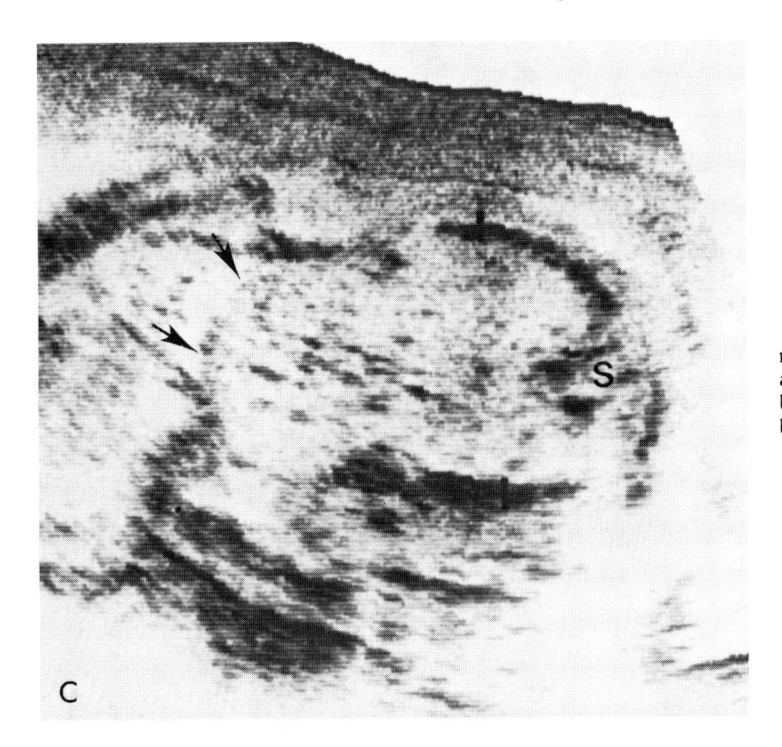

Figure 11. (Continued). C, This represents a more typical appearance of an omphalocele, showing bowel loops within a covering membrane (arrows). Fetal spine (S).

In contradistinction, gastroschisis has a normal insertion of the umbilical cord, with the abdominal wall defect and herniation of bowel occurring most often on the right side of the umbilicus.[19] Consequently, there is no covering membrane. In both cases, transverse sections of the fetal abdomen show a small trunk with extrusion of contents to the outside. Careful scanning may define the membrane or sac surrounding these eviscerated contents and may also show the presence of a liver or spleen (Fig. 11); however, the sac in an omphalocele can be distended by ascites, and the floating loops of bowel give the appearance of gastroschisis (see Fig. 11B). Differentiation, then, of these two abnormalities can be difficult but is not critical, as management decisions for delivery of the fetus are the same for both. In each case, there are three reasons for electing cesarean section: (1) a vaginal delivery may traumatize the exposed bowel, (2) the eviscerated contents may cause birth dystocia, or (3) the abdominal contents may become infected by passage through the birth canal.[11, 19, 40] If immediate surgical management is required, the infant, having been delivered by cesarean section, can be handed directly to the surgical team in a sterile condition.

GENITOURINARY TRACT

The fetal kidneys are seen in the midabdomen on either side of the spine, the renal tissue itself being more echolucent than the echogenic central pyelocaliceal system. The kidneys are most easily identified when the fetus is spine up, and one or both kidneys will first be seen in 90 per cent of patients at 17 to 22 weeks' gestation.[33] Cystic abnormalities of the fetal kidneys are more easily seen by ultrasound than are solid lesions since there is greater contrast with the surrounding fetal structures.

Renal Agenesis. Potter's syndrome consists of bilateral renal agenesis, oligohydramnios, characteristic facies, and pulmonary hypoplasia.[9, 26–28] The findings of severe oligohydramnios between the sixteenth and twenty-eighth weeks of gestation should strongly suggest a renal abnormality (Fig. 12), because prior to the sixteenth week, the fetal kidneys contribute little to the production of amniotic fluid. After 28 weeks, preterm rupture of the membranes and/or placental dysfunction may lead to reduced amniotic fluid.[9] Unfortunately, with reduced amounts of fluid surrounding the fetus, the natural ul-

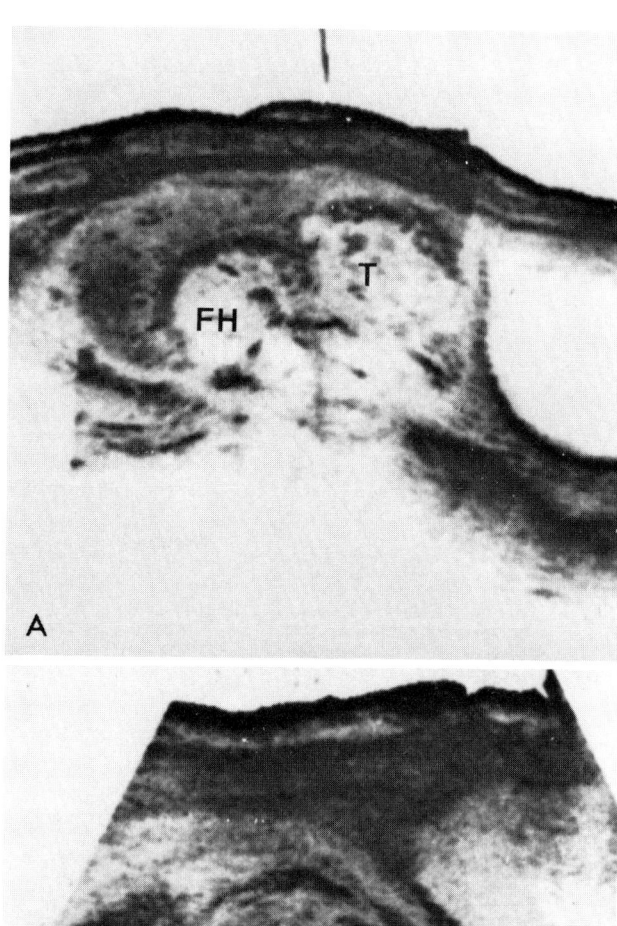

Figure 12. Severe oligohydramnios is present in this pregnancy of a fetus with Potter's syndrome. Neither fetal bladder nor kidney was present on this examination or on subsequent studies. Fetal head (FH); trunk (T); spine (S).

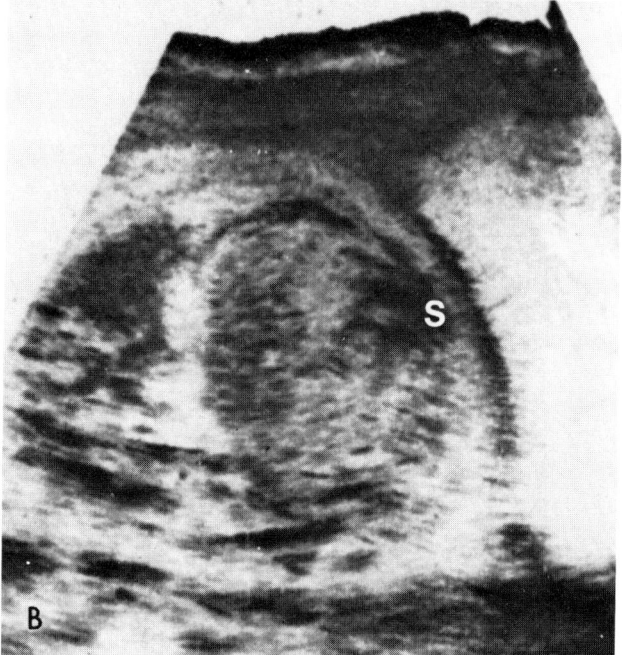

trasound window is lost, and identification of fetal structures, including the kidneys, may be difficult (see Fig. 12A). Often the presence or absence of the fetal bladder is a more helpful sign than recognition of the fetal kidneys. Normally, the fetal bladder will fill and empty over a 1 to 1½ hour cycle.[25] An alternative to waiting this period of time is to administer 60 mg of furosemide to the mother, which will also have a diuretic effect on the fetus.[28, 61]

Hydronephrosis. Hydronephrosis is the most common cystic abnormality readily identified by ultrasound in the fetal kidney. Usually obstruction occurs at the ureteropelvic junction. Hydronephrosis may be unilateral (Fig. 13) or bilateral (Fig. 14). Oligohydramnios is not usually an associ-

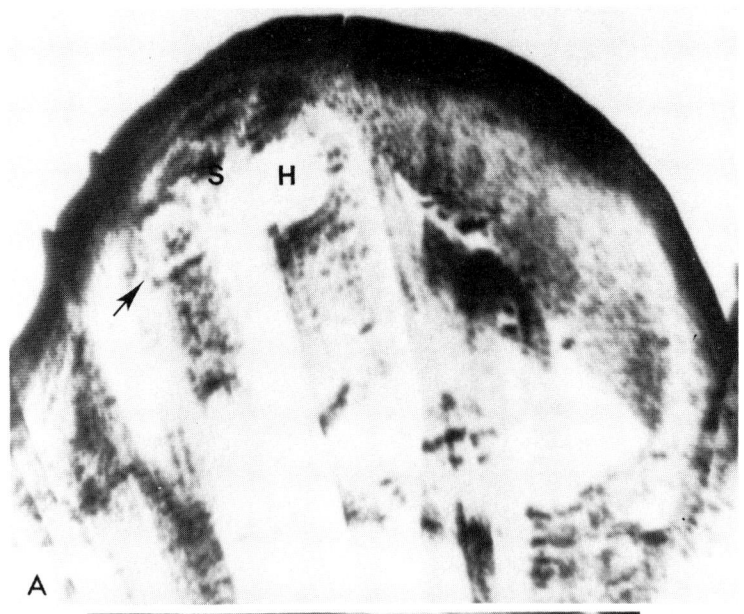

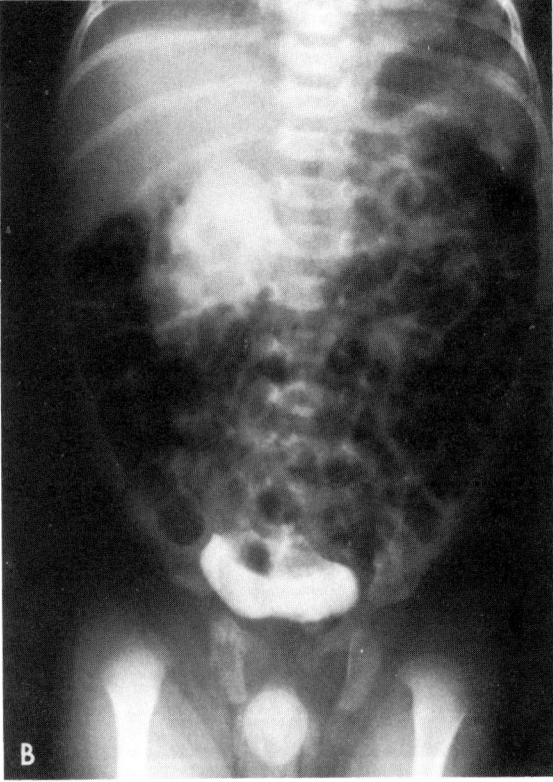

Figure 13. *A*, Cross section of the fetal abdomen shows a normal left kidney (*arrow*) and a hydronephrotic right kidney (H). The fetal spine (S) serves as a landmark for the posteriorly located kidneys. *B*, A postpartum intravenous pyelogram confirmed the antenatal ultrasonographic diagnosis of a right-sided hydronephrotic kidney.

ated feature.[21] The level of obstruction may also be at the ureterovesical junction, in which case there is hydronephrosis as well as dilated ureters. There may also be obstruction of the urethra, such as in posterior urethral valves. Here one finds a large bladder, hydroureters, hydronephrosis, and oligohydramnios (Fig. 15). If rupture of the renal collecting system occurs antenatally, the ultrasound appearance is that of fetal urinary ascites (Fig. 16).

Urinary ascites can be differentiated from the ascites of a hydropic fetus in that the features of placental enlargement,

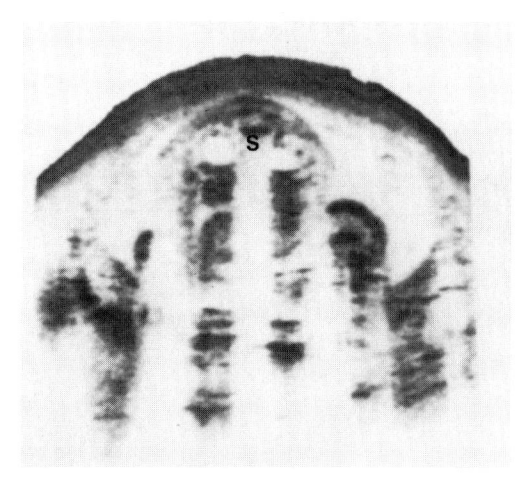

Figure 14. This ultrasound scan shows bilateral hydronephrosis. Again, the spine (S) serves as a landmark for the kidneys.

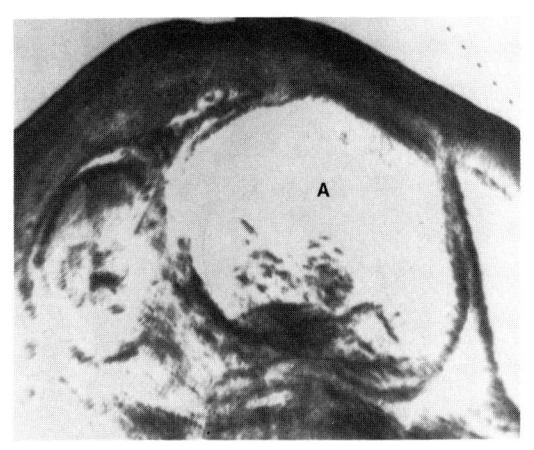

Figure 16. A sagittal scan of a fetus with marked urinary ascites (A) from rupture of the renal collecting system secondary to obstruction from posterior urethral valves. Note that the other signs of a hydropic fetus are not present.

polyhydramnios, and fetal soft tissue edema are lacking. When hydronephrosis is bilateral and severe, percutaneous antegrade contrast studies can be performed in utero to confirm the diagnosis as well as to attempt preservation of fetal renal function. Since preservation of renal function is of prime importance, methods of in utero drainage of the urinary tract, including fetal surgery, will become increasingly common in the future.

Multicystic Kidneys. Multicystic kidneys can be differentiated from hydronephrosis, which is the more commonly seen cystic abnormality in the fetus.[17, 46] The diagnosis of a multicystic kidney is suggested by the presence of multiple cysts (Fig. 17); however, these cystic structures may be large — up to 6 cm.[21] Similarly, hydronephrosis may produce large cystic lesions where little of the original renal structure can be identified. In these instances, differentiation between these two abnormalities may be impossible (Fig. 18).

Ten to 20 per cent of patients with multicystic kidneys will have other associated urinary tract anomalies, most frequently

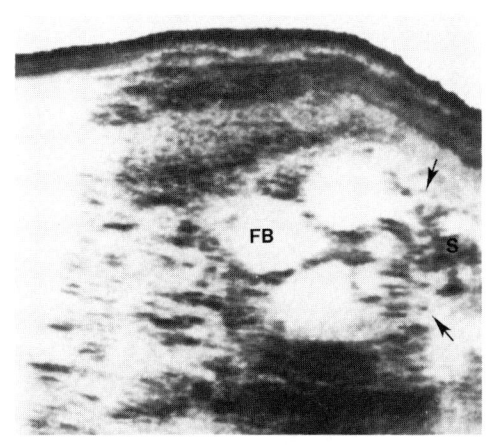

Figure 15. In this fetus with absence of the prostatic urethra, a large bladder (FB) is seen anteriorly with two dilated ureters to either side. Although markedly dilated urinary structures may be confused with obstructed bowel loops, in this case it was differentiated by tracing the ureters posteriorly to the renal fossa (*arrows*). Again the position of the spine (S) is a helpful landmark for posterior structures. The presence of oligohydramnios is also a helpful sign for diagnosing this abnormality.

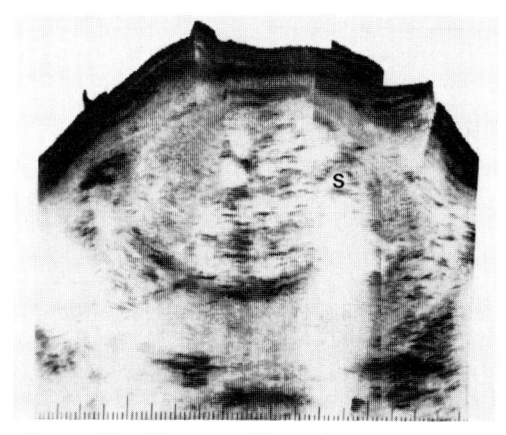

Figure 17. Many variable sized cysts are seen in a case of bilateral multicystic kidney. In this case, oligohydramnios is present. Spine (S).

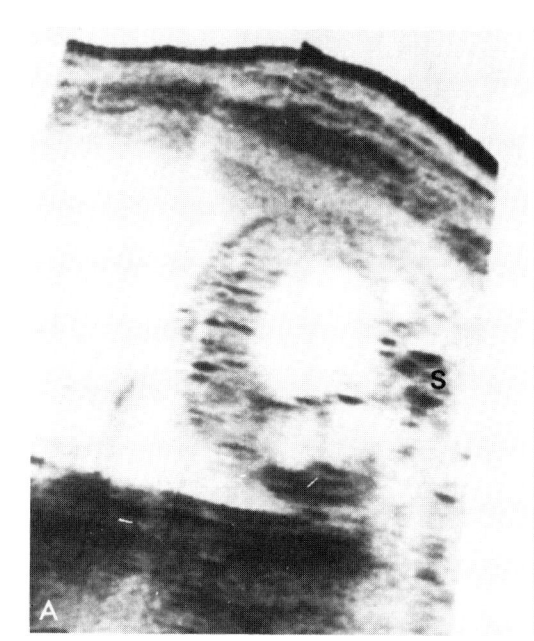

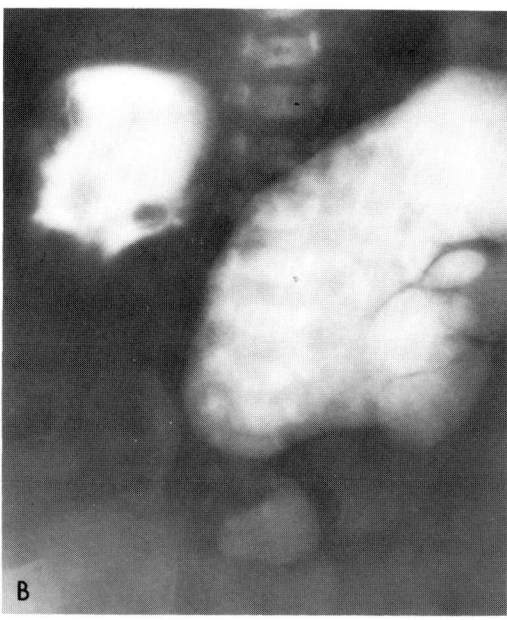

Figure 18. *A*, The prenatal scan of an infant with left hydronephrosis and right multicystic kidney shows multiple large and small cysts, which can be traced to either side of the fetal spine (S). Note that antenatal differentiation between these two cystic abnormalities of the kidney may be impossible. Amniotic fluid is present. *B*, While antenatal differentiation between hydronephrosis and multicystic kidneys may be difficult, the diagnosis can be established post partum by percutaneous antegrade pyelograms. Here, the left hydronephrotic kidney is identified by distribution of contrast material throughout the upper renal collecting system to the level of obstruction, whereas contrast material injected into the right multicystic kidney shows no communication.

hydronephrosis of the contralateral side (see Fig. 18).[46] Diagnosis in these cases can be made after birth with percutaneous antegrade pyelograms. Injection of contrast material into the cystic structures of the hydronephrotic kidney will show communication with a dilated renal pelvis, thus opacifying the entire upper collecting system to the level of the obstruction. Conversely, contrast material injected into a cyst of a multicystic kidney will show no communication with other cysts (see Fig. 18). Furthermore, at the time of antegrade studies, a percutaneous nephrostomy can be performed on the kidney that has been determined to be hydronephrotic.

Infantile Polycystic Kidney. The recurrence rate in patients with a previous history of an infant with polycystic kidney disease is 25 per cent.[51] This can be a difficult diagnosis to make by ultrasound since large cysts are not a usual feature of this disease.[21] The sonographic appearance is that of large and homogeneously echodense solid kidneys with an increased ratio of kidney circumference to abdominal circumference.[20, 21] The bladder, when seen, is usually small and there is no associated oligohydramnios. Large kidneys have also been reported in cases of Beckwith-Wiedemann syndrome, but in these cases there has been an associated omphalocele and no oligohydramnios.[60] Ultrasound

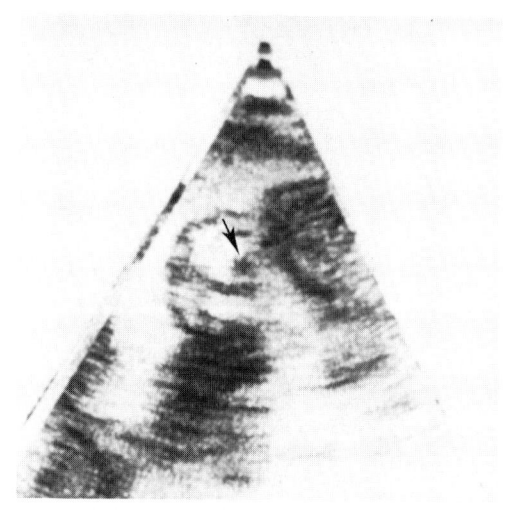

Figure 19. A scan of the fetal scrotum shows bilateral hydroceles. Identification of the testicle (*arrow*) within the scrotal sac is helpful for confirmation.

identification of solid renal tumors is also possible, but differentiation from large kidneys may be difficult.

Hydrocele. Hydroceles may be unilateral or bilateral.[5] Wnen large, their attachment to the perineum may be difficult to define.[42] Identification of testes with the fluid-filled scrotal sac is helpful for confirmation (Fig. 19).

FETAL ASCITES

Large amounts of fluid are easily imaged within the fetal abdomen (see Figs. 2, 8A, and 16). Bowel loops as well as the liver are outlined by the fluid (see Fig. 2).[34] Small amounts of fluid may be more difficult to identify and should not be confused with pseudoascites as described by Rosenthal, Filly, et al.[54] Ascites has usually been associated with Rh isoimmunization; however, there are many nonimmunologic causes of fetal ascites with or without associated fetal edema and/or placentomegaly. Some of these include alpha-thalassemia, chronic fetal maternal transfusion, congenital heart disease, fetal hydroproteinemia, urinary tract obstruction, syphilis, viral infections such as cytomegalovirus, and idiopathic forms.[44, 49, 50] In the case of Rh-isoimmunization, ultrason-

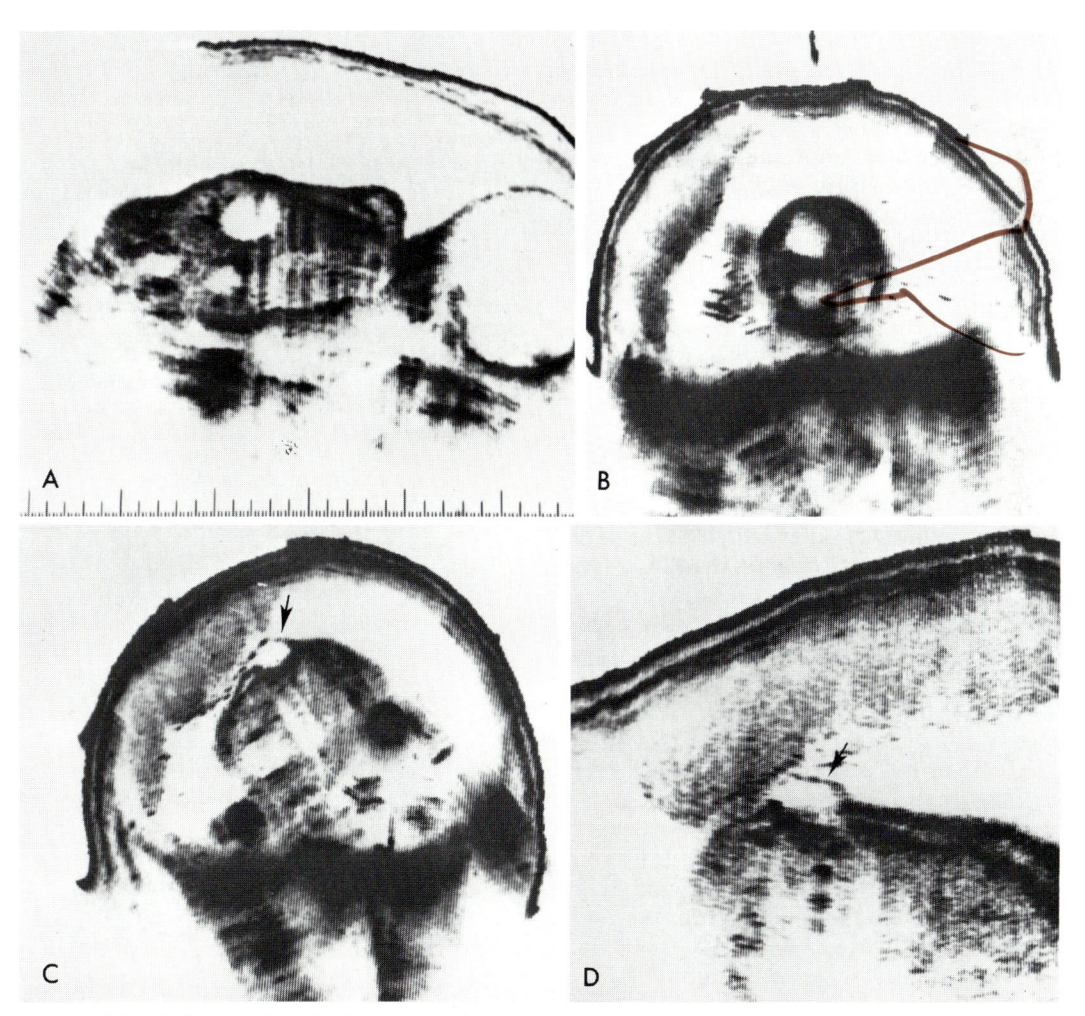

Figure 20. A fetus with multiple congenital anomalies serves as a reminder that one abnormality may be associated with others. Through attention to detail these abnormalities may be seen. A sagittal scan of the fetus shows hydranencephaly and "double bubble" of duodenal atresia. A, Polyhydramnios is present. B, A cross section of the same fetus shows the "double bubble" sign and polyhydramnios. A cross section (C) and a sagittal section (D) of the lower fetal spine demonstrates a meningomyelocele. (Courtesy of George R. Satterwhite, M.D., Willamette Falls Community Hospital, Oregon City, Oregon.)

CONCLUSIONS

Numerous fetal abnormalities can be identified by ultrasound. Most fetal malformations are serendipitous findings obtained by routine scanning for placental location, fetal number, and estimation of gestational size. Occasionally, as in the history of Rh isoimmunization or significant genetic history, specific fetal abnormalities are sought during ultrasound scanning. Management of the pregnancy may be greatly altered, depending upon the ultrasound findings. First, early termination of the pregnancy or fetal therapeutic procedures may occur. Second, the mode and timing of delivery may be changed, for example, in the case of omphalocele. In all these instances, immediate postpartum management is considerably helped by knowledge that an abnormal fetus is about to be delivered. If the mother can be referred from an outlying area to a regional medical center, potentially life-saving corrective procedures can be performed as soon as the infant is born. In addition, if the in utero diagnosis is uncertain, appropriate and sophisticated diagnostic studies will be available.

At the time of ultrasound examination, the specific abnormality may not have developed to the point where it may be recognized. Therefore, serial studies may be required. Also, a single abnormality may be associated with other congenital anomalies, which at the time of scanning may not be detectable. Certainly, many fetal abnormalities, especially if they are isolated, can be appropriately treated, both in utero and post partum, the result of which is a healthy infant. Others, however, especially in the event of multiple congenital anomalies, are less successfully treated, and the burden of caring for such infants raises moral and ethical questions (Fig. 20).[14, 22] Further, at current levels of diagnostic sophistication, antenatal treatment of recognized lethal anomalies may occur, thus adding to maternal risk as well as increased health cost. What has become clear, however, is that the fetus is assuming a role as patient separate from the mother, with identifiable diseases and the development of means by which to treat them.

REFERENCES

1. Bean, W. J., Calonje, M. A., Aprill, C. N., et al.: Anal atresia: a prenatal ultrasound diagnosis. J. Clin. Ultrasound, 6:111–112, 1978.
2. Bell, R. L.: Ultrasound of hemangioma of the neck in a newborn. J. Tenn. Med. Assoc., 71:289, 1978.
3. Bovicelli, L., Rizzo, N., Orsini, L. F., et al.: Ultrasonic real-time diagnosis of fetal hydrothorax and lung hypoplasia. J. Clin. Ultrasound, 9:253–254, 1981.
4. Boychuk, R. B., Lyons, E. A., and Goodhand, T. K.: Duodenal atresia diagnosed by ultrasound. Radiology, 127:500, 1978.
5. Conrad, A. R., and Rao, S. A. S.: Ultrasound diagnosis of fetal hydrocele. Radiology, 127:232, 1978.
6. Defoort, P., and Thiery, M.: Antenatal diagnosis of congenital chylothorax by gray scale sonography. J. Clin. Ultrasound, 6:47–48, 1978.
7. Dewbury, K. C., Aluwihare, A. P. R., Birch, S. J., et al.: Case reports. Prenatal ultrasound demonstration of a choledochal cyst. Br. J. Radiol., 53:906–907, 1980.
8. Donn, S. M., Martin, J. N., Jr., White, S. J.: Antenatal ultrasound findings in cystic adenomatoid malformation. Pediatr. Radiol., 10:180–182, 1981.
9. Dubbins, P. A., Kurtz, A. B., Wapner, R. J., et al.: Renal agenesis: Spectrum of in utero findings. J. Clin. Ultrasound, 9:189–193, 1981.
10. Duenhoelter, J. H., Santos-Ramos, R., Rosenfeld, C. R., et al.: Prenatal diagnosis of gastrointestinal tract obstruction. Obstet. Gynecol., 47:618, 1976.
11. Dunne, M. G., and Johnson, M. L.: The ultrasonic demonstration of fetal abnormalities in utero. J. Reprod. Med., 23:195–206, 1979.
12. Farrant, P.: The antenatal diagnosis of oesophageal atresia by ultrasound. Br. J. Radiol., 53:1202–1203, 1980.
13. Filly, R. A.: Detection of fetal malformations with ultrasonic B-scans. Birth Defects, 15(5A):45–49, 1979.
14. Fletcher, J. C.: The fetus as patient: Ethical issues (editorial). J.A.M.A., 246:772–773, 1981.
15. Fletman, D., McQuown, D., Kanchanapoom, V., et al.: "Apple peel" atresia of the small bowel: Prenatal diagnosis of the obstruction by ultrasound. Pediatr. Radiol., 9:118–119, 1980.
16. Frank, J. L., Hill, M. C., Chirathivat, S., et al.: Antenatal observation of a choledochal cyst by sonography. Am. J. Roentgenol., 137:166–168, 1981.
17. Friedberg, J. E., Mitnick, J. S., and Davis, D. A.: Antepartum ultrasonic detection of multicystic kidney. Radiology, 131:198, 1979.
18. Garrett, W. J., Kossoff, G., and Lawrence, R.: Gray scale echography in the diagnosis of hydrops due to fetal lung tumor. J. Clin. Ultrasound, 3:45–50, 1975.

19. Giulian, B. B., and Alvear, D. T.: Prenatal ultrasonographic diagnosis of fetal gastroschisis. Radiology, 129:473–475, 1978.
20. Grannum, P., Bracken, M., Silverman, R., et al.: Assessment of fetal kidney size in normal gestation by comparison of ratio of kidney circumference to abdominal circumference. Am. J. Obstet. Gynecol., 136:249–254, 1980.
21. Hadlock, F. P., Deter, R. L., Carpenter, R., et al.: Review. Sonography of fetal urinary tract anomalies. Am. J. Roentgenol., 137:261–267, 1981.
22. Harrison, M. R., Golbus, M. S., and Filly, R. A.: Management of the fetus with a correctable congenital defect. J.A.M.A., 246:774–777, 1981.
23. Henderson, S. C., Van Kolken R. J., and Rahatzad, M.: Multicystic kidney with hydramnios. J. Clin. Ultrasound, 8:249–250, 1980.
24. Henrion, R., and Aubry, J. P.: Fetal cardiac abnormality and real-time ultrasound study: A case of Ivemark syndrome. Contr. Gynecol. Obstet., 6:119–122, 1979.
25. Hobbins, J. C., Grannum, P. A. T., Berkowitz, R. L., et al.: Ultrasound in the diagnosis of congenital anomalies. Am. J. Obstet. Gynecol., 134:331–345, 1979.
26. Kaffe, S., Godmilow, L., Walker, B. A., et al.: Prenatal diagnosis of bilateral renal agenesis. Obstet. Gynecol., 49:478–480, 1977.
27. Kaffe, S., Rose, J. S., Godmilow, L., et al.: Prenatal diagnosis of renal anomalies. Am. J. Med. Genet., 1:241–251, 1977.
28. Keirse, M. J. N. C., and Meerman, R. H.: Antenatal diagnosis of Potter syndrome. Obstet. Gynecol., 52(Suppl):64s–67s, 1978.
29. Klein, M. D., Kosloske, A. M., and Hertzler, J. H.: Congenital defects of the abdominal wall. J.A.M.A., 245:1643–1646, 1981.
30. Kogult, M. S., et al.: Cervical teratoma in infants and children. South. Med. J., 70:122–123, 1977.
31. Krook, P. M.: Megacystic-microcolon-intestinal hypoperistalsis syndrome in a male infant. Radiology, 136:649–650, 1980.
32. Kurjak, A., Kirkinen, P., Latin, V., et al.: Diagnosis and assessment of fetal malformations and abnormalities by ultrasound. J. Perinat. Med., 8:219–235, 1980.
33. Lawson, T. L., Foley, W. D., Berland, L. L., et al.: Ultrasonic evaluation of fetal kidneys. Radiology, 138:153–156, 1981.
34. Lee T. G., Blake, S.: Prenatal fetal abdominal ultrasonography and diagnosis. Radiology, 124:475–477, 1977.
35. Lee, T. G., and Warren, B. H.: Antenatal ultrasonic demonstration of fetal bowel. Radiology, 124:471–474, 1977.
36. Lee, T. G., Knochel, J. Q.: Prenatal fetal thoracoabdominal ultrasonography. In Sanders, R. C., and James, E. (eds.): The Principles and Practice of Ultrasonography in Obstetrics and Gynecology. Edition 2. Baltimore, Williams and Wilkins Co., 1980.
37. Lees, R. F., Alford, B. A., Brenbridge, A. N. A. G., et al.: Case reports. Sonographic appearance of duodenal atresia in utero. Am. J. Roentgenol., 131:701–702, 1978.
38. Lehr, C., and DiRe, J.: Rare occurrence of a holoacardious acephalic monster: Sonographic and pathologic findings. J. Clin. Ultrasound, 6:259–261, 1978.
39. Leonard, C. O., Sanders, R. C., and Lau, H. L.: Prenatal diagnosis of the Turner syndrome, a familial chromosomal rearrangement and achondroplasia by amniocentesis and ultrasonography. Johns Hopkins Med. J., 145:25–30, 1979.
40. Lomas, F., Stafford-Bell, M., and Tymms, A.: Prenatal ultrasound in the diagnosis and management of fetal exomphalos. Case reports. Br. J. Obstet. Gynecol., 86:581–584, 1979.
41. Loveday, B. J., Garr, J. A., and Aitken, J.: The intrauterine demonstration of duodenal atresia by ultrasound. Br. J. Radiol., 48:1031, 1975.
42. Miller, E. I., and Thomas, R. H.: Fetal hydrocele detected in utero by ultrasound. Br. J. Radiol., 52:624–625, 1979.
43. Morgan, C. L., Trought, W. S., Sheldon, G., et al.: B-scan and real-time ultrasound in the antepartum diagnosis of conjoined twins and pericardial effusion. Am. J. Roentgenol., 130:578–580, 1978.
44. Morrison, J., and Brunello, L. P.: The antenatal diagnosis of hyperplacentosis, hydramnios and fetal ascites. J. Clin. Ultrasound, 5:338–340, 1977.
45. O'Brien, W. F., Cefalo, R. C., and Bair, D. G.: Ultrasonographic diagnosis of fetal cystic hygroma. Am. J. Obstet. Gynecol., 138:464–466, 1980.
46. Older, R. A., Hinman, C. G., Crane, L. M., et al.: In utero diagnosis of multicystic kidney by gray scale ultrasonography. Am. J. Roentgenol., 133:130–131, 1979.
47. Pawlowitzki, I. H., and Wormann, B.: Elevated amniotic alpha fetoprotein in a fetus with Turner's syndrome due to puncture of a cystic hygroma. Am. J. Obstet. Gynecol., 133:584–585, 1979.
48. Phillips, H. E., and McGahan, J. P.: Intrauterine fetal cystic hygromas: Sonographic detection. Am. J. Roentgenol., 136:799–802, 1981.
49. Price, J. M., Fisch, A. E., and Jacobson, J.: Ultrasonic findings in fetal cytomegalovirus infection. J. Clin. Ultrasound, 6:268, 1978.
50. Quagliarello, J. R., Passalaqua, A. M., Greco, M. A., et al.: Ballantyne's triple edema syndrome: Prenatal diagnosis with ultrasound and maternal renal biopsy findings. Am. J. Obstet. Gynecol., 132:580–581, 1978.
51. Reilly, K. B., Rubin, S. P., Blanke, B. G., et al.: Infantile polycystic kidney disease: A difficult antenatal diagnosis. Am. J. Obstet. Gynecol., 133:580–582, 1979.
52. Rento, J. J., Bailly, G., Toussaint, D., et al.: Cyste congenital du choledoque chez le nouveau-ne. J. Gynecol. Obstet. Biol. Reprod., 10:61–65, 1981.
53. Roberts, C.: Intrauterine diagnosis of omphalocele. Radiology, 127:762, 1978.
54. Rosenthal, S. J., Filly, R. A., Callen, P. W., et al.: Fetal pseudo-ascites. Radiology, 131:195–197, 1979.
55. Sabbagha, R. E., and Shkolnik, A.: Ultrasound diagnosis of fetal abnormalities. Semin. Perinatol., 4:213–227, 1980.
56. Sabbagha, R. E., Tamura, R. K., Dalcompo, S., et al.: Fetal cranial and craniocervical masses: Ul-

trasound characteristics and differential diagnosis. Am. J. Obstet. Gynecol., *138*:511–517, 1980.
57. Scott, J. S., and Wilson, J. K.: Hydramnios as an early sign of oesophageal atresia. Lancet, *2*:569–572, 1957.
58. Silver, T. M., Wicks, J. D., Spooner, E. W., et al.: Prenatal ultrasonic detection of congenital heart block. Am. J. Roentgenol., *133*:546–547, 1979.
59. Vezina, W. C., Morin, F. R., and Winsberg, F.: Megacystic-microcolon-intestinal hypoperistalsis syndrome: Antenatal ultrasound appearance. Am. J. Roentgenol., *133*:749–750, 1979.
60. Weinstein, L., and Anderson, C.: In utero diagnosis of Beckwith-Wiedemann syndrome by ultrasound. Radiology, *134*:474, 1980.
61. Wladimiroff, J. W.: Effect of furosemide on fetal urine production. Br. J. Obstet. Gynaecol., *82*:221–224, 1975.
62. Yaghoobian, J., Chaudary, R., and Pinck, R. L.: Antenatal diagnosis of omphalocele by ultrasound. J. Reprod. Med., *26*:274–275, 1981.
63. Yamaguchi, D. T., and Lee, F. Y. L.: Ultrasonic evaluation of the fetal heart. Am. J. Obstet. Gynecol., *134*:422–430, 1979.
64. Yiu-Chi, V., and Chiu, L.: Ultrasonographic evaluation of normal fetal anatomy and congenital malformations. CJCTDL, *5*:367–510, 1981.
65. Zimmerman, H. B.: Prenatal demonstration of gastric and duodenal obstruction by ultrasound. J. Can. Assoc. Radiol., *29*:138–141, 1978.

5

Ultrasonography of the Normal and Pathologic Fetal Skeleton

Roy A. Filly, M.D., and Mitchell S. Golbus, M.D.

Our ability to detect a structure with ultrasound is dependent not only on spatial resolution but subject contrast as well. Thus, a structure that possesses a high degree of intrinsic contrast can be consistently detected at a smaller size than one displaying poor intrinsic contrast. Ultrasonographers possess no agents to alter contrast of fetal organs, thus we are totally dependent on intrinsic (subject) contrast.

Obviously, there are other parameters in addition to subject contrast, which cannot be controlled. Ultrasound is a tomographic technique. Unfortunately, the fetus cannot cooperate by assuming an appropriate position for obtaining the best tomographic plane. We also cannot control maternal body habitus or the amount of amniotic fluid, both of which may dramatically alter ability to discern small fetal structures. Despite these problems, fetal bones are probably the easiest single type of fetal structure to image because of the extremely high contrast difference they exhibit compared to the soft tissues which surround them.

Since many of the fetal bones we wish to image are in the extremities, motion is also a problem. A slight motion of the thigh or upper arm results in a large excursion of the foot or hand. Real-time ultrasonography provides the most appropriate format for imaging fetal bones. The flexibility offered by such systems enables one to survey rapidly and sequentially. Additionally, fetal movements are viewed directly, which enables rapid reorientation of the transducer to the desired plane of interest.

A feature of critical importance is the fetal position. For example, the posterior elements of the fetal spine may be clearly imaged with the fetus in a prone or decubitus position, but are difficult to image when the fetus is supine. Similarly, the extremities are imaged to excellent advantage when floating or moving freely in the amniotic fluid. The same extremity tucked under the fetus can be quite difficult to assess. In the presence of normal or increased amounts of amniotic fluid one need only be patient: the fetus will likely change to a more advantageous imaging position.

THE NORMAL FETAL SKELETON

Fetal skeletal parts are among the earliest structures which can be specifically recognized on an ultrasonogram.[3, 4] The calvarium, for example, can be imaged from late first trimester onward. At only 15 to 16 weeks after conception, a large number of fetal bones are easily detected. By 18 to 19 weeks even phalanges can be visualized. Bones of only 2 to 3 mm in size can be imaged (some consistently) via ultrasonography. It is the ossification center (rather than the entire developing bone) that is imaged sonographically.[4] Many specific bony structures can be depicted. Bones in both the appendicular and axial skeleton are readily imaged.

The majority of bones of the appendicular skeleton can be imaged in the early to mid second trimester, although the phalanges of the toes may be quite difficult to perceive. As a general rule of appendicular skeletal imaging, the more proximal a bone the more readily it is identified. This rule is untrue of the hands and feet, where the metacarpals and metatarsals are more readily seen than the carpal or tarsal bones. This is because the metacarpals and metatarsals are ossified while the carpals and tarsals (except for the tarsal calcaneus and talus) are still cartilaginous. The tarsal calcaneus and talus ossify between the fifth and sixth months (Fig. 1). The remaining tarsals and carpals do not ossify until after

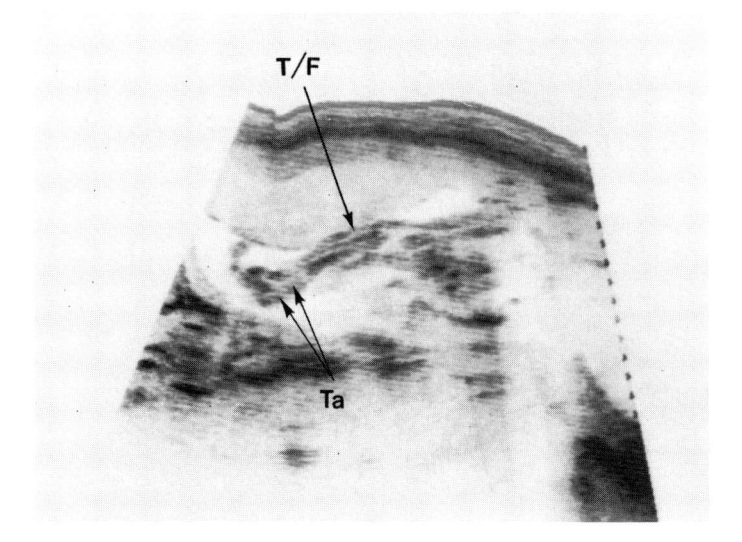

Figure 1. Ultrasonogram of the distal fetal leg demonstrates the tibia and fibula (T/F) and the ossified portion of the talus (Ta) and calcaneus.

birth.[5, 8] The metatarsals and metacarpals are well ossified at four months.

The scapula (Fig. 2), clavicle, humerus (Fig. 3), radius, ulna, metacarpals, and phalanges (Fig. 4) can be imaged in most cases. Interestingly, the clavicle may be difficult to see, presumably because of the flexed position of the fetal neck which draws the calvarium into a position which obscures the clavicle. Similarly, the femur (Fig. 5), tibia, fibula (Fig. 6), and metatarsals can be appreciated sonographically.

The simplest way to identify the long bones of the extremities is to scan the fetus in a plane that traverses the short axis of the limb. Sonograms obtained in such a plane through the upper arm or thigh will be seen to contain one bone whereas those through the forearm and calf will contain two bones (Figs. 3 and 7). In the lower leg, the more lateral bone is the fibula, and the more medial bone the tibia. This method is less precise in the forearm where the potential for pronation may cause the radius and ulna to "cross." In the normal fetus, the tibia and fibula and the radius and ulna end at the same point distally. This observation is important in assessing possible limb reduction abnormalities.

The hand can be assessed more critically than the foot. With patience one can usually discern all four fingers and the thumb (Fig. 4). The hand is frequently clenched in fist-like fashion, which can complicate the

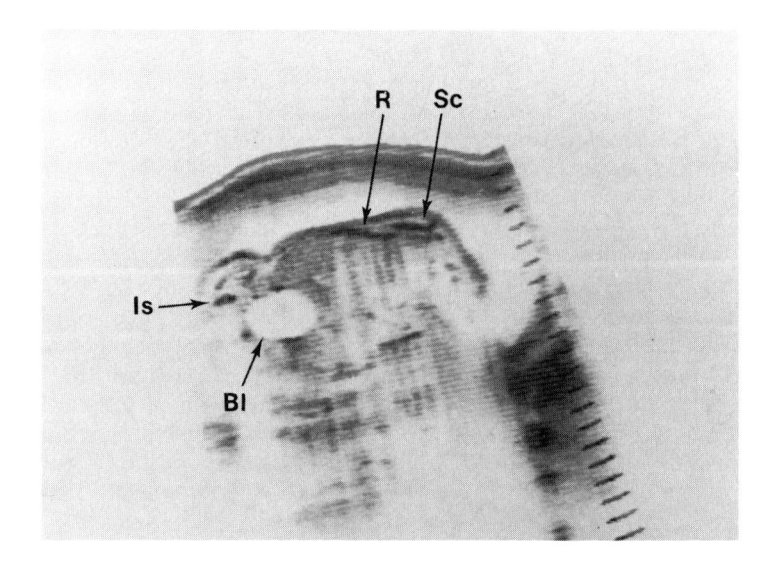

Figure 2. Coronal section through the fetal trunk demonstrates several bony structures (Is, ischium; R, ribs; Sc, scapula).

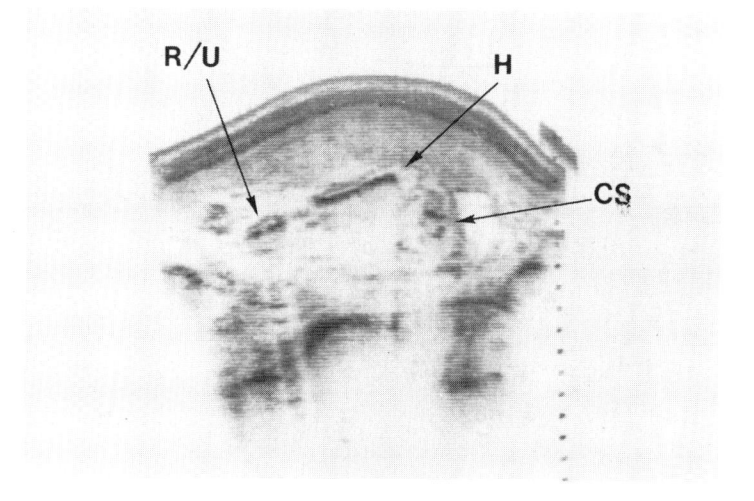

Figure 3. Longitudinal section of the fetal humerus (H). (R/U, radius and ulna; CS, cervical spine).

counting of fingers. However, even under this circumstance one can frequently make the necessary observations.

It is possible in late third trimester fetuses to identify the distal femoral epiphysis (Fig. 8) and the proximal tibial epiphysis. Ossification of these epiphyses as seen on radiographs is known to be an indicator of fetal maturity.[18] We are investigating the relationship of fetal maturity to sonographic identification of these ossification centers. Unfortunately, our preliminary data indicate that both of these ossification centers may appear before lung maturity is attained.

The major structures of the axial skele-

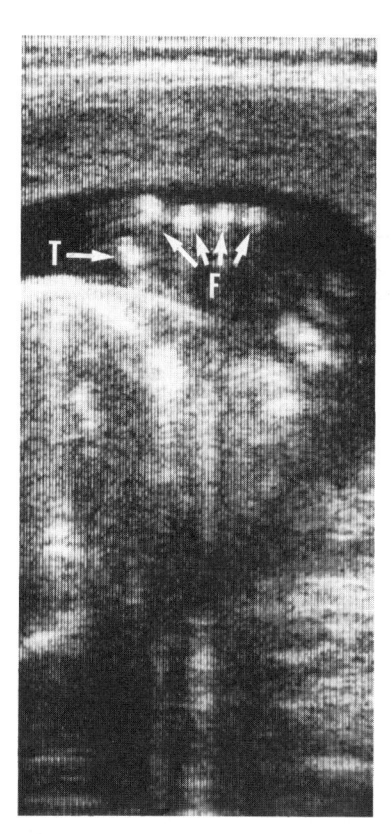

Figure 4. Real time sonogram of the fetal hand demonstrates the thumb (T) and four fingers (F).

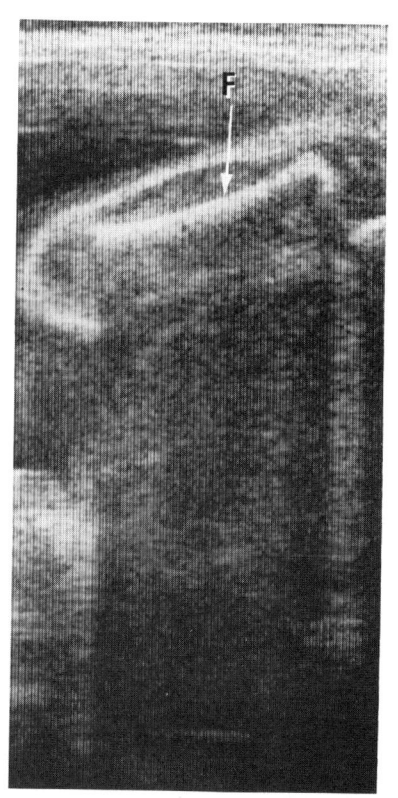

Figure 5. Real time sonogram performed to measure the femoral (F) length. The ischial ossification center is seen proximally.

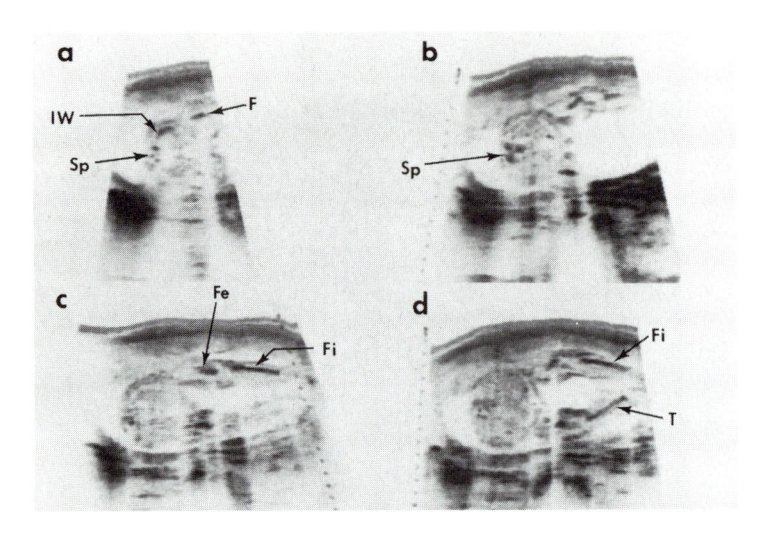

Figure 6. Multiple scans of a fetus demonstrate (a) the iliac wing (IW), sacral spine (Sp) and proximal femur (F); (b) the three ossification centers at the lumbar level (Sp). Images c and d demonstrate bones of the leg. (T, tibia; Fi, fibula).

ton are also routinely visualized. In the skull region one can perceive a number of bones in part or as a conglomerate. The greater wing of the sphenoid and petrous ridge are easily identified and define the anterior, middle, and posterior cranial fossae. The orbits can be visualized without difficulty unless the more anteriorly positioned orbit severely shadows the more posteriorly positioned orbit. Portions of the maxilla and mandible can be identified, as well as the bony nasal ridge. In late pregnancy, tooth buds are occasionally appreciated.

The ribs, spine, and pelvis can be easily imaged and serve as excellent anatomic landmarks. In the pelvis, the iliac ossification centers (Fig. 9) are easily observed from early second trimester onward (ossifies at 2½ to 3 fetal months). Ischial ossification appears at four months of fetal age (Fig. 2), but the pubic ossifications are not present until six fetal months.

The spine, an extremely important structure in fetal diagnosis, can fortunately be seen with great clarity in nearly all fetal positions. There is usually no difficulty in definitively evaluating the spine prior to 22 weeks after conception. The spine may be seen in both longitudinal and transverse planes (Figs. 10 and 11). While both planes are important, the transverse plane demonstrates the anatomy to best advantage. This latter observation is opposed to our earlier concepts.[3]

The fetal spine, as seen sonographically, is composed of three ossification centers, two posteriorly and one anteriorly. The dis-

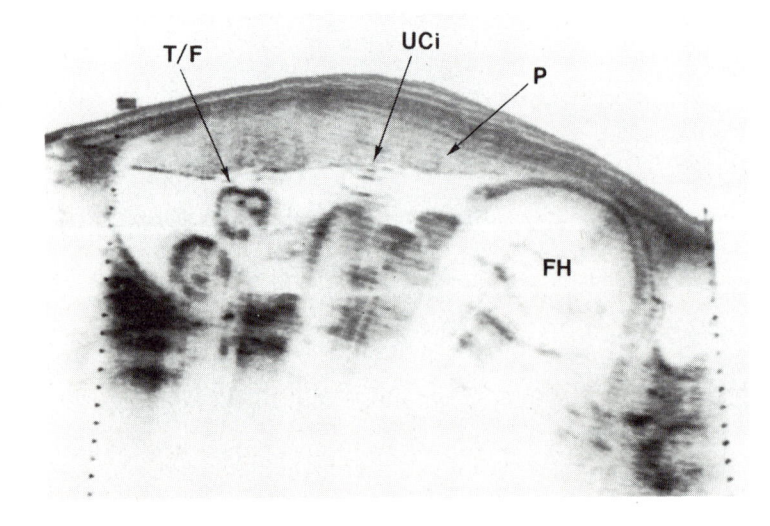

Figure 7. Typical appearance of a "two bone" portion of an extremity sectioned in short axis, in this case, the lower leg, demonstrating the tibia and fibula (T/F). (P, placenta; UCi, umbilical cord insertion into placenta; FH, fetal head).

tance between the posterior ossification centers is tantamount to the interpedicular distance. On longitudinal planes of section the posterior elements are seen as "parallel" bands of echoes. In fact, they are not precisely parallel since they flare in the upper cervical region and converge in the sacrum and, in addition, careful scanning usually discloses a slight widening in the lumbar area. Since the fetal spine is normally kyphotic one cannot visualize the entirety of the spine in a single longitudinal plane. This kyphosis associated with torsion of the fetal trunk also results in crossover from the posterior elements to the vertebral body in many instances. This can result in confusion concerning the spinal integrity. However, transverse scans resolve the confusion.

On planes transverse to the long axis, the three ossification centers of the spine can be seen clearly. Caution must be exercised to ensure that the spine is examined in its entirety in transverse planes. At the cephalic end, no problem arises since one encounters the calvarium. However, the caudal end is more difficult. We employ the ischial ossification centers as landmarks to ensure that the caudal end of the spine has been reached.

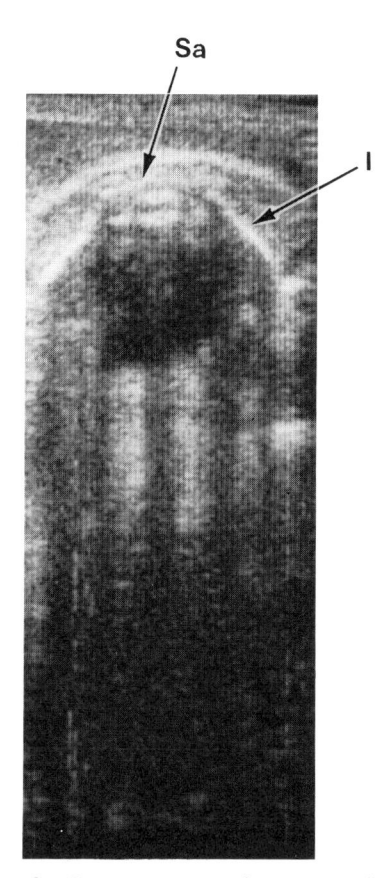

Figure 9. Transverse scan of the pelvis of a prone fetus demonstrates the sacrum (Sa) and iliac wing (I).

MEASURING FETAL EXTREMITIES

The length of the extremity bones can be accurately measured by ultrasound.[4] Ultrasonography has some significant advantages over radiography for measuring fetal bones. Ultrasound generates an image free of distortion and magnification.* Since no ionizing radiation is employed, multiple images may be generated to verify the accuracy of measurement.

A number of investigations have now determined normal values for length of the long bones of the extremities.[4, 9, 16] It is important to realize that there are differences in both the mean and standard deviations

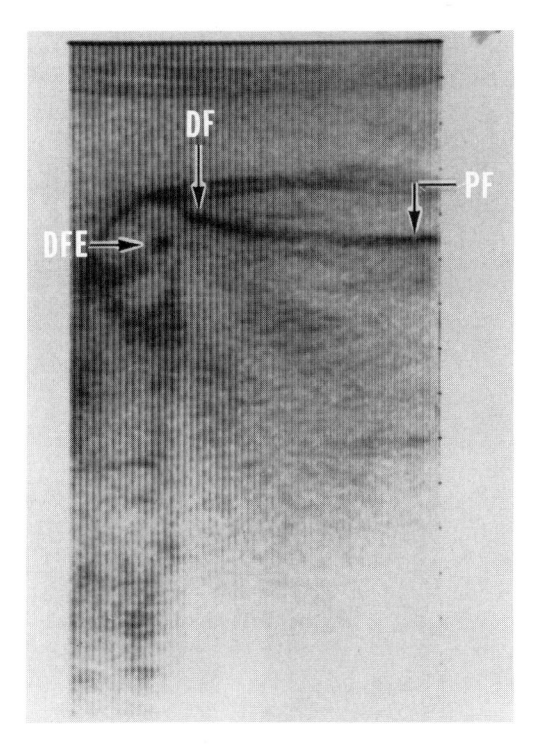

Figure 8. Demonstration of the distal femoral epiphysis (DFE). (DF, distal femur; PF, proximal femur).

---

*Mechanical sector scanners do produce some bone distortion in the far field. The bone appears to be slightly curved along the arc of the sector.

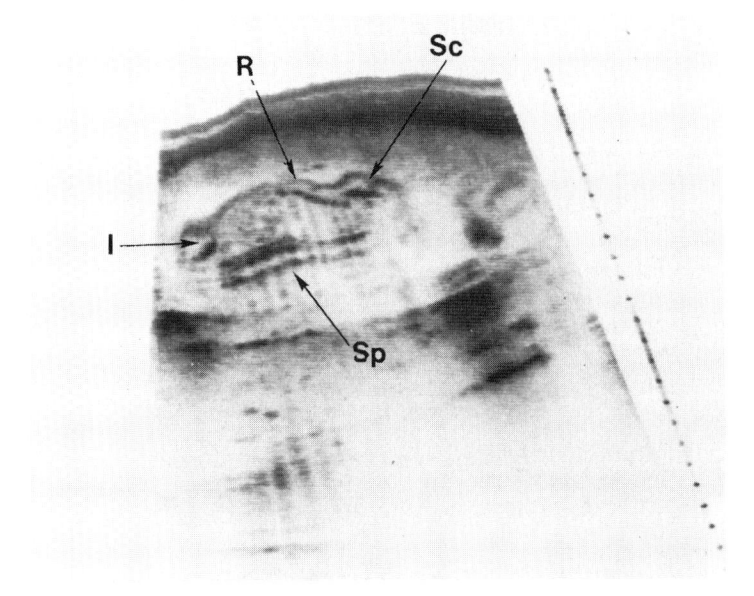

Figure 10. Longitudinally oriented scan of a portion of the fetal spine (Sp). Note that the posterior element ossification centers display a parallel organization. (I, iliac wings; R, ribs; Sc, scapula).

or confidence limits set by different authors. There are also differences in data analysis. We have plotted femoral length versus the biparietal diameter (instead of menstrual age) to serve as an internal control of size variability (Table 1).[4] We opted for biparietal diameter for several reasons. First, it is likely that femoral and calvarial size will vary in the same direction, resulting in "less" biologic variation. Employing the biparietal diameter will avoid serious errors that might be engendered by incorrect estimation of gestational age from faulty dates. Similarly, when comparing results of various authors, it is clear that a biparietal diameter of 40 mm may mean considerably different gestational ages to different investigators, whereas variation in the measurement of a biparietal diameter would tend to be very slight.

The method selected relates to the intended purpose of the measurement.[4, 13] If one wishes to employ the measurement for purposes of dating a pregnancy, charts that relate extremity length to age are desirable.[13] If one wishes to employ the measurement to ascertain fetuses affected by short limb dysplasias, charts that relate length of extremity to biparietal diameter are desirable.[4] Occasionally, a visualized femur demonstrates obvious morphologic aberration (Fig. 12).

We initially began measuring both humeral and femoral lengths. However, our

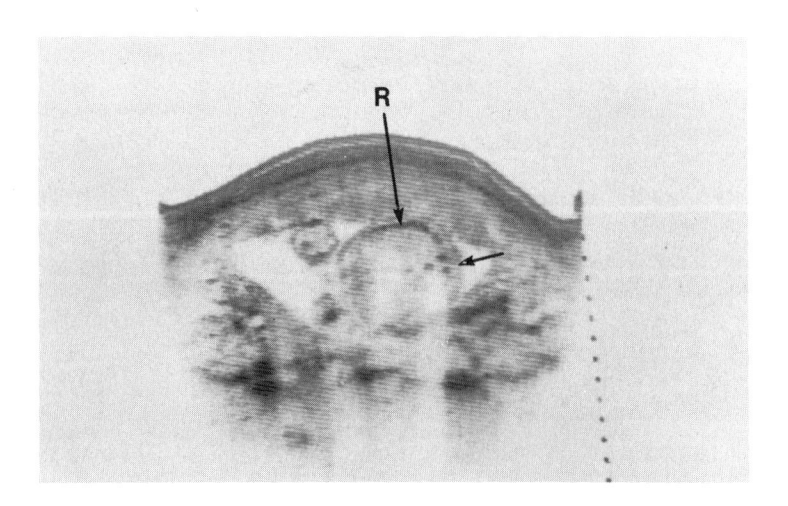

Figure 11. Transverse scan of the distal thoracic spine (*arrow*) demonstrates the typical triangular orientation of the three ossification centers which comprise the spine. The rib (R) documents that the image is at the thoracic spine level.

Table 1. *Femoral Length Versus Biparietal Diameter*

BIPARIETAL DIAMETER	PREDICTED FEMORAL LENGTH (MEAN)	LOWER 99% PREDICTION INTERVAL	BIPARIETAL DIAMETER	PREDICTED FEMORAL LENGTH (MEAN)	LOWER 99% PREDICTION INTERVAL
27	15	12	46	34	29
28	16	13	47	35	30
29	17	14	48	36	31
30	18	15	48	36	31
31	19	16	48	36	31
32	20	17	49	37	32
33	21	18	49	37	32
34	22	19	50	38	32
35	23	19	50	38	32
36	24	20	50	38	32
37	25	21	51	39	33
38	26	22	51	39	33
39	27	23	51	39	33
40	28	24	52	40	34
40	28	24	53	41	35
41	29	25	54	42	36
42	30	26	55	43	37
43	31	26	56	44	38
43	31	26	56	44	38
44	32	27	57	45	38
45	33	28	58	46	39
45	33	28	59	47	40
			60	48	41

early experience and that of others disclosed that the lengths of the humerus and femur of normal fetuses younger than 22 postmenstrual weeks were virtually identical.[9] The femur is more readily measured than the humerus, for several reasons. The fetus displays greater freedom of motion of the humerus than the femur. Fetal movement of the thigh is largely limited to flexion and extension in early pregnancy, while the upper arm is abducted and adducted in addition to being flexed and extended. Also, when the elbow and knee are in a flexed position, the proximal radius and ulna lie nearer the distal humerus than the proximal tibia and fibula lie to the distal femur. This results in less difficulty in determining the distal endpoint of the femur compared to the humerus. Also, the ischial ossification center serves as an excellent marker to assure that the true proximal end of the femur is recorded. The scapula does not serve this purpose as well for the humerus.

SHORT-LIMBED BONE DYSPLASIAS

Identification of short-limbed dysplasia by ultrasonic measurement of length of

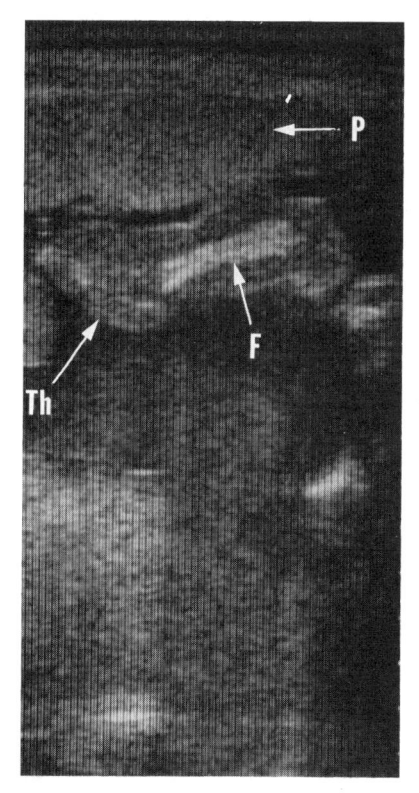

Figure 12. Abnormally short and thick femur (F) in a fetus with multiple anomalies. There is associated edema of the thigh (Th). (P, placenta).

fetal limbs has been accomplished in several centers.[2, 4, 7, 11, 12, 14] The methodology has varied slightly, but recently there has been a consensus of measurement of the ossified portion of the femoral diaphysis as an indication of overall length of extremity. Even syndromes that more severely affect the middle segment (mesomelic dwarfism affecting radius, ulna, tibia, and fibula) than the proximal extremity (rhizomelic dwarfism affecting femur and humerus) may be diagnosed by femoral measurements. For example, using femoral measurements, chondroectodermal dysplasia, a mesomelic dwarf syndrome, can be diagnosed earlier in gestation than can heterozygous achondroplasia, which is a rhizomelic dysplasia.

We have diagnosed seven short-limbed bone dysplasias in utero and have consulted on two addtional cases. These will form the basis of the following assessment. Three fetuses were the products of nonconsanguineous marriages between achondroplastic dwarfs. While many cases of this entity appear to be sporadic, indicating spontaneous mutation, family histories indicate that this disease is transmitted as an autosomal dominant trait. Thus, with both parents affected, the inheritance pattern produces a 25 per cent chance of an infant of normal stature, a 50 per cent chance of heterozygous achondroplasia, and a 25 per cent chance of homozygous achondroplasia (a severe form of the disease). The fourth fetus was the product of conception of an achondroplastic dwarf and a hypochondroplastic dwarf. A transmission pattern similar to that described above would be anticipated. The fifth fetus was at risk only for heterozygous achondroplasia, a 50 per cent chance based on the transmission pattern from one normal and one heterozygous achondroplastic parent.

The sixth and seventh fetuses were at risk, respectively, for Ellis–van Creveld syndrome (chondroectodermal dysplasia) and achondrogenesis. The eighth fetus was at risk for a short-limbed dysplasia not previously classified. These three entities have an autosomal recessive transmission pattern (i.e., 25 per cent risk of recurrence). Our last case, a fetus with thanatophoric dysplasia, was important since it was not clinically suspected, appearing spontaneously in a family without a prior family history of the disorder. This case will be considered in more detail later.

The measurements of these fetuses are demonstrated in Figures 13 and 14. All results have been radiologically or pathologically confirmed.

Although these observations are based on a small number of affected fetuses, the data clearly indicate that ultrasonography is accurate in the detection of short-limbed dwarfs. Other investigators have diagnosed another case each of achondrogenesis[2] and of chondroectodermal dysplasia.[11] Two cases of diastrophic dwarfism,[12, 14] a case of camptomelic dysplasia,[7] and a case of thanatophoric dysplasia[7] have similarly been identified in the second trimester.

There appears to be a basic difference in growth patterns among dwarf fetuses. This observation broadens our concepts of the natural history of certain dwarf syndromes. Fetuses with achondrogenesis, chondroectodermal dysplasia, diastrophic dysplasia, and thanatophoric dysplasia have all been diagnosed prior to 22 weeks' gestational age.[2,4,7,11,12,14] The three fetuses with heterozygous achondroplasia did not demonstrate recognizably short femurs until later in the second trimester.[4]

There are two important observations in the achondroplastic group. The first is that all the heterozygotes display a remarkably similar long bone growth pattern. Second, this experience with heterozygous achondroplasia indicates that, as other dwarf syndromes are investigated, an early femoral measurement that falls within the normal range cannot be taken as unequivocal evidence that the fetus is not affected.

Because homozygous achondroplasia manifests abnormally short femurs earlier than heterozygous achondroplasia (a result which was anticipated),[1, 4] we may be capable of genotyping achondroplasia with this simple ultrasonic measurement. Homozygous achondroplasia is a more severe dwarfism with skeletal manifestations similar to, but more pronounced than, the heterozygous form.[6] The homozygous variety is usually lethal after birth because of the smallness of the thorax. Macrocephaly may be pronounced. The implications for an affected mother with her small pelvis and potential for developing low back problems can well be imagined when faced with the likelihood of a nonsurviving child. By

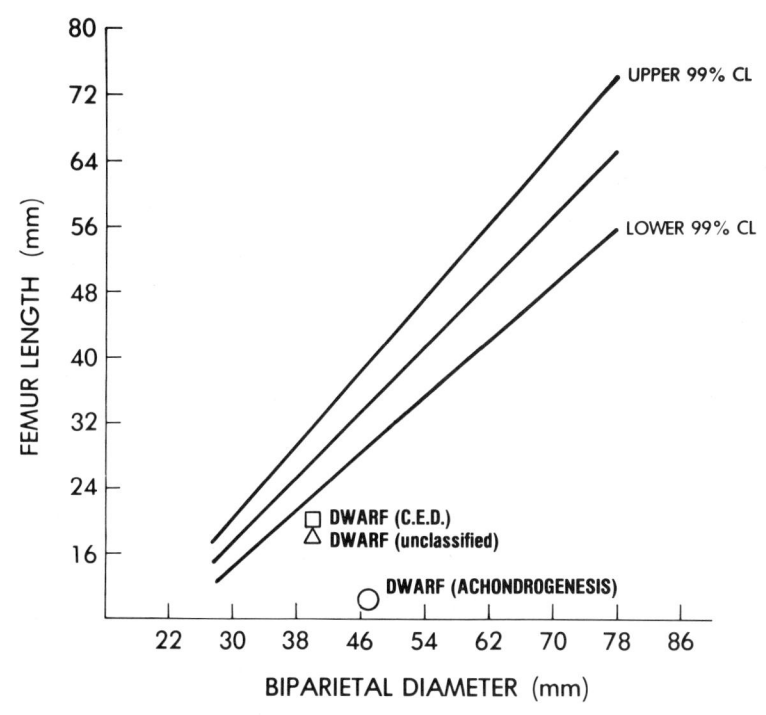

Figure 13. Graph demonstrating the relationship of biparietal diameter to femur length in normal fetuses. Prediction intervals were calculated at a 99 per cent confidence limit. Three dwarf fetuses demonstrate abnormally short femurs early in pregnancy.

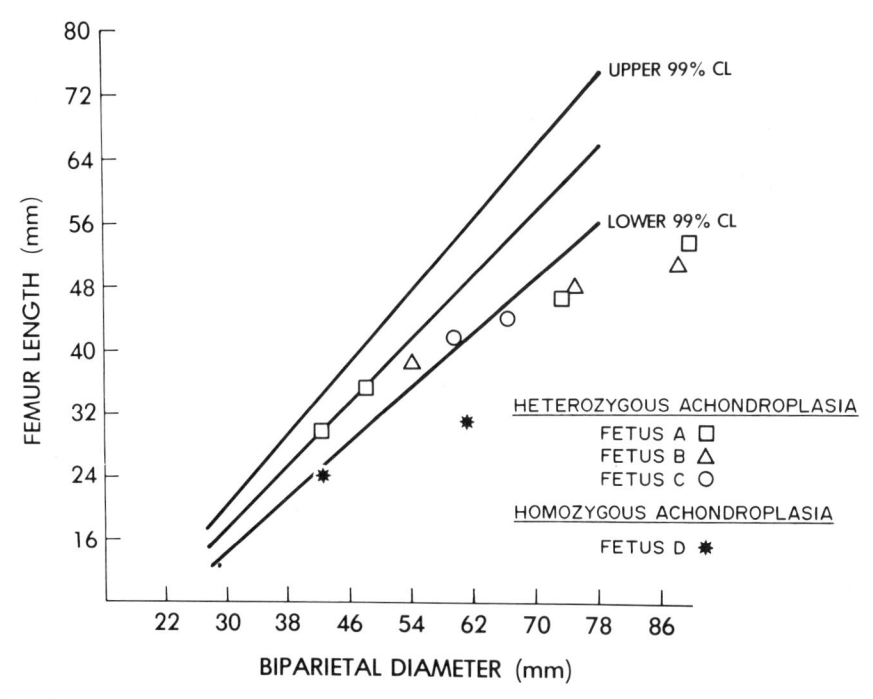

Figure 14. Same graph as in Figure 12 demonstrates the growth pattern of three heterozygous achondroplastic dwarfs and one homozygous achondroplastic dwarf.

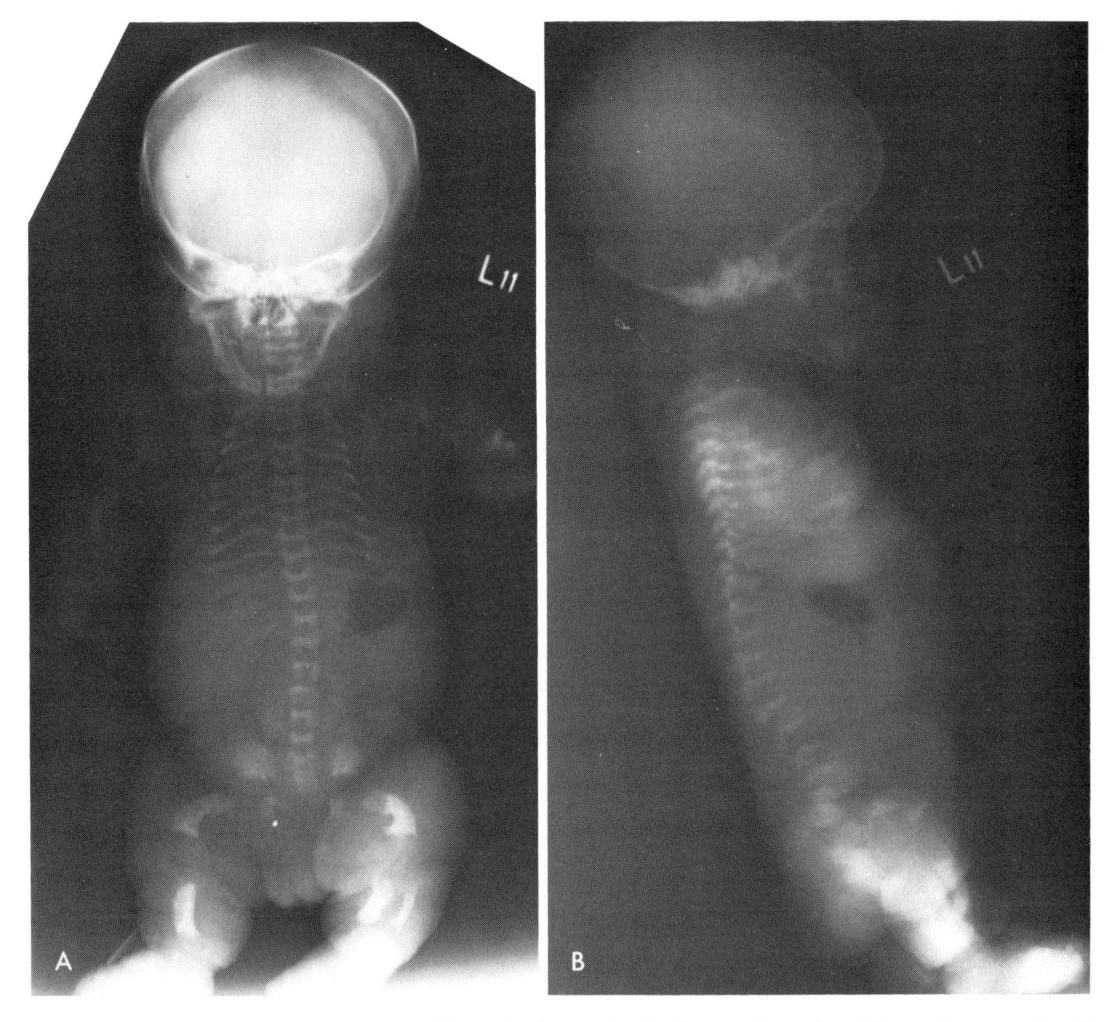

Figure 15. A and B, Anteroposterior and lateral radiographs of a thanatophoric dwarf detected sonographically in late gestation. Note the bowing and severe shortening of the long bones, the large head size, small thorax and characteristically narrow sacrosciatic notches, and flattened vertebral bodies.

contrast, heterozygous fetuses are usually highly desired by the parents (one or both of whom are similarly affected).

We have recently observed an unsuspected severe short-limbed dysplasia (thanatophoric dysplasia) late in gestation (Fig. 15). The sonographic observations included a large head size (biparietal diameter of 10 cm), severely shortened and bowed extremities (Fig. 16), a small thorax, five fingers on each hand, and markedly thickened soft tissues in the extremities (Fig. 17) and chest (Fig. 18). Additionally, the spine and calvarium demonstrated an entirely normal sonographic appearance.

A number of dysplasias may demonstrate marked limb shortening and a small thorax. These include homozygous achondroplasia, achondrogenesis, congenital hypophosphatasia, asphyxiating thoracic dysplasia, short rib–polydactyly syndrome, and the congenital recessive form of osteogenesis imperfecta. Importantly, all of these conditions, with the occasional exception of asphyxiating thoracic dysplasia, are fatal in the neonatal period.

A basic difference in approach occurs when a short-limbed dysplasia is incidentally discovered as opposed to when it is sought in a fetus genetically at risk. In the latter case, if short limbs are found, one can be absolutely confident that the dysplasia will be the one that the fetus is at risk to develop. A distinction between various forms of dysplasia is not required. By contrast, in the incidentally discovered dys-

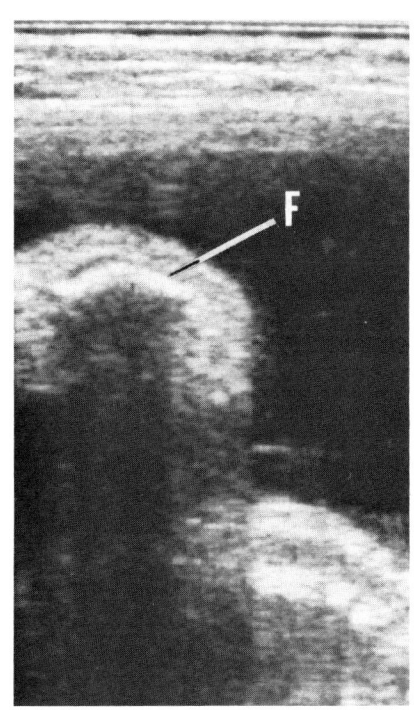

Figure 16. Markedly shortened and bowed femur (F). Compare with Figure 15A.

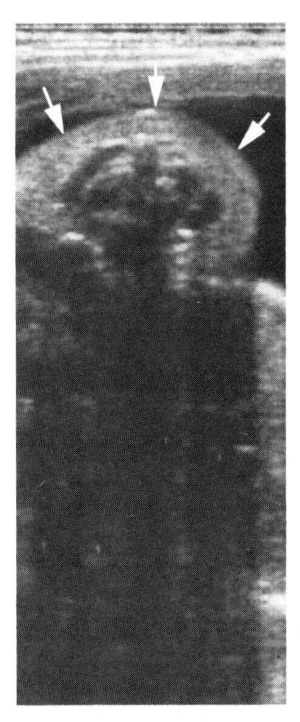

Figure 17. Marked soft tissue thickening (*arrows*) in the extremity of a thanatophoric dwarf. Compare with Figure 15A.

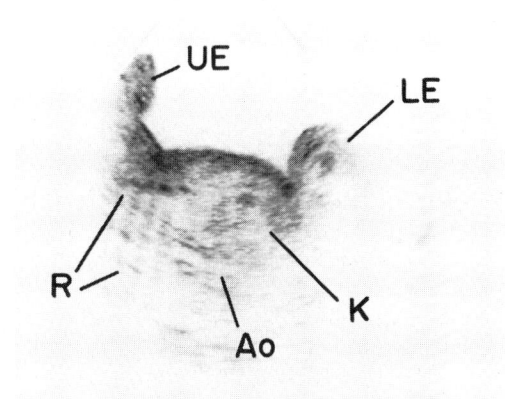

Figure 18. Markedly small thorax demarcated by the ribs (R). Compare with Figure 15A. This strongly suggests a poor prognosis.(Ao, abdominal aorta; K, kidney; UE, upper extremity; LE, lower extremity).

plasia it is important to gather all the information one can to help classify the disorder. For example, the observations in the above case lead one to strongly consider thanatophoric dysplasia. Homozygous achondroplasia is ruled out genetically. Achondrogenesis and congenital hypophosphatasia are characterized by markedly diminished ossification of the calvarium and/or spine. The extremities in congenital hypophosphatasia are thinned and generally not bowed. The likelihood of short rib–polydactyly syndrome is reduced since five fingers were easily demonstrated. Finally, asphyxiating thoracic dysplasia produces a less dramatic degree of limb shortening. In addition to these negative features, the large head size and marked subcutaneous tissue thickening spoke in favor of thanatophoric dysplasia. Most significant is the fact that all of these features indicated a high probability that the neonate would not be viable.

In conclusion, it appears that fetal femoral measurement is an accurate means of identifying many short-limbed dysplasias; that the growth patterns of different classes of dwarfs differ; and that this difference may make it possible to accurately discriminate homozygous from heterozygous offspring of achondroplastic dwarfs in the second trimester. Additionally, these and subsequent observations will add to our knowledge of the natural history of short-limbed dysplasias.

LIMB REDUCTION ABNORMALITIES

Ultrasonography offers an opportunity to assess fetuses who are genetically at risk for limb reduction abnormalities. We must confine the examination group to those with a genetic risk because detailed examination of all four extremities is beyond the scope of a routine sonographic evaluation of a pregnancy. Even in fetuses at a potential genetic risk, one may anticipate a low yield of positive cases. We have done detailed examinations of approximately 15 such pregnancies and have yet to find a limb reduction defect (all predicted normals have, however, been confirmed).

Limb reduction defects have been classified according to the embryonic somatic origin of the limb.[15] Table 2 is a general guide to nomenclature but these basic terms are frequently altered by numerous modifiers. Aplasias and hypoplasias of major long bones occur in the following descending order of frequency: fibula, radius, femur, ulna, and humerus.

Very few such abnormalities have been recognized sonographically. We have diagnosed amelia in a fetus with the amniotic band syndrome (Fig. 19), and Hobbins and Mahoney have diagnosed a phocomelic extremity in a fetus at risk for Robert's syndrome.[7] The amniotic band syndrome is not genetically heritable, while Robert's syndrome is transmitted in an autosomal recessive fashion. This latter syndrome includes cleft lip, microcephaly, phocomelia, and occasionally renal dysplasia.

Despite the fact that only a few such cases have been recognized to date, we anticipate that ultrasonography will be quite useful in the prenatal diagnosis of limb reduction abnormalities. Visualization of the

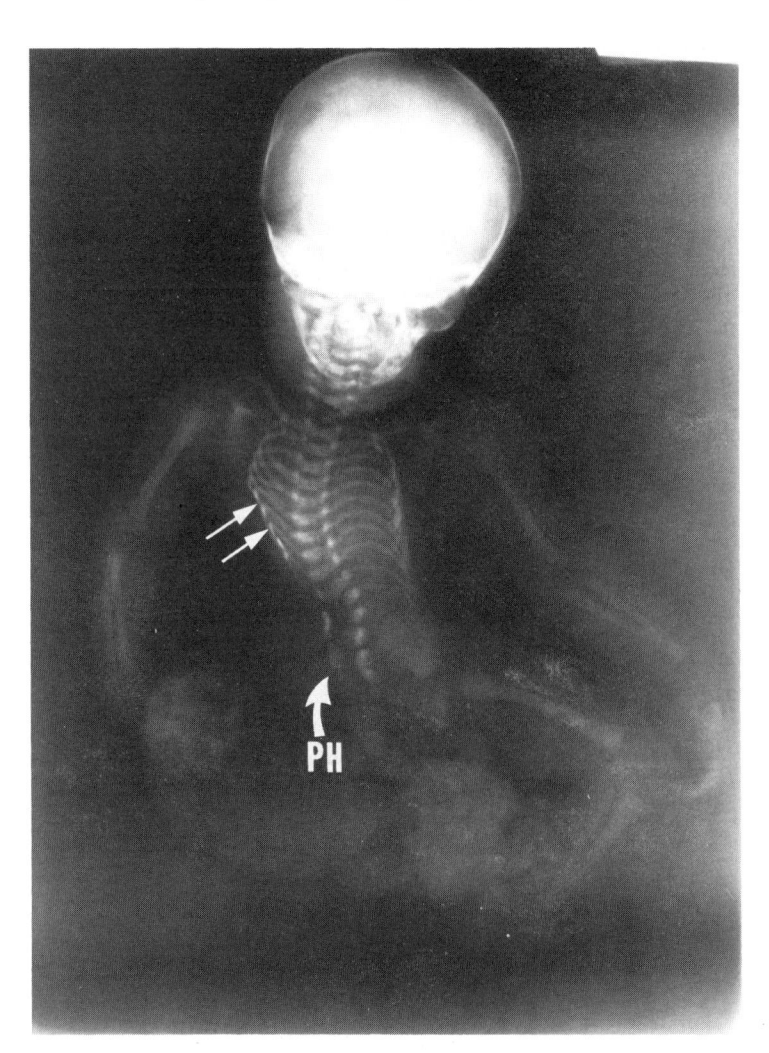

Figure 19. Amelia in a fetus with amniotic band syndrome. As the band entrapped the fetus, it created a linear defect in the ribs (*arrows*) and hypoplasia of the pelvis (PH), as well.

fetal extremities can be quite detailed and complete with the exception of the toes. Virtually any pregnancy at risk for a limb reduction abnormality should be examined in an ultrasonographic center interested in such diagnoses.

A number of syndromes may be associated with a limb reduction defect. For example, Robert's syndrome (autosomal recessive), Holt-Oram syndrome (autosomal dominant), thrombocytopenia–absent radius (TAR) syndrome (autosomal recessive), and Fanconi anemia (autosomal recessive) are all characterized by radial limb reduction abnormalities.

Although it may not be possible to detect minor degrees of thumb hypoplasia or to

Table 2. *Limb Reduction Abnormalities*

Amelia	Complete absence of extremity
Hemimelia	Absence of extremity below the elbow or knee; may be complete or incomplete
Ulnar paraxial hemimelia	Aplasia, partial aplasia, or hypoplasia of the ulna and ulnar digits
Radial paraxial hemimelia	Aplasia, partial aplasia, or hypoplasia of the radius and thumb; associated with clubbed hand
Acheiria	Absence of the hand
Adactylia	Absence of the fingers; may be complete or incomplete
Phocomelia	Intercalary deficiency of the mid extremity with preservation of the proximal and distal portions (seal flipper deformity)

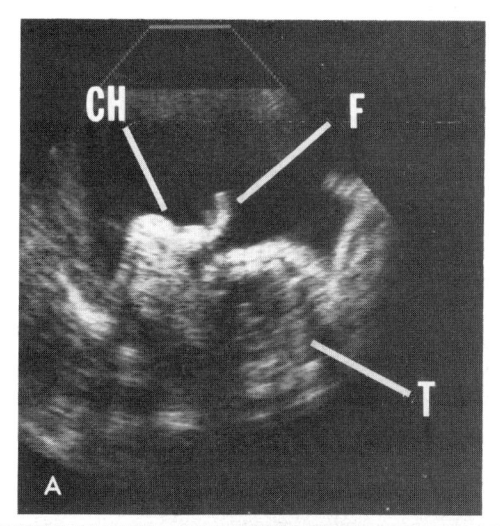

Figure 20. *A*, Sonogram demonstrating a club hand deformity (CH). This led to more detailed evaluation which disclosed four fingers and absent radius. F, finger; T, thorax. *B*, Confirmatory radiograph.

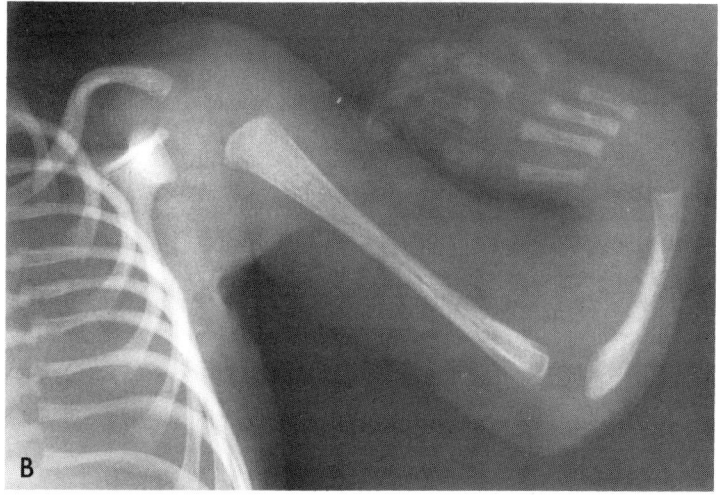

determine the integrity of each finger, major limb reduction defects should be visible. Absence or hypoplasia of the radius is usually associated with bowing and shortening of the ulna, as well. When the radius is hypoplastic, it does not end at the same distal level as the ulna. This feature appears to be easily assessed. In addition, the hand is markedly deviated in the radial direction (at nearly 90 degrees to the forearm) when the radius is hypoplastic or absent. This complex should be readily visible on sonographic evaluation.

The observation of a club hand has recently enabled us to correctly categorize an unsuspected case of limb reduction (Fig. 20). Radial aplasia and a missing thumb were noted bilaterally as well as bilateral absence of the tibias.

We are confident that ultrasonography will have great utility in the assessment of limb reduction abnormalities in the future. As interest in this type of diagnosis grows, more and more of these rare heritable disorders will come to examination, and we are certain that many bone hypoplasias and aplasias will be recognized.

The identification of polydactyly is not dissimilar from identification of limb reduction abnormalities. Both types of abnormality require the same type of detailed examination of the distal extremity. We have observed hexadactyly in our case of chondroectodermal dysplasia and polydactyly of the foot in a fetus with multiple congenital anomalies (Fig. 21).

BONE SYNDROMES RESULTING IN FRACTURES OF FETAL BONES OR HYPOMINERALIZATION

Ultrasonography may significantly contribute to the diagnosis of disorders which result in hypomineralization of bone. Such disorders include achondrogenesis, hypophosphatasia, and osteogenesis imperfecta. For example, Johnson and coworkers have demonstrated a fracture of the fetal femur in a case of osteogenesis imperfecta (Fig. 22).[17] We have recently diagnosed a similar case in a fetus genetically at risk by demonstrating marked bowing of the femur (Fig. 23). Cooperberg and coworkers have noted the inability to demonstrate the fetal spine in a case of achondrogenesis.[2] In this latter syndrome there is virtually no ossification of the spine even though other bones in the axial skeleton possess sufficient bone calcium to be perceived. While such positive findings, as noted above, are encouraging, care must be exercised since it is unclear to what extent a bone must be calcified to behave in a "normal" fashion on an ultrasonogram. A hypomineralized bone may possess sufficient calcium to generate a high amplitude reflection and an acoustic shadow. We have consulted on a case of possible hypophosphatasia in which the fetal bones behaved normally with regard to acoustic characteristics and yet the fetus was affected.

Achondrogenesis could potentially be diagnosed by virtue of the severe spinal hypomineralization, but it is well documented that this diagnosis can be confirmed early in gestation by the extreme limb shortening in this syndrome. Similarly, homozygous recessive osteogenesis imperfecta can be diagnosed by measuring the femoral

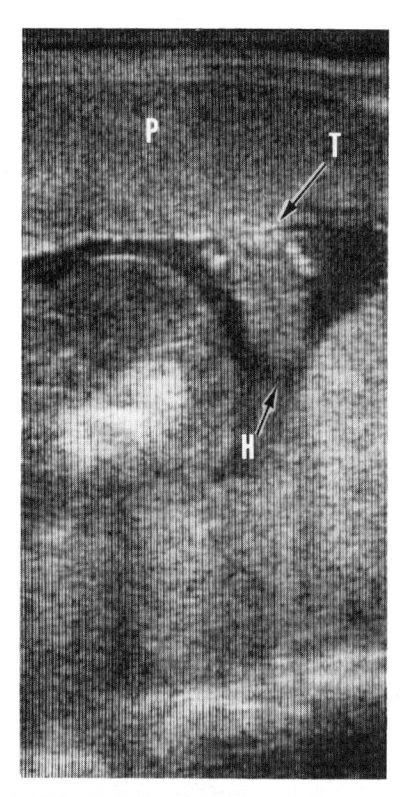

Figure 21. Polydactyly, in this case eight toes (T), in a fetus with multiple congenital anomalies. (H, heel; P, placenta).

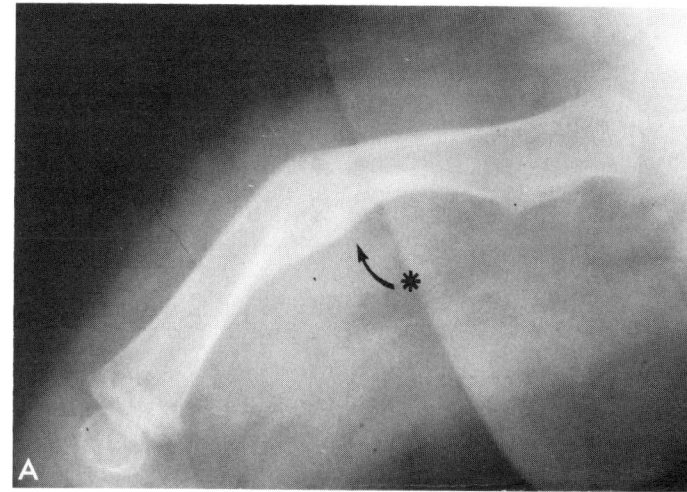

Figure 22. Femoral fracture (*above*) in a live born child with osteogenesis imperfecta (dominant form) which was detected in utero (*below*). (* = fracture site). (Reproduced from Clinics in Diagnostic Ultrasound, *8*:210, 1981 with permission.)

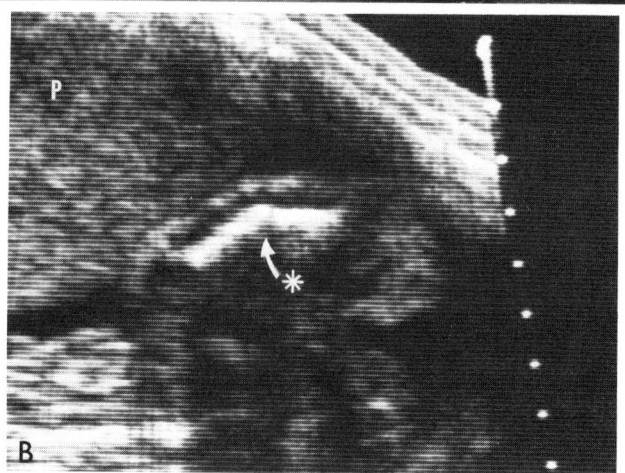

Figure 23. Markedly bowed femur (F) in a fetus genetically at risk for dominant osteogenesis imperfecta. While many bone dysplasias may cause bowing of the long bones, we can be confident that this fetus will manifest the one for which it is genetically at risk.

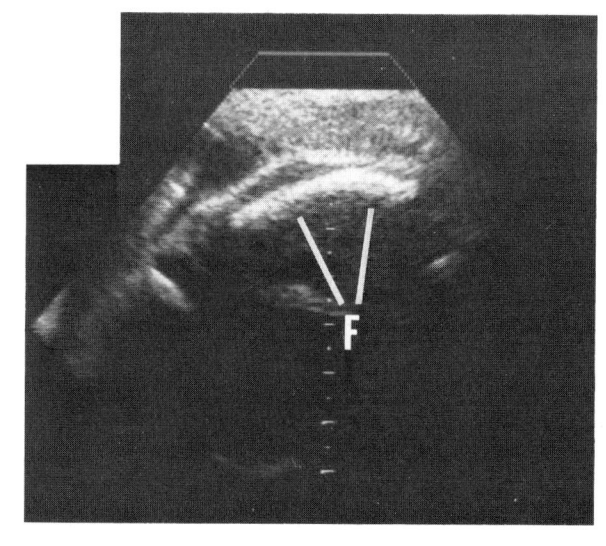

length which is dramatically shortened in this abnormality.[10] Diagnosis of the autosomal dominant form of the disease will probably be based on demonstration of fracture deformities or excess callus formation, and such deformities possibly may be sonographically visible only late in gestation.

In summary, it seems clear that ultrasonography may play a role in confirming disorders such as autosomal dominant osteogenesis imperfecta and hypophosphatasia, but it is probably not capable of definitively excluding these disorders in patients at risk. Care should be exercised in this regard until more fetuses have been studied and followed to delivery.

REFERENCES

1. Bowie, J.: Personal communication.
2. Cooperberg, P.: Personal communication.
3. Filly, R. A., and Callen, P. W.: Normal fetal anatomy as visualized with gray scale ultrasonography. In Sanders, R. C., and James, E. (eds.): The Principles and Practice of Ultrasonography in Obstetrics and Gynecology. Edition 2. New York, Appleton-Century-Crofts, 1980, pp. 91–110.
4. Filly, R. A., Golbus, M. S., Carey, J. C., et al.: Short-limbed dwarfism: Ultrasonic diagnosis by mensuration of fetal femoral length. Radiology, 138:653, 1981.
5. Greulich, W. W., and Pyle, S. I. (eds.): Radiologic Atlas of Skeletal Development of the Hand and Wrist. Edition 2. Stanford, California, Stanford University Press, 1959.
6. Hall, J. C., Dorst, J. P., Tayki, H., et al.: Two probable cases of homozygosity for the achondroplasia gene. Birth Defects, 5:24–34, 1969.
7. Hobbins, J. C., and Mahoney, M. J.: The diagnosis of skeletal dysplasias with ultrasound. In Sanders, R. C., and James, A. E. (eds.): The Principles and Practice of Ultrasonography in Obstetrics and Gynecology. Edition 2. New York, Appleton-Century-Crofts, 1980, pp. 191–203.
8. Hoerr, N. L., Pyle, S. I., and Francis, C. C. (eds.): Radiographic Atlas of Skeletal Development of the Foot and Ankle. Springfield, Illinois, Charles C Thomas, 1962.
9. Jeanty, P., Kirkpatrick, C., Dramaix-Wilmet, M., et al.: Ultrasonic evaluation of fetal limb growth. Radiology, 140:165, 1981.
10. Kazazian, H.: Personal communication.
11. Mahoney, M. J., and Hobbins, J. C.: Prenatal diagnosis of chondroectodermal dysplasia (Ellis-Van Creveld syndrome) with fetoscopy and ultrasound. N. Engl. J. Med., 297:258, 1977.
12. Mantagos, S., Weiss, R. R., Mahoney, M., et al.: Prenatal diagnosis of diastrophic dwarfism. Am. J. Obstet. Gynecol., 139:111, 1981.
13. O'Brien, G. B., Queenan, J. T., and Campbell, S.: Assessment of gestation age in the second trimester by real-time ultrasound measurement of the femur length. Am. J. Obstet. Gynecol., 139:540, 1981.
14. O'Brien, G. D., Rodeck, C., and Queenan, J. T.: Early prenatal diagnosis of diastrophic dwarfism by ultrasound. Br. Med. J., 280:1300, 1980.
15. O'Rahilly, R.: Morphologic patterns in limb deficiencies and duplications. Am. J. Anat., 89:135, 1951.
16. Queenan, J. T., O'Brien, G. B., and Campbell, S.: Ultrasound measurement of the fetal limb bones. Am. J. Obstet. Gynecol., 138:297, 1980.
17. Rumack, C. M., Johnson, M. L., and Zunkel, D.: Antenatal diagnosis. Clin. Diag. Ultrasound, 8:210, 1981.
18. Schreiber, M. H., and Morettin, L. B.: Antepartum prediction of fetal maturity. Radiol. Clin. North Am., 5:21, 1967.

6

Ultrasound Evaluation of the Normal and Abnormal Fetal Neural Axis

Charles E. Fiske, M.D., and Roy A. Filly, M.D.

Among the various fetal anomalies which can be diagnosed by ultrasound, probably none are more devastating in their clinical consequences and therefore important in early recognition than neural tube defects. Each year in the United States, approximately 6000 infants born are afflicted with one of these congenital anomalies. Earlier in the development of sonographic prenatal diagnosis, only defects producing gross anatomical distortions were detected. Recent rapid technologic advances now allow early and accurate diagnosis of a variety of neural tube malformations. As a result, the ultrasonographer, by observation and diagnosis, frequently initiates the decision-making process involving the obstetrician and prospective parents regarding difficult options. Consequently, it is incumbent upon the ultrasonographer to provide accurate and reliable information upon which those decisions can be based. Knowledge of normal and abnormal developmental neuroanatomy is essential in making these determinations. This chapter reviews normal fetal developmental neuroanatomy as demonstrated by ultrasound and discusses the ultrasonographic features of the more common neural tube defects.

NORMAL DEVELOPMENTAL ANATOMY OF THE FETAL BRAIN

Fetal neuroanatomy was one of the first areas of investigational interest in the diagnosis of fetal anomalies. This was a result of two facts: the fetal head was examined routinely to obtain a biparietal diameter for the determination of fetal age; and neural tube anomalies are among the most common congenital defects. At first, only gross abnormalities such as anencephaly and advanced hydrocephalus were discovered prenatally. As instrumentation improved, more and more intracranial structures became recognizable early in development. Initially many anatomic errors were made when interpreting intracranial structures, because of the unusual circumstance that the "fluid" and "solid" areas of the brain did not behave in a standard fashion. It was not appreciated initially that the lateral ventricles are largely filled with choroid plexus which is highly echogenic, whereas developing neural tissue is remarkably echopenic. In addition, the dramatic changes that occur as brain development progresses had never been observed in vivo, and postmortem examination of the brain can be at variance with its appearance during life.

A series of key observations led to the clear delineation of normal developmental neuroanatomy as viewed by ultrasound. The first was the realization that the normal choroid plexus and subarachnoid cisterns were very echogenic. This enabled the ultrasonographer to locate the lateral ventricles with certainty. The second observation was the delineation of the brainstem, cerebral peduncles, and sylvian fissures by tracing the normal pulsating cerebral arterial vasculature.[9] The third observation was the correct identification of the slit-like appearance of the third ventricle separating the thalamic nuclei. By employing the landmarks of the lateral ventricles, brainstem, sylvian fissures, and third ventricle established by these observations, one can build a logical framework to identify many discrete neural structures.

As the neonatal brain came under study in recent years, much greater understanding of the appearance of the fetal brain has emerged. Examinations of the neonatal brain were routinely performed on preterm infants as young as 26 to 27 weeks of development. Investigators then began to compare sonographic neuroanatomy learned from the neonatal brain, which can be imaged with great clarity, with that of the developing fetal brain as seen in utero. Based on these observations, the following analysis of fetal intracranial anatomy is presented.

The developing fetal skull can be recognized as early as 8 to 9 weeks after conception. At this point in time the cranial contents consist almost entirely of fluid-filled cerebral vesicles which later become the lateral ventricles. The majority of the solid brain tissue is made up of the thalamus and the corpus striatum which develop caudally and peripherally in the walls of the cerebral vesicles (Fig. 1). The lateral ventricles de-

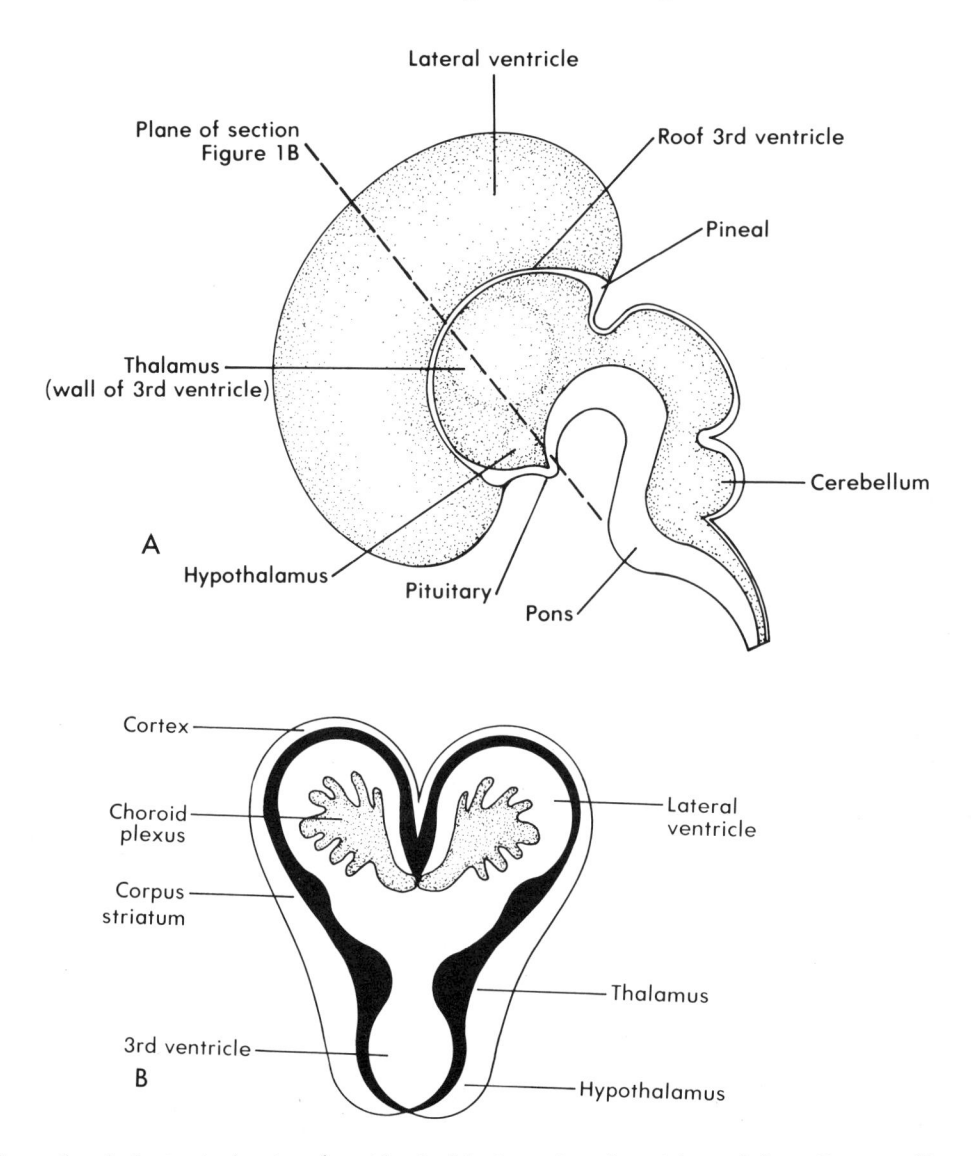

Figure 1. *A*, Anatomic drawing of a midsagittal brain section of an eight week fetus. Recognizable anatomic structures are already present including lateral ventricles, thalamus, and brainstem. *B*, Anatomic drawing of a coronal plane of section through the brain of an eight week fetus as marked in *A*. Note the relative size of the lateral and third ventricles compared to the surrounding brain substance. Choroid plexus fills the majority of the lateral ventricular volume, while the overlying developing cortex is relatively thin. Thalamus and corpus striatum will further expand cephalad toward the middle.

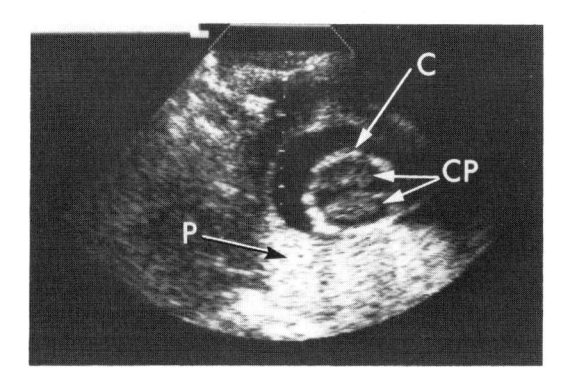

Figure 2. Axial scan of a 12 week fetus. The choroid plexus (CP) is the most prominent intracranial structure at this stage of development. Notice that the brain mantle (the space between the choroid and the calvarium, C) is remarkably echopenic. P, placenta.

velop from the vesicles as the midbrain structures grow cephalad toward the midline. By the twelfth week the lateral ventricles are recognized sonographically as cavities filling the majority of the cranial vault and containing the echogenic choroid plexus (Fig. 2). The choroid is the easiest structure to recognize at this stage in fetal development because of its high echogenicity. It appears likely that the germinal matrix is also highly echogenic at this stage of pregnancy and contributes to the appearance described above. The mantle of the developing cerebral cortex surrounding the lateral ventricle is difficult to delineate because of its low echogenicity, but a demarcation between lateral ventricle and cerebral mantle can be identified as the linear echogenic walls of the lateral ventricle become progressively more visible.

By 15 weeks these boundaries are more clearly defined. The echogenic choroid completely fills the lateral ventricles in their transverse dimension, while not quite filling them in their anterior-posterior dimension. It is important to note that the anterior horns of the lateral ventricles do not possess choroid plexus and are thus "fluid" in appearance as opposed to the body and atrium of the ventricle which appear "solid" because of the presence of choroid (Fig. 3). The occipital horns, also devoid of choroid, are not developed at this stage of gestation. Several midline echoes may be seen at this time. In a cephalad position the invaginated cortex and mesenchyme which later give rise to the falx form a midline echo. Also at this stage, the thalami, having grown from the vesicle walls to meet in the midline, form the lateral walls of the third ventricle which is seen as a single midline linear echo centrally located within the calvarium.

By 17 weeks there has been rapid proliferation of cerebral cortex which is recognized by progressive separation of the lateral wall of the lateral ventricle from the calvarium. The choroid plexus still predominantly fills the ventricles. Lateral ventricular structure can often be recognized as distinct body and frontal horns. Nonetheless, the relative volume of the anterior horns diminishes such that they become less prominently visible. The thalamus can be recognized on either side of the linear

Figure 3. An axial scan of the calvarium in a normal 17 week fetus. At this stage the lateral ventricles begin to shrink in size with growth of the overlying cortex. Choroid plexus (CP) fills the full width of the ventricle in the midbody portion. However, choroid does not extend into the frontal horns (FH). It is important at this stage in development not to mistake the fluid-filled frontal horns as being abnormally dilated.

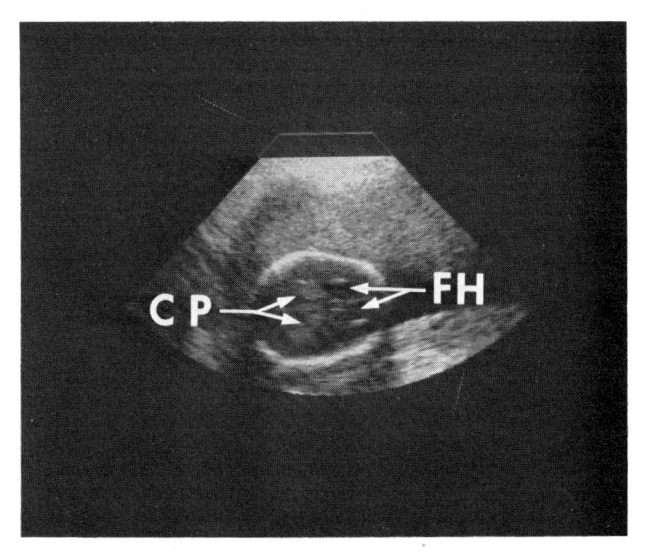

echo representing the third ventricle. The cerebral peduncles are seen directly caudal to the third ventricle and demarcate the region of the midbrain and brainstem. The aqueduct of Sylvius is seen as an extension of the third ventricle into the mid portion of the brainstem where it is recognizable as a bright echo positioned midway between the peduncles and toward the posterior aspect of the midbrain. The echogenic ambient cisterns demarcate the margins of the midbrain.

With a knowledge of the anatomy discussed above, one can accurately define the level of a transverse axial scan of the fetal head. A scan demonstrating a crossed appearance is likely to be obtained at the base of the skull (Fig. 4A). A scan that demonstrates the thalami on either side of the third ventricle will be an appropriate plane of section to measure the biparietal diameter (Fig. 4B). At the most rostral level the lateral walls of the lateral ventricles will be seen on either side of the falx/interhemispheric fissure complex (Fig. 4C).

By 20 weeks the lateral ventricles take on the characteristic pattern which is recognized throughout the remainder of gestation and in the neonate. Axial scans commonly demonstrate anterior horns, bodies, and atria of the ventricles. The temporal horns can be clearly demarcated if the appropriate transducer direction is utilized.

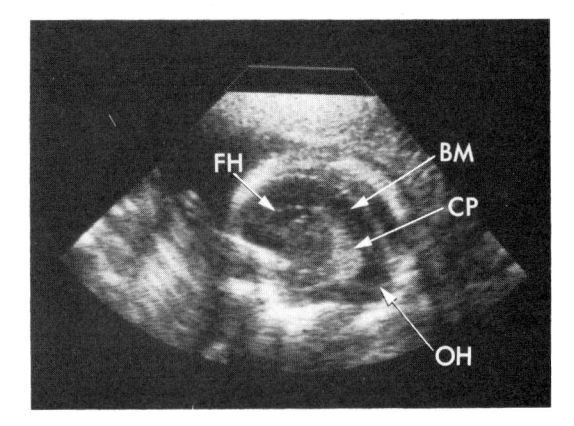

Figure 5. Parasagittal sonogram of the calvarium in a 20 week fetus. The semicircle of the choroid plexus (CP) outlines the basal ganglia region and clearly demarcates the body, atrium, and temporal horn of the lateral ventricle. The frontal horn (FH) and the developing occipital horn (OH) are devoid of choroid. The brain mantle (BM) remains relatively echopenic.

Distribution of choroid plexus in a semicircular arc around the basal ganglia extending into the roof of the temporal horn is similar to that seen in the neonate in the parasagittal plane of section (Fig. 5). The lateral ventricular size in relation to the transverse intracranial dimensions greatly decreases, though the choroid plexus continues to fill the ventricle in its transverse axis.

On axial scans taken parallel to Reid's baseline, a complex of two or three parallel

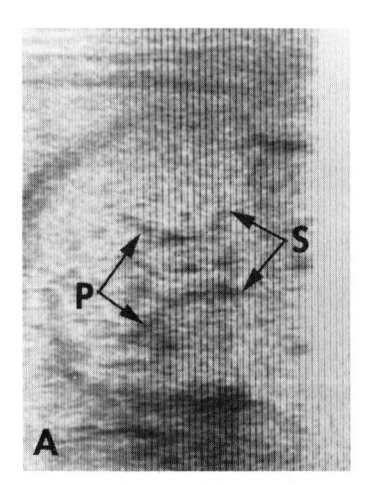

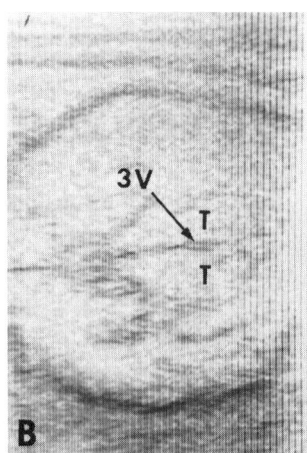

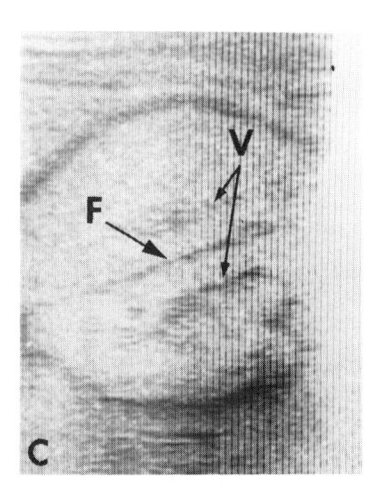

Figure 4. Three axial scans of the fetal head at planes of section from the base of the skull extending rostrally. A, Transverse axial scan at the base of the fetal skull demonstrates the typical "cross" appearance secondary to the greater wing of the sphenoid anteriorly (S) and the petrous ridges posteriorly (P). B, At a slightly higher level, the appropriate plane of section for measuring a biparietal diameter is obtained. The thalamus (T) and third ventricle (3V) can be seen at this plane of section. C, At the most rostral plane of section, three parallel lines can be frequently seen. The midline reflection is secondary to the falx/interhemispheric fissure (F), while the lateral reflections are due to the lateral walls of the lateral ventricles (V).

linear echoes is identified immediately anterior to the third ventricle in the region of the anterior third of the lateral ventricular bodies. The two parallel linear echoes (initially interpreted incorrectly as the walls of the third ventricle) represent one of two anatomic complexes: either the lateral walls of the frontal horns separated by the corpus callosum or, if present, a large cavum septum pellucidum. In a slightly more caudal transverse plane, three parallel linear echoes are seen which represent the junction of the frontal horns with the foramen of Monro laterally and the column of the fornix medially.

Pulsating vasculature outlines the brainstem and basilar cisterns in axial scans. The tentorium is seen at its incisura, with the brainstem anterior to it. The sylvian fissure is easily identified in this plane and the pulsating middle cerebral artery branches demarcate its surface. Caudal to the incisura, the cerebellar vermis is recognized as a strongly echogenic midline structure in the posterior fossa.

At this point in time the morphologic development of the mesencephalon and the diencephalon is nearly complete but continues to increase in size. With rapid growth the telencephalon (cerebral ventricles and overlying cortex) changes appearance as the mantle of cortex is thrown into convolutions along its surface. The lateral ventricles decrease in size as the cortex and ventricles compete for available space within the confines of the cranial vault.

Between 24 weeks and term, the brain undergoes little structural change other than increased cortical convolutions which can be recognized in scans near the convexities. Ventricles become slit-like in size and the cavum septum pellucidum is often recognized as a fluid-filled space between the anterior portion of the lateral ventricular bodies (Fig. 6).

The majority of fetal anomalies that affect the nervous system are apparent before 24 menstrual weeks. Some are recognizable even earlier. In the following sections we will discuss individually the more common neural tube anomalies and evaluate specific features that allow their correct diagnosis.

PATHOLOGY OF THE FETAL BRAIN

Anencephaly

This severe defect is the most common anomaly affecting the central nervous system and has an overall incidence of 1 in 1000 births and a female to male ratio of 4 to 1. The recurrence risk is estimated at 4 per cent, and rises to 10 per cent after two successive affected fetuses.[3] The increased familial recurrence rate which has been established probably accounts for geographic differences in incidence (for example, occurrence greater in the United Kingdom than in the United States).

Even though anencephaly means absence of the brain, functioning neural tissue is always present. The telencephalon (the cerebral hemispheres) is usually ab-

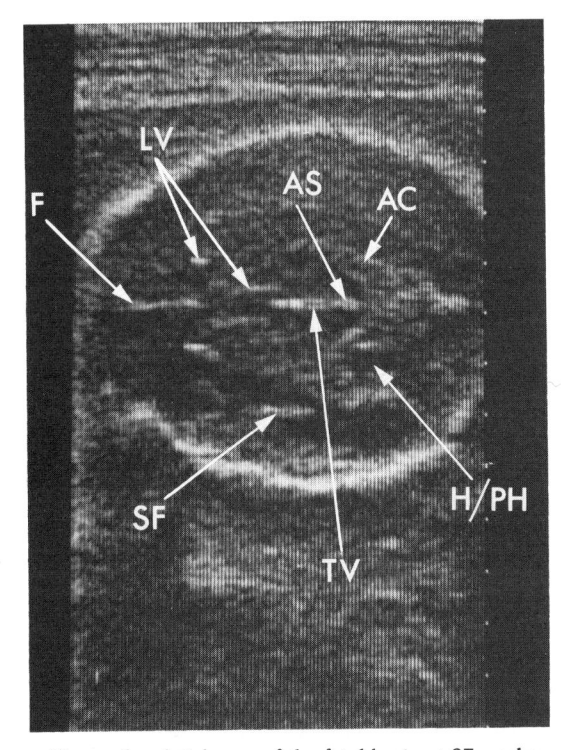

Figure 6. Axial scan of the fetal brain at 27 weeks. This scan corresponds to a plane of section 15 degrees above the canthomeatal line. Notice that the falx (F), the third ventricle (TV), and the aqueduct of Sylvius (AS) are all seen as midline linear echoes. Portions of the anterior horns and the anterior third of the bodies of the lateral ventricle (LV) are also seen as linear echoes anterior to the third ventricle. The echogenic ambient cisterns (AC) demarcate the midbrain. Adjacent to the ambient cistern is the complex of echoes produced by the hippocampal and parahippocampal gyri (H/PH). SF, sylvian fissure overlying the echogenic gray matter of the insular cortex.

sent while the brainstem and portions of the mesencephalon (midbrain) are usually present. Absence of the cranial vault (acrania) is a constant finding, although portions of the cranial bones, especially the occipital bones and the orbits, are usually present. Rachischisis is a frequent accompaniment.

Anencephaly results from a failure of the neural tube to completely close at its cephalic end. This occurs between the second and third weeks of development when the neural folds at the cranial end of the neural plate normally fuse to form the forebrain. The defect is covered by a thick membrane of angiomatous stroma but never bone or normal skin.

Most often anencephaly is discovered ultrasonographically at the time of attempted biparietal diameter determination for fetal age. More frequently, it is being discovered in patients referred for an elevated amniotic fluid alpha-fetoprotein. The specific diagnosis is based most heavily on the abnormal bony anatomy (Figs. 7 and 8). The inability to identify a cranial vault by 12 to 14 weeks is highly suggestive of anencephaly. Failure to identify normal bony structure and brain tissue cephalad to the orbits is the most reliable feature of this anomaly.

Common associated anomalies include spinal defects which occur in 50 per cent of anencephalics. Spina bifida, meningocele, and myelomeningocele can consistently be demonstrated by ultrasonography. Other associated anomalies include cleft palate, umbilical hernia, and equinovarus. Anencephaly rarely occurs in a twin. Polyhydramnios is present in 40 to 50 per cent of cases but does not usually occur until after 26 weeks of gestation. Occasionally oligohydramnios is encountered.

A distinction should be made between anencephaly and other conditions which may be confused with it. When severe, microcephaly may mimic the appearance of anencephaly. However, if one can identify either a cranial vault, no matter how small, or cortical brain tissue, classic anencephaly is excluded. Amniotic band syndrome involving the head may present a confusing picture because portions of the cranial vault (often large portions) may be absent. This anomaly is fortunately rare. Classic anencephaly demonstrates symmetric absence of calvarium. With the amniotic band syndrome the calvarium is destroyed asymmetrically. The rare occurrence of holoacardious anencephalic twin is a true anencephalic aberration lacking any cranial structure.[15] This condition occurs in twins only; confusion with anencephaly, which is rare in twins, is not usually a problem since dramatic abnormalities in the thorax and abdomen usually accompany the holoacardious anencephalic twin monster which are not seen in simple anencephaly.

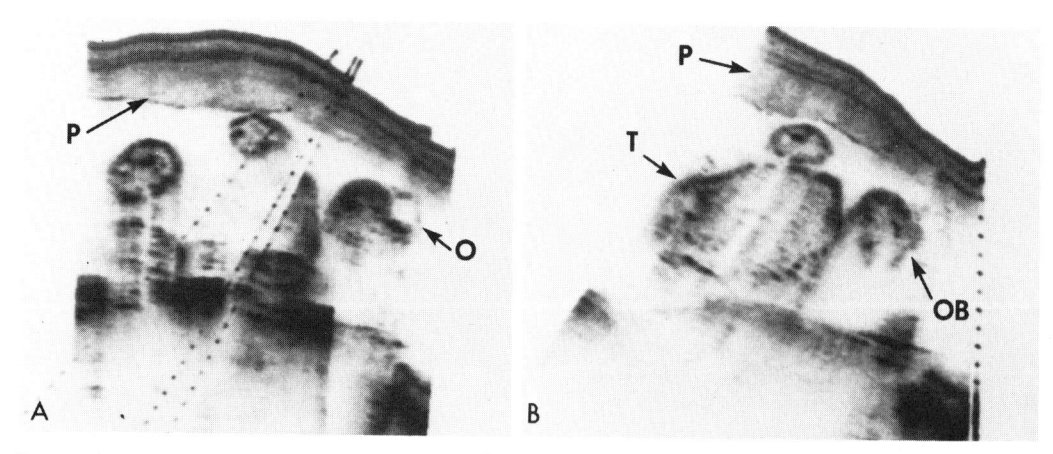

Figure 7. A, Parasagittal sonogram of the gravid uterus demonstrating the key diagnostic feature of anencephaly. The frontal bone should be easily seen sloping away from the orbit (O) in this plane. Its absence confirms acrania—the hallmark of anencephaly. B, The abnormal bone formation of the basiocciput (OB) is seen posterior to the orbit. Some vestiges of brain tissue can be seen. P, placenta; T, torso of fetus.

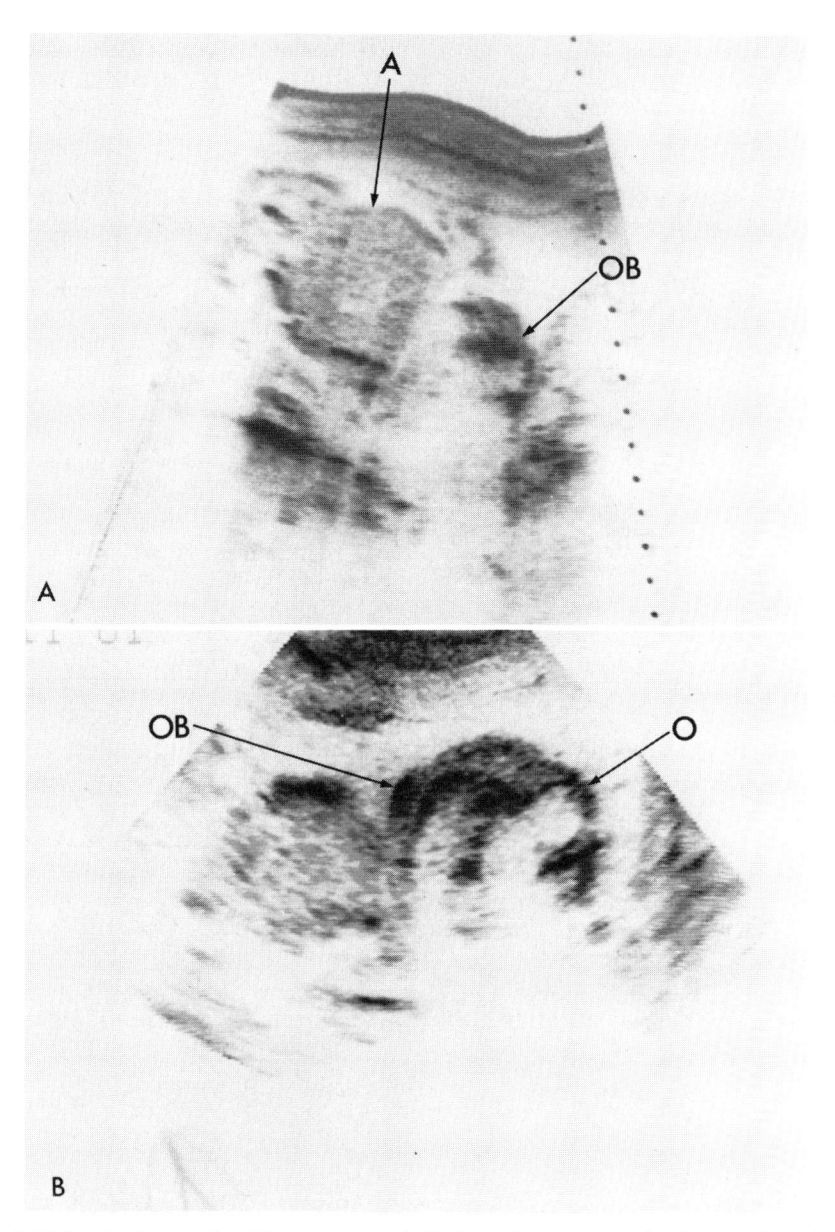

Figure 8. *A,* Midsagittal scan of a different anencephalic fetus demonstrates the distinguishing features of this anomaly. Recognizable intracranial structures or calvarium are not identified above the base of the skull. A, abdomen; OB, basiocciput. *B,* A scan through the region of the head reveals absence of the cranium and prominent appearing orbits (O). OB, basiocciput.

Hydrocephalus

The clinical diagnosis of hydrocephalus in utero is possible only after gross ventricular dilatation has resulted in an enlarged fetal head. Initially, ultrasound was only slightly more successful by confirming a large biparietal diameter in the hydrocephalic fetus. Diagnosing gross dilatation of the lateral ventricles using ultrasound then became commonplace in the third trimester.[6] However, as we have already demonstrated, ventricles can now be identified as early as 12 weeks in gestation. Consequently, it is now possible to diagnose hydrocephalus early in gestation, but caution must be exercised so as not to confuse normally developing ventricles with those which are abnormally enlarged.

When the ventricles are first identified at 12 weeks, the choroid plexus fills their entire transverse dimension. This is an important relationship because in second trimester hydrocephalus, the first recognizable aberration is a relative shrinkage of the normally prominent choroid plexus within the body of the lateral ventricle. The apparent lateral ventricular size may seem prominent even in the normal second trimester fetus, but as long as choroid plexus can be seen filling the lateral ventricular body in its transverse dimension, hydrocephalus is not likely present. This relationship holds true until approximately 20 to 24 weeks at which time the appearance of the choroid is less reliable in determining ventricular dilatation. Importantly, the head size (biparietal diameter) may not be enlarged when the ventricles are definitely dilated. This feature may be true at any stage of pregnancy and is almost universally true in early hydrocephalus.

In general, diagnosing hydrocephalus in the third trimester is not difficult (Figs. 9 and 10). By this stage in development the ventricles are normally slit-like in appearance in both the axial and coronal planes. Detection of early ventricular dilatation before obvious hydrocephalus develops can be more difficult.

Considerable work has been done using measurements of frontal horns and lateral ventricular widths to define the normal limits for ventricular size at different stages in development. A set of ratio measurements comparing the distance of the lateral wall of the lateral ventricle from the midline to the hemispheric width (LVW/HW ratio) has been proposed as a method to diagnose hydrocephalus.[17] However, the ratio measurement accuracy suffers not only from technical difficulties which alter considerably the ratio value depending on the plane of section in which the scan is performed but also from a very wide standard deviation which renders it insensitive to identification of early dilatation. The first manifestation of lateral ventricular dilatation (beginning at approximately 22 weeks and beyond) is medial displacement of the medial wall of the lateral ventricle toward the midline.[5] This sign of ventricular dilatation occurs before the ratio measurement is affected by displacement of the lateral ventricular wall away from the midline (Fig. 11). After occipital horn dilatation, which occurs first in early hydrocephalus, displacement of the medial wall of the lateral ventricle toward the midline in the axial plane is the most reliable indicator of early ventricular dilatation in the third trimester.

Communicating (nonobstructive) hydrocephalus is the more common form of hydrocephalus which is secondary either to an

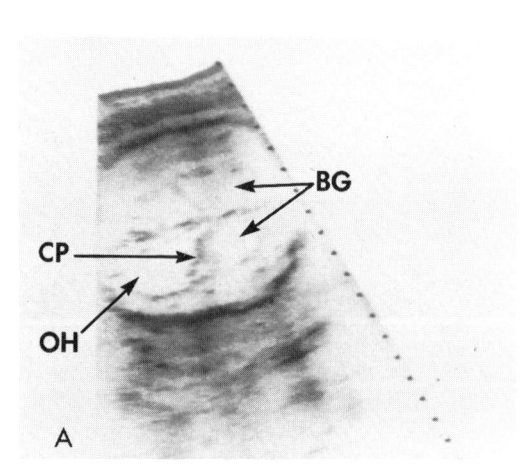

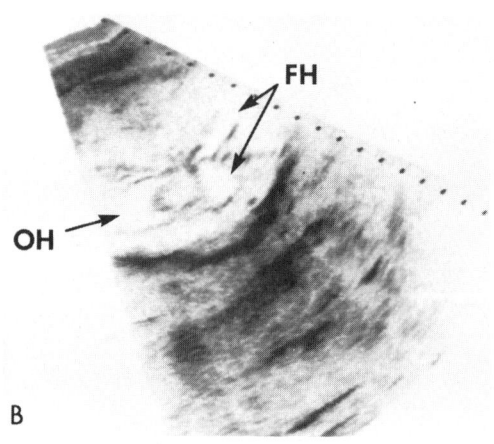

Figure 9. *A*, Axial scan of the calvarium demonstrates moderately severe dilatation of the occipital horn (OH). CP, choroid plexus; BG, basal ganglia. *B*, An axial scan above Reid's baseline demonstrates dilatation of the occipital horns (OH) and frontal horns (FH). The frontal horns angle back toward the midline to meet the anterior thirds of the bodies of the lateral ventricles. Immediately posterior to the septum pellucidum (unlabelled) one can see the brightly echogenic "V" formed by the choroid as it penetrates the foramen of Monroe.

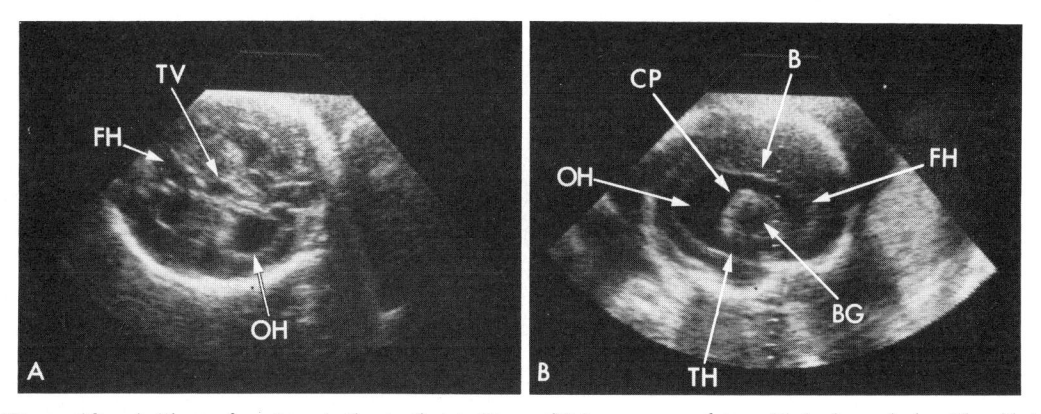

Figure 10. *A*, Plane of section similar to that in Figure 9*B* in a younger fetus with hydrocephalus. The dilated frontal (FH) and occipital horns (OH) are clearly demarcated, as is the dilated third ventricle. Unlabelled are the echogenic shrunken choroid in the atria of the lateral ventricles and the basal ganglia flanking the third ventricle. *B*, The parasagittal scan of the same fetus demonstrates the entirety of the lateral ventricle (a very useful view and easily recognized by anyone who has examined a newborn hydrocephalic infant through the anterior fontanelle). FH, frontal horn; B, body of lateral ventricle; CP, choroid plexus extending from the roof of the temporal horn, through the atrium and onto the floor of the ventricular body, ending at the foramen of Monro; OH, occipital horn; TH, temporal horn; BG, basal ganglia.

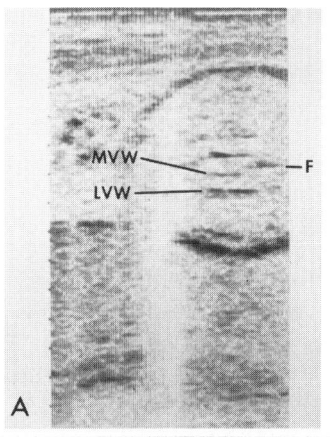

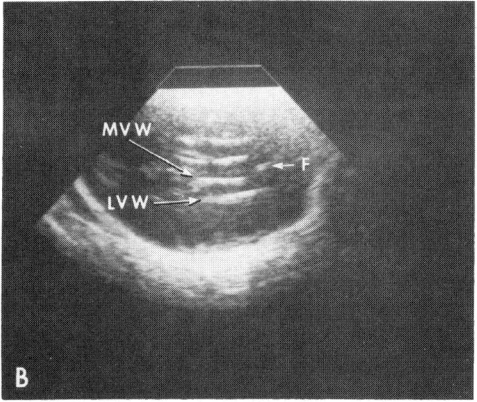

Figure 11. *A*, The medial wall (MVW) of the lateral ventricular bodies is visible on this axial in utero scan. Although the LVW/HW ratio is normal, the visible medial wall signifies early ventricular enlargement. *B*, Scan confirming mild ventricular dilatation in the newborn. F, falx cerebri.

abnormality of the arachnoid villi blocking the flow of cerebrospinal fluid into the dural venous channels or overproduction of cerebrospinal fluid by the choroid plexus beyond the ability of the arachnoid villi to absorb it. The recurrence rate for communicating hydrocephalus is from 1 to 4 per cent. The less common noncommunicating (obstructive) hydrocephalus is secondary either to aqueductal stenosis (a condition that may occur as an X-linked recessive trait) or impedance of cerebrospinal fluid flow through the foramina of the fourth ventricle (Magendie and Luschka). As a general rule, obstructive (and to a lesser degree nonobstructive) hydrocephalus is usually progressive as the fetus develops. It is now becoming recognized that mild to moderate ventricular dilatation (early hydrocephalus) may not progress. These fetuses tend to have less severe anomalies, most commonly midline defects such as absence of the septum pellucidum (Fig. 12) or corpus callosum. Nonprogressive early hydrocephalus does not, therefore, carry the poor prognosis attached to either severe or progressive hydrocephalus and does not usually have associated spinal anomalies.

Abnormalities associated with hydrocephalus include spina bifida, meningocele, and encephalocele (Fig. 19). It is therefore important to thoroughly examine the fetus for these associated anomalies once hydrocephalus has been identified. Arnold-

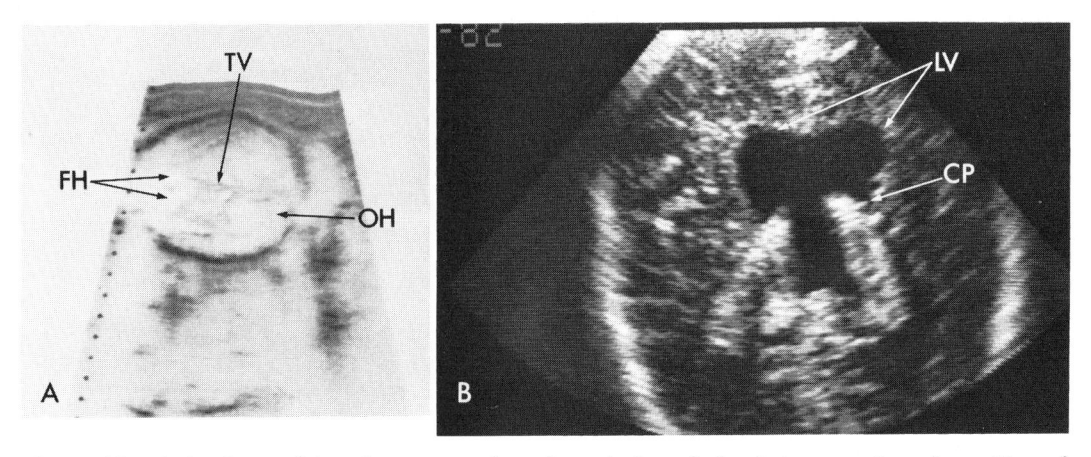

Figure 12. *A*, Axial scan of the calvarium reveals moderate hydrocephalus. Later scans showed no evidence for progression in the degree of hydrocephalus. FH, frontal horns; OH, occipital horns; TV, third ventricle. *B*, Coronal scan angled posteriorly toward the occipital horns in the immediate newborn period. The lateral ventricles are enlarged. In addition there is midline fusion of the lateral ventricles with absence of the normal septum pellucidum. LV, midbody lateral ventricle; CP, choroid plexus within lateral ventricle.

Chiari malformation is also associated with hydrocephalus although this determination preterm is difficult. Determining the level of obstruction is highly useful when progression can be unequivocally established early in gestation. This is especially true now that intrauterine shunt therapy is being attempted to treat hydrocephalus in the fetus.

Microcephaly

Microcephaly is an uncommon condition which is of clinical importance when there is coexistent micrencephaly and mental retardation. The true incidence of microcephaly is not known because many affected fetuses spontaneously abort or are stillborn. Estimates of the incidence of this anomaly range from 1 in every 6200 to 8500 births.

Etiologies for microcephaly can be divided into three groups: (1) inherited microcephaly, which is considered to be an autosomal recessive trait associated with parental consanguinity or the Meckel-Gruber syndrome (polydactyly, encephalocele, polycystic kidneys, and microcephaly); (2) chromosomal abnormalities, as seen in trisomies; and (3) environmental damage resulting from prenatal radiation or viral infection. While it is clear that some of these causes may result in sonographically demonstrable involvement early in pregnancy (Meckel-Gruber syndrome), others may occur later in pregnancy (viral infection).

True microcephaly has been best defined as an abnormally small head having a biparietal measurement more than 3 standard deviations below the mean (Fig. 13). If the fetal head measurement lies between 2 and 3 standard deviations below the mean, no strong correlation exists with either microcephaly or mental retardation. This determination obviously requires an accurate menstrual history to be reliable. Other helpful indicators include an abnormal head to body ratio associated with normal body growth (thus excluding growth

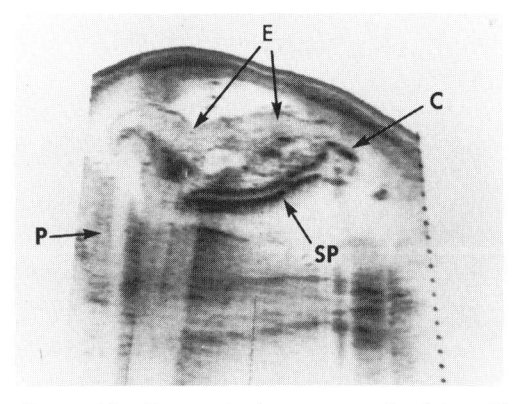

Figure 13. Parasagittal sonogram of a fetus with multiple congenital anomalies associated with microcephaly. The very small calvarium (C) is seen attached to the cervical portion of the spine (SP). E, marked body wall edema; P, placenta.

retardation). Head area measurement is useful to exclude the abnormal biparietal diameter associated with craniosynostosis in which biparietal diameter may measure less than 2 standard deviations below the norm while brain size is still normal. Abnormal intracranial morphology is further supporting evidence for microcephaly; however, normal intracranial anatomy may be present. The diagnosis of microcephaly in borderline cases is extremely difficult in the latter stages of pregnancy. If the intracranial anatomy appears normal when the calvarial size is borderline, this diagnosis should be offered most cautiously.

Hydranencephaly

Hydranencephaly is congenital absence of the cerebral hemispheres. The midbrain including the basal ganglia is present, as is the cerebellum. The abnormality is thought to represent the end result of bilateral internal carotid artery occlusion early in development.[14] The cerebral hemispheres consequently fail to develop and are reduced to a thin gliomatous layer of tissue surrounding a large collection of cerebrospinal fluid which occupies the majority of the cranial vault.

The sonographic appearance is typical (Fig. 14). The cranial vault is usually enlarged and contains a nearly circumferential fluid-filled space surrounding the midbrain and basal ganglia. No midline echo is seen because of the absence of the falx. However, the third ventricle can be delineated. At the base of the brain a small rounded soft tissue density is identified in the midline which retains the typical appearance of the brainstem and portions of the basal ganglia and sometimes occipital lobes. The tentorium can be seen to sweep posteriorly, dividing the largely fluid-filled anterior and middle cranial fossae from the posterior cranial fossa. Polyhydramnios may be an associated finding. The amount of remaining brain tissue is variable and depends on the volume of infarcted tissue.

Holoprosencephaly

Holoprosencephaly is a defect in the formation of midline structures resulting in a

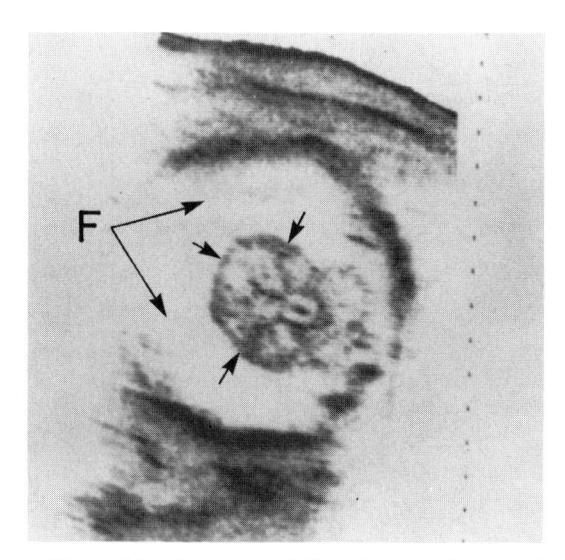

Figure 14. Axial scan of the calvarium of a typical case of hydranencephaly. The telencephalon is largely absent, being replaced by fluid (F) which surrounds the preserved lower brain centers (arrows). No falx echo is seen. If one compares the preserved brain centers with Figure 6, one can clearly identify the third ventricle, basal ganglia, aqueduct of Sylvius and the preserved hippocampal and parahippocampal gyri. Posterior to these structures the normal cerebellar hemispheres are noted.

single enlarged midline ventricle with associated facial anomalies. This is a rare condition but because of the intracranial anatomic aberrations is recognizable in utero. This defect results from failure of the mesoderm to interact with the ectoderm and entoderm during the fifth week of development to form the prosencephalon. Consequently there is failure of formation of the diencephalon and in lateral expansion and cleavage of the telencephalon to form the cerebral hemispheres.

Holoprosencephaly is recognized most commonly as a large cystic space within the cerebral hemispheres which is median or paramedian in location (Fig. 15). This fluid-filled structure represents a large central ventricle which expands into the parietal-occipital regions or on occasion into the frontal lobe region. Because the hemispheres fail to develop normally, lateral ventricular structures and midline falx are absent which helps differentiate this anomaly from subarachnoid cyst or the Dandy-Walker syndrome. Associated facial anomalies include cyclopia, ethmocephaly, and cleft lip. Association with the trisomy 13-15 syndrome and a familial occurrence have been described.

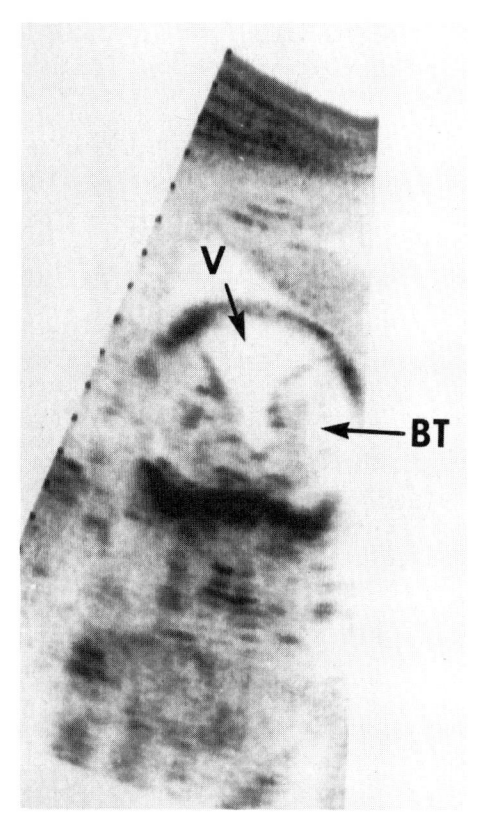

Figure 15. Coronal scan of the calvarium of a fetus with holoprosencephaly. The large third ventricle communicates directly with a large median ventricle (V) flanked by the brain tissue (BT).

Miscellaneous

Other cystic intracranial malformations are among the more recognizable lesions in the fetus. It has already been demonstrated that hydrocephalus, holoprosencephaly and hydranencephaly are recognizable because the lesions are fluid filled. This is also the case in the Dandy-Walker syndrome which is cystic dilatation of the fourth ventricle often associated with hydrocephalus. The posterior fossa is enlarged and fluid-filled because of obstruction to the outflow of cerebrospinal fluid from the fourth ventricle. Distinction between Dandy-Walker cyst and subarachnoid cyst of the posterior fossa is difficult.[4] Agenesis of the corpus callosum is an associated anomaly but has yet to be diagnosed prenatally.

Intracranial teratoma has been successfully diagnosed prenatally in an infant with an enlarged head and unrecognizable intracranial structures.[8] The importance in recognizing normal anatomy is stressed as the key in making this diagnosis. Extracranial teratoma or epignathus has also been diagnosed; however, normal intracranial anatomy accompanied this malformation.[11]

Vascular anomalies have the potential of being diagnosed prenatally though none has yet been reported. Cooperberg has diagnosed such a case but has not yet reported it. An aneurysm of the vein of Galen (arteriovenous malformation) can be identified as a fluid-containing structure near the midline posteriorly (in the region of the straight sinus). This entity may, however, be confused with posterior fossa cysts and holoprosencephaly. Large arteriovenous malformations may result in hydrops fetalis.

Finally intracranial hemorrhage has been diagnosed in the fetus. The appearance is similar to that in the neonate. Earlier and more frequent prenatal diagnosis of these and other entities is sure to be reported in the future as investigators continue to pay closer attention to intracranial morphology.

PATHOLOGY OF THE FETAL CALVARIUM, SPINE, AND MENINGES

The incidence of neural tube defects in the United States is approximately 2 in 1000 pregnancies. The recurrence risk is 1 in 20 if there has been one previously affected fetus and rises to 1 in 10 after the second affected fetus.[17] Since 90 per cent of neural tube defects are a first time occurrence, it becomes impractical to screen every pregnancy for the presence of such anomalies using ultrasound.[2] However, a group at special risk can be identified. This group constitutes those patients noted to have elevation of the serum or amniotic fluid alpha-fetoprotein.

Alpha-fetoprotein is a glycoprotein synthesized by the fetal liver. The amniotic fluid displays a unimodal concentration curve first appearing in the sixth week of gestation, peaking at 14 to 16 weeks, and declining thereafter until delivery.[7] Low concentrations of alpha-fetoprotein normally enter the amniotic fluid primarily through fetal urination. Alpha-fetoprotein also enters the maternal circulation in measurable quantities in serum. When portions of the fetal body are not covered by normal integument (as in neural tube defects), the alpha-fetoprotein levels in both the maternal circulation and the amniotic fluid are elevated. Presumably, the alpha-fetoprotein leaks across the fetal capillaries supplying the membranes (or in the case of ruptured meningocele sacs, the surface tissues) which are not covered by normal integument. Unfortunately, 10 per cent of neural tube defects are completely covered with normal skin so that no elevation in the alpha-fetoprotein results. Problems exist also with false-negative results in small defects and false positive results seen with inaccurate dates, twins, fetal death, and amniotic fluid contaminated with fetal blood. Non-neural tube defects not covered by normal skin, such as omphalocele, will also result in elevation of the alpha-fetoprotein.

Patients having a fetus with a neural tube defect present in one of two ways. The patient may be at increased risk because of a prior affected fetus or a known elevated serum or amniotic fluid alpha-fetoprotein. In these patients there is an obviously high suspicion and care is taken to carefully examine the regions where the defects occur. The second and statistically more common patient is the one in whom a neural tube defect is an incidental finding on sonograms performed for other indications.

Sonography is a pivotal examination in the patient presenting with an elevated alpha-fetoprotein level or in whom a question has been raised regarding the presence of a neural tube abnormality on a routine examination. When performed carefully, it is highly accurate in confirming a fetal anomaly or normalcy. In a recently completed study at our institution, patients with borderline and markedly elevated levels of alpha-fetoprotein were examined sonographically for evidence of neural tube defects. Only one of the patients with borderline elevation of alpha-fetoprotein level demonstrated an abnormality. The remainder, diagnosed as normal, delivered normal fetuses. In the group with markedly elevated alpha-fetoprotein level (5 standard deviations or more above the mean), two fetuses were correctly diagnosed as normal. The remainder had varying anomalies including neural tube defects, omphalocele, cystic hygroma, and fetal demise. All were correctly diagnosed in utero.

The normal ultrasonographic appearance of the developing fetal spine is fully covered in chapter 3. In this section we review the appearance of the more common neural tube defects affecting the bony calvarium and spine.

Encephalomeningocele

This condition occurs in approximately 1 in 2000 births. Encephalomeningoceles result from failure of the surface ectoderm to separate from the neuroectoderm. This results in a mesodermal (bony calvarium) defect which allows herniation of either the meninges alone or the brain and meninges both through the bony defect. The most common site of occurrence is the occipital midline (75 per cent) followed by the frontoethmoidal (13 per cent) and parietal (12 per cent) locations.[17]

Encephalomeningoceles are recognized as spherical fluid- or brain-filled sacs extending off of the bony calvarium in the occipital or frontal location or as a bony defect in these regions (Figs. 16 and 17). When intact, identification of the meningoencephalocele sac is not usually difficult. In the suspect gestation with elevated alpha-fetoprotein, a systematic and detailed approach should be employed to evaluate the calvarium for these defects in the typical locations described above.

Absence of brain tissue within the meningocele sac is the single most favorable prognostic feature for survival which can be determined by ultrasound. Associated anomalies include hydrocephalus, agenesis of the corpus callosum, Dandy-Walker syndrome, and Meckel syndrome. Lesions having a similar appearance to encephalomeningocele include cystic hygroma (Fig. 18) and hemangioma (which tend to have multiple septations inside a fluid-filled structure) and teratoma which more often occurs in the nasal region and is usually solid and irregular.

Myelomeningocele—Spina Bifida

Myelomeningocele is a more common and severe defect than meningocele and

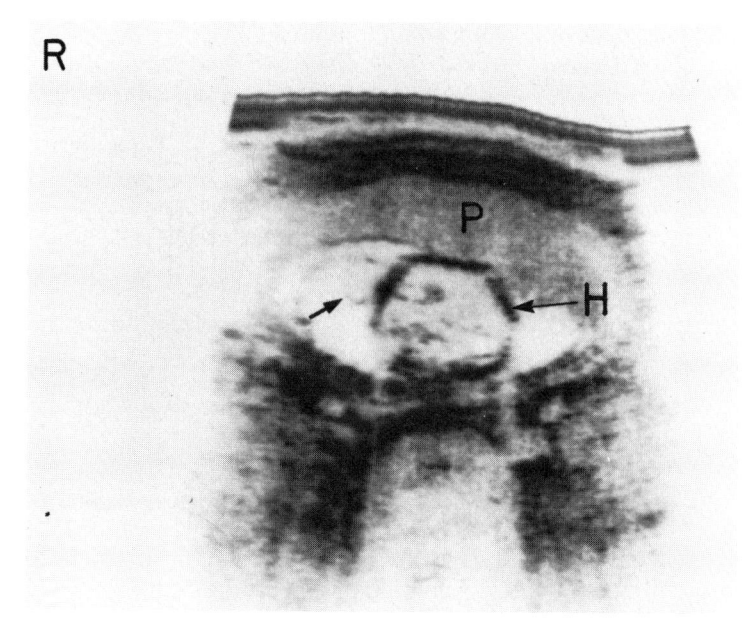

Figure 16. Axial scan of a fetal head (H) showing a small midline encephalocele (arrow). P, placenta; R, right.

has an incidence of 1 in 1000 births. It may occur anywhere along the spine but is most common in the lumbar region. The malformation results from failure of closure of the neural tube at three to four weeks resulting in an exposed neural plate. The defect is variable in size and content ranging from spina bifida cystica (small defect containing only meninges) to myelomeningocele which is a longer segment and contains spinal cord and nerve roots. Neurologic defects range from minor anesthesia to complete paraparesis or death.[1]

The fetal spine is easily and clearly evaluated by 16 to 17 weeks of development. As discussed elsewhere in this volume, the

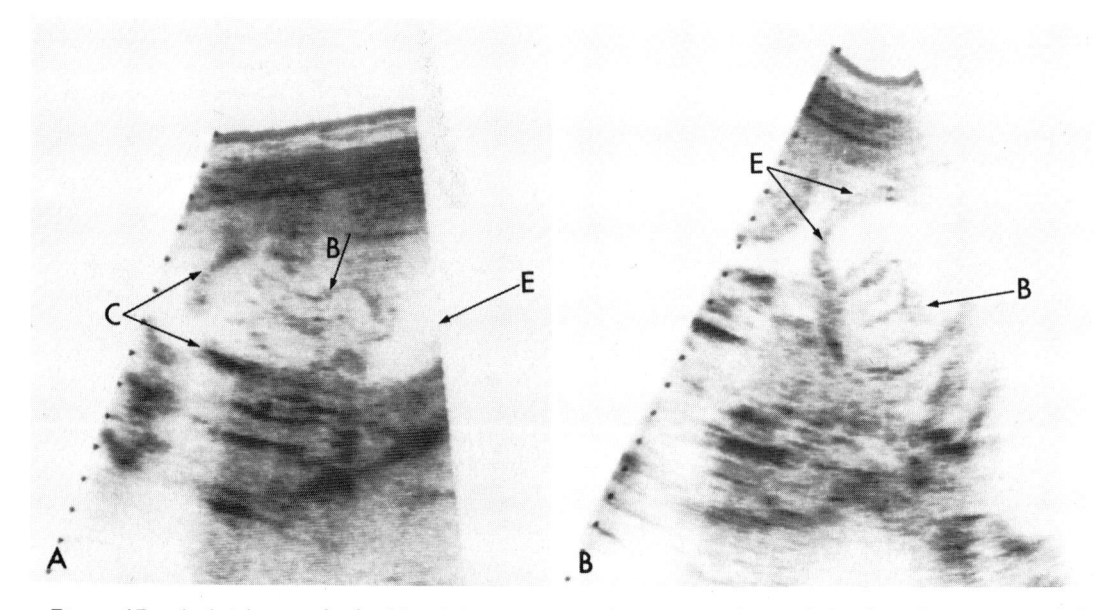

Figure 17. *A,* Axial scan of a fetal head demonstrates a large occipital encephalocele with a majority of the brain herniating through the defect in the bony calvarium. C, calvarium; B, brain; E, encephalocele. *B,* Oblique scan in the same fetus shows to better advantage the brain substance herniating into the meningeal sac. E, encephalocele; B, brain.

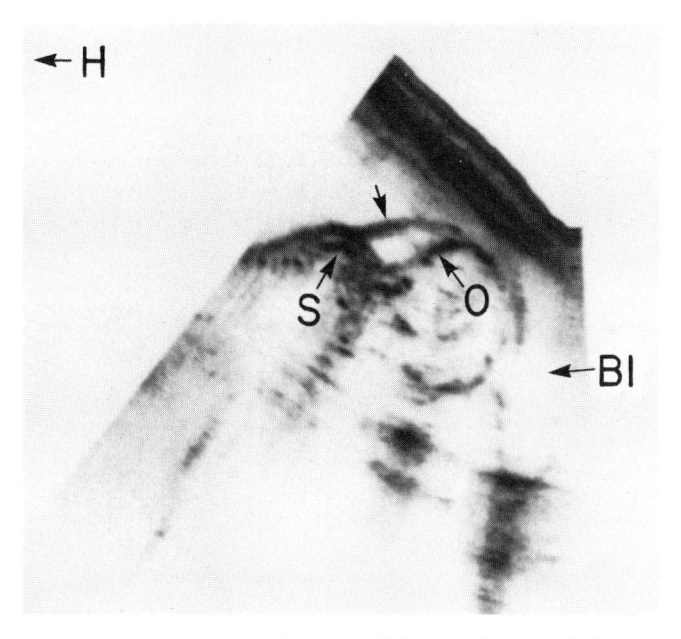

Figure 18. Oblique scan demonstrates a cystic hygroma of the neck (*arrow*) which must be distinguished from an encephalomeningocele. In this case the distinction is easy, since this lesion lies between the scapula (S) and the *lateral* aspect of the occiput (O). B, maternal bladder; H, direction of maternal head.

normal posterior ossification centers are seen as two closely spaced parallel lines of echos which widen normally in the cervical region. The distance between the posterior ossification centers is tantamount to the interpedicular distances. In the transverse plane of section three ossification centers are identified, all within close proximity surrounding the spinal cord. In spina bifida, which is the bony accompaniment to myelomeningocele, there is separation on the transverse and longitudinal scans of the posterior ossification centers. Normally in transverse planes the posterior ossification centers parallel each other or angle toward one another. Spina bifida can be diagnosed when the posterior ossification centers splay outwardly or display a "U" shape and are further apart than the ossification centers above or below the defect (Fig. 19). The latter is noted on longitudinal images. The cleft in the soft tissues can be seen often. Defects recognized in this form are easily diagnosed if more than three segments are involved. If two or less segments are involved, the diagnosis becomes more difficult. These features must be utilized to make the diagnosis if the sac

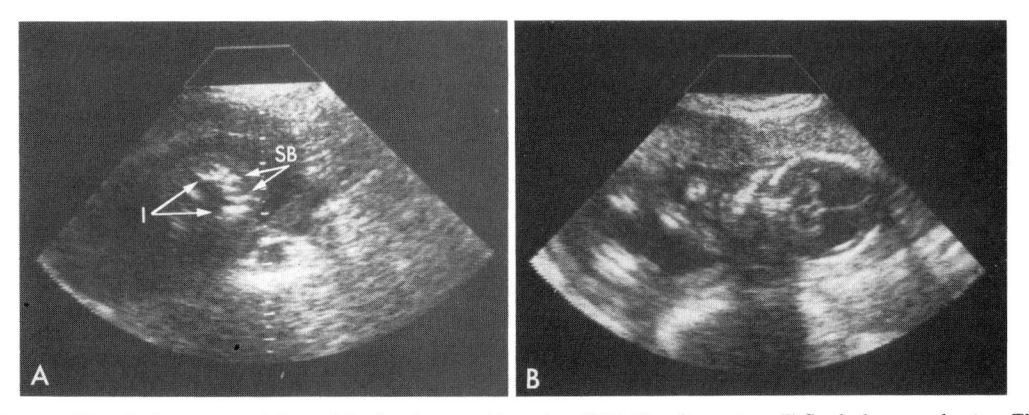

Figure 19. *A*, Open spine defect of the lumbosacral junction (SB). The iliac wings (I) flank the sacral spine. The posterior ossification centers of the spine are flared in a typical "U" appearance. *B*, Associated hydrocephalus in the same fetus. The gestational age is approximately 20 weeks.

is not intact. If the sac is intact, the anomaly then is more easily recognized as a cystic extension off the dorsal aspect of the spine which in real-time may have a shimmering quality with fetal motion.

As with encephalomeningoceles associated anomalies should be looked for and include hydrocephalus, encephalocele, and Arnold-Chiari II malformation.

REFERENCES

1. Babcock, D. S., and Han, B. K.: Cranial sonographic findings in meningomyelocele. Am. J. Roentgenol., *136*:563–569, 1981.
2. Campbell, S.: Early prenatal diagnosis of neural tube defects by ultrasound. Clin. Obstet. Gynecol., *20*:351–359, 1977.
3. Cunningham, M. E., and Walls, W. I.: Ultrasound in the evaluation of anencephaly. Radiology, *118*:165–167, 1976.
4. Dempsey, P. J., and Hobb, H. J.: In utero diagnosis of the Dandy-Walker syndrome: Differentiation from extra-axial posterior fossa cyst. J. Clin. Ultrasound, *9*:403–405, 1981.
5. Fiske, C. E., Filly, R. A., and Callen, P. W.: Sonographic measurement of lateral ventricular width in early ventricular dilation. J. Clin. Ultrasound, *9*:303–307, 1981.
6. Freeman, R., K., McQuown, D. S., Secrist, L. J., et al.: The diagnosis of fetal hydrocephalus before viability. Obstet. Gynecol., *49*:109–112, 1977.
7. Goldberg, M. F., and Daisley, G. P.: Interpreting elevated amniotic fluid alpha-fetoprotein levels in clinical practice: Use of the predictive value positive concept. Am. J. Obstet. Gynecol., *133*:126–132, 1979.
8. Hoff, N. R., and Mackay, I. M.: Prenatal ultrasound diagnosis of intracranial teratoma. J. Clin. Ultrasound, *8*:247–249, 1980.
9. Johnson, M. L., Dunne, M. G., Mack, L. A., et al.: Evaluation of fetal intracranial anatomy by static and real-time ultrasound. J. Clin. Ultrasound, *8*:311–318, 1980.
10. Johnson, M. L., Mack, L. A., Rumack, C. M., et al.: B-mode echoencephalography in the normal and high risk infant. Am. J. Roentgenol., *133*:375, 1979.
11. Kang, K. W., Hissong, S. L., and Langer, A.: Prenatal ultrasonic diagnosis of epignathus. J. Clin. Ultrasound, *6*:330–331, 1978.
12. Kim, M. S., and Elyadcrani, M. K.: Sonographic diagnosis of cerebroventricular hemorrhage in utero. Radiology, *142*:479–480, 1982.
13. Kurtz, A. B., Wapner, R. I., Rubin, C. E., et al.: Ultrasound criteria for in utero diagnosis of microcephaly. J. Clin. Ultrasound, *8*:11–16, 1980.
14. Lee, T. G., and Warren, B. H.: Antenatal diagnosis of hydranencephaly by ultrasound: Correlation with ventriculography and computed tomography. J. Clin. Ultrasound, *5*:271–273, 1977.
15. Lehr, C., and DiRe, J.: Rare occurrence of a holoacardious acephalic monster: Sonographic and pathologic findings. J. Clin. Ultrasound, *6*:259–261, 1978.
16. Morgan, C. L., Hanley, A., Christakos, A., et al.: Antenatal detections of fetal structural defects with ultrasound. J. Clin. Ultrasound, *3*:287–290, 1975.
17. Robinson, H. P., Hood, V. D., Adam, A. H., et al.: Diagnostic ultrasound: Early detection of fetal neural tube defects. Obstet. Gynecol., *56*:705–710, 1980.

7

Evaluation of Normal Fetal Growth and the Detection of Intrauterine Growth Retardation

Russell L. Deter, M.D., Frank P. Hadlock, M.D., and Ronald B. Harrist, Ph.D.

During the course of its development in utero, the fetus undergoes significant anatomic changes which we characterize as growth. These changes may be in the size, shape, or relative position of different anatomic structures,[11] but in the past primary attention has been given to changes in size. Measures of size include weight, volume, surface area, the area of anatomic planes, circumferences, and diameters. Monitoring how such parameters change during pregnancy has become the primary means for evaluating fetal growth.

Monitoring fetal growth is of major concern in the management of any pregnancy because of the consequences associated with decreased growth in utero (Fig. 1). Numerous studies have shown that fetuses with evidence of intrauterine growth retardation are at increased risk for problems in the perinatal and newborn periods as well as for long-term sequelae. These problems include premature delivery, asphyxia, and death in utero in the perinatal period[52] and hypocalcemia, hypoglycemia, polycythemia, meconium aspiration, intracerebral hemorrhage, irritability, and convulsions in the newborn period.[1] Long-term effects such as reduced somatic growth,[23,36] hyperactivity, shortened attention span, seizures, speech problems, poor coordination, discipline problems, learning disabilities, and mental retardation[23,35] have been reported. The seriousness of these problems makes it essential that every effort be made to detect and treat intrauterine growth retardation whenever it occurs.

Monitoring the growth process in utero has several objectives. The first is the detection of abnormal growth patterns as early in pregnancy as possible. Since many growth abnormalities are caused by fetal malnutrition (inadequate nutrients or oxygen[3]), early detection allows early treatment and thus minimizes damage to the fetus. A second objective is to determine if the growth abnormality is progressive and, if so, to quantitate the degree. Because in utero treatment modalities are limited, one must determine when the risks of remaining in the uterus outweigh the risks of premature delivery. In making this decision, adequate characterization of the magnitude of the growth abnormality is essential. Finally, one would like to obtain a description of the abnormal growth process. Although not realized as yet, it may be possible to correlate etiologies, outcomes, or responses to treatment with specific abnormal growth patterns. Such correlations require the availability of well-documented growth patterns and, if proven, would be of significant value in the obstetric management of these patients.

NORMAL GROWTH

Choice of Growth Parameter

The detection and characterization of abnormal fetal growth obviously require the availability of an adequate description of normal fetal growth to serve as a reference. As mentioned earlier and discussed in more detail elsewhere,[11] the definition of "growth" is not as obvious as one might think. In considering a growth problem, it is essential that an appropriate parameter, or set of parameters, be chosen. With respect to the fetus, it seems reasonable to

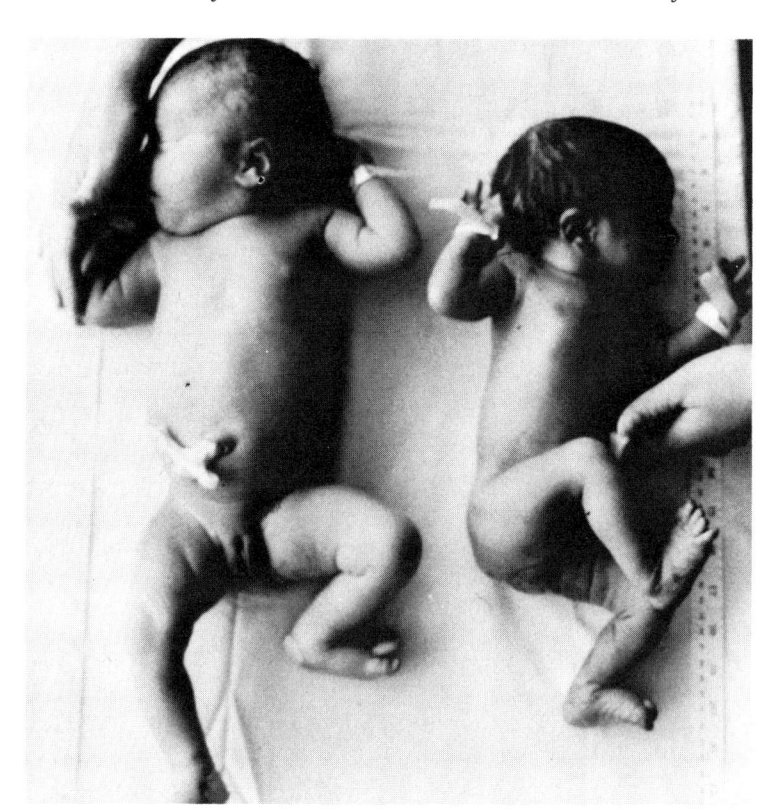

Figure 1. Two infants of the same gestational age. The one on the left is normal; the infant on the right is growth retarded. The growth-retarded infant demonstrates decreased weight, length, and subcutaneous tissue.

choose parameters that characterize the size of different parts of the body. As discussed previously,[11] there are many parameters from which to choose. Since the fetus is a three-dimensional object of complex geometry, the most logical parameters would be the three-dimensional measures of weight, volume, and surface area. Methods for measuring such parameters using the two-dimensional images obtained with ultrasound are available.[6, 11] However, with the exception of those for weight, these methods are currently too time-consuming for clinical use. However, continued development of computer-assisted image analysis may change this situation in the near future.

Because of the two-dimensional character of the ultrasonic images used in fetal evaluations, more practical parameters would be a two-dimensional measure such as profile area or one-dimensional measures such as circumference and diameter. Such measures require appropriate and reproducible selection of the anatomic plane on which the measurements will be made. As this single plane is used to represent an object with complex three-dimensional geometry, measurement variability will be significantly affected if the measurements are not made on the same plane in different individuals. In choosing between profile area, circumference, and diameter measures, one should consider the sensitivity of the measure to changes in shape, its ease of measurement, and the accuracy obtainable. Areas and circumferences are much less sensitive than diameters to change in shape but are more difficult to measure, particularly if hand methods are employed. The simplicity of the measurement process makes diameter measurements inherently more reliable, but well-defined anatomic landmarks must be available to specify the dimension to be measured. Selection in any given case depends on the anatomic situation and the purpose of the measurement.

An example of the importance of the measure chosen can be found in the data on head growth evaluation. Although head volumes can be determined (Deter, unpublished), most studies of head growth have utilized measurements of various two-dimensional or one-dimensional parameters.[11] Because the head is a large complex structure, there are many planes identifiable by the internal anatomy of the brain[32, 37] which could be chosen for measurement.

When the plane used is not standardized, variations in the values obtained at different stages of pregnancy are seen in measurements of head area (HA), head circumference (HC), and fronto-occipital diameter.[11] The effects of plane choice have been studied in greatest detail for biparietal diameter (BPD). Differences as large as 1 cm were seen between measurements made at the optimal level and those made elsewhere.[29]

The sensitivity of diameter measurements to changes in shape has been documented for biparietal diameter in which the presence of dolicocephaly or brachycephaly resulted in significant errors in estimates of menstrual age derived from measurements of biparietal diameter.[27] The effect of changes in shape on measurements of head circumference has not been investigated but would be expected to be considerably less important. Comparisons of the reproducibility (intra-observer error) of measurements of biparietal diameter and head circumference [mean per cent difference between two measurements: -0.36 ± 1.69 S.D.% (BPD); -0.57 ± 2.12 S.D.% (HC)] have documented the greater reliability of the former (Deter, unpublished).[10]

Evaluation of the Growth Process

Having selected the parameter and the means for measuring it, one is now ready to proceed with the evaluation of the growth process. At the initial examination, the data collected can only be compared to the range of normal values obtained at the same time in pregnancy in previous investigations. In such comparisons two factors are of primary importance. The first is the quality of the gestational age specification. For virtually all parameters of fetal growth, the range of normal values varies with gestational age, and what changes occur depend on the parameter being measured.[11] Therefore, proper evaluation of specific values requires accurate dating if a proper choice of the normal range is to be made. The second factor concerns selection of the appropriate set of normal data for the population under study. As has been demonstrated recently for measurements of head and abdominal circumference,[13] estimates of normal variability obtained by different investigators can be different. Because of this, normative values must be evaluated to determine which are most appropriate for the population being studied. This usually requires comparison of a preliminary set of data from one's own institution with published standard curves. If reasonable agreement is obtained with a given standard curve, these data can be used. However, periodic checks should be made to be certain that the original sample was not biased or that the population characteristics have not changed. If appropriate standards cannot be found, then they must be developed as indicated in the subsequent discussion.

Standard Growth Curves

The reliability of standard growth curves depends on the population studied, the accuracy of the measurements, and the appropriateness of the analysis. Basically there are two types of fetal growth studies, longitudinal and cross-sectional,[11] each with its own strengths and weaknesses. Longitudinal growth studies, in which individual fetuses are examined serially throughout pregnancy, give actual fetal growth curves, provided reliable dating is available (see Fig. 2). Such curves allow one to determine if one or more populations are present and provide the information needed for calculating estimates of the population growth curves and their variability.[11] In these latter calculations, the representativeness of the sample studied is crucial. Obtaining such a sample can be difficult because of the time and effort associated with longitudinal studies. However, recent investigations[15] have indicated that sample sizes as small as 20 fetuses can give reliable biparietal diameter, head and abdominal circumference growth curves, provided measurements are made at three-week intervals between 14 weeks and delivery.

An alternative solution to this sampling problem is the use of cross-sectional studies of fetal growth to obtain estimates of population growth curves. In such studies, a large number of fetuses are measured only once during pregnancy, and an estimate of the population growth curve is obtained from these data using mathematic fitting

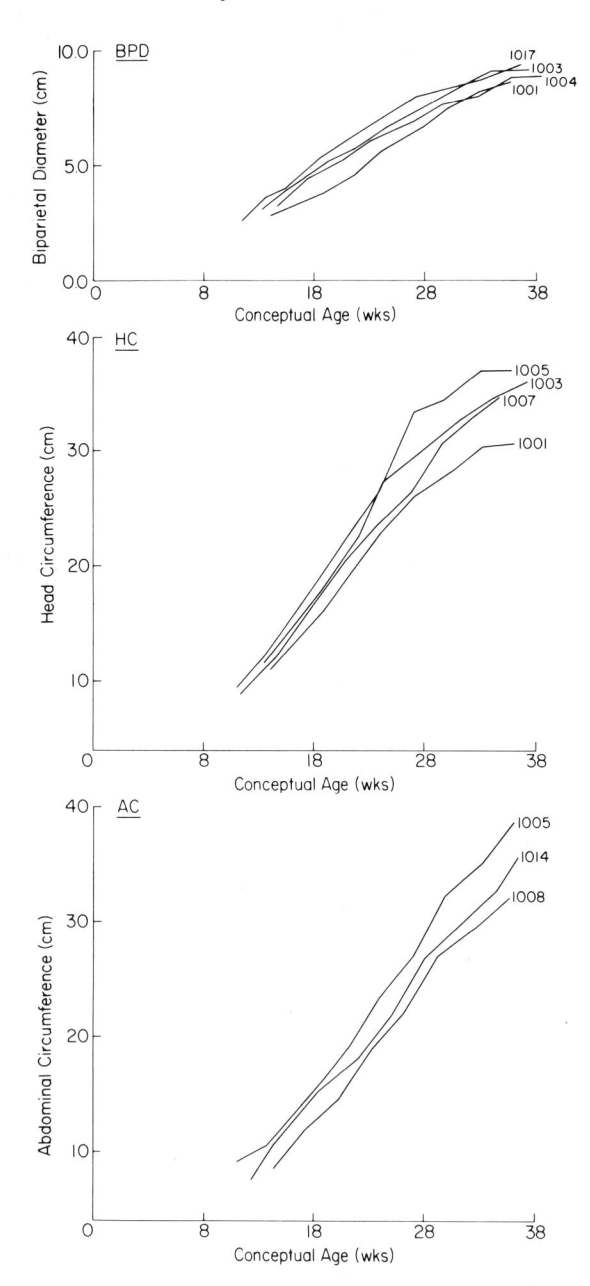

Figure 2. Individual fetal growth curves. Examples of growth curves for biparietal diameter, head circumference, and abdominal circumference for individual fetuses. The data used to construct these curves were obtained from serial ultrasound examinations of normal fetuses with known dates of conception.[5] The curves for all 20 fetuses studied were confined to the region demarcated by the outer curves in these subfigures. (*From* Deter, R. L., Harrist, R. B., Hadlock, F. P., et al.: The use of ultrasound in the assessment of normal fetal growth: A review. J. Clin. Ultrasound, 9:481–493, 1981, with permission.)

procedures.[11, 15] These estimates are reliable provided the sample size is adequate, the sample is uniformly distributed throughout the time interval studied, and there are no sources of systematic variability which affect certain fetuses more than others. In fact, as indicated previously,[15, 28] growth curves obtained under these conditions can be expected to be very similar to average longitudinal growth curves derived from representative samples (Fig. 3). Such results strongly indicate that an appropriate estimate of the true population growth curve has been obtained and that potential sources of error in both the longitudinal and cross-sectional studies are not significant.[28]

Presentations of growth curve data tend to focus on the expected or average (depending on how the data is analyzed) values at different stages in pregnancy. *However, it is the normal variability associated with these values which is actually more important in evaluating measurements from individual patients.* Estimates of this variability can be obtained from standard deviation or percentile calculations using data collected at specified time points or through regression analysis. However, the former method is very sensitive to sample size (maximal errors in standard deviation estimates increase from 39 to 188 per cent as the sample size decreases from 25 to 5[49]) whereas the latter requires variance homogeneity to be valid since it provides only an "average" value for the entire time period studied. A more powerful approach involves plotting the values of the difference between the expected values and their corresponding observed values (often called deviations) as a function of gestational age.[16] Such plots allow evaluation of the magnitude and regularity of the variability along the time line and permit detection of points of change in variability (Fig. 4). With this information, appropriate normal ranges can be determined even when variability heterogeneities of different types are present as shown recently for head and abdominal circumferences.[13] Such analyses also provide a means for quickly comparing the variability of different data sets (Fig. 4), which is important in choosing the appropriate normative data for evaluating individuals from a specific population.

Definition of the Boundary Between Normal and Abnormal Parameter Values

It is conventional to set the boundary between normal and abnormal values arbitrarily based on some concept of the "normal range." As illustrated in ultrasonographic studies of intrauterine growth retardation, boundaries such as the third percentile, the tenth percentile, and twenty-fifth percentile, and two standard deviations below the mean have been used depending on the investigation and the parameter being evaluated.[14] Percentile values make no distribution assumptions whereas standard deviations imply that

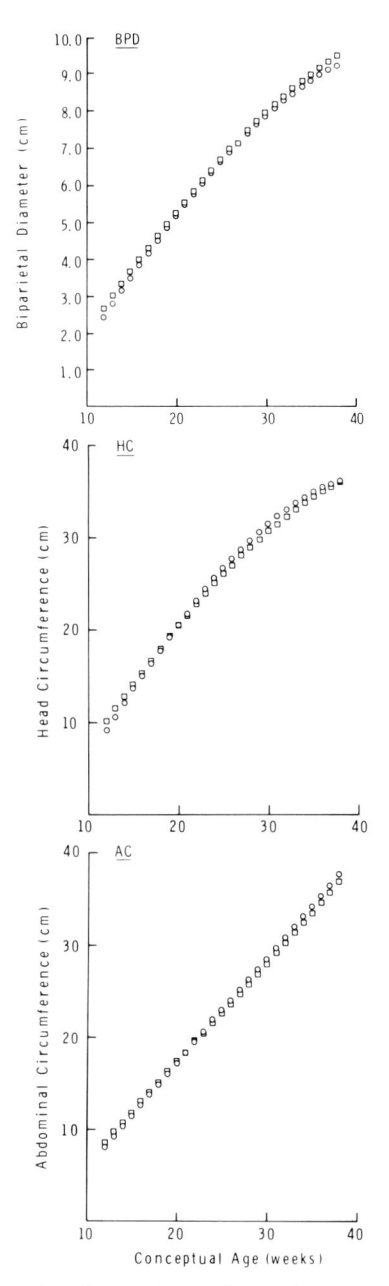

Figure 3. Comparisons of growth curves derived from cross-sectional and longitudinal studies of fetal growth. Average longitudinal growth curve (○) and the cross-sectional growth curve (□) for three fetal parameters (BPD,HC,AC). The average longitudinal curves were constructed from 20 individual curves derived from data obtained in serial ultrasound examinations of normal fetuses with known dates of conception.[5] The cross-sectional curves were derived from measurements on 533 (BPD) or 252 (HC,AC) normal fetuses.[13,28] No fetus was measured more than once in these studies. The values presented in each subfigure are the predicted values calculated from the mathematic function which optimally modeled each specific set of experimental data. (A reproduced from Hadlock, F. P., Deter, R. L., Harrist, R. B., et al.: Fetal biparietal diameter: A critical re-evaluation of the relation to menstrual age by means of real-time ultrasound. J. Ultrasound Med., 1:97–104, 1982, with permission. B and C reproduced from Deter, R. L., Harrist, R. B., Hadlock, F. P., et al.: Fetal head and abdominal circumferences: A critical re-evaluation of the relation to menstrual age using dynamic image ultrasonography. J. Clin. Ultrasound, 1982, in press, with permission.)

the parameter is normally distributed. Use of such boundaries (except the 25th percentile) implicitly assumes that it is more important to minimize false positive (normal fetuses considered to be abnormal) than false negatives (abnormal fetuses considered to be normal) in those situations in which there is a significant overlap in parameter values between the normal and abnormal populations. As both false negatives and false positives are significant in the detection of abnormal fetal growth, a more logical approach would be one that establishes the boundary between normal and abnormal values so that the number of both false negatives and false positives is minimized. This can be done using linear discriminant analysis, a statistical procedure that determines the parameter value (or values) which separates two classes of objects with minimal misclassification (Fig. 5).[7] To date, linear discriminant analysis has not been used to determine appropriate boundary values for any of the pa-

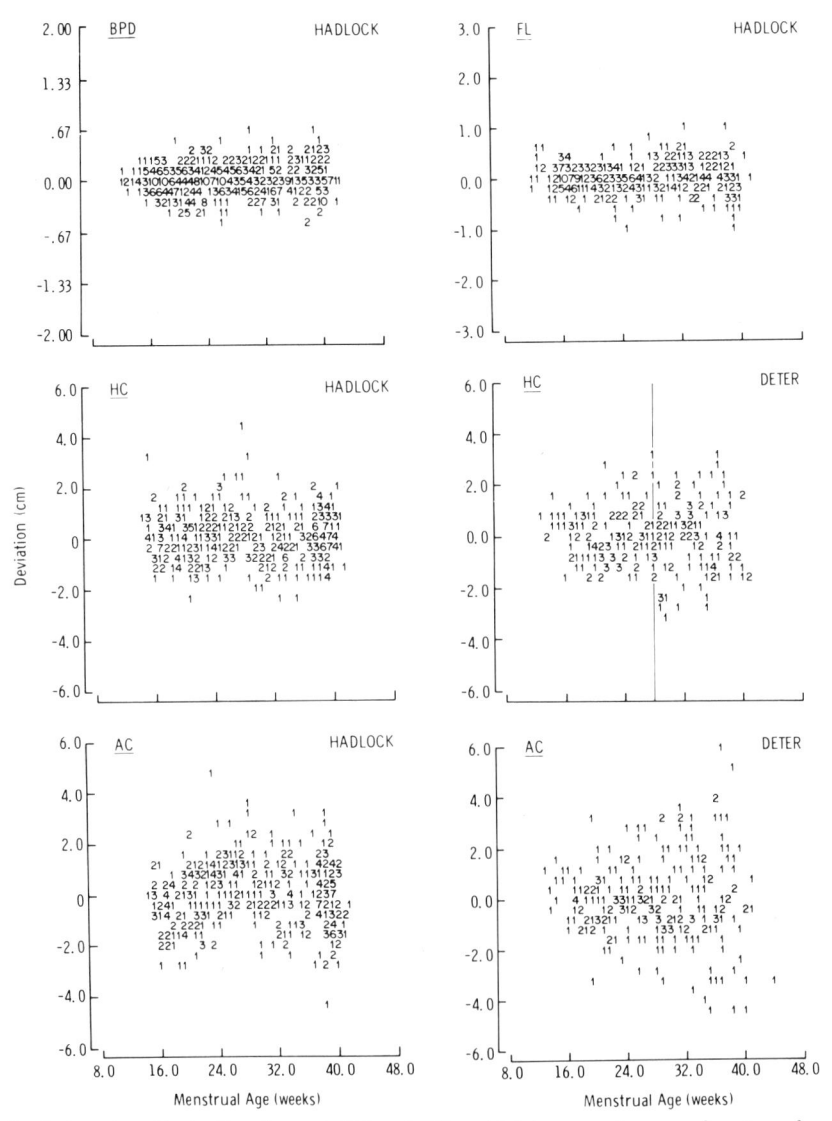

Figure 4. Deviation plots illustrating the variability of different fetal parameters as a function of menstrual age. Distributions of deviations (predicted values-observed values) as a function of menstrual age derived from the cross-sectional studies of Hadlock et al.[28,30,31,33] and Deter et al.[13] The number of measurements were 533 (BPD), 400 (HC and AC), and 338 (FL) in the studies of Hadlock et al. and 252 (HC and AC) in those of Deter et al. Note that the deviation scale factors for BPD and FL differ from those for HC and AC. The numerals indicate the number of deviations having the value indicated at the menstrual age specified. (*From* Deter, R. L., Harrist, R. B., Hadlock, F. P., et al.: Fetal head and abdominal circumferences: A critical re-evaluation of the relation to menstrual age using dynamic image ultrasonography. J. Clin. Ultrasound, 1982, in press, with permission.)

Figure 5. Weight criteria for separating clinically intrauterine well nourished (CIWN) infants from clinically intrauterine malnourished (CIMN) infants determined by linear discriminant analysis. Linear discriminant analysis is used to determine criteria for optimally separating CIWN (△) and CIMN (●) infants on the basis of their birth weights.[35] The broken line indicates the weight values at different menstrual ages (38 to 45 weeks) determined from the discriminant function which minimizes misclassification. Use of these criteria resulted in accurate classification of 89.1 per cent of the infants, with 1 (2.2 per cent) of the CIWN infants and 4 (8.7 per cent) of the CIMN infants being misclassified. For comparison, the 10th percentile values (solid line) given by Brenner et al.[2] are plotted at the bottom of the figure. Using these criteria to separate the CIWN and CIMN infants, 82.6 per cent were correctly classified, 1 (2.2 per cent) of the CIWN infants and 7 (15.2 per cent of the CIMN being misclassified.

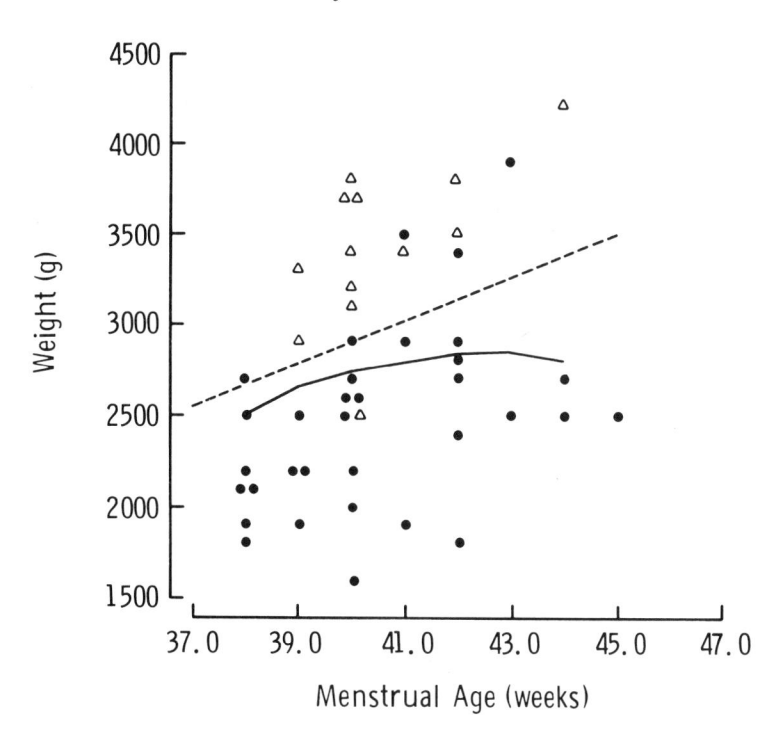

rameters employed prenatally to detect abnormally growing fetuses. Until such values are available, the traditional (though arbitrarily chosen) statistical boundaries of two standard deviations below the mean or the third percentile will have to be used. However, it should be kept in mind that the use of such boundaries may lead to an underestimation of the number of fetuses with growth abnormalities (Fig. 5).

ABNORMAL GROWTH

Types of Fetal Growth Retardation

Development of an appropriate procedure for detecting fetal growth retardation obviously depends on an appropriate definition of growth retardation. As reviewed previously,[14] almost all studies of the use of ultrasound in the prenatal detection of intrauterine growth retardation have assumed that a birth weight below the 10th percentile was the appropriate criterion for identifying the growth-retarded fetus. Although this criterion is widely used in Pediatrics, there is no evidence that it optimally separates normal and growth-retarded fetuses,[14] and it classifies 7 per cent of normal populations, as defined by conventional statistical parameters (third percentile, two standard deviations below the mean), as abnormal. This criterion also does not define a homogeneous population of growth-retarded fetuses as pointed out by Miller.[42] Small-for-dates infants have been found to be (1) short [crown-heel length (CHL) below the third percentile] but well nourished (as indicated by the Pondral Index,[42] $PI = Wt/CHL^3 \times 100$ above the third percentile), (2) malnourished (PI below the third percentile) but of normal length (CHL above the third percentile) or (3) malnourished and short. Diakoku et al.[9] extended this type of study by using the PI, CHL, HC, and weight to identify fetuses with growth abnormalities. These authors found that only 47 per cent of those fetuses showing other evidence of abnormal growth had birth weights below the 10th percentile. Hill et al.[35] have confirmed this finding in a group of 33 infants judged to be malnourished at birth on the basis of a decrease in subcutaneous tissue and muscle mass. Only 78.8 per cent of these infants had birth weights below the 10th percentile (Brenner weight tables[2]). As these results clearly indicate, *an eval-*

uation of weight alone is not adequate for determining whether or not a fetus has a growth problem. The significance of growth abnormalities not manifesting themselves as low birth weights is underlined by the results of the 14 year follow-up study carried out by Hill et al.[35] on intrauterine malnourished infants. Eleven per cent of the children with permanent neurologic impairment had birth weights above the 10th percentile while this figure was 20 per cent in those children with transient neurologic abnormalities.

Growth Profile

It is clear from the study of newborn infants[9, 35, 41, 42, 51] that intrauterine growth retardation can manifest as a decrease in weight, length, head circumference, chest circumference, abdominal circumference, subcutaneous tissue, and muscle mass (singly or in various combinations). For this reason, evaluation of a growth profile[14] would be required if intrauterine growth retardation in all its forms were to be detected. To date no ultrasonographic study using such a profile has been carried out.[14] Instead, investigators have employed a variety of one- and two-dimensional parameters, usually singly but in pairs on a few occasions, in an effort to detect growth-retarded fetuses. The results of these studies are seriously compromised by the postnatal criterion used to define the infant with intrauterine growth retardation (i.e., birth weight below the 10th percentile in most cases); but even if this were disregarded, major problems still exist. With virtually all the parameters used, there is a significant incidence (15 to 75 per cent) of normal fetuses with abnormal ultrasound parameter values and abnormal fetuses with normal parameter values.[14] Use of parameter pairs improved detection, but such studies have been carried out with only a small number of fetuses.[4, 8, 38] In no instances have evaluations of fetal weight, length, or soft tissue mass been used to detect fetuses with intrauterine growth retardation.

On the basis of the results obtained both prenatally and postnatally, we do not feel that there is a well-documented, reproducible method for reliably detecting intrauterine growth retardation prenatally with ultrasound. The methods used to date will detect many cases, but by no means all, and in too many instances they will indicate intrauterine growth retardation when it does not exist. The actual magnitudes of these errors cannot be established from the available data because of the inadequacies of the postnatal evaluations, but they are very likely to be unacceptably high. This situation is most certainly worse than currently thought in view of the findings of Hill et al.[35] that intrauterine malnutrition, manifesting itself *only* as a decrease in soft tissue mass, is associated with a significant incidence of neurologic abnormalities which are both permanent (6 per cent) and transient (36 per cent).

In view of this situation we would like to propose the use of the following growth profile in the hope that it will prove more effective in detecting growth retardation, in reducing the number of false positives, and in providing new insights into the nature and etiology of growth problems:

Growth Profile
Head Size
Trunk Size
Soft Tissue Mass
Length
Weight
Body Proportionality

Ultrasound Assessment of Growth Profile

Menstrual Age. As indicated previously, any assessment of fetal growth requires accurate dating of the stage in pregnancy at which measurements are made. As described elsewhere in this book (see chapter 2), there are a variety of ways by which menstrual age can be determined, each having its own errors. A number of these involve the use of ultrasound (such as measurement of crown-rump length, biparietal diameter, femur length, and head circumference). With respect to growth studies, one can say that those methods providing the most accurate data at the earliest point in the pregnancy are to be preferred.

Head Size. *Choice of Parameter.* To characterize the size of the fetal head, there are a variety of one-, two-, and three-dimensional parameters that could be used.[11] Volume would be the most logical size parameter for a complex three-dimensional object such as the head. Although this is possible, measurement of this parameter involves either time-consuming serial sectioning and analysis (Deter, unpublished) or grossly oversimplified shape assumptions.[40] Two-dimensional parameters such as surface area or profile area could also be used, but the former requires serial sections and is sensitive to movement[6] whereas the latter has not been shown to be superior to one-dimensional parameters and requires more complex instrumentation for reliable measurements. For these reasons most evaluations of head growth have focused on the use of one-dimensional parameters such as diameters or circumferences.[11] Because of the simplicity of their measurements, diameters have been used primarily, particularly biparietal diameter. However, as shown recently for biparietal diameter,[27] diameter measurements are rather sensitive to changes in profile shape (brought about by changes in the shape of the head as a whole) and require well-defined anatomic landmarks within the profile to be measured reproducibly.[29] Profile circumference measurements, on the other hand, are much less sensitive to shape changes and do not require the presence of profile landmarks except for plane selection. These advantageous characteristics of the head circumference far outweigh the extra effort required for its measurement. For these reasons we feel that the head circumference is the most appropriate parameter for evaluating head growth.

Measurement Procedure. To measure the head circumference, a plane through the head must be chosen. The ideal plane would be one that can be readily identified ultrasonically. It would also be helpful if the circumference measurement made on this plane corresponded to the measurements of head circumference made postnatally as this would allow continuous monitoring of head growth in utero and ex utero. The head circumference measured postnatally is on a horizontal plane located just above the ear which contains both frontal and occipital bones of the skull.[43] This plane has been identified ultrasonically by virtue of the skull characteristics and the internal brain structures present at that level.[13, 30, 32] As shown in Figure 6, the head profile characteristics are its oval shape, the prominent skull bone profiles seen on all sides of the profile, and the presence of a peak (parietal eminence) in the

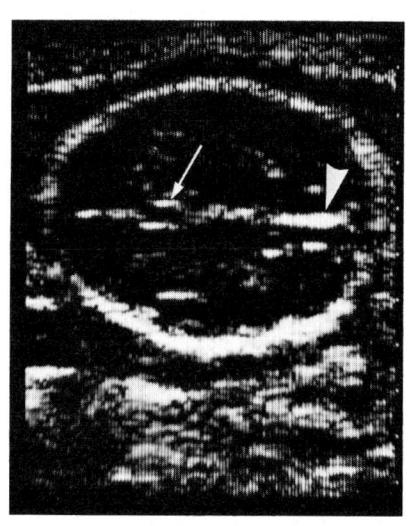

Figure 6. Head profile used in measurement of head circumference. Anatomic characteristics of the head profile on which head circumferences are measured. This plane is identified by its oval shape as well as the cavum septum pellucidum (*arrow*) anteriorly and the falx cerebri (*arrowhead*) posteriorly located in the midline of the profile. (*From* Deter, R. L., Harrist, R. B., Hadlock, F. P., et al.: Evaluation of sources of error in the measurement of the fetal head and abdominal circumferences. J. Clin. Ultrasound, 1982, in press, with permission.)

middle of the sides parallel to the long axis. The important brain structures are the corpus callosum[32] (or cavum septum pellucidum[37]) anteriorly and the falx cerebri posteriorly seen in the midline.[32] The latter is particularly important since this plane is above the level of the cerebellar tentorium and the absence of the falx indicates that the plane has been tilted downward so that it passes below the tentorium. Proof that the head circumference measured on this plane is actually maximal and assessment of the errors associated with measurements made on other planes are not yet available. However, as indicated previously, such studies have been carried out for biparietal diameter.[29] It has been shown that maximal values for biparietal diameter are obtained using this plane and that significant errors do occur when other planes are used.

Measurement of the head circumference can be made with a map measurer, light pen, electronic planimeter, or other means (Fig. 7). In all cases the length of the outside perimeter is measured. If a map measurer is used, a correction for the degree of demagnification usually must be introduced to obtain a true value. Other measuring devices can be programmed to

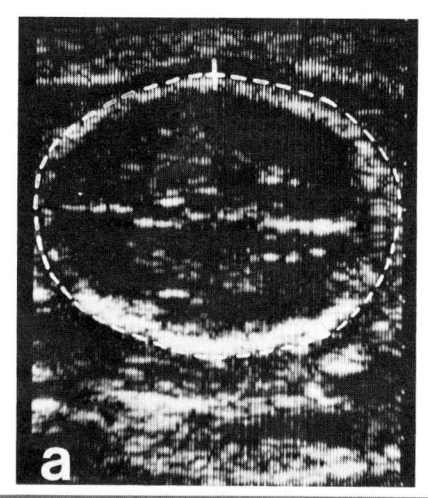

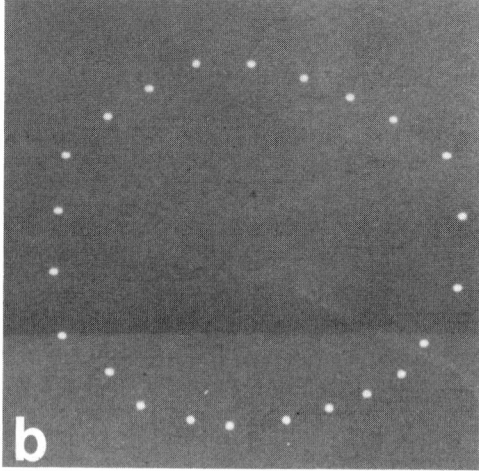

Figure 7. Measurement of head circumference. *A*, The outer boundary of the profile is delineated by a broken line and a starting point (vertical line) is chosen. Using a map measurer or electronic planimeter, the length of the broken line is measured by following this line around the profile. *B*, The broken line is replaced by a series of boundary points placed at the edge of the profile (displayed on a television monitor) with a light pen (the image has been removed to show the points more clearly). Boundary points can also be specified using an acoustic pen. These points should be placed so that the profile boundary will be closely approximated by a set of straight lines connecting the points. When this condition is met, the length of the profile circumference can be calculated by summing the lengths of the connecting lines. These lengths are determined from the coordinates of the points they connect.

compensate automatically for image demagnification. With the map measurer, intra-observer errors of -0.57 (± 2.12 S.D.) per cent and inter-observer errors of 1.2 (± 4.35 S.D.) per cent have been reported by experienced investigators.[10]

Attempts have been made to simplify the procedure of measuring head circumference through the use of the "ellipse approximation."[8] This method assumes that the head circumference profile is an ellipse and that its circumference can be determined from diameter measurements and the appropriate mensuration formula. Since such methods are dependent on shape, erroneous results could be obtained if the shape assumption is not valid. An evaluation of the errors inherent in the use of this method has not been made in a sample of significant size.

Data Evaluation. Data sets specifying the normal variability of head circumference at different stages in pregnancy have been published by several investigators as summarized by Deter et al.[13] However, inadequate samples, poor analysis of data, and the inclusion of multiple measurements on the same fetus, a procedure known to reduce estimates of variability,[18] significantly reduce the usefulness of most of these results. Only the data of Hadlock et al.[30] and Deter et al.[13] are free of these methodologic problems and thus can be considered reliable (Table 1). The mean values at different menstrual ages are very similar but differences exist in the ranges of normal. In the data set of Hadlock et al.,[30] the normal range is considered to be a constant (estimated by twice the standard deviation of the regression) throughout pregnancy and has a value of ± 1.8 cm. The use of a single variability estimator is justified by the reasonably uniform distribution of deviations along the time line (see Fig. 4). The data set of Deter et al.,[13] however, indicates that a change in the normal range occurs at 28 weeks (< 28 weeks: ± 1.5 cm; ≥ 28 weeks: ± 2.5 cm). This change in variability was seen in the deviation plot (Fig. 4) derived from the cross-sectional data[13] and in the individual fetal head circumference growth curves (Fig. 2) obtained in a longitudinal study.[15] The differing results observed by Hadlock et al. and Deter et al. have not been explained and at present are assumed to result from differences in populations. However, both data sets were generated from middle to upper class Caucasian populations seen in two very similar hospitals in the same city. These observations point out the need for evaluating each specific patient population to determine whether or not published normative data can be used with that population.

Detection of growth retardation affecting the head is possible using either individual values or growth rates for head circumference. An abnormal value for the former in-

Table 1. *Head Circumference: Normal Values*

	DETER ET AL.[13]			HADLOCK ET AL.[30]		
MENSTRUAL AGE (WKS)	Lower Limit* (cm)	Predicted Value† (cm)	Upper Limit‡ (cm)	−2 S.D.∥ (cm)	Predicted Value§ (cm)	+2 S.D.∥ (cm)
12	5.8	7.3	8.8	5.1	7.0	8.9
13	7.2	8.7	10.2	6.5	8.9	10.3
14	8.6	10.1	11.6	7.9	9.8	11.7
15	9.9	11.4	12.9	9.2	11.1	13.0
16	11.3	12.8	14.3	10.5	12.4	14.3
17	12.6	14.1	15.6	11.8	13.7	15.6
18	13.9	15.4	16.9	13.1	15.0	16.9
19	15.2	16.7	18.2	14.4	16.3	18.2
20	16.4	17.9	19.4	15.6	17.5	19.4
21	17.7	19.2	20.7	16.8	18.7	20.6
22	18.9	20.4	21.9	18.0	19.9	21.8
23	20.0	21.5	23.0	19.1	21.0	22.9
24	21.2	22.7	24.2	20.2	22.1	24.0
25	22.3	23.8	25.3	21.3	23.2	25.1
26	23.4	24.9	26.4	22.3	24.2	26.1
27	24.4	25.9	27.4	23.3	25.2	27.1
28	24.4	26.9	29.4	24.3	26.2	28.1
29	25.4	27.9	30.4	25.2	27.1	29.0
30	26.3	28.8	31.3	26.1	28.0	29.9
31	27.2	29.7	32.2	27.0	28.9	30.8
32	28.1	30.6	33.1	27.8	29.7	31.6
33	28.9	31.4	33.9	28.5	30.4	32.3
34	29.7	32.2	34.7	29.3	31.2	33.1
35	30.4	32.9	35.4	29.9	31.8	33.7
36	31.1	33.6	36.1	30.6	32.5	34.4
37	31.7	34.2	36.7	31.1	33.0	34.9
38	32.3	34.8	37.3	31.9	33.6	35.5
39	32.9	35.4	37.9	32.2	34.1	36.0
40	33.4	35.9	38.4	32.6	34.5	36.4

* <28 weeks: predicted value −1.5 cm.
  >28 weeks: predicted value −2.5 cm.
† $HC = -10.3676 + 1.5021 (MA) - .0002136 (MA)^3 [R^2 = 97.3\%]$.
‡ <28 weeks: predicted value +1.5 cm.
  >28 weeks: predicted value +2.5 cm.
§ $HC = -10.339 + 1.481 (MA) - .0002259 (MA)^3 [R^2 = 98.3\%]$.
∥ 2 S.D. = 1.9 cm.

dicates that a growth abnormality occurred during some time interval prior to the examination but does not specify when it occurred or if it is continuing. To determine the current status, the growth rate must be determined using data collected in sequential ultrasound examinations. The appropriate interval between scans depend on the rate of growth at that point in pregnancy, the rate of change in the growth rate, and the magnitude of the errors associated with measurements of head circumference. If the same investigator makes all measurements, the latter can be as high as 4 per cent (2 S.D.) for each measurement.[10] Growth rates for weekly intervals can be obtained directly from Table 2, whereas those for longer intervals can be estimated by averaging the weekly growth rates over the interval studied. This average growth rate is considered to be the growth rate at the mid-point of the interval. Such values may have questionable validity if the growth rate changes significantly over the interval.

Evaluation of both individual values and growth rates depends upon accurate knowledge of the menstrual age since the normal ranges for both measures are not constant throughout pregnancy (see Tables 1 and 2). The ranges given for individual values were obtained in cross-sectional studies, whereas those for growth rates were derived from longitudinal studies of individual fetuses.[15] These ranges encompass approximately 95 per cent of the values

Table 2. *Head Circumference: Normal Growth Rates*

	DETER ET AL.[15]		
MENSTRUAL AGE INTERVAL (WKS)	−2 S.D.[†] (cm/wk)	Predicted Value* (cm/wk)	+2 S.D.[†] (cm/wk)
12–13	1.4	1.6	1.8
13–14	1.3	1.5	1.7
14–15	1.3	1.5	1.7
15–16	1.3	1.5	1.7
16–17	1.3	1.5	1.7
17–18	1.2	1.4	1.6
18–19	1.2	1.4	1.6
19–20	1.2	1.4	1.6
20–21	1.1	1.3	1.5
21–22	1.1	1.3	1.5
22–23	1.2	1.3	1.4
23–24	1.1	1.2	1.3
24–25	1.1	1.2	1.3
25–26	1.1	1.2	1.3
26–27	1.0	1.1	1.2
27–28	1.0	1.1	1.2
28–29	0.9	1.0	1.1
29–30	0.9	1.0	1.1
30–31	0.8	0.9	1.0
31–32	0.8	0.9	1.0
32–33	0.7	0.8	0.9
33–34	0.6	0.8	1.0
34–35	0.5	0.7	0.9
35–36	0.5	0.7	0.9
36–37	0.4	0.6	0.8
37–38	0.4	0.6	0.8
38–39	0.3	0.5	0.7
39–40	0.1	0.4	0.7

* Data represent first derivative values of the function

$$HC = -13.84 + 1.68 \times (MA) - 2.67 \times 10^{-4} (MA)^3$$

which describes the average longitudinal growth curve. These values are calculated as follows:

$$\frac{dHc}{dMA} = 1.68 + 3(-2.67 \times 10^{-4}) MA^2$$

The values given are mid-week values (i.e., 12–13 week interval: derivative value at 12.5 weeks).

[†] Values calculated as follows:

$$2 \text{ S.D.} = \left(\frac{2}{9}\left[\sum_{i=1}^{19}(a_{1i} - 1.68)^2 + 9(MA)^4 \right.\right.$$
$$\times \sum_{i=1}^{19}(a_{3i} + 2.67 \times 10^{-4})^2 + 6(MA)^2$$
$$\left.\left.\times \sum_{i=1}^{19}(a_{1i} - 1.68)(a_{3i} + 2.67 \times 10^{-4})\right]\right)^{\frac{1}{2}}$$

where a_{1i} and a_{3i} are coefficients of the individual HC growth curves.[15]

obtained in normal pregnancies. As discussed earlier, use of such criteria to separate normal and abnormally growing fetuses may underestimate the number of fetuses with growth abnormalities if there is significant overlap in the values characterizing these two populations. The results obtained postnatally by Hill,[35] Daikoku,[9] and McLean[41] indicate that this is indeed the case at term. However, until there is sufficient data on abnormally growing fetuses throughout pregnancy to allow selection of criteria by discriminant analysis, we recommend the use of these criteria.

Trunk Size. *Choice of Parameter.* As it is well established from postnatal studies that trunk growth can be affected in growth-retarded fetuses,[41,51] it is essential that a measure reflecting the growth of this part of the fetus be monitored in any evaluation of fetal growth. As reviewed previously,[11] several such parameters can be evaluated with ultrasound. Using a line of reasoning similar to that presented for the head circumference, we have concluded that at present a circumference measurement on a well-defined plane would be the most appropriate measure.[11] Specifying such a plane in the chest is a problem because unequivocal landmarks detectable with ultrasound are difficult to define. Also the presence of the ribs presents image problems as the fetus becomes larger. The alternative to a measurement of chest circumference is a measurement of abdominal circumference. Campbell and Wilkin[5] suggested use of a plane perpendicular to the long axis of the fetus which contains a profile of the umbilical vein for such measurements (Fig. 8).

Use of this anatomic plane has several distinct advantages. First, it is anatomically well defined. Perpendicularity to the long axis of the fetus can be established by requiring that the abdominal, aortic, and vertebral profiles be as round as possible (the trunk, aorta, and vertebral column approximate cylinders aligned parallel to the long axis of the fetus). This orientation can be further checked by examining the profile of the umbilical vein itself (Fig. 9). Since this structure runs diagonally from the umbilicus to the root of the liver,[56] a plane perpendicular to the fetal long axis will intersect it only over a short segment. Therefore, umbilical vein profiles in appropriately ori-

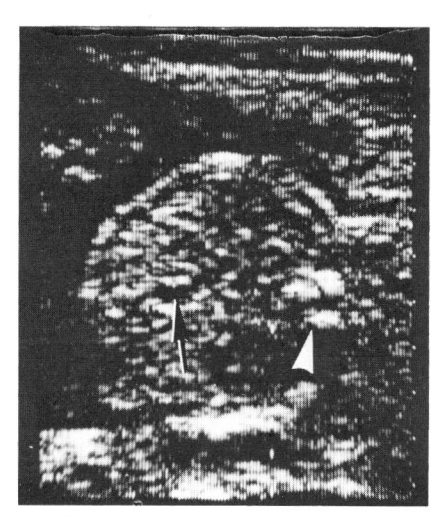

Figure 8. Abdominal profile used in measurement of abdominal circumference. Scan demonstrating the anatomic characteristics of the plane on which abdominal circumference is measured. The perpendicularity of the plane with respect to the long axis of the fetus is indicated by the circular shape of the vertebral profile (*arrowhead*) and the abdominal profile itself. The appropriateness of the location is indicated by the presence of a small oval profile of the umbilical vein (*arrow*). (*From* Deter, R. L., Harrist, R. B., Hadlock, F. P., et al.: Evaluation of sources of error in the measurement of the fetal head and abdominal circumferences. J. Clin. Ultrasound, 1982, in press, with permission.)

ented planes are short and slightly ovoid. The level for measurement as defined by Campbell was simply where a profile of the umbilical vein was present in the image. However, owing to its length and position, profiles of the vein can be found anywhere in the anterior half of the abdominal profile, depending on the location of the plane along the long axis. In fact, movement of the vein profile through this region as one moves the transducer along the fetal long axis is one means of identifying it. As this part of the abdomen approximates a cylinder, the exact position of the vein profile may not be critical, but this remains to be demonstrated by experiment. In our measurements, we try to choose a level at which the umbilical vein profile is located at a point approximately one third of the distance across the abdominal profile (see Figs. 8 and 9*B*).

The second advantage to use of this measurement is that it will reflect changes in liver size. It is well established that the liver is unusually large in the fetus[46] and is significantly affected by growth retardation.[3,25] In view of its role in maintaining blood glucose levels by glycogen mobilization when malnutrition occurs,[26] one might expect the liver to be the first organ to change when conditions leading to growth retardation are present. The preliminary results of our longitudinal study of fetuses at risk for intrauterine growth retardation suggest that this may indeed be the case as the abdominal circumference is usually the first parameter to show a decrease in growth rate. For these reasons there is a strong possibility that measurements of abdominal circumference may be among the most sensitive indicators of impending intrauterine growth retardation.

A third advantage to the use of measurements of abdominal circumference derives from the fact that a substantial literature indicates that measurements of abdominal circumference, together with biparietal diameter, provide the best estimates of fetal weight.[11,12] As discussed later, weight estimates are important in the evaluation and management of fetal growth abnormalities. With the availability of measurements of abdominal circumference, estimates of fetal weight can be obtained.

The only disadvantages associated with the use of measurements of abdominal circumference are those resulting from the absence of bone at the boundary of the abdomen. Because of this, the boundary can be difficult to identify, particularly if the fetus is against the placenta or uterine wall, and significant distortions in profile shape can occur since there is little resistance to deforming forces. The first problem can usually be overcome by (1) carefully positioning the transducer so that boundary echoes are maximized (bringing the sound in perpendicular to the surface) and (2) moving the fetus to a position where most of the boundary is in contact with amniotic fluid to increase the acoustic contrast at the profile edge. The second problem is not significant if the abdominal circumference is measured directly since the circumference measurement is relatively independent of shape.

Measurement Procedure. As with the head circumference, measurement of the abdominal circumference can be done with a map measurer, light pen, or electronic planimeter (Fig. 10). Electronic planimeters can give statistically different results on the same photographs if not func-

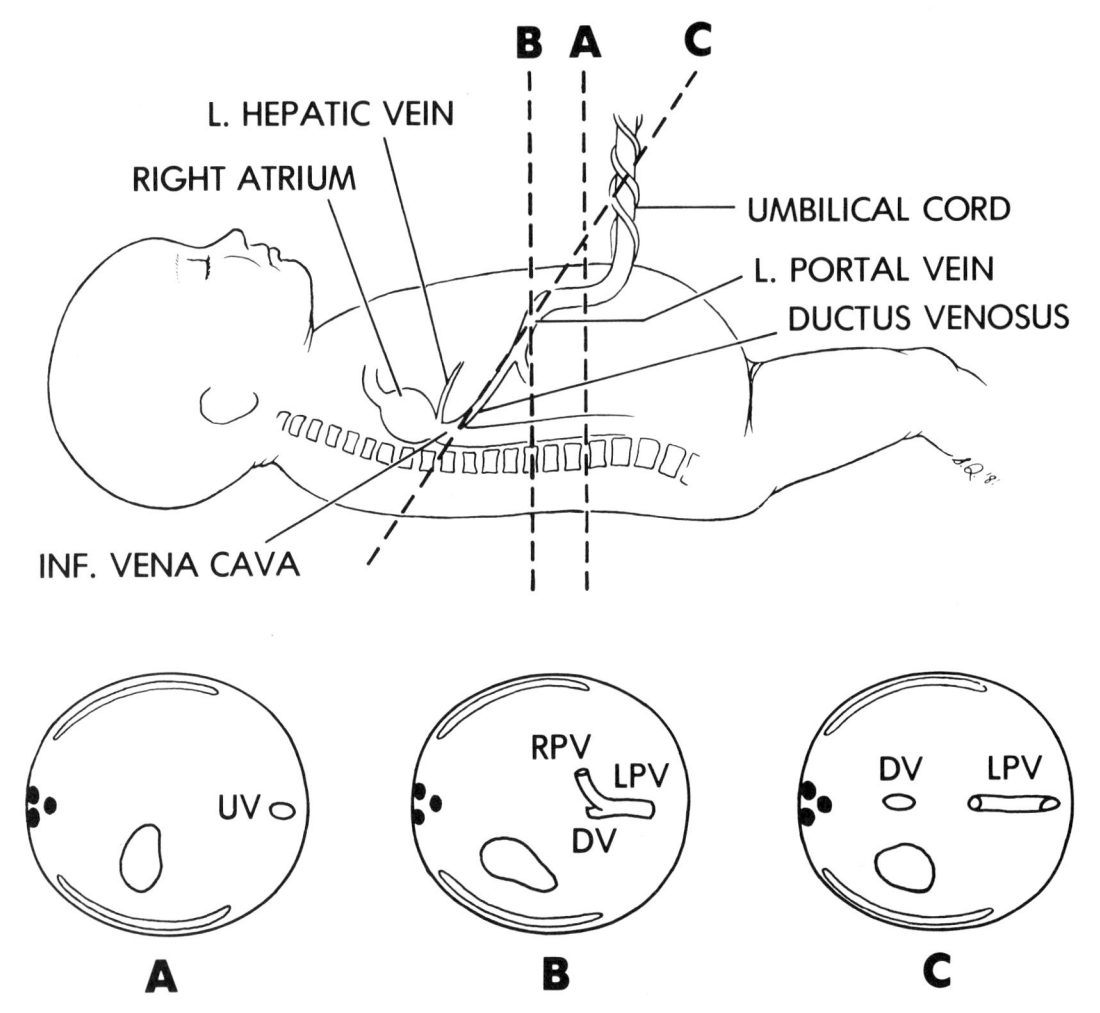

Figure 9. Diagrammatic illustration of the umbilical venous blood supply to the fetus. The approximate plane of section for measurement of the abdominal diameter or circumference may be chosen on the basis of the appearance of the umbilical blood supply to the fetus. In section A the scan is made at too low a level as the umbilical vein (UV) sectioned along its short axis is adjacent to the anterior abdominal wall. In section C the plane is angulated so that a long segment of the umbilical segment of the left portal vein (LPV) is seen. The appropriate plane of section (B) demonstrates a short tubular segment of the umbilical segment of the left portal vein approximately one-third of the way posterior from the anterior abdominal wall. DV, ductus venosus.

tioning properly.[10] With the map measurer, intra-observer errors of −0.5 (±2.6 S.D.) per cent and inter-observer errors of 2.4 (±1.6 S.D.) per cent have been reported by experienced investigators.[10] Again, simplification of the measurement process through use of the ellipse approximation has been reported,[45] but there has been no evaluation of the errors associated with the use of this method.

Data Evaluation. Normal variability in abdominal circumference at various stages in pregnancy has been evaluated by several investigators as summarized by Deter et al.[13] As with the head circumference, serious methodologic problems raise questions about the validity of normal range data from all investigations except those of Hadlock et al.[31] and Deter et al.,[13] even though the mean values obtained by all investigators are similar. The data of Deter et al.[13] and Hadlock et al.[31] are presented in Table 3. The range remains constant (2 S.D. = ±2.5 cm) in the data of Hadlock et al. but varies continuously (from 0.8 cm at 12 weeks to 4.8 cm at 40 weeks) in the data of Deter et al. These relationships of variability to menstrual age are better seen in the deviation plots presented in Figure 4. The progressive change in variability found by Deter et al. can be eliminated if the deviations are expressed as a percentage of the expected value (Fig. 11). Further evaluation of this transformed data indicated that 94.1 per cent of the deviations are within ±13 per cent of the expected value. At present we have no explanation for the difference in variability seen in these two data sets except for differences in population.[13] However, both populations were middle class Caucasians from the same city (Houston, Texas). The existence of such differences illustrates again the need for checking a specific population to determine which set of normative data is appropriate for that population.

As discussed for head circumference, abnormal growth of abdominal circumference can be detected by evaluating individual values or growth rates. The use of individual values requires good dating because the normal range varies with menstrual age. This is not the case for growth rates, since our longitudinal studies[15] indicate linear growth throughout pregnancy and thus constant growth rate variability. These results justify the use of a single normal range [(±2 S.D.) of 1.00 to 1.28 cm per week] at all stages of pregnancy. Again, as with the head circumference, arbitrary use of individual value or growth rate normal ranges encompassing approximately 95 per cent of the values obtained in normal pregnancies may lead to a underestimation of the number of fetuses with growth abnormalities. Discriminant analysis will have

Table 3. *Abdominal Circumference: Normal Values*

	DETER ET AL.[13]			HADLOCK ET AL.[31]		
MENSTRUAL AGE (WKS)	Lower Limit* (cm)	Predicted Value† (cm)	Upper Limit‡ (cm)	−2 S.D.‖ (cm)	Predicted Value§ (cm)	+2 S.D.‖ (cm)
12	5.4	6.3	7.1	3.1	5.6	8.1
13	6.4	7.4	8.3	4.4	6.9	9.4
14	7.4	8.4	9.5	5.6	8.1	10.6
15	8.3	9.5	10.8	6.8	9.3	11.8
16	9.3	10.6	12.0	8.0	10.5	13.0
17	10.2	11.7	13.3	9.2	11.7	14.2
18	11.2	12.8	14.5	10.4	12.9	15.4
19	12.1	13.9	15.7	11.6	14.1	16.6
20	13.1	15.0	17.0	12.7	15.2	17.7
21	14.0	16.1	18.2	13.9	16.4	18.9
22	15.0	17.2	19.5	15.0	17.5	20.0
23	16.0	18.3	20.7	16.1	18.6	21.1
24	16.9	19.4	22.0	17.2	19.7	22.2
25	17.9	20.5	23.2	18.3	20.8	23.3
26	18.8	21.6	24.4	19.4	21.9	24.4
27	19.8	22.7	25.7	20.4	22.9	25.4
28	20.7	23.8	26.9	21.5	24.0	26.5
29	21.7	24.9	28.2	22.5	25.0	27.5
30	22.6	26.0	29.4	23.5	26.0	28.5
31	23.6	27.1	30.6	24.5	27.0	29.5
32	24.6	28.2	31.9	25.5	28.0	30.5
33	25.5	29.3	33.1	26.5	29.0	31.5
34	26.5	30.4	34.4	27.5	30.0	32.5
35	27.4	31.5	35.6	28.4	30.9	33.4
36	28.4	32.6	36.9	29.3	31.8	34.3
37	29.3	33.7	38.1	30.2	32.7	35.2
38	30.3	34.8	39.3	31.1	33.6	36.1
39	31.2	35.9	40.6	32.0	34.5	37.0
40	32.2	37.0	41.8	32.9	35.4	37.9

* Predicted value $-.13$ (predicted value).
† $AC = -6.9300 + 1.0985 \, (MA) \; [R^2 = 95.5\%]$.
‡ Predicted value $+.13$ (predicted value).
§ $AC = -10.4997 + 1.4256 \, (MA) - .00697 \, (MA)^2 \; [R^2 = 97.9\%]$.
‖ 2 S.D. = 2.5 cm.

to be used to identify the optimal criteria when sufficient data on abnormally growing fetuses are collected.

Soft Tissue Mass. *Choice of Parameter.* The pathologic studies of Greunwald[25] and more recently the postnatal investigations of Miller,[42] McLean,[41] Diakoku,[9] and Hill[35] have shown that growth retardation can manifest itself as a loss of subcutaneous tissue, muscle mass, or both. This can occur with or without other evidence of growth retardation and is associated with both temporary and long-term neurologic sequelae.[35] In a 14 year follow-up study of newborns classified as intrauterine malnourished based on the loss of subcutaneous tissue, Hill et al.[35] found that the incidence of permanent neurologic disabilities was 27.3 per cent and the incidence of temporary disabilities was 84.8 per cent, many of the latter being multiple and lasting for several years. An incidence of 0 per cent for permanent disabilities and 38.4 per cent for temporary disabilities was seen in the well-nourished controls. Of the infants with permanent disabilities, 11.1 per cent had normal weights and lengths at birth while this value was 20 per cent for those with transitory disabilities. These results clearly demonstrate that this degree of intrauterine malnutrition is not benign, and a means for detecting it in utero must be developed. For this purpose, we propose the use of the thigh circumference (Fig. 12).

The choice of this parameter is based on

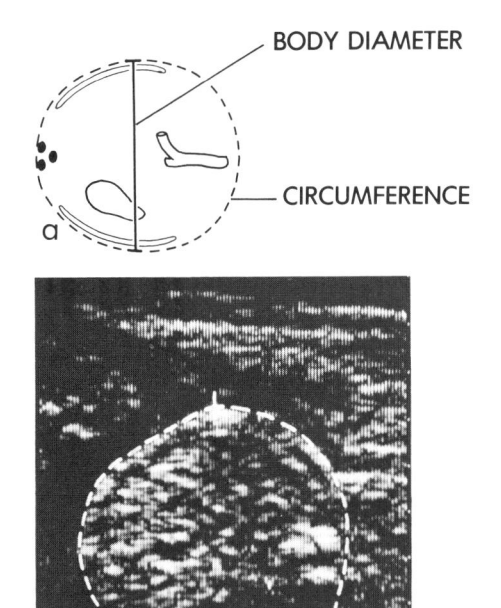

Figure 10. *A*, Diagram of the method of measuring abdominal diameter and circumference. Body diameter is measured transversely across the fetus from the center of the outer body wall to the center of the opposing body wall. The abdominal circumference is measured at the outer perimeter at the approximate anatomic plane. *B*, Procedure for measurement of circumference. The outer boundary of the profile (broken line) is delineated and a starting point (vertical line) chosen. The circumference is measured with a map measurer or electronic planimeter by following the broken line around the profile. Light and acoustic pen techniques can also be used (see Fig. 7).

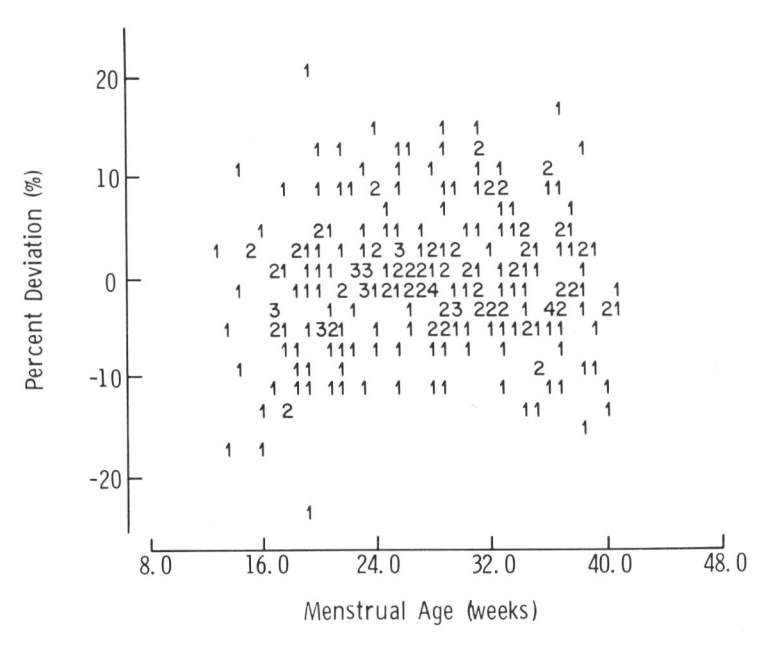

Figure 11. Elimination of dependence of variability in abdominal circumference on menstrual age by expressing deviations in abdominal circumference as a percentage of expected abdominal circumference values. This variability in abdominal circumference seen in the deviation plot (Fig. 4) of Deter et al.[13] can be eliminated by transformation of the data. To obtain the values presented here, the predicted abdominal circumference at each time point was calculated using the optimal linear function obtained in the mathematic fitting procedure. Each deviation was then expressed as a percentage of the appropriate predicted abdominal circumference value and plotted along the time line. (*From* reference 13, with permission.)

Figure 12. Thigh profile used in measurements of thigh circumference. *A*, Anatomic characteristics of the thigh profile on which thigh circumference measurements are made. This profile is identified by the relatively round profile of the femur (*arrow*) and the well-defined profile boundary (*arrowhead*). *B*, Circumference measurement procedure. The outer boundary of the profile is delineated (broken line) and a starting point (vertical line) chosen. The circumference is measured using a map measurer or electronic planimeter by following the broken line around the profile. Light and acoustic pen techniques can also be used.

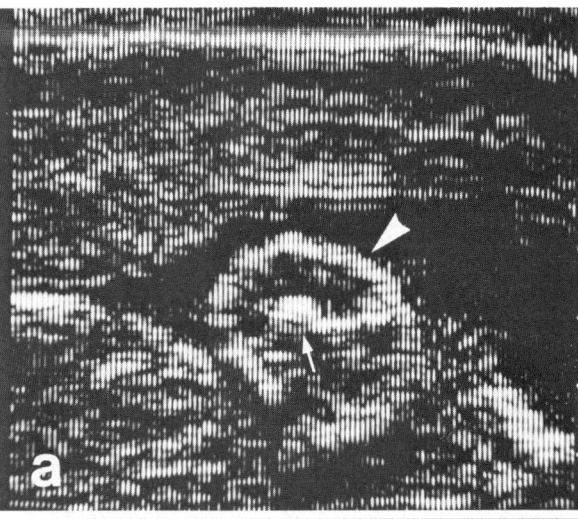

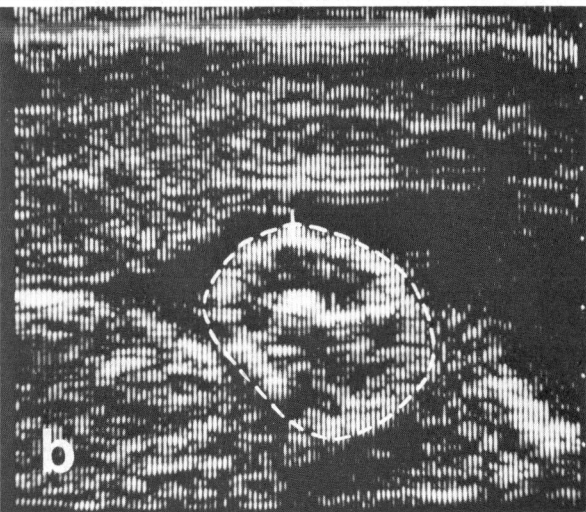

the anatomic fact that its measurement reflects the subcutaneous tissue and muscle mass of the leg primarily, and it was found to be significantly decreased in small-for-dates infants studied postnatally.[41] The skinfold thickness, a measure of the amount of subcutaneous tissue present[17] which is frequently evaluated in the inguinal area, was also found to be significantly smaller in infants judged to be malnourished.[41]

Measurement Procedure. Thigh circumferences (ThC) can be determined with ultrasound (Fig. 12B), although specification of a reproducible procedure is still a subject of current investigation. The procedure presently in use is applied to either leg as comparisons of right and left thigh circumference measurements made at birth (Hill, unpublished) in 56 clinically intrauterine well nourished infants (CIWN) and 13 clinically intrauterine malnourished infants (CIMN) showed no significant differences [mean difference CIWN: −0.10 (±0.40 S.D.) cm; CIMN: 0.02 (±0.41 S.D.) cm]. To obtain the appropriate profile for measurement, the long axis of the femur is first imaged. The transducer is then rotated to obtain a cross-sectional profile of the mid-thigh. As the transducer is moved along the long axis of the femur, changes in the bone profile are seen (Fig. 13). Bone profiles in the upper part of the thigh are polygonal but at a position above the midpoint of the femur, the profiles become round. This transition point is used as the level of measurement even though there may be some variability in its location among different individuals. The transducer is positioned so that the bone profile is as round as possible and the boundary of the thigh profile is well defined. The outer

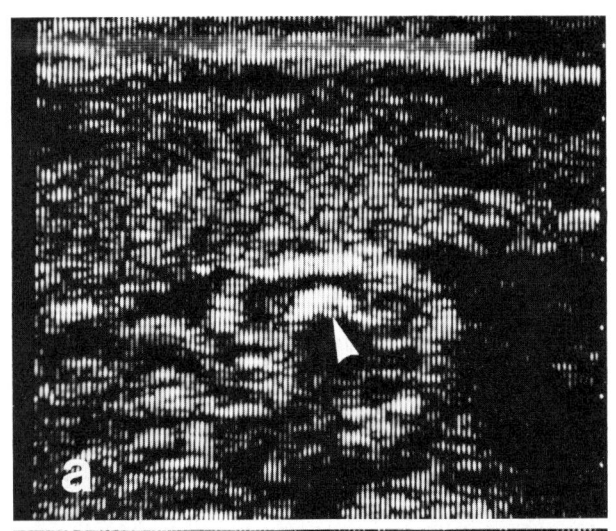

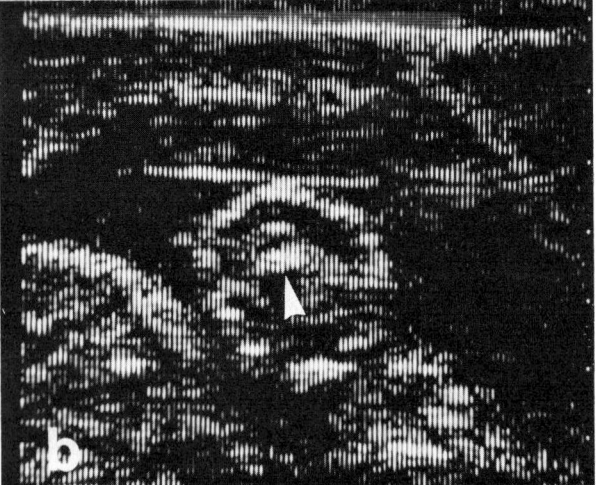

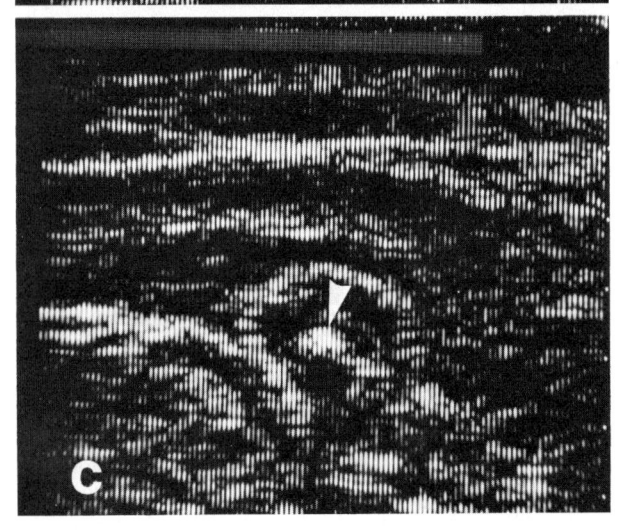

Figure 13. Appearance of thigh circumference profiles at various points along the length of the thigh. *A*, Changes in thigh circumference profiles can be seen as the acoustic plane is moved along the long axis of the thigh. The principal characteristic of this profile taken in the upper part of the thigh near the hip joint is the polygonal-shaped profile of the femur (*arrowhead*). *B*, A profile located distal to that shown in Figure 13A but probably proximal to the midpoint of the thigh. The thigh profile is somewhat smaller than that seen more proximally and the femur profile (*arrowhead*) is more rounded. *C*, A profile located in the distal part of the thigh. The thigh profile is smaller than those presented in Figure 13, *A* and *B*, but the femur profile (*arrowhead*) is still relatively round as seen in Figure 13B.

boundary of the thigh profile is then measured with a map measurer as done for the head and abdominal circumferences.

Data Evaluation. At present there are no thigh circumference growth curves available except that published by Usher and McLean for the 24 to 44 week period (Table 4).[53] These measurements were obtained postnatally at mid-thigh, and their relationship to measurements made on ultrasound images is not known. Previous studies of prenatal and postnatal measurements[3, 10] have demonstrated a close correlation with certain parameters (biparietal diameter, head circumference) and systematic errors with others (abdominal circumference). Therefore, these thigh circumference data should be used with caution when interpreting ultrasound measurements. Ultrasound studies of thigh circumferences as a function of gestational age during the second and third trimester are in progress at our institution.

As two standard deviation values for individual measurements are the only ones available, these criteria will have to be used to separate normal fetuses from abnormally growing fetuses. The data of McLean and Usher[41] indicate that approximately 18 per cent of the fetuses considered to be small-for-dates or "wasted" will have thigh circumference values in the normal range during the 36 to 42 week period.

Length. ***Choice of Parameter.*** It is well established from pediatric studies of growth-retarded infants that many of these infants can be abnormally short.[9, 35, 41, 42, 51] The percentage of such infants has been found to vary between 33 and 54 per cent, depending on the criteria used to classify infants as having intrauterine growth retardation. As shown by both Hill et al.[35] and Daikoku et al.,[9] infants with abnormal weights are much more likely to have abnormal lengths. These observations clearly indicate that an assessment of skeletal growth should be part of any comprehensive evaluation of fetal growth.

While crown-heel lengths are used in studies of the newborn, prenatal evaluations of fetal length[11] have been limited to the crown-rump length because of the complex and frequently changing positions of the legs. Prenatal studies have been limited to the 6 to 14 week period for the most part because fetal movement and flexion of the head, body, or both make accurate measurements of crown-rump length beyond this stage very difficult. Therefore, the use of fetal length itself to evaluate skeletal growth is not possible. As an alternative, we propose the use of the femur length. The femur is well imaged ultrasonically (Fig. 14A) from 12 weeks (menstrual age) on and the length values obtained by different investigators at various stages of pregnancy are quite similar.[33] Postnatal studies have shown that the length of the femur is related to crown-heel length in a consistent manner[20] and that the length of the leg bones does decrease in infants with other evidence of intrauterine growth retardation.[57] However, it should be pointed out that as yet there are no data demonstrating that growth retardation can be detected prenatally from measurements of the femur length, although dwarfism has been diagnosed.[21, 33]

Measurement Procedure. Measurement of the femur length requires selection of an image containing the longest dimension of the femur. Such an image can be obtained by positioning the sound plane parallel to the long axis of the thigh, imaging the femur, and moving the transducer until a femur profile having the maximum length is seen (Fig. 14A). The ends of this profile should be sharply defined. Frequently there is evidence of curvature in these femur profiles (Fig. 14A). Femur lengths are measured along a line connecting the mid-points of the profile ends using hand-held or electronic calipers (Fig. 14B). It is current practice to ignore bone curvature if it is present even though this practice obviously introduces an error in the measurement. The magnitude of these

Table 4. *Thigh Circumference: Normal Values*

MENSTRUAL AGE (WKS)	USHER AND MCLEAN[53]		
	−2 S.D. (cm)	Mean (cm)	+2 S.D. (cm)
24–26	6.5	8.5	10.5
27–28	8.4	9.6	10.8
29–30	8.8	10.0	11.2
31–32	9.4	11.6	13.8
33	11.0	12.6	14.2
34	11.1	12.7	14.3
35	11.4	13.9	16.4
36	11.6	13.9	16.6
37	12.2	15.0	17.8
38	12.9	15.6	18.3
39	13.8	16.2	18.6
40	13.7	16.5	19.3

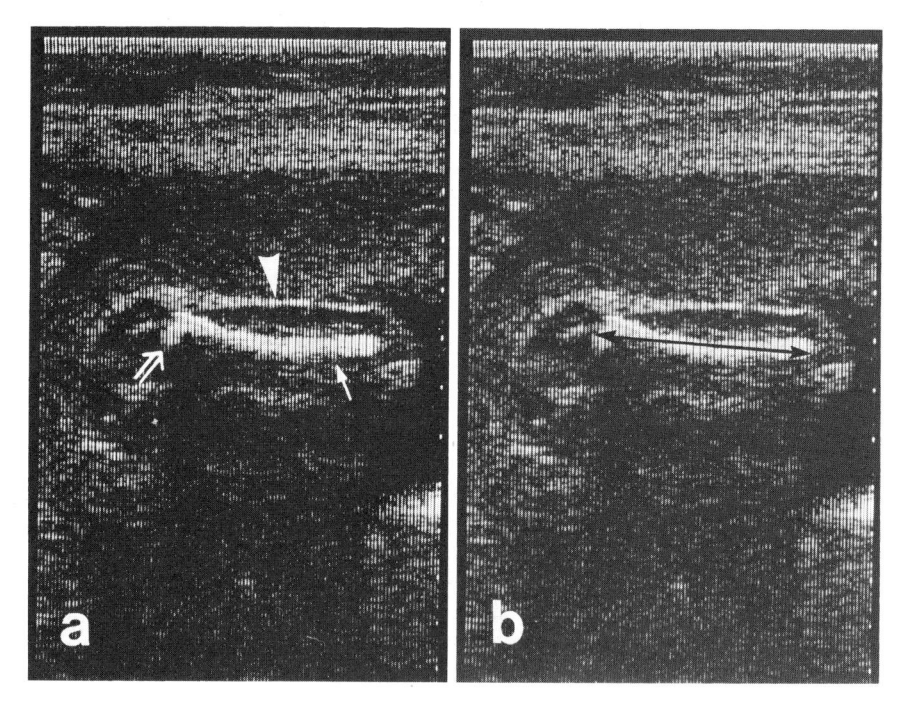

Figure 14. Femur profile used in measurements of femur length. *A,* Anatomical characteristics of the femur profile used for measurements of femur length. The very echogenic bone profile (*arrow*) is seen within the boundaries of the thigh profile (*arrowhead*). What appears to be the head of the femur (*double arrows*) is seen at the proximal end of the bone. Note the curvature of the shaft in this example. *B,* Femur length measurement procedure. The straight line distance (*double-headed arrow*) between the ends of the bone profile is measured ignoring bone curvature. (*From* General Electric Ultrasound Symposium, Vol. 1, no. 6, 1982, with permission.)

errors is not known, but they may contribute significantly to the substantial variability seen in femur length, particularly in the third trimester.[33] For femur length measurements, inter-observer errors of −0.33 (±2.16) mm have been reported by experienced investigators.[33]

Data Evaluation. Use of individual femur length values as a measure of skeletal growth requires data on normal variability at different stages in pregnancy. In Table 5, we present such a data set determined from the measurements made by Hadlock et al.[33] Variability in femur length is constant with menstrual age, having a normal range (twice the standard deviation of the regression) of 0.6 cm.

To date longitudinal studies of femur length growth have been limited to that by O'Brien and Queenan.[44] These authors studied 149 patients serially (at least two measurements were made per pregnancy), but the number of measurements made on each patient and the interval between measurements were not given. Growth rates based on paired measurements were calculated, and their means and 2 S.D. ranges are given in Table 6. However, as the intervals between paired measurements were not indicated, the reliability of these data is open to question. Intervals which were too long when the growth rate was changing significantly would give nonrepresentative values.

As with other parameters, the data to determine the appropriate criteria for separating normal and abnormally growing fetuses are not available. Therefore, we suggest that two standard deviations below the mean be used, despite its limitations, until better criteria can be established.

Weight. *Choice of Procedure.* Fetal weight has been the primary parameter used in identifying infants with intrauterine growth retardation,[1, 14, 24, 39] and it is well known that the outcome of the pregnancy is related to the weight of fetus.[47, 54] For these reasons estimating fetal weight from parameters determined by ultrasound has been the objective of a great many investigations.[11] Although a number of procedures have been proposed, comparison of the results obtained[12, 48, 50, 55] has indicated that currently the best method is that developed by Warsof.[55] The Warsof procedure was derived from meas-

Table 5. *Femur Length: Normal Values*

MENSTRUAL AGE (WKS)	HADLOCK ET AL.[33]		
	−2 S.D.* (cm)	Predicted Value† (cm)	+2 S.D.* (cm)
12	0.2	0.8	1.4
13	0.5	1.1	1.7
14	0.9	1.5	2.1
15	1.2	1.8	2.4
16	1.5	2.1	2.7
17	1.8	2.4	3.0
18	2.1	2.7	3.3
19	2.3	3.0	3.6
20	2.7	3.3	3.9
21	3.0	3.6	4.2
22	3.3	3.9	4.5
23	3.6	4.2	4.8
24	3.8	4.4	5.0
25	4.1	4.7	5.3
26	4.3	4.9	5.5
27	4.6	5.2	5.8
28	4.8	5.4	6.0
29	5.0	5.6	6.2
30	5.2	5.8	6.4
31	5.5	6.1	6.7
32	5.7	6.3	6.9
33	5.9	6.5	7.1
34	6.0	6.6	7.2
35	6.2	6.8	7.4
36	6.4	7.0	7.6
37	6.6	7.2	7.8
38	6.7	7.3	7.9
39	6.9	7.5	8.1
40	7.0	7.6	8.2

* 2 S.D. = 0.6 cm.
† FL = −3.9322 + .43834 (MA) − .0037387 (MA)^2 [R^2 = 97.7%].

Table 6. *Femur Length: Normal Growth Rates*

MENSTRUAL AGE (WKS)	O'BRIEN AND QUEENAN[44]		
	−2 S.D. (cm/wk)	Mean (cm/wk)	+2 S.D. (cm/wk)
17	.21	.32	.42
19	.14	.30	.45
21	.17	.30	.44
23	.13	.26	.40
25	.11	.25	.39
27	.08	.22	.36
29	.07	.21	.35
31	.03	.20	.36
33	.02	.18	.33
35	.04	.17	.31
37	.00	.16	.32
39	.03	.16	.28

urements of biparietal diameter and abdominal circumference made just before delivery, and the birth weights. Mathematic fitting procedures were used to obtain a function relating the biparietal diameter and abdominal circumference to the birth weight. Two forms of this function have been published but the one giving the best results[12,50] is as follows (weight in kg, biparietal diameter and abdominal circumference in cm):

$$Log_{10} Wt. = -1.7492 + 0.166(BPD) + 0.046(AC) - 0.002646(AC)(BPD)$$

Weight estimates for different biparietal diameter and abdominal circumference values are given in Table 7. Estimates obtained using this function have been found to be relatively unbiased, to be more uniform over different weight classes, and to have a random error of ±8.8 per cent (1 S.D.).[12]

Data Evaluation. Normal weight ranges at different stages in pregnancy have been published by a number of investigators but, as discussed previously,[14] significant differences exist among these data sets. Sex, race, and parity differences have also been found.[2] These results document the need for selecting a set of normal ranges which is appropriate for the specific population being studied.

It has been customary in the past to use an evaluation of individual values to detect growth abnormalities, although data on growth rates at different stages of pregnancy are available.[2] The 10th percentile has been considered to be the boundary between normal and abnormal values,[1,14,24,39] although to our knowledge there are no published reports demonstrating that this criterion optimally separates normal infants from those with evidence of growth problems. In fact, a recent postnatal study by Hill et al.[35] demonstrated, by discriminant analysis, that infants considered to be intrauterine malnourished at birth were optimally separated from those classified as intrauterine well nourished by weight criteria which represented the 15th to 25th percentiles (based on the normal values of Brenner et al.[2]), depending on menstrual age. These results document the need for the use of more objective means for finding appropriate criteria to define the boundary between normal and abnormal values. However, until such data are available, con-

Table 7. Estimated Fetal Weights for Different Biparietal Diameters and Abdominal Circumferences (From Warsof,[55] with permission.)

Table 7. Estimated Fetal Weights for Different Biparietal Diameters and Abdominal Circumferences (Continued)

sistency and conventional statistical practice would dictate the use of 2 standard deviations from the mean or the third percentile as the appropriate criteria. Of course, the use of these criteria will further exacerbate the problem of classifying individuals as normal, based on their weight, when there is other evidence of a growth abnormality.[9, 35] These situations suggest that parameters such as weight may not be the most appropriate for detecting growth retardation because there is too much overlap between normal and abnormal values.

Body Proportionality. *Choice of Parameter.* Growth abnormalities frequently manifest themselves as changes in the relationships between different fetal parameters. This disproportionate growth has been detected postnatally through comparisons of weight (Wt) to length (L) [Wt/L, Wt/L^2, Wt/L^3], head circumference/length, and length/head circumference.[9, 35, 42, 51] The Pondral Index ($Wt/L^3 \times 100$) has been used to identify growth-retarded infants with normal birth weights[9] but when used to separate CIWN from CIMN infants, false-positive and false-negative rates of 10.9 and 19.6 per cent were found.[35] In this latter study, weight/length gave the optimal results, correctly categorizing 91.3 per cent and giving false-positive and false-negative rates of 2.2 and 6.5 per cent, respectively. Two investigations have examined more than one of these parameters in the same patient population. The first[51] compared weight/length, head circumference/length, and head circumference/abdominal circumference in well nourished and malnourished infants and found statistically significant differences for weight/length and head circumference/length but not head circumference/abdominal circumference. In the second study,[9] $Wt/L^3 \times 100$ and length/head circumference were evaluated. There were no abnormal length/head circumference values in the newborns with abnormal $Wt/L^3 \times 100$ values, but 44.4 per cent of those considered short (crown-heel length below the third percentile) did have abnormal length/head circumference values. These results indicate that although abnormalities in body proportions occur in fetuses with growth abnormalities, there is at present no unequivocally superior parameter and the patterns of change with all parameters are not well defined.

Proportionality parameters (head circumference/abdominal circumference, head profile area/thoracic profile area, and head profile area/abdominal profile area) have also been used in prenatal attempts to detect small-for-dates fetuses with ultrasound.[14] While such parameters are abnormal in a significant number of small-for-dates fetuses, they are also abnormal in many fetuses with normal birth weights and are normal in fetuses who are small-for-dates. Their usefulness may be further compromised by a marked individual variability such has been shown for the head circumference/abdominal circumference.[11, 15] These results again indicate that while potentially important in the evaluation of fetal growth, proportionality parameters must be studied further in order to determine how they should be used.

Based on our assessment of the current literature, we propose use of weight/femur length, head circumference/abdominal circumference, and possibly thigh circumference/femur length as measures of body proportionality. Profile circumferences are preferred over profile areas for the reasons discussed previously and femur length is the logical substitute for crown-heel length as indicated in our previous discussion. Weight/femur length would appear to be the parameter most likely to identify fetuses with loss of subcutaneous tissue based on the postnatal studies of Hill et al.,[35] although the ratio of thigh circumference to femur length could be more effective if the thigh circumference is in fact an appropriate measure of soft tissue mass. The ratio of head to abdominal circumference has already been shown to be useful in differentiating "symmetric" from "asymmetric" intrauterine growth retardation,[4, 8] although our experience strongly suggests that this is the case only when the value for either the head circumference or abdominal circumference is outside the normal range. For example, a high normal head circumference value and a low normal abdominal circumference value will give an abnormal head circumference/abdominal circumference value which is associated with normal weight estimates and does not persist as the pregnancy progresses. Other possible parameters such as the head circumference/femur length and the abdominal circumference/femur length should also be examined to see if they will provide any additional insight into the nature of growth abnormalities.

Data Evaluation. At present there are no normal growth curve data for any of the above parameters except the head circumference/abdominal circumference.[4, 11] Normal ranges based on cross-sectional studies have been published by Campbell and Thom[4] and confirmed by us (see Table 8). However, use of such data in specific cases is open to serious question because of the extreme individual variability found among individuals in longitudinal studies of normal fetal growth.[15] An appropriate means for dealing with this variability has not been developed, and the degree of overlap between the values for normal and abnormally growing fetuses has not been determined. Because of the latter, the optimal boundary for separating normal and abnormal values is also not known. For these reasons, head circumference/abdominal circumference values must be interpreted cautiously until more information is available.

Use of Growth Profile

From the foregoing discussion, it should be clear that definitive statements concerning the application of the growth profile in individual cases cannot be made at this time. Additional data on normal growth must be collected, more extensive

Table 8. *Ratio of Head Circumference to Abdominal Circumference: Normal Values*

	DETER ET AL.			HADLOCK ET AL.		
MENSTRUAL AGE (WKS)	−2 S.D.[†] (cm)	Predicted Value* (cm)	+2 S.D.[†] (cm)	−2 S.D.[§] (cm)	Predicted Value[‡] (cm)	+2 S.D.[§] (cm)
12	1.16	1.29	1.41	1.12	1.22	1.31
13	1.15	1.28	1.40	1.11	1.21	1.30
14	1.14	1.27	1.39	1.11	1.20	1.30
15	1.13	1.26	1.38	1.10	1.19	1.29
16	1.12	1.25	1.37	1.09	1.18	1.28
17	1.11	1.24	1.36	1.08	1.18	1.27
18	1.10	1.22	1.35	1.07	1.17	1.26
19	1.09	1.21	1.34	1.06	1.16	1.25
20	1.08	1.20	1.33	1.06	1.15	1.24
21	1.07	1.19	1.32	1.05	1.14	1.24
22	1.06	1.18	1.30	1.04	1.13	1.23
23	1.05	1.17	1.29	1.03	1.12	1.22
24	1.04	1.16	1.28	1.02	1.12	1.21
25	1.03	1.15	1.27	1.01	1.11	1.20
26	1.02	1.14	1.26	1.00	1.10	1.19
27	1.01	1.13	1.25	1.00	1.09	1.18
28	1.00	1.12	1.24	.99	1.08	1.18
29	.99	1.11	1.23	.98	1.07	1.17
30	.97	1.10	1.22	.97	1.07	1.16
31	.96	1.09	1.21	.96	1.06	1.15
32	.95	1.08	1.20	.95	1.05	1.14
33	.94	1.07	1.19	.95	1.04	1.13
34	.93	1.05	1.18	.94	1.03	1.13
35	.92	1.04	1.17	.93	1.02	1.12
36	.91	1.03	1.16	.92	1.01	1.11
37	.90	1.02	1.15	.91	1.01	1.10
38	.89	1.01	1.13	.90	1.00	1.09
39	.88	1.00	1.12	.89	.99	1.08
40	.87	.99	1.11	.89	.98	1.08

* HC/AC = 1.42104 − .0106229(MA) [R^2 = 58.9%].
[†] 2 S.D. = 0.12.
[‡] HC/AC = 1.32293 − .0084471(MA) [R^2 = 67.2%].
[§] 2 S.D. = 0.10.

comparisons between normal and abnormal growth processes must be made, and correlations between prenatal and postnatal assessments must be carried out. However, some general comments may be helpful.

Because of its comprehensive design and foundation in the pediatric assessment of growth-retarded infants, we anticipate that the growth profile will be capable of detecting most growth-retarded fetuses, particularly if evaluation takes place more than once during pregnancy. Unfortunately, there are no available data on which to base decisions concerning the number of examinations needed and the menstrual ages at which such examinations should be made. However, since growth retardation has been detected as early as 17 weeks,[19] an initial examination in the second trimester would seem appropriate. For high-risk patients, a reasonable procedure would be to date the pregnancy at 10 to 12 weeks, then evaluate growth at 6-week intervals between 18 and 30 weeks and at 3-week intervals between 30 weeks and delivery. If abnormalities are seen, the interval between examinations should be shortened but, due to measurement errors and growth rates, intervals of less than 2 weeks are not likely to give reliable data.

From the theoretical point of view, an abnormal value for any of the parameters of the growth profile is potentially a sign that a growth problem exists. However, it should be pointed out that depending on the criterion used for separating abnormal from normal values, there is a finite probability (of differing magnitude) that such a value can be obtained in an otherwise normal fetus. Also, these values only indicate that abnormal growth occurred *some time* in the past, and the process may or may not be continuing. The preliminary results of our longitudinal study of fetuses at high risk for growth retardation indicate that the growth pattern in such fetuses is more erratic than that seen in normal pregnancies and may show periods of both normal and abnormal growth rates. However, persistent abnormal growth rates are seen as the growth problem becomes more serious. From these observations we conclude that while growth retardation may be detected by either abnormal individual values or abnormal growth rates, the significance of such a finding varies. Persistent abnormal growth rates associated with abnormal individual values indicate a serious problem. Abnormal individual values at a single examination may have the same significance but could also be due to a serious growth problem in the past from which the fetus has now recovered. A single abnormal growth rate value may signal the beginning of a growth problem but, if transitory, may only be the result of instability in the control system regulating fetal growth.

Finally, there is the question of judging the severity of the growth abnormality. Until long-term outcomes can be correlated with abnormal growth profile patterns, making such evaluations will involve a great deal of speculation. Although it is clear that decreased weight is associated with increased mortality and morbidity,[47,55] malnutrition sufficient to cause only loss of soft tissue mass can produce significant neurologic difficiencies in some individuals.[35] These latter results, if confirmed, would indicate that *any* persistent growth abnormality is significant and should be treated vigorously. However, based on our experience to date, we believe that (1) multiple abnormal parameters indicate a more serious problem than a single abnormal parameter, (2) abnormal skeletal growth indicates a chronic and therefore a more potentially detrimental process, and (3) the risk for a bad outcome significantly increases when the weight estimate and/or head circumference become abnormal. Subsequent research may require us to change these guidelines, but at present they are serving as the basis for our interpretations of growth profile data.

ACKNOWLEDGMENT

This work was supported in part by a grant (No. 6-248) to Dr. Deter from the March of Dimes Birth Defects Foundation.

REFERENCES

1. Bard, H.: Intrauterine growth retardation. Clin. Obstet. Gynecol., *13*:511–525, 1970.
2. Brenner, W. E., Edelman, D. A., and Hendrick, C. H.: A standard of fetal growth for the United States of America. Am. J. Obstet. Gynecol., *126*:555–564, 1976.
3. Campbell, S.: Fetal growth. *In* Beard, R. W., and Nathanielsz, P. W. (eds.): Fetal Physiology and Medicine. Philadelphia, W. B. Saunders Co., 1976, pp. 271–300.

4. Campbell, S., and Thoms, A.: Ultrasound measurement of the fetal head to abdomen circumference ratio in the assessment of growth retardation. Br. J. Obstet. Gynecol., 84:165–174, 1977.
5. Campbell, S., and Wilkin, D.: Ultrasonic measurement of fetal abdominal circumference in the estimation of fetal weight. Br. J. Obstet. Gynaecol., 82:689–697, 1975.
6. Cook, L. F., and Cook, P. N.: Volume and surface area estimators. Automedica, 4:13–23, 1981.
7. Cornfield, J.: Discriminant functions. Rev. Internat. Stat. Inst., 35:142–153, 1967.
8. Crane, J. P., and Kipta, M. M.: Prediction of intrauterine growth retardation via ultrasonically measured head/abdominal circumferences ratios. Obstet. Gynecol., 54:497–601, 1979.
9. Daikoku, N. H., Johnson, J. W. C., Graf, C., et al.: Patterns of intrauterine growth retardation. Obstet. Gynecol., 54:211–219, 1979.
10. Deter, R. L., Hadlock, F. P., Harrist, R. B., et al.: Fetal head and abdominal circumference. I. Evaluation of measurement errors. J. Clin. Ultrasound, 10:357–363, 1982.
11. Deter, R. L., Harrist, R. B., Hadlock, F. P., et al.: The use of ultrasound in the assessment of normal fetal growth. J. Clin. Ultrasound, 9:481–483, 1981.
12. Deter, R. L., Hadlock, F. P., Harrist, R. B., et al.: Evaluation of three methods for obtaining fetal weight estimates using dynamic image ultrasound. J. Clin. Ultrasound, 9:421–425, 1981.
13. Deter, R. L., Harrist, R. B., Hadlock, F. P., et al.: Fetal head and abdominal circumferences. II. A critical re-evaluation of the relationship to menstrual age. J. Clin. Ultrasound, 10:365–372, 1982.
14. Deter, R. L., Harrist, R. B., Hadlock, F. P., et al.: The use of ultrasound in the detection of intrauterine growth retardation — a review. J. Clin. Ultrasound, 10:9–16, 1982.
15. Deter, R. L., Harrist, R. B., Hadlock, F. P., et al.: Longitudinal studies of fetal growth with dynamic image ultrasonography. Am. J. Obstet. Gynecol., 143:545–554, 1982.
16. Draper, N. R., and Smith, H.: Applied Regression Analysis. New York, John Wiley and Sons, Inc., 1966, pp. 86–103.
17. Durnin, J. V. G. A., and Rahaman, M. M.: The assessment of the amount of fat in the human body from measurements of skin fold thickness. Br. J. Nutr., 21:681–689, 1967.
18. Elston, R. C., and Grizzle, J. E.: Estimation of time-response curves and their confidence bands. Biometrics, 18:148–159, 1962.
19. Fancourt, R., Campbell, S., Harvey, D., et al.: Follow-up study of small-for-dates babies. Br. Med. J., 1:1435–1437, 1976.
20. Fazekas, I. G., and Kosa, F.: Forensic Fetal Osteology. Budapest, Akademiai Kiado, 1978, p. 256.
21. Filly, R. A., Golbus, M. S., Carey, J. C., et al.: Short-limbed dwarfism: Ultrasonographic diagnosis by mensuration of fetal femoral length. Radiology, 138:653–656, 1981.
22. Fitzhardinge, P. M., and Steven, E. M.: Small-for-date infant. II. Neurological and intellectual sequelae. Pediatrics, 50:50–57, 1972.
23. Fitzhardinge, P. M., and Steven, E. M.: The small-for-date infant. I. Later growth patterns. Pediatrics, 49:671–681, 1972.
24. Frigoletto, R. D., and Rothchild, S. B.: Altered fetal growth: An overview. Clin. Obstet. Gynecol., 20:915–923, 1977.
25. Gruenwald, P.: Chronic fetal distress and placental insufficiency. Biol. Neonate, 5:215–265, 1963.
26. Guyton, A. C.: Textbook of Medical Physiology. Edition 4. Philadelphia, W. B. Saunders Company, 1971, p. 918.
27. Hadlock, F. P., Deter, R. L., Carpenter, R. J., et al.: Estimating fetal age: Effect of head shape on BPD. Am. J. Roentgenol., 137:83–85, 1981.
28. Hadlock, F. P., Deter, R. L., Harrist, R. B., et al.: Fetal biparietal diameter: A critical re-evaluation of the relation to menstrual age by means of real-time ultrasound. J. Ultrasound Med., 1:97–104, 1982.
29. Hadlock, F. P., Deter, R. L., Harrist, R. B., et al.: Fetal biparietal diameter: Rational choice of plane of section for sonographic measurement. Am. J. Roentgenol., 138:871–874, 1982.
30. Hadlock, F. P., Deter, R. L., Harrist, R. B., et al.: Fetal head circumference: Relation to menstrual age. Am. J. Roentgenol., 138:649–653, 1982.
31. Hadlock, F. P., Deter, R. L., Harrist, R. B., et al.: Fetal abdominal circumference as a predictor of menstrual age. Am. J. Roentgenol., 139:367–370, 1982.
32. Hadlock, F. P., Deter, R. L., and Park, S. K.: Ventricular and vascular anatomy of the fetal brain: Real-time sonography in utero. Am. J. Nucl. Radiol., 1:507–512, 1980.
33. Hadlock, F. P., Harrist, R. B., Deter, R. L., et al.: Femur length as a predictor of menstrual age: Sonographically measured. Am. J. Roentgenol., 138:875–878, 1982.
34. Hill, M.: Statistics for Comparative Studies. New York, Halsted Press, 1974, pp. 118–147.
35. Hill, R. M., Verinaud, W. M., Deter, R. L., et al.: The effect of intrauterine malnutrition on the human infant. J. Pediatr., in press.
36. Holmes, G. E., Miller, H. C., Hassanein, K., et al.: Postnatal somatic growth in infants with atypical fetal growth patterns. Am. J. Dis. Child., 131:1078–1083, 1977.
37. Johnson, M. L., Dunne, M. G., Mack, L. A., et al.: Evaluation of the fetal intracranial anatomy by static and real-time ultrasound. J. Clin. Ultrasound, 8:311–318, 1980.
38. Kurjak, A., Kirkinen, P., and Latin, V.: Biometric and dynamic ultrasound assessment of small-dates infants: Report of 260 cases. Obstet. Gynecol., 56:281–284, 1980.
39. Low, J. A., and Galbraith, R. S.: Pregnancy characteristics of IUGR. Obstet. Gynecol., 44:122–126, 1974.
40. Martinez, D. A., and Barton, J. I.: Estimation of fetal body and fetal head volumes: Description of technique and nomograms for 18 to 41 weeks of gestation. Am. J. Obstet. Gynecol., 137:78–84, 1980.
41. McLean, F., and Usher, R.: Measurements of liveborn fetal malnutrition infants compared with similar gestation and with similar birth weight normal controls. Biol. Neonate, 16:215–221, 1970.

42. Miller, H. C., and Hassanein, K.: Diagnosis of impaired fetal growth in newborn infants. Pediatrics, 48:511–522, 1971.
43. Nelson, W. E., Vaughan, V. C., III, and McKay, R. J. (eds.): Textbook of Pediatrics. Edition 9. Philadelphia, W. B. Saunders Co., 1969, p. 54.
44. O'Brien, G. D., and Queenan, J. F.: Growth of the ultrasound fetal femur length during normal pregnancy. I. Am. J. Obstet. Gynecol., 141:833–837, 1981.
45. Ott, W. J.: Clinical application of fetal weight determination by real-time ultrasound measurements. Obstet. Gynecol., 57:758–762, 1981.
46. Park, W. W.: Photographic Atlas of Fetal Anatomy. Baltimore, University Park Press, 1975, p. 202.
47. Paul, R. H., Koh, K. S., and Manfared, A. H.: Obstetric factors influencing outcome in infants weighing 1001 to 1500 grams. Am. J. Obstet. Gynecol., 133:503–508, 1979.
48. Poll, V. and Kasby, C. B.: An improved method of fetal weight estimation using ultrasound measurements of fetal abdominal circumference. Br. J. Obstet. Gynaecol., 86:922–928, 1979.
49. Remington, R. D., and Schork, M. A.: Statistics with Applications to the Biological and Health Sciences. Englewood Cliffs, New Jersey, Prentice Hall, Inc., 1970, p. 165.
50. Shepard, M. J., Richards, V. A., Berkowitz, R. L., et al.: An evaluation of two equations for predicting fetal weight by ultrasound. Am. J. Obstet. Gynecol., 142:47–54, 1982.
51. Unrusti, J., Yoshida, P., Welasco, L., et al.: Human fetal growth retardation I. Clinical features of sample with intrauterine growth retardation. Pediatrics, 50:547–558, 1972.
52. Usher, R. H.: Clinical and therapeutic aspects of fetal malnutrition. Pediatr. Clin. North. Am. 17:169–184, 1970.
53. Usher, R., and McLean, F.: Intrauterine growth of liveborn caucasian infants at sea level: Standards obtained from measurements in 7 dimensions of infants born between 25 and 44 weeks of gestation. J. Pediatr. 74:901–910, 1969.
54. Usher, R. H., and McLean, F. H.: Normal fetal growth and the significance of fetal growth retardation. In Davis, J. S., and Dobbing, J. (eds.): Scientific Foundations of Pediatrics. London, Heinemann, 1974, pp. 69–80.
55. Warsof, S. T.: Ultrasonic Estimation of Fetal Weight for the Detection of Intrauterine Growth Retardation by Computer Assisted Analyses. Thesis. New Haven, Yale University School of Medicine, 1977.
56. Warwick, R., and Williams, P. L. (eds.): Gray's Anatomy. 35th British Edition. Philadelphia, W. B. Saunders Co., 1973, p. 613.
57. Wilson, M. G., Meyers, H. I., and Peters, A. H.: Postnatal bone growth of infants with fetal growth retardation. Pediatrics, 40:213–222, 1967.

8

The Placenta

Peter Grannum, M.D., and John C. Hobbins, M.D.

Recent advances in the technology of ultrasound now afford physicians a more detailed look at the intrauterine environment. Knowledge of normal anatomy and the ability to identify anatomic landmarks within the fetus have enabled obstetricians to make the diagnosis of structural abnormalities in the fetus.[13] In addition to a detailed examination of the fetus, scanning techniques have now been defined for the placenta. For example, a grading classification has been devised for the maturational process occurring within the placenta during the gestational period.[9] This, along with the diagnosis of placenta previa and abruptio placentae, will be discussed in detail below.

PLACENTAL GRADING CLASSIFICATION

At approximately the tenth to twelfth week of gestation, structures of the placenta can be clearly identified (Fig. 1). Prior to that time, the placenta appears as a conglomeration of high level echoes. In a study that reviewed 120 placental scans taken at varying times in normal pregnancies, a classification of the maturational process of the placenta was devised (Fig. 2).[9] A summary of the progressive changes is listed in Table 1. The classification describes four basic patterns from Grades 0 through III. In the original study placental examinations were done on the static scanner. Petrucha et al. have more recently confirmed the four basic appearances and the fact that grading can be adequately performed using a dynamic scanner.[21]

In describing the maturational process, reference will be made to the three basic areas of the placenta: (1) the chorionic plate, (2) the substance of the placenta, and (3) the basal layer.

Grade 0 Placenta (Fig. 3). This configuration represents the appearance of all placentas in the first and second trimesters. With reference to the three structures of the placenta, the grade 0 placenta is represented by: (1) a smooth chorionic plate, (2) the substance of the placenta devoid of any echogenic densities, and (3) a basal area devoid of densities.

Grade I Placenta (Figs. 4 and 5). (1) The chorionic plate shows subtle undulations (this may not always be possible to detect if the fetus is closely positioned to the plate). (2) Linear echogenic densities are randomly dispersed within the substance of the placenta; their long axis is parallel to the long axis of the placenta, i.e., roughly parallel to the chorionic plate, and they measure 2 to 4 mm in length. (3) The basal area is devoid of echogenic densities.

Grade II Placenta (Figs. 6 and 7). (1) In this configuration the chorionic plate may appear markedly indented, but again this may be difficult to recognize if the fetus is closely positioned to the placenta. (2) The substance of the placenta maintains the presence of the linear echogenic densities described under Grade I placenta. They may, however, be larger or more numerous. In addition, linear echogenic densities (comma-like densities) may extend from the chorionic plate into the placental substance. They do not represent a continuous connection from the chorionic plate to the basal layer.[21] (3) The basal area shows the presence of basal echogenic densities that have their long axis parallel to the long axis of the placenta, and may measure 6 mm in length or greater. They can be dense enough to cast acoustic shadows of their own. They should not be confused with reverberation from the anterior abdominal wall.

Grade III Placenta (Fig. 8). This configuration represents the so-called "mature placenta."[12, 26] (1) The chorionic plate is

142 The Placenta

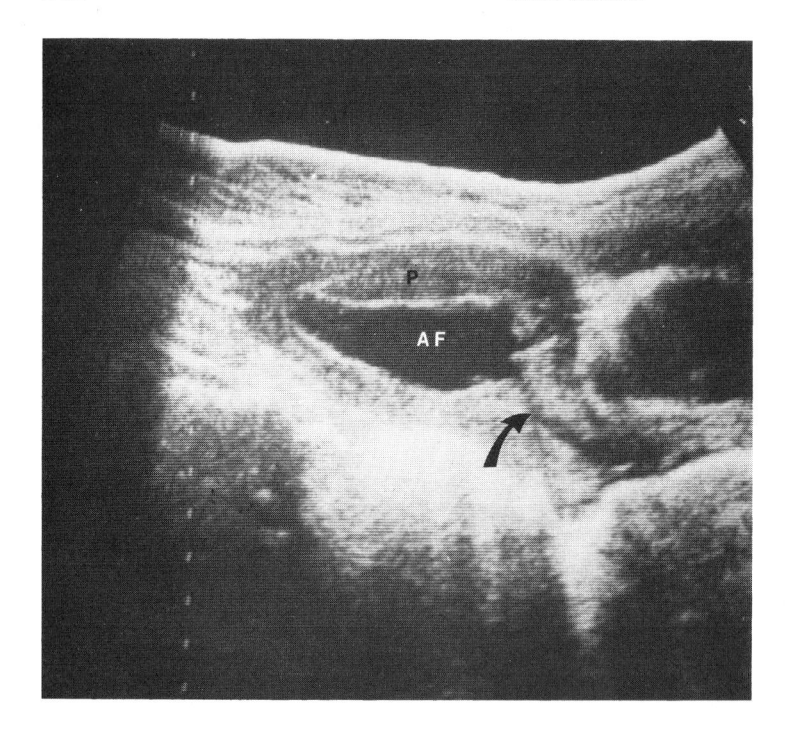

Figure 1. A 12-week intrauterine pregnancy showing the placenta and chorionic plate, amniotic fluid, and endocervical canal. P, placenta; AF, amniotic fluid; arrow, endocervical canal. (*From* Grannum, P.: The placenta. Clin. Diag. Ultrasound, *3*:41–55, 1979, with permission.)

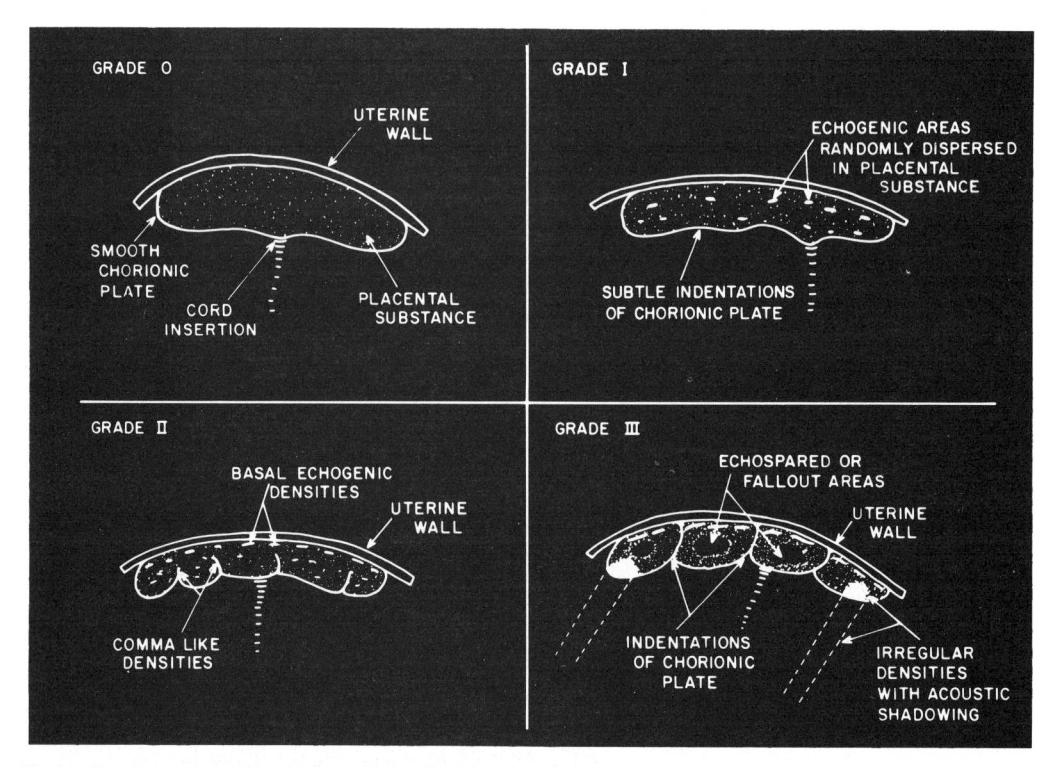

Figure 2. Diagrammatic version of the grading classifications of the placenta Grades 0 through III. (*From* Grannum, P. A. T., Berkowitz, R. L., and Hobbins, J. C.: The ultrasonic changes in the maturing placenta and their relation to fetal pulmonic maturity. Am. J. Obstet. Gynecol., *133*:915–922, 1979, with permission.)

Table 1. *Summary of Placental Grading**

	GRADE 0	GRADE I	GRADE II	GRADE III
Chorionic plate	Straight and well-defined	Subtle undulations	Indentations extending into but not to the basal layer	Indentations communicating with the basal layer
Placental substance	Homogeneous	Few scattered echogenic areas	Linear echogenic densities (comma-like densities)	Circular densities with echo-spared areas in center; large irregular densities which cast acoustic shadowing
Basal layer	No densities	No densities	Linear arrangement of small echogenic areas (basal stippling)	Large and somewhat confluent basal echogenic areas; can create acoustic shadows

* *From* Grannum, P. A. T., Berkowitz, R. L., Hobbins, J. C.: The ultrasonic changes in the maturing placenta and their relation to fetal pulmonic maturity. Am. J. Obstet. Gynecol., *133*:915–922, 1979, with permission.

more markedly indented. (2) The linear echogenic densities from the chorionic plate now extend all the way to the basal area *without a break*, presumably dividing the placenta into cotyledons. The densities randomly dispersed in the substance of the Grades I and II placentas persist. Large irregular echogenic densities (large enough to cast acoustic shadows) may be present in the substance of the placenta and situated more closely to the chorionic plate. The central portions of the demarcated cotyledonary areas may appear sonolucent ("fall out areas") which, as described by Crawford,[4] represent the central portions of the cotyledons devoid of villi. (3) The echogenic densities in the basal area as noticed in the Grade II placenta persist but may be more confluent and dense enough to cast acoustic shadows.

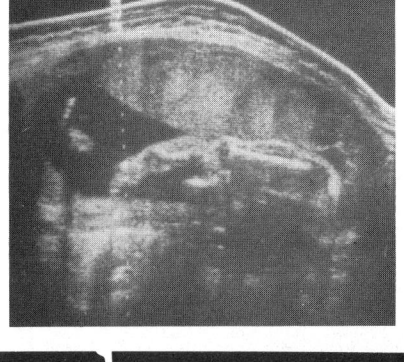

Figure 3. Grade 0 placenta. Note the homogeneous texture of the placental substance, the smooth contour of the chorionic plate, and the basal layer devoid of echogenic densities. (*From* Grannum, P., Berkowitz, R. L., and Hobbins, J. C.: The ultrasonic changes in the maturing placenta and their relation to fetal pulmonic maturity. Am. J. Obstet. Gynecol., *133*:915–922, 1979, with permission.)

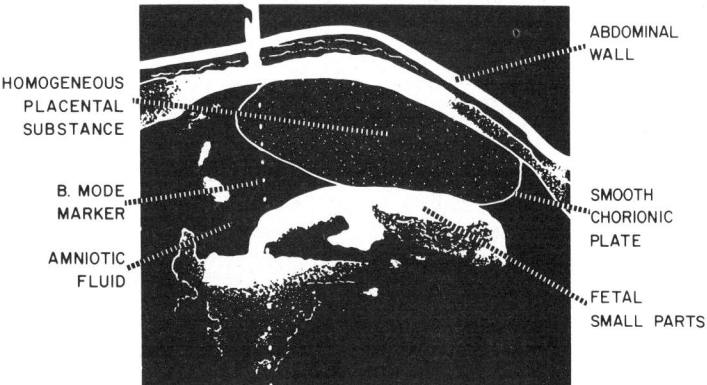

Figure 4. Grade I placenta. The placental substance shows finely displaced echogenic densities. The basal layer remains clear of echogenic densities. (*From* Grannum, P., Berkowitz, R. L., and Hobbins, J. C.: The ultrasonic changes in the maturing placenta and their relation to fetal pulmonic maturity. Am. J. Obstet. Gynecol., *133*:915–922, 1979, with permission.)

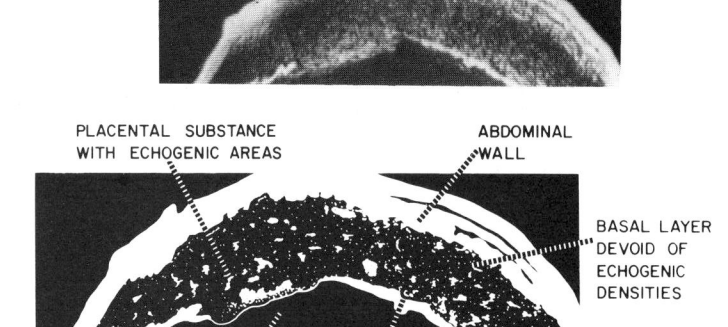

It is not unusual for two portions of the placenta to have different grades (Fig. 8). The highest grade should be assigned. Many factors are thought to be associated with the maturation of the placenta, most notably the deposition of calcium as well as fibrin. It has long been known that calcium is deposited in the decidua, fibrin, and villa of normal term placentas.

TECHNIQUE FOR SCANNING THE PLACENTA

In scanning the placenta, it is vitally important that the direction of the sound waves be perpendicular to the chorionic plate. The grading classification depends on this method for its accuracy. In the fundally or laterally positioned placenta, incorrect results may be obtained if this method is not adhered to.

The gain settings must be adjusted appropriately if a high degree of accuracy is to be achieved in assigning grades. Figure 9*A* demonstrates a placenta whose basal layer area has not been highlighted. The placenta may be assigned a lesser grade, such as Grade I, when in fact if basal echogenic densities were present it would have been a Grade II (Fig. 9*B*).

The posterior placenta may be difficult to scan because of acoustic shadowing from the fetus (Fig. 10). Scanning over the small

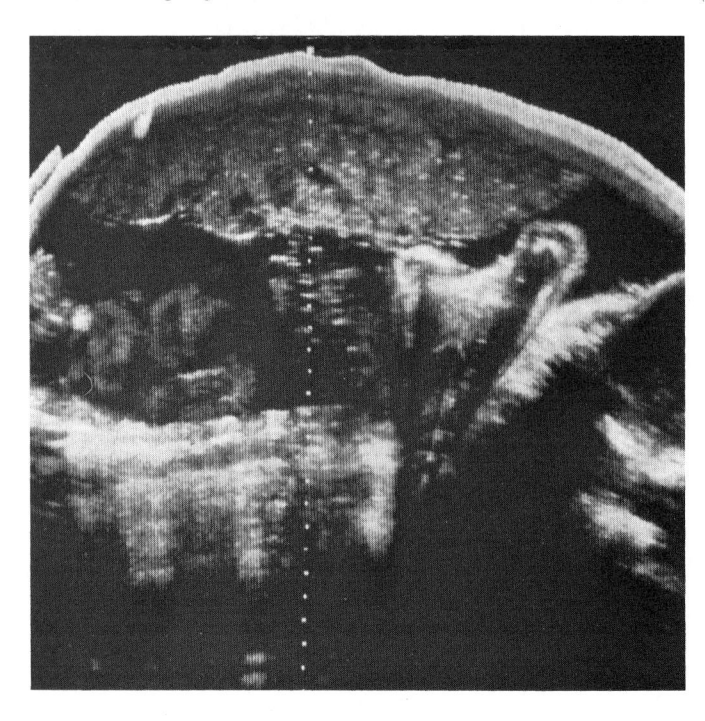

Figure 5. Grade I placenta showing randomly dispersed echogenic densities in the substance of the placenta.

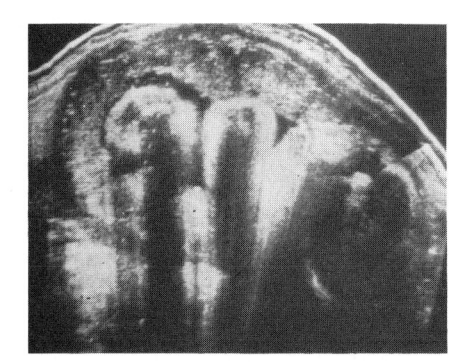

Figure 6. Grade II placenta. The basal layer shows presence of basal echogenic densities. (*From* Grannum, P., Berkowitz, R. L., and Hobbins, J. C.: The ultrasonic changes in the maturing placenta and their relation to fetal pulmonic maturity. Am. J. Obstet. Gynecol., *133*:915–922, 1979, with permission.)

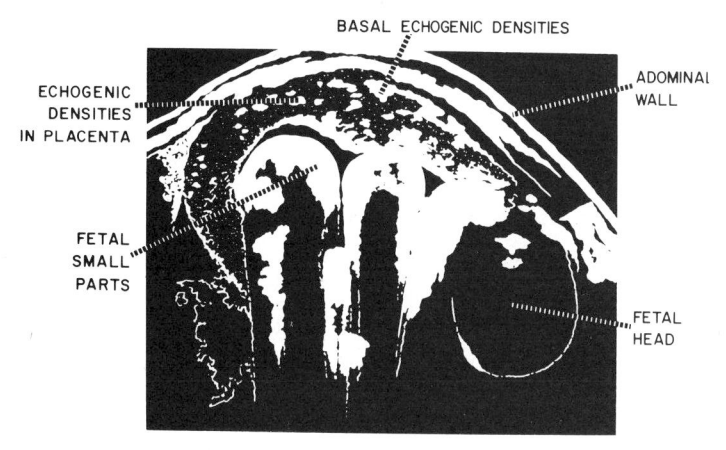

Figure 7. Grade II placenta demonstrating basal echogenic densities and "comma-like" densities.

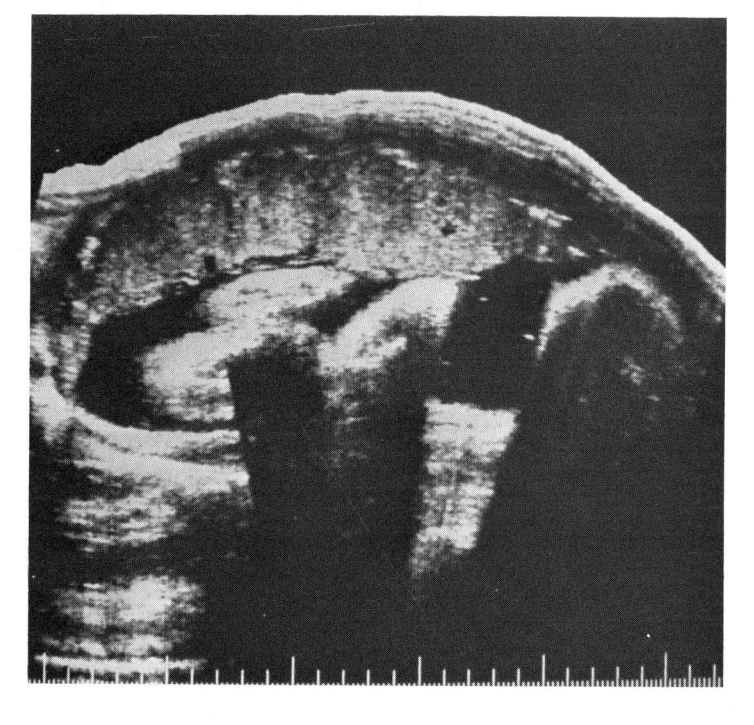

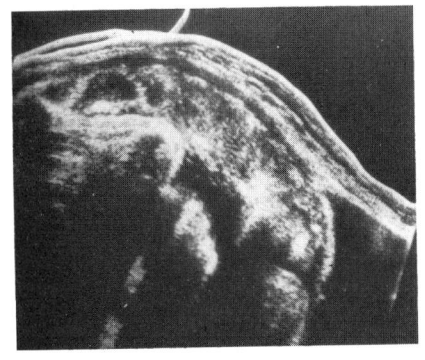

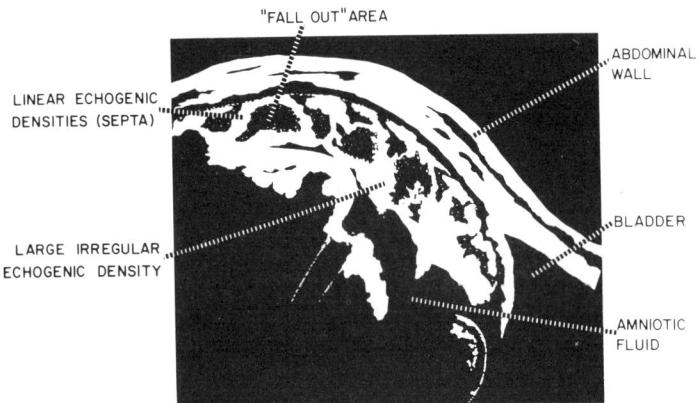

Figure 8. Grade III placenta. Note the appearance of the "fall-out" area in the cotyledons, divided by intercotyledonary septa, as well as the irregular densities. (*From* Grannum, P., Berkowitz, R. L., and Hobbins, J. C.: The ultrasonic changes in the maturing placenta and their relation to fetal pulmonic maturity. Am. J. Obstet. Gynecol., *133*:915–922, 1979, with permission.)

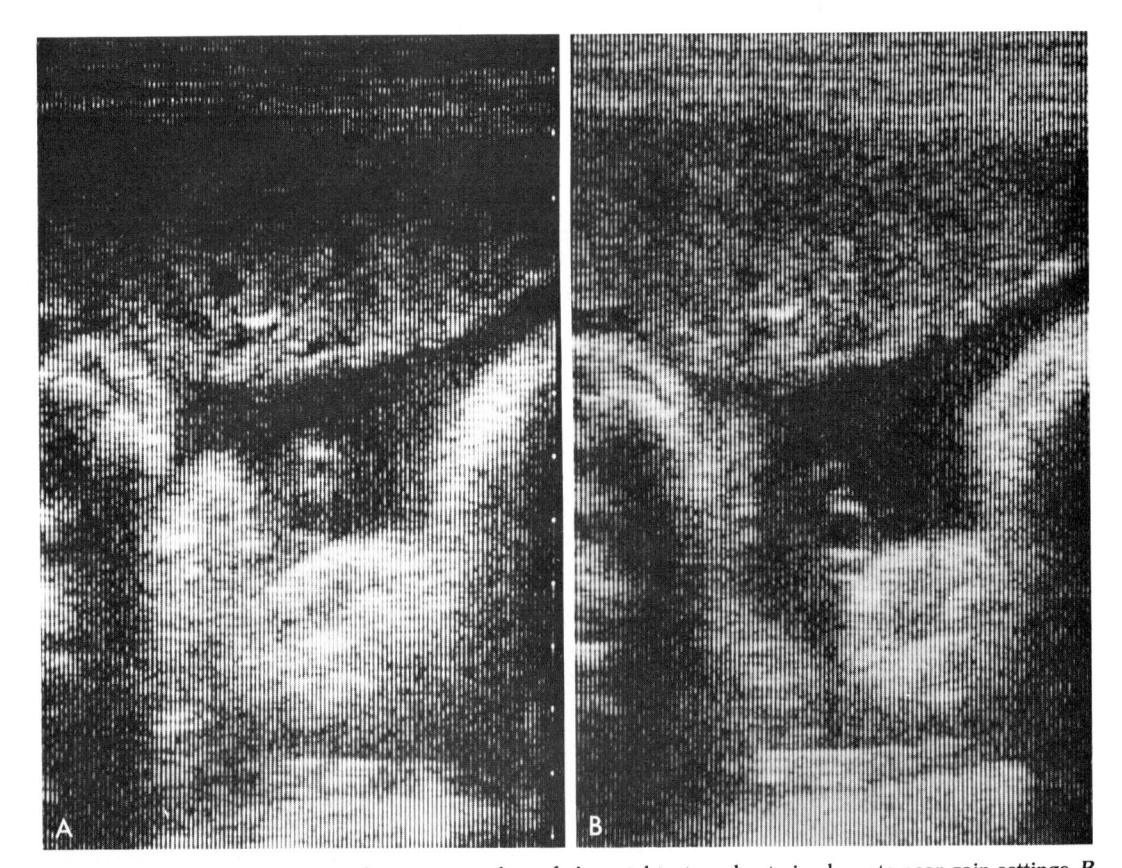

Figure 9. *A*, Anterior placenta demonstrating loss of placental texture due to inadequate near gain settings. *B*, Same placenta correctly examined.

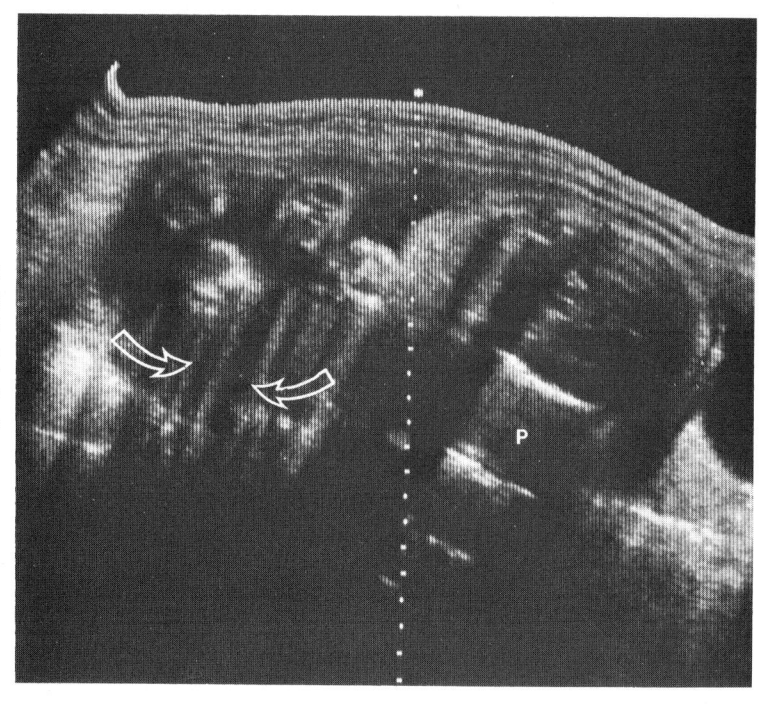

Figure 10. Posterior placenta (P). Note acoustic shadowing from the fetus (*arrows*). (*From* Grannum, P., Berkowitz, R. L., and Hobbins, J. C.: Ultrasonographic evaluation of the placenta. Perinatol. Neonatol. 6:1, 35–47, 1982, with permission.)

parts of the fetus will allow greater portions of the placenta to be assessed. In general, more than a third of the placenta should be seen in order to attempt grading.

PLACENTAL GRADING AND GESTATIONAL AGE

In normal pregnancies, Grade 0 represents the initial appearance of the placenta. As gestation advances, the placenta will mature to a Grade I at approximately 31 weeks of gestation.[20] In 40 per cent of normal patients, the placenta will maintain this configuration until term; in 45 per cent the placenta will mature to a Grade II at approximately 36 weeks and maintain this appearance until term. In the remaining 15 per cent the placenta will mature to a Grade III configuration at 38 weeks and maintain this appearance until delivery. Other investigators, Hohler (unpublished data and personal communication)[14] and Platt,[21] have confirmed similar results.

Preliminary results of postdate patients indicate that the placenta matures considerably after the fortieth week of pregnancy. Seven per cent of patients will go past the forty-second week of pregnancy, and the postmaturity syndrome will develop in 15 per cent of them. At the forty-second week of pregnancy, 55 per cent of patients will have Grade II placentas, and 45 per cent will have Grade III placentas. Presence of a Grade I placenta after the forty-second week of pregnancy seriously challenges the patient's dates.

There is no meaningful correlation between biparietal diameters and placental grading. In a preliminary study comparing placental grades and biparietal diameter,[9] the range of biparietal diameter for Grade I was 7.6 to 9.6 cm, Grade II 8.1 to 9.8 cm, and Grade III 8.7 to 9.5 cm. Petrucha et al. have reported similar results.[21]

PLACENTAL THICKNESS

In general, placental thickness increases linearly until the thirty-third week of pregnancy. After this time there is a gradual decrease in placental thickness, which is mediated by the degree of placental maturation. For example, the mean thickness for a Grade I placenta is 3 to 8 cm, Grade II 3.6 cm, and Grade III 3.4 cm.[9]

Although placental thickness may not be diagnostic of a particular complication of pregnancy, it can be helpful in its management. Placental thickness greater than 4 cm is most often a normal finding, but is also seen in patients with gestational dia-

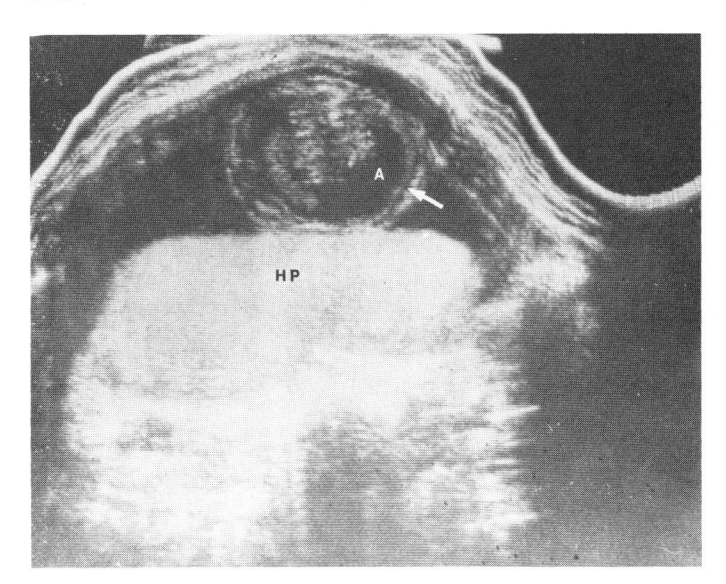

Figure 11. Severe Rh sensitization at 31 weeks' gestation showing cross-section of the fetal abdomen with ascites, subcutaneous edema, amniotic fluid, and a thick hydropic placenta. SE, subcutaneous edema; A, ascites; HP, hydropic placenta. (*From* Grannum, P.: The placenta. Clin. Diag. Ultrasound, 3:41–55, 1979, with permission.)

betes, nonimmune hydrops, congenital anomalies, and Rh-sensitization. The fetus with nonimmune hydrops demonstrates the greatest placental thickness. In assessment of the Rh-sensitized patient, placental thickness should be observed and included as part of the ultrasound examination. An increase in the thickness of the placenta is usually associated with increasing severity of disease (Fig. 11). On the other hand, patients with preeclampsia, intrauterine growth retardation, and juvenile diabetes with proliferative retinopathy have thin placentas. In our experience a glucose screen is recommended in patients whose placentas have matured beyond the Grade 0 stage and measure more than 4 cm in thickness. The results invariably indicate gestational diabetes.

PLACENTAL SURFACE AREA

Bleker et al. have shown that the surface area of the placenta increases linearly throughout pregnancy in 15 per cent of pa-

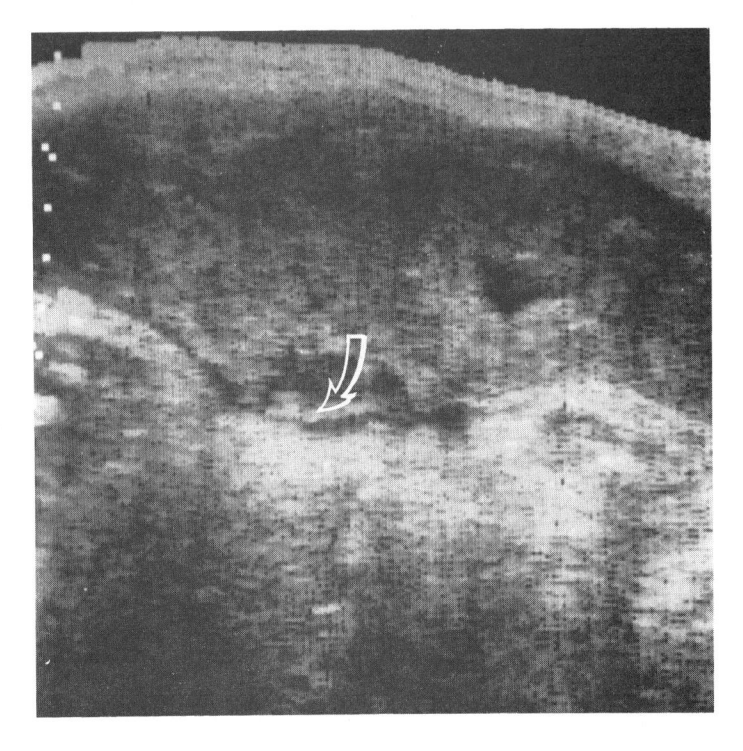

Figure 12. Cord insertion. Note echo-spared areas representing the insertion of the cord into the placenta (*arrow*).

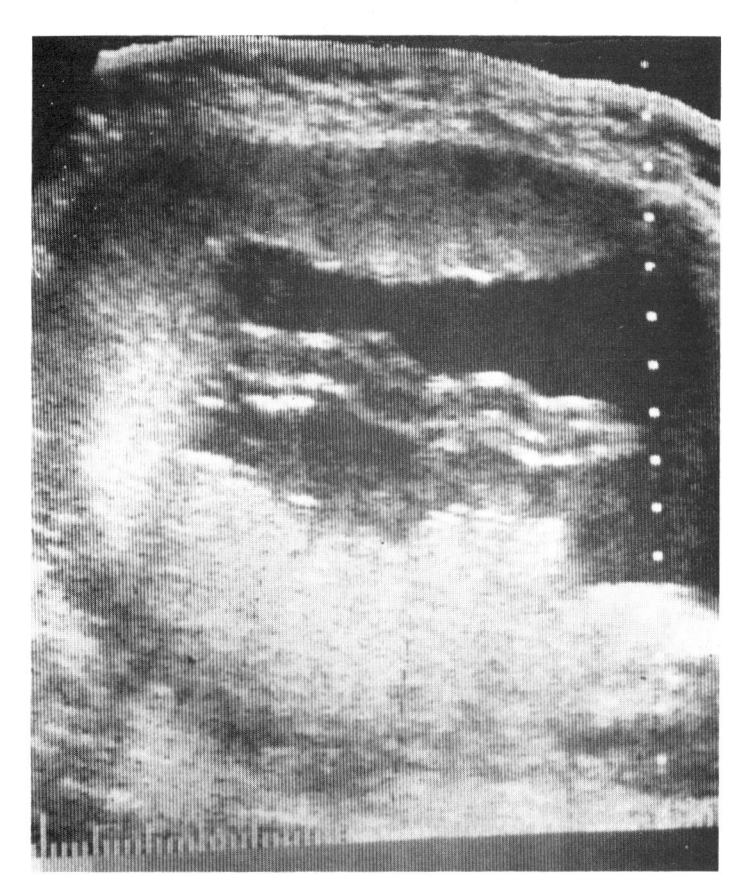

Figure 13. Cord insertion showing vessels traced into the placental substance.

tients. The remaining 85 per cent show a plateauing after 34 to 35 weeks of gestation.[1] Hoogland et al.[15] have suggested measuring placental surface area as a screening tool for intrauterine growth retardation. They measured the surface area of the placenta by taking serial transverse and longitudinal sections of the placenta from which the surface area was computed. The preliminary results indicated that if the surface area was 187 sq cm or less at 150 days' gestation, there was a 50 per cent chance of intrauterine growth retardation.

CORD INSERTION

Amniocentesis has become a routine obstetric procedure. When there is an anterior placenta which must be transversed, it is important to identify the site of cord insertion. Although the site of insertion is usually central, eccentric to markedly eccentric cord insertions occur with varying frequency, 48 to 75 per cent according to several authors.[17, 18, 22] Marginal or velamentous insertions of the cord occur in 5 to 6 per cent of cases.[7] In order to improve the safety of amniocentesis, identification of the cord insertion site is necessary.

The appearance of the insertion site on ultrasound is often that of echo-spared areas adjacent to the chorionic plate, having a V shape in the thickest portion of the placenta (Fig. 12). Meticulous longitudinal scanning may demonstrate the cord as it

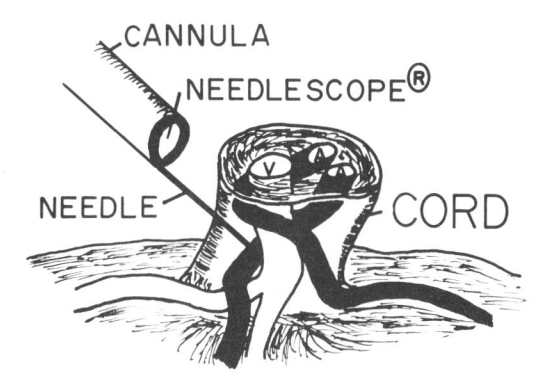

Figure 14. Fetoscopy showing technique for blood drawing. (*From* DeVore, G. R., Venus, I., Hobbins, J. C., et al.: Fetoscopy. *In* Rocker, I., and Lawrence, K. M. (eds.): Fetoscopy. New York, Elsevier/North Holland, 1981, with permission.)

enters the site of insertion on the placenta (Fig. 13). When fetoscopy is being performed,[5] it is vitally important to identify the cord as it enters the placenta since blood is drawn directly from the umbilical cord at that site (Fig. 14).

PLACENTAL GRADING AND FETAL PULMONIC MATURITY

Since the placenta is an integral part of the intrauterine unit, it is not surprising to find a correlation between the maturational processes of the placenta and the fetus. In a study correlating placenta grades and pulmonic maturity of the fetus, it became apparent that the processes are interrelated. Grade I is associated with a 67 per cent positive lecithin/sphingomyelin (L/S) ratio, Grade II 87.5, and Grade III 100 per cent (Table 2).[9]

The most striking result is that in normal pregnancies (35 weeks or greater) there is a 100 per cent correlation between Grade III placentas and mature L/S ratios. Petrucha et al. reported similar results.[21] This group reported a 91 per cent correlation of mature L/S ratios with a Grade I placenta, 97 per cent with a Grade II placenta, and 100 per cent with a Grade III placenta. Furthermore, of significance is the absence of the respiratory distress syndrome with all Grade III placentas.

Placental grading, then, can be very helpful if carefully applied to the high risk patient in whom fetal pulmonic maturity becomes the issue for further management, and amniocentesis is difficult or hazardous.

Table 2. *Acceleration* or Delay† of Time of Appearance in Gestation of Mature L/S Ratio Associated with Maternal, Fetal, or Placental Disease‡*

	L/S RATIO		
	NO.	ACCEL.	DELAY
Maternal disease			
"Chronic" toxemia	48	+	
Hypertensive renal disease	18	+	
Hypertensive cardiovascular disease	15	+	
Sickle cell disease	2	+	
Narcotics addiction	10	+	
Dibetes mellitus			
Classes A, B, and C	33		+
Classes D, E, and F	4	+	
Chronic, nonhypertensive glomerulonephritis	4		+
Fetal disease			
Hydrops fetalis	2		+
Smaller of nonparasitic monochorial twins	2		+
Placental disease			
Circumvallate placenta	1	+	
Chronic retroplacental bleeding	7	+	
Placental insufficiency, unspecified	1	+	
Premature rupture of membranes longer than 24 hr.	11	+	

* Acceleration refers to an L/S ratio of 2 or more which is identified prior to week 35 of gestation.

† Delay refers to an L/S ratio of 2 or more which is identified after week 35 of gestation.

‡ *From* Carroll, B.: Ultrasonic features of preeclampsia. J. Clin. Ultrasound, 8:483, 1980, with permission.

PLACENTAL GRADES AND OBSTETRIC OR MEDICAL COMPLICATIONS

The maturational process of the placenta as described in normal patients prevails in the complicated pregnancy. However, the timing of the maturational process can be affected by medical or obstetric complication. For example, pregnancies compromised by pregnancy-induced hypertension[2] or intrauterine growth retardation result in an acceleration of the maturational process of the placenta. In our experience it is not unusual to see a Grade III placenta prior to the thirty-fifth week in pregnancies compromised by intrauterine growth retardation and/or preeclampsia. This finding may precede the diagnosis of the complication, and it should lead to a close follow-up of the patient for the duration of the pregnancy.

The mean gestational period for the appearance of a Grade I placenta is 31 weeks.[20] If a Grade 0 placenta is recognized after the thirty-second week of pregnancy, one should consider the possibility of gestational diabetes. A glucose screen is then advised. Rh-sensitization also causes a delay in the maturational process of the placenta.[10]

The effect of these medical or obstetric complications on the timing of the maturational process of the placenta, either accelerated or delayed, is similar to the effect on the maturation of other organ systems in the fetus such as pulmonic maturity (see Table 2).[24]

PLACENTA PREVIA

The most common cause of vaginal bleeding in the second and third trimesters of pregnancy is placenta previa. Ultrasound has become the diagnostic modality of choice.[8, 16, 17] The diagnosis of placenta previa is made by assessing the relationship of the lower margins of the placenta to the internal os. Partial distention of the bladder, with urine acting as an acoustic window, allows visualization of this area (Fig. 15). Overdistention of the bladder may distort the true relationship of the lower margins of the placenta and the internal os by approximating the anterior lower uterine segment to the posterior uterine wall. Hence, an anterior or posterior placenta may appear to be more closely positioned to the internal os than it really is.[25]

It is much easier to delineate an anterior placenta previa (Fig. 16) than a posterior placenta previa since the posterior placenta is often obscured by shadowing from the fetus (see Fig. 10). Hence, defining the lower margins of the placenta and the internal os can be difficult. Two techniques can be used to assist us: elevation of the presenting part by abdominal palpation[25] and measurement of the distance between the presenting part and the sacral promontory. If the distance is greater than 1.5 cm, posterior placenta previa should be strongly suspected (Fig. 17).

Scans done during the second trimester (16 to 20 weeks) may reveal an incidence of 20 per cent total placenta previas, whereas at term the incidence is 0.5 per cent.[19] This apparent change, sometimes referred to as "placental migration," is the result of the development of the lower uterine segment. It is more likely to occur in patients in whom the placenta also has a fundal attachment. Patients with total placenta previas at 20 weeks with significant portions of placenta on either side of the cervix are more likely to have a persistent placenta previa in the third trimester. If the diagnosis of a total placenta previa is made at 20 weeks, a repeat scan at 28 weeks, or sooner if bleeding occurs, should be performed. If the placenta is still situated in the lower uterine segment at this stage, scans should be performed later in

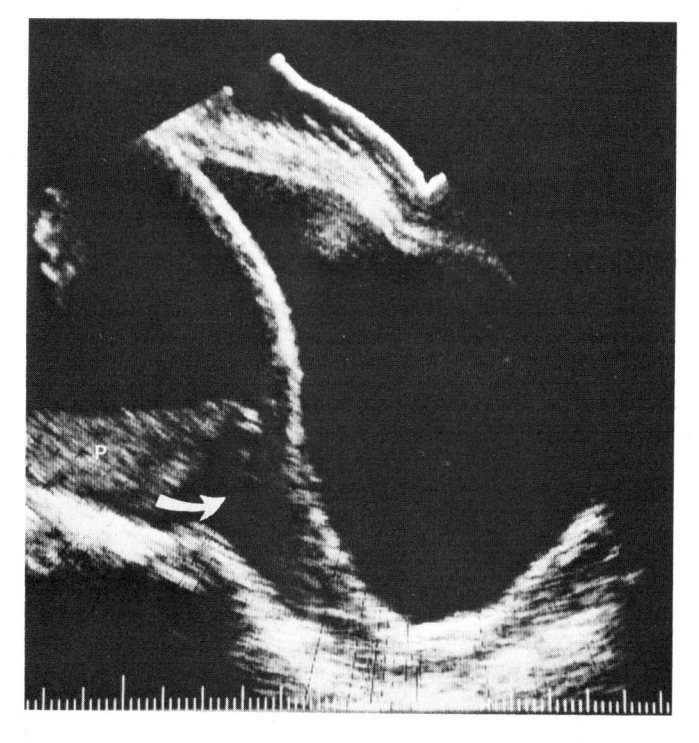

Figure 15. Posterior placenta previa (P) demonstrating the area of the internal os (*arrow*).

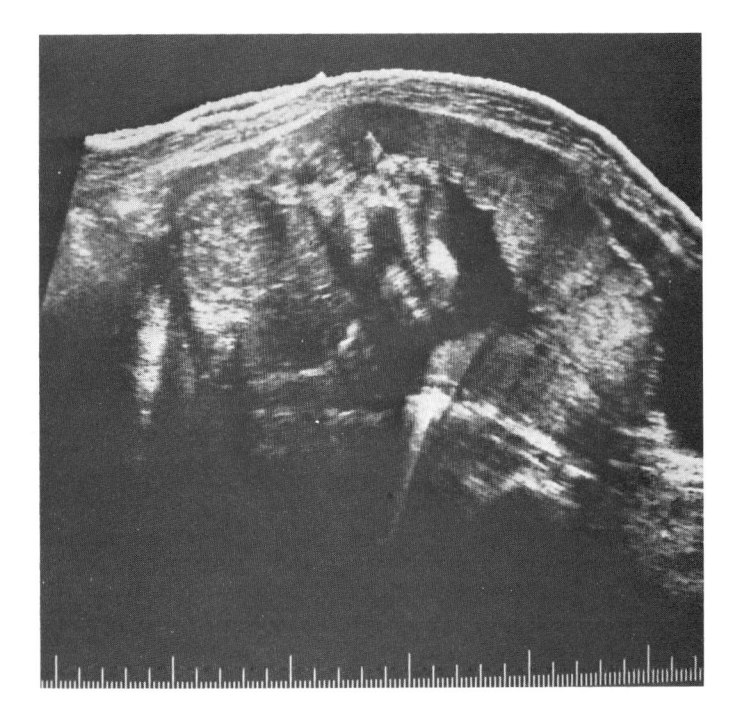

Figure 16. Anterior placenta previa.

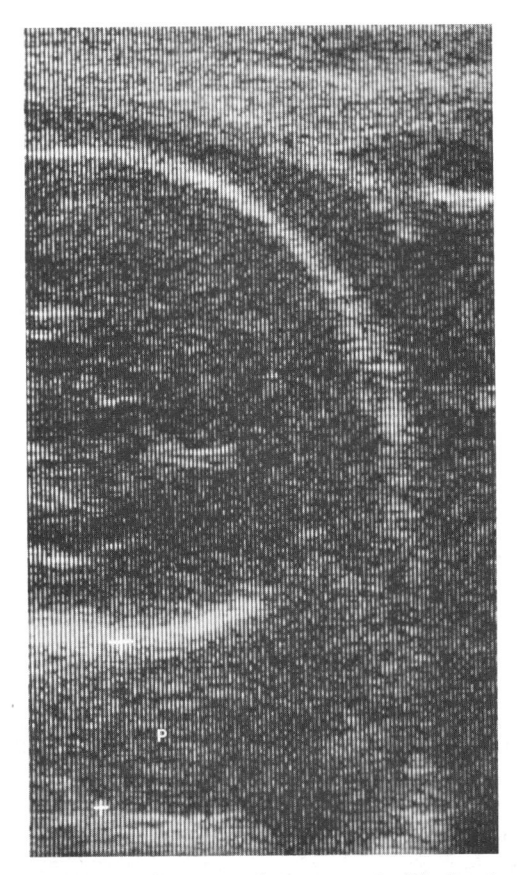

Figure 17. Posterior placenta previa (P) showing distance between sacral promontory and presenting part of greater than 1.5 cm.

the pregnancy since further "migration" is still possible.

ABRUPTIO PLACENTAE

Ultrasound can be useful in the diagnosis and conservative management of this condition. If the separation cannot be seen on ultrasound it does not preclude the diagnosis. Clinical diagnosis still represents the diagnostic modality of choice.

The two findings noted on ultrasound are the presence of a retroplacental clot (Fig. 18) and an extramembranous clot (Figs. 18 and 19). The retroplacental clot appears as a transonic area between the basal area of the placenta and the uterine wall. It is unusual to see this separation as clearly as it is indicated in Figure 18. Serial ultrasound scans can be used to follow the progress of the abruption by measuring the size of the area of placental separation or the retroplacental clot. As the clot becomes more organized, it becomes more echogenic, which aids in separating old clot from fresh clot. In the laterally positioned placenta, the large uterine veins and sinuses should not be confused with a massive abruptio placentae (Fig. 20).[11]

Rupture of the uteroplacental veins at

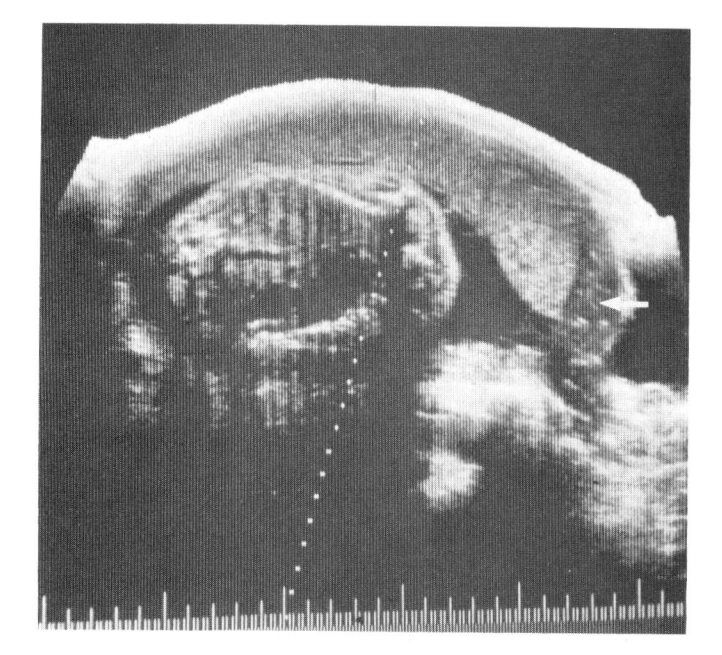

Figure 18. Abruptio placentae. Note the presence of a retroplacental and an extramembranous clot (*arrow*).

the margins of the placenta is sometimes seen (Fig. 21). If the plaenta is low lying, a retromembranous clot from this entity can simulate placenta previa, especially after it has become echogenic, representing an organized clot. Correct adjustment of the gain controls will help to distinguish between these two entities.

MULTIPLE PREGNANCY

Twins, the most common manifestation of a multiple gestation pregnancy, may either be monozygotic or dizygotic. Monozygotic twins, a random occurrence, results when a single fertilized ovum replicates during the early stages of devel-

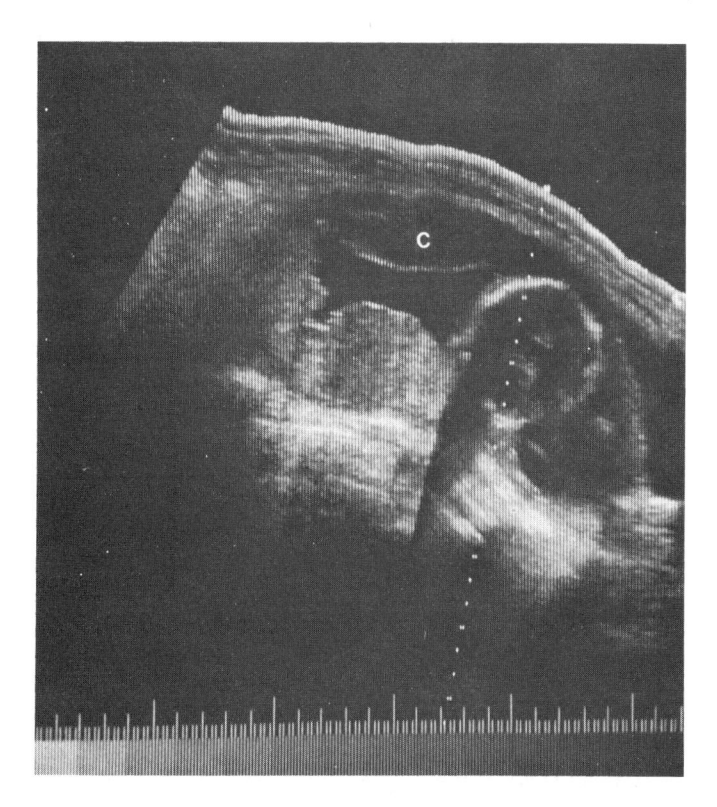

Figure 19. Abruptio placentae demonstrating large extramembranous clot (C).

154   The Placenta

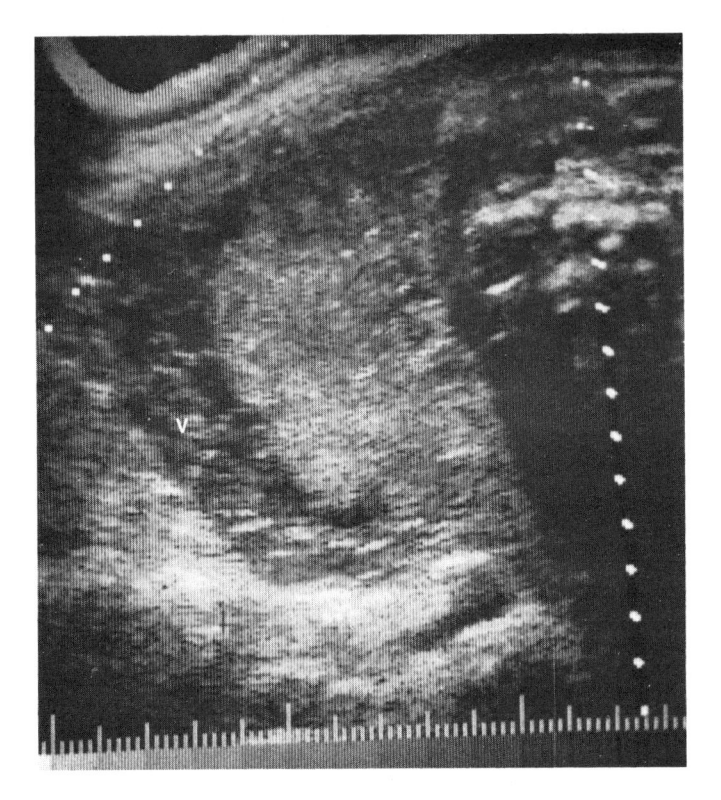

Figure 20. Large uterine veins (V) visible in laterally positioned placenta should not be confused with abruptio placentae.

opment resulting in fetuses of the same genetic makeup. Dizygotic twins are the result of fertilization of two separate ova in which genetic similarity is no greater than in any other pair of siblings.

If the two ova of dizygotic twins are implanted at widely separated sites within the uterus there will be two separate and discrete placentas, each having its own amniotic sac.[7] This type of placentation is that of the dichorionic-diamniotic type. If, however, the two ova implant adjacent to one

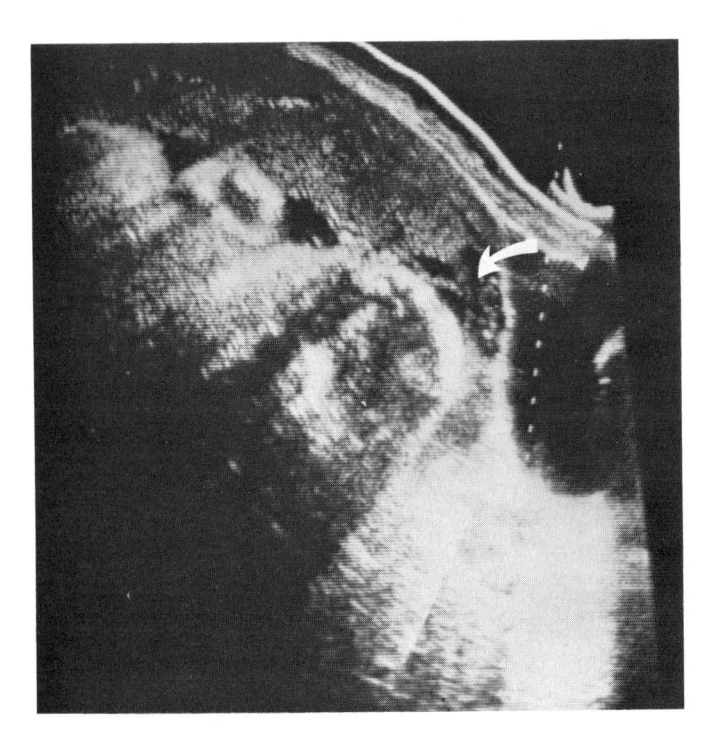

Figure 21. A 36-week pregnancy with an anterior placenta with bleed from the margins of the placenta with retromembranous clot. (*arrow*). (*From* Grannum, P.: Case No. 7. Vaginal bleeding in the third trimester. Clin. Diag. Ultrasound, *3*:175, 1979, with permission.)

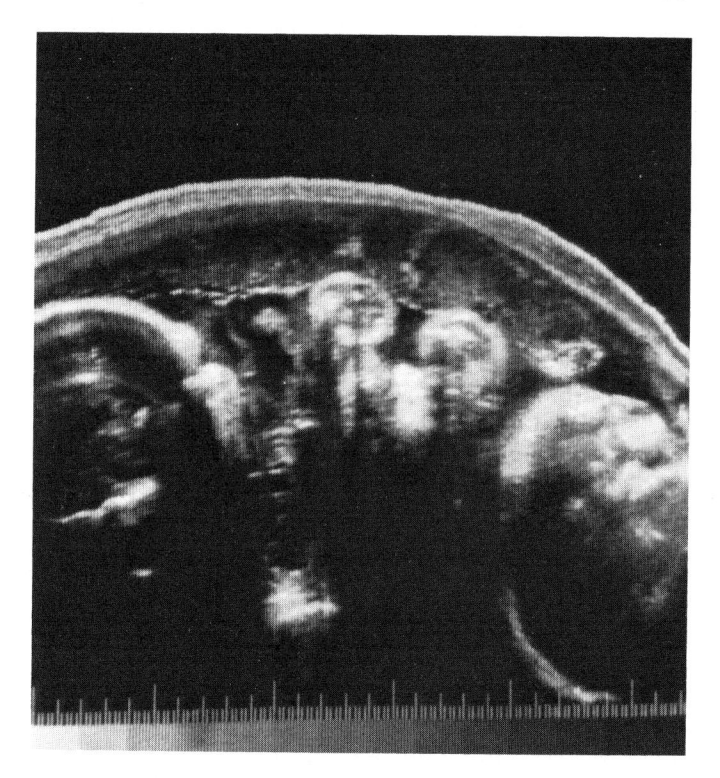

Figure 22. Multiple pregnancy demonstrating an apparent single placenta.

another there will be two amniotic sacs but the two placentas will show varying degrees of fusion, forming what appears to be a single placenta (Fig. 22). Careful examination will reveal this also to be a dichorionic-diamniotic gestation.

With monozygotic twins the form of placentation depends upon the stage at which replication occurs.[7] If the single fertilized ovum divides during the first three days after fertilization two separate embryos will develop, each having its own placenta

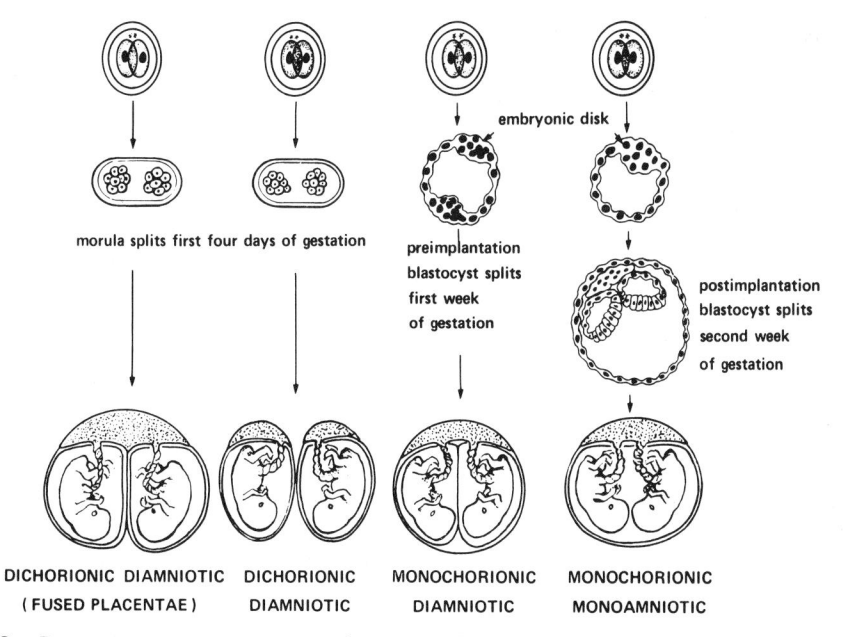

Figure 23. Diagrammatic representation of the development and placentation of monozygotic twins. (*From* Fox, H.: Pathology of the Placenta. Philadelphia, W. B. Saunders Co., 1978, with permission.)

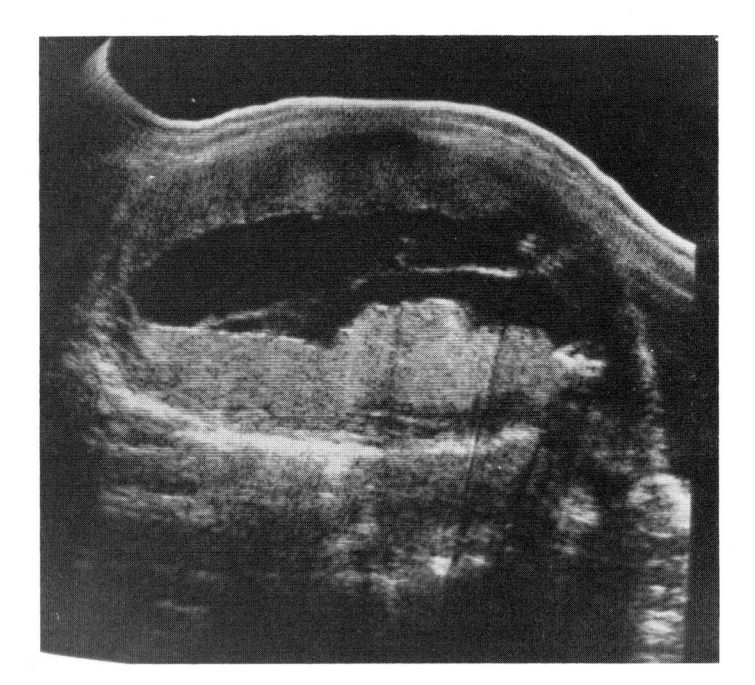

Figure 24. Multiple pregnancy with twins demonstrating two separate placentas, one anterior, the other posterior. Dividing membranes are seen. (*From* Grannum, P., Berkowitz, R. L., and Hobbins, J. C.: Ultrasonography in the antepartum patient. *In* Bolognese, R., Schwarz R. J., and Schneider, J. (eds.) Perinatal Medicine. Edition 2. Baltimore, Williams and Wilkins, 1981, with permission.)

and amniotic sac, and thus will be dichorionic-diamniotic.[3] If division of the fertilized ovum occurs between the third and eighth day after fertilization when the trophoblast but not the amniotic cavity has differentiated, the twins will develop a single placenta with two amniotic sacs and thus have a monochorionic-diamniotic placenta (Fig. 23).[3] If division of the fertilized ovum occurs between the eighth and thirteenth day after fertilization (the time of amniotic cavity differentiation) there will be one placenta and one amniotic sac, thus a monochorionic-monoamniotic gestation.[7]

The twin-to-twin transfusion syndrome, which may occur in 15 to 20 per cent of monozygotic twin pregnancies,[23] is characterized by discordant growth of the two fetuses as a result of communication between their circulatory symptoms. One twin will deliver a portion of its blood to the other twin with each beat of the heart. The recipient will become cardiac-overloaded and polycythemic. The donor twin develops intrauterine growth retardation. Careful antepartum monitoring and timely delivery are essential for good fetal outcome. Discordant growth can also be seen if there is inequality in the size of the placenta serving each twin. Presence of two separate placentas does not preclude the possibility of discordant growth since local factors in each placenta may interfere with the potential for normal growth in one of the twins (Fig. 24). Also it is not unusual to have a different grade in the two placentas in this situation.

If division occurs on or after the thirteenth day after fertilization the result will be conjoined twins.

ACKNOWLEDGMENT

We would like to extend our appreciation to Ingeborg Venus for her editorial assistance.

REFERENCES

1. Bleker, O. P., Kloosterman, G. J., Breur, W., et al.: The volumetric growth of the human placenta: A longitudinal ultrasonic study. Am. J. Obstet. Gynecol., *127*:657, 1977.
2. Carroll, B.: Ultrasonic features of pre-eclampsia. J. Clin. Ultrasound, *8*:483, 1980.
3. Corner, G. W.: The observed embryology of human single-ovum twins and other multiple births. Am. J. Obstet. Gynecol., *70*:933–951, 1955.
4. Crawford, J. M.: Vascular anatomy of the human placenta. Am. J. Obstet. Gynecol., *84*:1543, 1962.
5. DeVore, G. R., Venus, I., Hobbins, J. C., et al.: Fetoscopy: General clinical approach. *In* Rocker, I., and Lawrence, K. M. (Eds.): Fetoscopy. New York, Elsevier/North-Holland, 1981.
6. Earn, A. A.: The effect of congenital abnormalities of the umbilical cord and the placenta on the newborn and mothers—A survey of 5,676 consecutive deliveries. J. Obstet. Gynaecol. Br. Emp., *58:*456–459, 1951.
7. Fox, H.: Pathology of the Placenta. Philadelphia, W. B. Saunders Co., 1978, pp. 426–457.

8. Gottesfeld, K. R., Thompson, H. E., Holmes, J. H., et al.: Ultrasonic placentography—a new method for placental localization. Am. J. Obstet. Gynecol., 96:538–547, 1966.
9. Grannum, P. A. T., Berkowitz, R. L., and Hobbins, J. C.: The ultrasonic changes in the maturing placenta and their relation to fetal pulmonic maturity. Am. J. Obstet. Gynecol., 133:915–922, 1979.
10. Grannum, P., Berkowitz, R. L., Silverman, R., et al.: Correlation of ultrasound classification of placental maturity with L/S ratios in non Rh-sensitized pregnacies. Society for Gynecological Investigation, 26th Annual Meeting, San Diego, 1979.
11. Hadlock, F. P., Deter, R. L., Carpenter, R., et al.: Hypervascularity of the uterine wall during pregnancy: Incidence, sonographic appearance, and obstetric significance. J. Clin. Ultrasound, 8:399–403, 1980.
12. Hobbins, J. C., and Winsberg, F.: Ultrasonography in Obstetrics and Gynecology. Baltimore, Williams and Wilkins, 1977.
13. Hobbins, J. C., Mahoney, M. J., Berkowitz, R. L., et al.: Use of ultrasound in the diagnosis of congenital anomalies. Am. J. Obstet. Gynecol., 135:331–346, 1979.
14. Hohler, C.: Personal communication.
15. Hoogland, H. J.: Ultrasonographic Aspects of the Placenta. The Netherlands, Koninklijke Drukkerij G. J. Thieme, BV, Nijmegen, Alphen a/d Rijn. 1980.
16. Kobayashi, M., Hellman, L. M., and Fillisti, L.: Placental localization by ultrasound. Am. J. Obstet. Gynecol., 106:279–285, 1970.
17. Kohorn, E. I., Walker, R. H. S., Morrison, J., et al.: Placental localization. Am. J. Obstet. Gynecol., 103:868–877, 1969.
18. Krone, H. A., Jopp, H., and Schellerer, W.: Die Bedeutung anamnestischer Befunde für die verschiedenen Formen des Nabelschnursatzes. Zeitschrift Geburts. Gynäkol., 163:205–213, 1964.
19. Lee, R. G., Knochel, J. Q., Melendez, M. G., et al.: Fetal elevation: A new technique for placental localization in the diagnosis of previa. J. Clin. Ultrasound, 9:467–471, 1981.
20. Levine, L. R.: Placental grades and gestational age. Doctoral Thesis, New Haven, Connecticut, Yale University School of Medicine, March 1981.
21. Petrucha, R., Golde, S., and Platt, L.: Realtime ultrasound of the placenta in assessment of fetal pulmonic maturity. Am. J. Obstet. Gynecol., 142:463–467, 1982.
22. Purola, E.: The length and insertion of the umbilical cord. Ann. Chir. Gynecol., 57:621–622, 1968.
23. Strong, S. J., and Corney, G.: The Placenta in Twin Pregnancies. Oxford, Pergamon Press, 1967.
24. Whitfield, C. R., and Sproule, W. B.: Fetal lung maturation. Br. J. Hosp. Med., 12:678–686, 1974.
25. Williamson, D., Bjorgen, J., Barer, B., et al.: The ultrasonic diagnosis of placenta previa: Value of the post-void scan. J. Clin. Ultrasound, 6:1, 58, 1978.
26. Winsberg, F.: Echographic changes with placental aging. J. Clin. Ultrasound, 1:52–55, 1973.

9

Fetal Behavior and Condition

Jason C. Birnholz, M.D.

Every ultrasound examination of the fetus should address the interrelated topic areas of structure, growth, and condition. Imaging structure implies the detection and classification of congenital anomalies. Growth, assessed typically from morphologic features, relates to the metabolic and thermodynamic competence of the fetus and fetoplacental unit. Condition refers to the immediate or short-term risk of fetal morbidity and mortality. Measures of fetal condition are used in conjunction with equivalent risks for the newborn, at the same gestational age, to assess the need and urgency of elective delivery.

The way in which ultrasonic imaging subserves these three topics represents a graded conceptual transition from static, anatomic diagnosis to dynamic monitoring of physiologic and pathophysiologic processes. Condition is inferred from fetal behavior, generally, and from dynamic and organizational properties of individual patterns of movement, specifically. This line of research is new so that present descriptions are preliminary. Fetal behavior will be considered in its applied context of helping the clinician to assess the condition of the fetus. This review is intended as a practical guide to that end; primary sources should be consulted for literature survey.

ERYTHROBLASTOSIS FETALIS AND CONGESTIVE HEART FAILURE

Assessing the condition of the fetus is important in every examination in the third trimester, but it is particularly relevant whenever a "high risk" situation is identified. Erythroblastosis fetalis provides an example in which management is predicated upon serial indication of condition. Erythroblastosis is due usually to Rh factor isoimmunization and occasionally to anti-Kell (or other irregular antibody) reactions. This disorder is also one of the best examples of an essentially normal fetus reacting to a hostile environment.

The management standard has been serial monitoring of amniotic fluid bilirubin level (ΔOD), after the pioneer work of Liley. Initial ultrasound efforts attempted to define the presence of ascites, which was taken as a priori evidence of the fetus's poor condition and the need for a blood transfusion or delivery of the child. Ascites is, in fact, a poor prognostic indicator, and our own experience has shown that more sensitive signs of deterioration must be sought so that a transfusion protocol can be initiated before ascites has developed. Rhesus factor sensitization involves two pathophysiologic processes that may be disjointed: liver disease (with ascites due to hypoalbuminemia) and severe anemia (with high output congestive failure). The former is recognized by ascites (without skin edema) and hepatomegaly (Fig. 1). The liver is infiltrated and very firm, and the liver margin is, typically, blunted. Congestive failure would involve chronic, passive hepatic congestion, ascites, pleural effusions, and, ultimately, skin edema (the combination being hydrops fetalis). That is the case, although the liver does not become particularly enlarged, and the margins remain sharp (Fig. 2). The fetal myocardium is not particularly distensible; however, the right atrium can enlarge selectively. Right atrial dilatation is the earliest and most consistent morphologic sign of congestive failure in utero.

Hydrops is, essentially, the only morphologic indication of poor fetal condition. In certain situations, such as Rh sensitization, ascites alone indicates a poor prognosis. Right atrial distention implies a need for further investigation but does not of itself imply that the condition of the fetus has deteriorated. This theme recurs in the common case of intrauterine growth retardation.

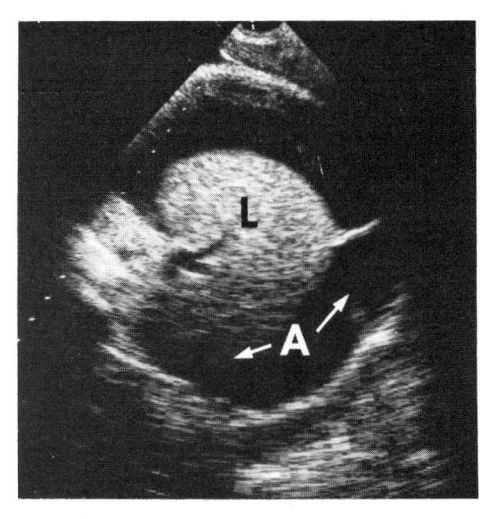

Figure 1. There is large amount of ascites (A) without associated skin edema. The liver (L) is rounded; the hepatic veins are not distended. This is a case of erythroblastosis caused by Kell factor sensitization.

RETARDATION OF GROWTH AND "STRESS"

Retardation of growth is discussed in chapter 7. In this chapter, I will consider the specific case of progressive failure of placental competence, which will cause declining rate of fetal (weight) growth. This situation poses a risk of fetal death and is associated with a well-known range of morbidity for newborns. Nevertheless, the point to be understood is that retardation of growth per se does not indicate delivery in the mid or late third trimester, unless, possibly, the growth rate falls below 5 gm per day. Retardation of growth indicates a high risk for which other signs of stress or deteriorating condition should be sought.

Retardation of growth (in the specific category implied here) may be thought of as a chronic fetal compromise equivalent to malnutrition. One wants to detect hypoxia, acidosis, or both (or their effects), since they will cause acute deterioration, with risk of fetal death. Serial estriol determinations (usually urine samples every 24 hours from the mother) provide a means of establishing the trend of functional capacity of the fetoplacental unit. Assuming appropriate steroid production from the adrenal glands of the fetus, falling estriol values indicate progressive placental failure. Although one assumes that fetal distress will be highly likely when placental function falls below some threshold, it should be understood that this test provides inferential data about the actual condition of the fetus. Norepinephrine levels in the amniotic fluid correlate well with fetal oxygenation, but currently available assays are too lengthy and laborious for routine clinical use. In the particular case of retardation of growth, the pathophysiologic conditions of hypoxia and acidosis must be distinguished from predisposing or moderating clinical factors.

HEART RATE

Average heart rate signifies little about fetal condition unless the variation from the norm is extreme. Fetal cardiac activity can be identified between 6 and 6½ weeks with time motion (T-M), Doppler, or electronically scanned imaging systems. The average heart rate may be in the 100 to 120 bpm range at that time, but it increases to about 145 bpm relatively soon thereafter. Average heart rate will remain within 135 to 155 bpm (with progressive but very slight decrement) throughout the remainder of the pregnancy.

The fetus has practically no capability for adjusting stroke volume. Cardiac output depends, principally, upon heart rate; for this reason, bradycardia is a particularly bad sign. Bradycardia is a very late sign of fetal compromise, and by the time it has occurred, the probability of neonate survival is already extremely low. The one exception is bradycardia due to atrioventricular block, which is often associated with

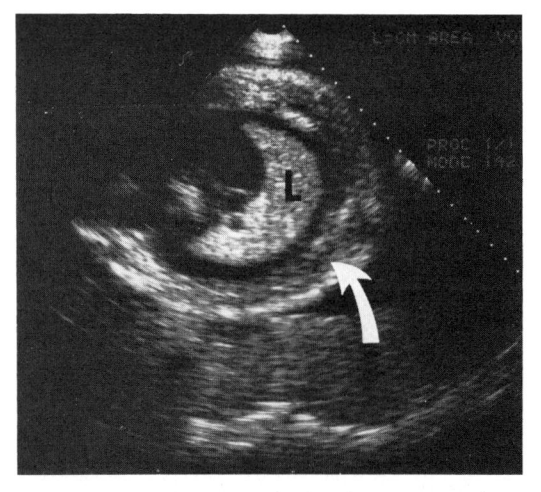

Figure 2. Ascites and thick subcutaneous edema (*arrow*) are present but the liver (L) edges are sharp in this patient with congestive failure due to atrial tachycardia.

maternal collagen vascular disease. In those cases, there will be a 2:1 to 4:1 differential of atrial and ventricular beats, ventricular pulsations will be particularly forceful, and there will be no other signs of fetal compromise.

Persistent slight increases in average heart rate can be associated with mild acceleration of growth. Ventricular filling is impaired at rates above 180. Two possibilities are primary atrial tachycardia and secondary increase in atrial rate in the fetus with severely depressed myocardial function (such as viral myocarditis). In any case, tachycardia always requires further investigation and cannot be ascribed to stress alone. Conversely, one cannot be reassured by normal average heart rate that the condition of the fetus is normal.

During the past 20 years, applied clinical study of beat-to-beat timing or rate variations with fetal movements (the nonstress test) and with naturally occurring or pharmacologically induced contractions has been conducted.

NON-STRESS TEST (NST)

- BASELINE FETAL CARDIAC ACCELERATION WITH FETAL MOVEMENT REFLECTS NORMAL FUNCTIONING OF THE FETAL HEART AND IS CONSIDERED A GOOD PROGNOSTIC SIGN (REACTIVE NST)

- REACTIVE (NORMAL) NST -- DETECTION OF AT LEAST 2 (4-5) FETAL HEART RATE ACCELERATIONS, 15 BPM ABOVE BASELINE, LASTING 15 SEC., IN A 20 (30) MIN. TEST PERIOD

Although average heart rate may remain 140 bpm over prolonged periods of time, there is short-term modulation of vagal tone. Abnormal patterns in the short term or beat-to-beat timing intervals have been defined and correlated with newborn outcome; therefore, these tests are the most widely used and best understood of the current methods for evaluating fetal condition.[26] These tests, particularly the nonstress test, provide a standard for judging the utility of newer ultrasound indicators of fetal risk.

CONTRACTION STRESS TEST (CST)

- UTERINE CONTRACTIONS ↓ UTERINE AND INTERVILLOUS BLOOD FLOW → STRESS → FETOPLACENTAL UNIT

- FAILURE TO TOLERATE STRESS MANIFEST BY REPETITIVE UNIFORM LATE DECELERATIONS RELATED TO FETAL MYOCARDIAL HYPOXIA (POSITIVE TEST)

- SPONTANEOUS OR OXYTOCIN INDUCED CONTRACTIONS (3 PER 10 MINUTE PERIOD, EACH LASTING 40-60 SEC IN DURATION)

- FALSE POSITIVE RATE – HIGH (30-60%)
- FALSE NEGATIVE RATE – LOW (<1%)

Variability of heart rate is more useful than average heart rate for evaluating fetal condition because it provides information about physiologic control mechanisms. In any physiologic monitoring situation, organization or control factors will be perturbed earlier or more thoroughly than the function of the end effector itself. Therefore, measurement of the pre-ejection period (that is, timing the cardiac electromechanical coupling interval) has been suggested as an alternative (or supplement) to variability of heart rate for clinical management.[10] The pre-ejection period is shortened when hypoxia is present. In that particular case, the observed effect may be caused by increased production of catecholamines by the fetus, and the specific physiologic observation represents a second or higher order effect of hypoxia. To search for first-order effects so that analysis under clinical usage can be simplified and to identify variables that may be studied directly with ultrasound imaging systems alone is our goal.

GENERAL BODY MOVEMENTS

One of the clinical adages of obstetric practice is that the mother's perception of less fetal movement during the third trimester is an ominous prognostic sign. Relations between the mother's perception of fetal movement and fetal well being have been emphasized as guidelines for practice.[20, 27] Ultrasound imaging studies show that expectant mothers feel only a small percentage of fetal movements, chiefly forceful kicks and extension of the head and neck. Perceived movements are also decreased, adventitiously, when oligohydramnios restricts fetal activity and when polyhydramnios "insulates" the fetus within the uterus. Leaving aside issues of type and quality of movement, and excluding maternal-fetal sedation, undoubtedly a third trimester fetus who is completely immobile during ultrasonic inspection with a high-speed imaging device (and who remains so in successive studies during the following 12 to 24 hours) is seriously compromised.[11] These same fetuses also exhibit poor body tone.[16] If a gestational norm is established for specific or total body movements, decreased frequency and slow, sluggish, or torpid activity represent lesser degrees of clinical deterioration. The following description from the 19th century remains valid even after technical translation to direct intrauterine visualization:

> After the movements have been distinctly felt, they sometimes diminish without appreciable cause, both in frequency and intensity, and then altogether disappear, which circumstances demand the most serious attention of the accoucher, as it is in general an unfortunate symptom.[4]

Rhesus factor sensitization provides an example of the relationship of fetal body movements and condition. The severely compromised fetus will exhibit few or no movements, and there will be no aversive movements as a transfusion needle is guided into the peritoneal space. Body movements will have returned to baseline normal by the second to third day after transfusion, if the administered blood is absorbed.

Passive observation of movements may be supplemented by interactive studies, as suggested in the following paragraph of the text just quoted:

> I prefer placing a hand upon one of the sides of the abdomen, and striking with the other on a point opposite, for the foetus then rarely fails to move briskly as though to resist the impulse.[4]

Likewise, observations may be continued while the examiner attempts to percuss or ballot the limbs, torso, or head. An intense, noxious stimulus should provoke an aversive reaction in the intact fetus. Conversely, lack of responsiveness emphasizes the severity of compromise when immobility or rare, isolated movements have been found.

The fetus will have developed a wide repertory of specific body movements by 20 weeks (Fig. 3). Subsequent development will result in smoother execution of individual movements and progressive coordination of collected patterns of activity. A recurrent general theme in motor development is the achievement of some milestone, its apparent loss as inhibitory mechanisms are developed, and its later reappearance in a persistent and organized form. Neuromotor regression to a gestationally earlier standard of movement competence will probably precede declining frequency and strength of movement, although further study of that possibility is still necessary.

BREATHING MOVEMENTS

The beginning and regulation of respiration are signal issues in fetal physiology. Clinical interest in ultrasonically observed breathing movements has been prompted by the possibility that this dynamic feature may provide information about fetal well being.[21]

Forceful diaphragmatic movements, such as hiccups, may be visible externally, and the notion of antenatal "breathing" was reported nearly a century ago.[1] Nevertheless, respiratory or respiratory-like activity was not accepted generally as a feature of normal antenatal development until the detailed studies of Dawes and collaborators reported initially in the early 1970s.[8]

Breathing movements have several diaphragmatic and chest wall components. Ul-

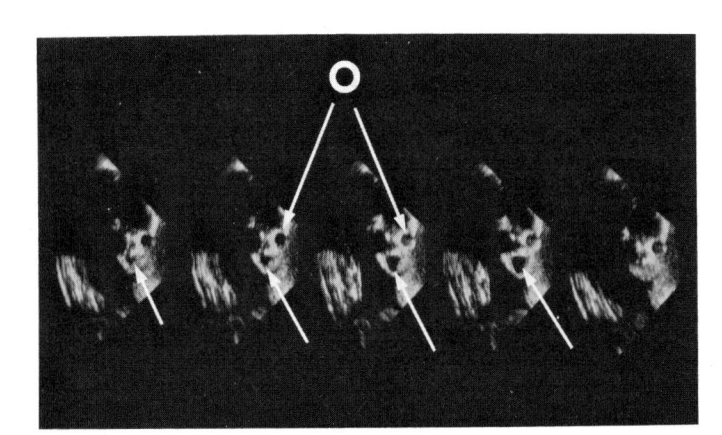

Figure 3. This sequence of views shows yawning at 19 weeks of gestational age. Mouth movements (*arrows*) are among the earliest occurring complex activity patterns. O, orbit.

trasonic monitoring should be directed primarily toward recognizing craniocaudal movements of the diaphragm (or liver or kidneys) in views oriented in a sagittal fetal plane. Radial (expansile) movements of the abdominal wall or chest can be seen (and are documented readily with T-M or Doppler methods) but are secondary to diaphragmatic excursions, have lower amplitude, and may vary in phase relationship to diaphragmatic movements depending upon behavioral state (Fig. 4). Breathing activity should be reserved for a series of diaphragmatic excursions, since single diaphragmatic movements (unassociated with yawning) may follow swallowing. Short segments of fairly regular movements of the diaphragm may be seen between 16 and 20 weeks' gestational age. They become less frequent (? active inhibition) during the next four to six weeks and then recur with progressive incidence, duration, and regularity in the final trimester. Breathing movements should be distinguished from hiccups, which are regular, forceful, and slower. Breathing episodes may be irregular in amplitude and timing (aperiodic) or regular in both of those features. They usually vary in rate from 60 to 100 per minute but may occur in short bursts of high frequency, low amplitude vibrations, particularly before 30 weeks' gestation.

The incidence of breathing movements decreases when the fetus is hypoxic.[15, 17] Episodes of breathing movements (and conversely the incidence of periods of apnea) have an innate periodicity (per gestational age level) and are affected further by numerous extrinsic factors including the mother's sedation, alcohol consumption, cigarette smoking, and the time since and the content of her last meal. Detailed investigation of the time statistics of breathing show that phases of apnea are sufficiently common and lengthy that continuous periods of monitoring more than an hour are needed in the third trimester to define a baseline estimate of average time spent in breathing activity.[3] Nevertheless, the simple occurrence of breathing can be informative, and it is commonly held that the presence of breathing is reassurring about fetal condition, but no conclusion should be drawn from apnea unless monitoring conforms to statistically necessary sampling minima, which may be difficult to achieve in routine clinical practice.

Breathing movements are provoked in the fetal lamb by stimulating the chest wall.[7] The overall incidence of human fetal breathing time, however, does not appear to be changed by vigorous external stimulation.[25] Increased breathing activity has been reported after oral and intravenous glucose loading of the mother,[18, 30] although extended time sampling may have contributed to those findings. Inasmuch as glucose loading may potentiate lactic acidosis in the hypoxic fetus, it may be prudent to limit glucose administration to an oral dose of 25 or 30 gm if it is used in the fasting, high-risk subject to increase diagnostic yield. One report noted an increase in fetal breathing movements when fasting subjects drank mineral water alone,[19] possibly because of increased auditory noise in the fetal environment.

The proportion of inspiratory to expiratory phases of breathing may provide information about vagal tone and represents one of the potential directions of more detailed physiologic analysis. Gasping is a grossly perceivable alteration in that ratio and in the timing of individual breaths, which may represent fetal distress. Gasping is a preterminal event in fetal lambs,[5] and whether or not it is due to hypoxia in the human fetus, its presence is significant because of the high probability of meconium aspiration. Gasping movements occur (as a vagal reflex) when the umbilical cord is stimulated inadvertently during third trimester amniocentesis (along with bradycardia) and when the diaphragm is pierced during the course of fetal transfusion or other intrafetal needle procedures. In any case, the "quality" of breathing movements, like the "presence" and "type," represents an additional feature of classification that may be sought observationally in clinical use.

EYE MOVEMENTS

The brain is extremely sensitive to hypoxemia. The clinical problem of detecting fetal hypoxia may be translated to an equivalent situation of diagnosing (and grading) alterations in central nervous system function. Fetal eye movements are important in that context because they are initiated in the midbrain, and their neural paths do not involve peripheral reflex arcs. The eyes may be seen ultrasonically in nearly all cases after 15 weeks' gestational age, except with prone cranial position throughout the observation period.[2] The typical scan position is a lateral coronal plane (Fig. 5), which is obtained most expeditiously with sector scanning instruments having unconstrained probe placement. Frontal coronal or base equivalent views (Fig. 6) may be obtained when cranial position is supine or semisupine, although it is sufficient to visualize either eye alone for diagnosis (rapid eye movements are conjugate).

The developmental sequence of eye movements begins with isolated, relatively slow excursions, which are observed, sporadically, at or before 16 weeks' gestational age. Individual movements become more brisk between 20 and 24 weeks but remain single. Beginning about 23 to 24 weeks, these rapid movements become linked into a series of three or more darting movements, typically irregular in direction and duration. Between 25 and 35 weeks, episodes of rapid eye movement increase in incidence and duration, and nystagmoid rapid eye movements may be seen late in the third trimester. Slow sustained eye movements also may be seen at any time and should be considered separate from rapid eye movements (REMs).

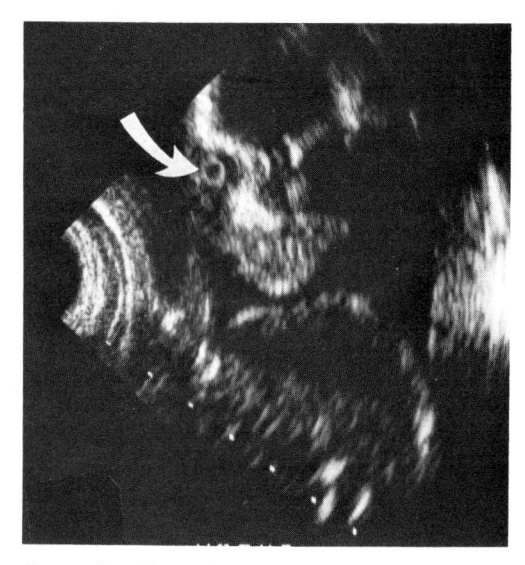

Figure 5. The right eye (*arrow*) is shown in this lateral coronal facial view.

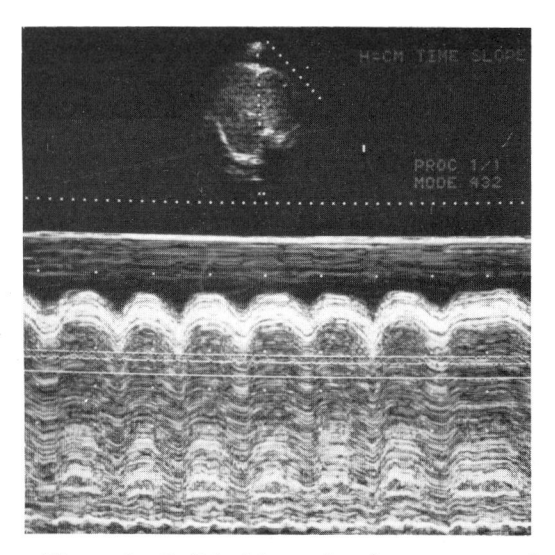

Figure 4. Radial abdominal wall components of breathing movements can be documented in T-M tracings. The central movements are nearly regular in timing. The inspiratory phase is longer than the expiratory component.

Simple but complete ultrasound observational descriptions of eye movement patterns are possible because the lens of the eye is constrained to move within a plane, but T-M quantitation is difficult because movements may include a combination of translational and rotational events. Clinically relevant information may be extracted from the presence of REMs during some observational period, but like breathing movements, additional, quantitative factors are necessary for physiologic research. Rapid eye movements are decreased (and eventually eliminated) with progressive hypoxia. Like breathing movements, REMs are also suppressed with maternal sedation and fasting, but the magnitude of those effects is less pronounced than for diaphragmatic movement. Rapid eye movement is so much more common than breathing movements between 25 and 35 weeks that one can obtain a reasonable idea of its presence (and derive negative information from its absence) with relatively short observation periods, that is, 5 minutes or less. Progressively longer phases of eye inactivity after 35 weeks' gestational age correspond to the development of deep sleep, which will be discussed later. The incidence of REMs is increased in newborn infants of diabetic pregnancy[28] and in fetuses of diabetic pregnancy throughout the third trimester.

HEARING AND HABITUATION

The fetal sensorium becomes functional in the third trimester.[13] Responses to audible sound are, perhaps, most obvious to expectant mothers who will often volunteer information about changes in fetal activity at concerts or sporting events when intensity of background sound increases. Many early studies have confirmed fetal hearing and several quantitative changes in heart rate as an end point of sensory effect. Ultrasound imaging provides additional ways of defining stimulus-response patterns.

In our own work, my co-workers and I have used a buzzer-like device that produces a noise stimulus (with predominant 100 Hz components rather than a pure tone source), with rapid rise time, and with output intensity of approximately 125 db at the skin surface of the mother. The buzzer is placed directly over an ear, and the face is observed after a single 0.5 second duration burst of noise. There is no response before 25 weeks' gestational age, inconsistent reaction between 25 and 27 weeks, and consistent startle reaction with aversion of head after 28 weeks. Presumably, stimuli that are less intense or that have a prolonged rise time will elicit an orienting rather than a defensive reaction,[12] which would be more difficult to evaluate in clinical context. The startle reaction is elicited in the healthy fetus anytime after 28 weeks. This time corresponds to a reported lack of correlation of blink-startle reaction with gestational age in newborn infants[9] and obviates one of the interpretative difficulties that may complicate analysis of breathing or eye movements. The defensive startle reaction also appears to be independent of behavioral state before testing.

Lack of any hearing response (under the previously mentioned test conditions) implies either deafness or serious depression of the central nervous system. Nonreactivity after a baseline demonstration of hearing is a priori evidence of impending fetal death, which has been observed in some cases of fetuses with hydrops who were not delivered promptly.

There are several individual components to the startle reaction. Observing the face particularly the eyelid area (Fig. 7), permits the examiner to score as separate reactions head-body aversion and involuntary blinking (or clenching of the cheek muscles). After 30 weeks (and often between 28 and 30 weeks), stimulation with a burst of serial tones separates these components. The blink reaction persists throughout the stimulus, whereas the body's response is lost after two to four repetitions. This behavior is referred to as habituation. Our own protocol uses a ten-burst sequence, with separate pulses spaced between one and two seconds.

Several of the signs of fetal compromise noted in this chapter have been the suppression of some motor activity. It may be expected that the control or organization of these movements would be affected earlier, since these activities may involve higher levels of the central nervous system. Habituation provides an example of a control mechanism. Our preliminary evidence shows that loss of auditory startle habituation is one of the earliest and most dependable signs of compromised fetal condition. Infants delivered by cesarean section

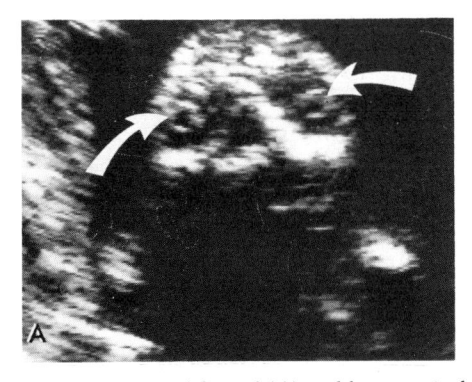

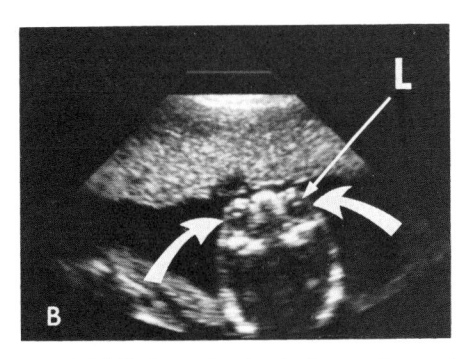

Figure 6. Supraorbital frontal (A) and base equivalent cranial (B) views showing both eyes (*arrows*) simultaneously. L, lens.

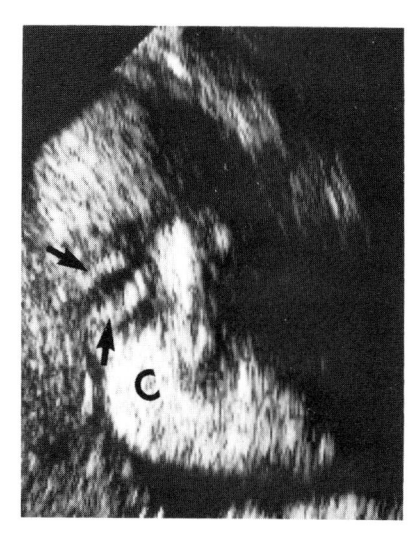

Figure 7. Lateral coronal views directed anterior to the eye will show the lids (*arrows*) and cheek (C). In this magnification view, the right lids are parted slightly.

within a few hours of demonstrating lack of habituation have had lower Apgar scores and other indicators of compromised condition. Conversely, high-risk subjects with intact habituation delivered shortly after testing have had uniformly satisfactory postnatal indicators of well being.

BEHAVIORAL STATE AND SYNTHESIS

Behavioral state describes a functional level of the central nervous system as it relates to its environment.[22] A specific behavioral state will include a combination of particular and recurrent physiologic components. The behavioral states of a full-term newborn infant are deep sleep, active (or REM) sleep, and arousal, which is subclassified into levels such as drowsy, alert-quiet, crying. The importance of the state concept is that the newborn is basically different, physiologically, in each of these states, and factors such as peripheral reflex responses, motor activity, and autonomic competence depend upon the state at observation. These considerations are relevant to fetal evaluation. Is an inactive fetus compromised or just sleeping? Can ultrasonic data be extended to resolve this potential difficulty?

The full-term newborn spends a certain amount of time in each behavioral state, and these proportions evolve during the first few years of development. Variations in these proportions may predict delayed neuromotor development.[29] Babies with Down's syndrome spend less time in active sleep than their peers,[24] re-emphasizing the diagnostic link between the function of the central nervous system and observation of control or organizational factors cited earlier. Hypoxic or acidotic newborns also spend less time in active sleep than anticipated (with deep sleep increased proportionately).

The coalescing or association of individual physiologic processes into separate and definable states occurs in the latter part of the third trimester. Before 30 weeks' gestation, the fetus appears to exist in an amorphous state in which there is great lability of individual state determinants. Observational signs of early organization and state definition are elicited from 32 weeks, and electroencephalographic signs of organization are found shortly thereafter. There are no established conventions for ultrasonic classification of a behavioral state, although the particular combination of eye and diaphragm movements provide a partial description. Deep sleep includes regular breathing and absence of eye movements. Active sleep includes aperiodic breathing and REMs. Alertness may occur when there are slow eye movements, since orienting responses to low intensity sound stimuli are elicited then. Deep sleep develops after 35 weeks, normally, but its development is accelerated in the presence of fetal stress. An apparent deep sleep pattern before 33 weeks (or prolonged deep sleep pattern without cycling later) may represent an analog of coma.[2]

Rapid eye movements alone cannot be equated to active or REM sleep, which is a behavioral state, although the practitioner may wish to regard the presence of REMs as an indication that a fetus can enter the REM state. This is an important and potentially unifying concept, because heart rate and other forms of physiologic variability are an integral feature of the REM state.[6, 14, 23, 31] The examiner may use the presence of REMs as equivalent to a reactive nonstress test as an indicator of fetal well being. We have found that fetal REM activity and its absence are more specific diagnostically than the nonstress test and at least as sensitive, although that remains to be proven conclusively.

SUMMARY

The human fetus has a wide range of sensory and motor behaviors, which mature with gestational age and which are altered by adverse intrauterine environmental conditions. Examiners should become familiar with individual motor patterns readily observed during routine ultrasound studies and attempt to use deviations from those norms as indicators of compromised clinical condition. Trends in this field are conceptual extensions from specific movements to an appreciation of control mechanisms and behavioral state and progression from passive observation to interactive stimulus-response testing.

REFERENCES

1. Ahlfeld, F.: Uber bister noch nicht beschriebene intrauterine bewegunzen des kindes. Verh. Dtsch. Ges. Gyn., 2:203–209, 1888.
2. Birnholz, J. C.: The development of human fetal eye movement patterns. Science, 213:679–681, 1981.
3. Campbell, K., MacNeill, I., and Patrick, J.: Time series analysis of human foetal breathing activity at 30–39 weeks gestation. J. Biomed. Eng., 2:108–111, 1980.
4. Cazeau, P.: A Theoretical and Practical Treatise on Midwifery (5th American Edition, Bullock, W.R., ed.) Philadelphia, Linday and Blakiston, 1872, p. 252.
5. Chapman, R. L. K., Dawes, G. S., Rurak, D. W., et al.: Intermittent breathing before death in fetal lambs. Am. J. Obstet. Gynecol., 131:894–898, 1978.
6. Clapp, J. F., III, Szeto, H. H., Abrams, R., et al. Physiologic variability and fetal electrocortical activity. Am. J. Obstet. Gynecol., 136:1045–1050, 1980.
7. Condorelli, S., and Scarpelli, E. M.: Fetal breathing: Induction in utero and effects of vagotomy and barbiturates. J. Pediatr., 88:94–101, 1976.
8. Dawes, G. S., Fox, H. E., Leduc, B. M., et al.: Respiratory movements and rapid eye movement sleep in the fetal lamb. J. Physiol., 210:119–143, 1972.
9. Finnström, O.: Studies on maturity in newborn infants. III. Neurological examination. Neuropadiatrie, 3:72–96, 1971.
10. Hawrylyshyn, P. A., Bernstein, A., and Organ, L. W.: Fetal preejection period. Obstet. Gynecol., 59:747–754, 1982.
11. Ianniruberto, A., and Tajani, E.: Ultrasonographic study of fetal movements. Semin. Perinatol., 5:175–181, 1981.
12. Kearsley, R. B.: The newborn's response to auditory stimulation: A demonstration of orienting and defensive behavior. Child Dev., 44:582–590, 1973.
13. Liley, A. W.: The foetus as a personality. Aust. N.Z. J. Psychiatry, 6:99–105, 1972.
14. Mann, L. I., Duchin, S., and Weiss R. R.: Fetal EEG sleep stages and physiologic variability. Am. J. Obstet. Gynecol., 119:533–538, 1974.
15. Manning, F. A., and Platt, L. D.: Human fetal breathing movements and maternal hypoxia. Obstet. Gynecol., 53:718, 1979.
16. Manning, E. A., Platt, L. D., and Sipos, L. : Antenatal fetal evaluation: Development of a fetal biophysical profile. Am. J. Obstet. Gynecol. 136:787–795, 1980.
17. Martin C. B., Murata, Y., Ikenoue T., et al.: Effect of alterations on PO_2 and PCO_2 on fetal breathing movements in rhesus monkeys. Gynecol. Invest., 6:74, 1975.
18. Natale, R., Richardson, B., and Patrick, J.: Effect of intravenous glucose infusion on human fetal breathing activity. Obstet. Gynecol., 59:320–324, 1981.
19. Neldam, S., Hornnes, P. J., and Icuhl, C.: Effect of maternal triglyceride ingestion on fetal respiratory movements. Obstet. Gynecol., 59:640–642, 1982.
20. Pearson, J. F., and Weaver, J. B.: Fetal activity and fetal well being: An evaluation. Br. Med. J., 1:1305–1307, 1976.
21. Platt, L. D., Manning, E. A., LeMay, M., et al.: Human fetal breathing movements: Relationship to fetal condition. Am. J. Obstet. Gynecol., 132:514, 1978.
22. Prechtl, H.F.R.: The behavioral states of the newborn infant. Brain Res., 76:185–203, 1974.
23. Prechtl, H. F. R., Farpel, J. W., Weinmann, H. M., et al.: Postures, motility and respiration of low-risk pre-term infants. Dev. Med. Child Neurol., 21:3–27, 1979.
24. Prechtl, H. F. R., Theorell, K., and Blair, A. W.: Behavioral state cycles in abnormal infants. Dev. Med. Child Neurol., 15:606–615, 1973.
25. Richardson, B., Campbell, K., Carmichael, L., et al.: Effects of external physical stimulation on fetuses near term. Am. J. Obstet. Gynecol., 139:344–352, 1981.
26. Rochard, F., Schifrin, B. S., Goupil, F., et al.: Nonstressed fetal heart rate monitoring in the antenatal period. Am. J. Obstet. Gynecol., 126:699, 1976.
27. Sadovsky, E., and Polishuk, W. Z.: Fetal movements in utero. Obstet. Gynecol., 50:49–55, 1977.
28. Schulte, F. J., Larson, U., Parl, U., et al.: Brain and behavioral maturation in newborn infants of diabetic mothers. Neuroped. 1:36–43, 1969.
29. Thoman, E. B., Denenberg, V. H., Sievel, J., et al.: State organization in neonates: developmental inconsistency indicates risk for developmental dysfunction. Neuropediatrics, 12:45–54, 1981.
30. Trudinger, B. J., and Knight, P. G.: Fetal age and patterns of human fetal breathing movements. Am. J. Obstet. Gynecol., 137:724, 1980.
31. VanGeijn, H. P., Jongsma, H. W., de Haan, J., et al.: Heart rate as an indicator of the behavioral state. Am. J. Obstet. Gynecol., 136:1061–1066, 1980.

10

The Role of Ultrasound in Prenatal Diagnostic Procedures

Mitchell S. Golbus, M.D.

Major advances in genetic counseling and medical genetics have occurred in the last decade. The development of techniques for the intrauterine detection of certain genetic diseases in the fetus is an important example of such progress. Prenatal diagnosis has evolved over the past few years from an experimental procedure offered in a limited number of centers to one of proven safety and efficacy annually offered to thousands of families at dozens of centers. The overall safety of amniocentesis in the early second trimester of pregnancy has been confirmed by several published series.[7, 10, 23, 31] The scheme of genetic counseling for prenatal diagnosis of genetic defects is depicted in Figure 1.

AMNIOCENTESIS

The timing of amniocentesis is a function of when amniotic fluid can consistently and safely be obtained, the time required for analysis of fluid or cell culture, and societal and the legal limits on how late in pregnancy selective abortion may be performed. Obtaining amniotic fluid in the first trimester requires a transvaginal approach and is associated with a significant risk of uterine infection and subsequent abortion. Fluids from pregnancies less than 12 menstrual weeks' gestation contain very few cells, and there is a low rate of successful cultures. Fuchs[6] has shown that at 15 menstrual weeks there is 125 ml of amniotic fluid, and that this volume increases 50 ml per week for the next 13 weeks. Analysis of our data from amniocenteses done between 15 and 20 weeks indicates that the time required for cell culture and analysis is not a function of the gestational age when the fluid is obtained. We therefore perform amniocentesis at 16 menstrual weeks, which allows sufficient time to repeat the amniocentesis if a cell culture fails and also often allows a diagnosis before quickening. Several studies have indicated that therapeutic abortions performed after quickening cause more serious psychiatric problems than those performed before quickening.[1]

The procedure itself is straightforward. After the abdomen is aseptically prepared, 1 per cent lidocaine is used as a local anesthetic. A 22 gauge, 3½ inch long spinal needle with stylet is used to obtain 25 ml of amniotic fluid (Fig. 2). To avoid contaminating the sample with maternal tissue, one must have the stylet in place when the needle is advanced. One syringe is used to draw the initial 0.5 ml of fluid to be sure it is clear of blood; a second syringe is used to obtain the specimen. As we have gained experience, we have lowered the incidence of "dry taps" to less than 1 per cent.

Ultrasonography before amniocentesis has been advocated by some investigators to ensure an uncomplicated amniotic fluid aspiration and to minimize potential risks to the fetus.[12, 29] The value of preliminary ultrasonography, however, has not been well documented. Much of the data is conflicting and based on dissimilar patient series.[4, 8, 13, 18, 22, 34] A few prospective studies comparing alternated patients have been reported and will be discussed later in this chapter.

Fetal and placental trauma have been reported during amniocentesis in the third trimester of pregnancy.[3, 5, 26] Ultrasonography should help avoiding such complications by identifying fetal position, pools of amniotic fluid, and placental location. Real-time ultrasonography demonstrates that fetal movements are so abrupt in the second trimester of pregnancy that prediction of fetal position from one moment to the next is much less accurate than in the third trimester. Rapid fetal movement is likely the reason for the rarity of fetal trauma during early second trimester amniocentesis. Although there are several reports of infants with minor scars, presumably due to needle scratches during genetic amniocentesis, there have been few reports of severe traumatic injury, and some of these were associated with fetuses having multiple congenital defects.[2, 9, 20]

Most investigators who have asked questions about the role of ultrasound in an amniocentesis program have either compared their experience before and after acquiring a sonography machine or compared the experience of some members of their group to

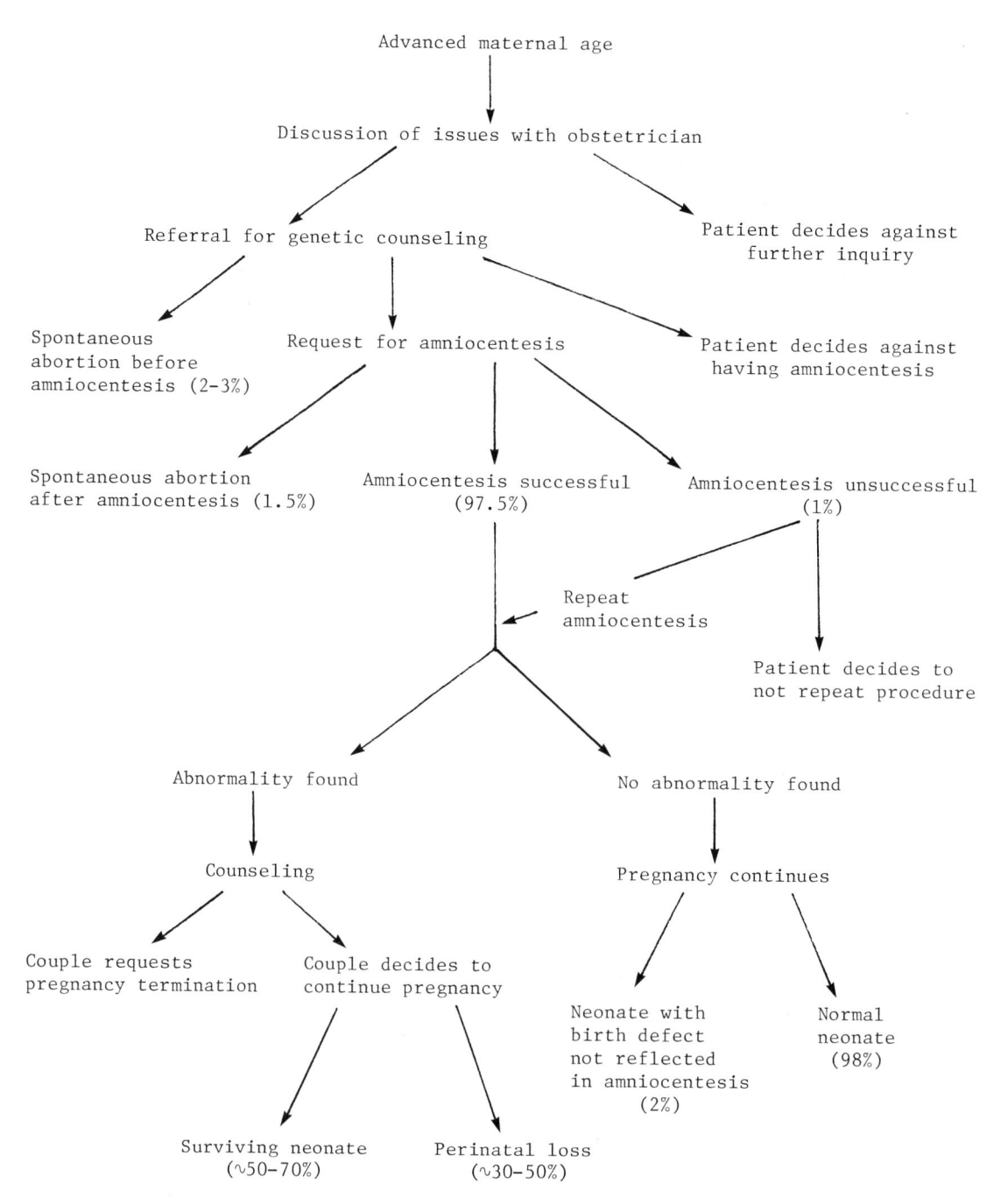

Figure 1. Scheme of genetic counseling for prenatal diagnosis of genetic defects.

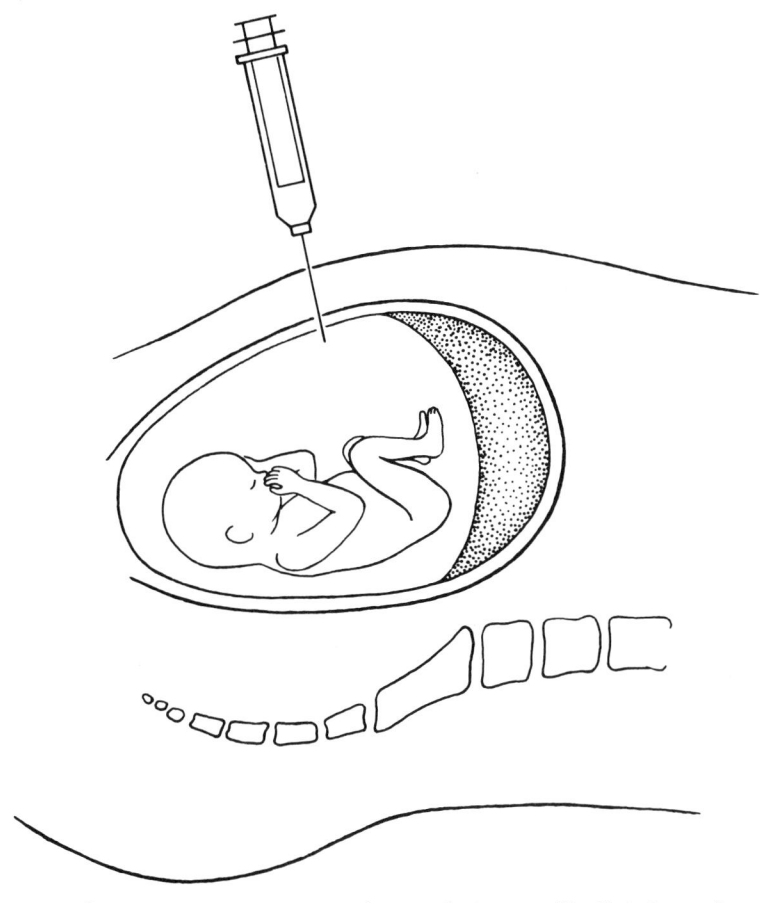

Figure 2. Technique of genetic amniocentesis in early second trimester. Needle is inserted so as to avoid fetus and placenta.

that of other members of the group.[4, 8, 13, 18, 22, 34] These studies are open to the criticism that any differences noted may be because of experience or because of different abilities among the various members of the group.

There have been two prospective studies of sonography for amniocentesis. One series, by our group, alternately assigned 150 patients to a control group or to an ultrasound group who underwent examination with a real-time scanner immediately before amniocentesis.[21] In this study, ultrasonography did not reduce the failure rate, the incidence of multiple needle insertions, or the proportion of amniotic fluid samples containing blood (Table 1). The second study involved 82 patients nonrandomly assigned to a control or sonography group and found no difference in the incidence of multiple punctures.[16] This is not to say that ultrasonographic information is in any way spurious. Certainly, the recognition of twins (see later) and the assessment of fetal viability are pertinent for appropriate genetic counseling. Both of the preceding studies involved experienced operators and addressed only the ease with which clear amniotic fluid could be obtained. One issue not addressed, for example, is our finding that 1.2 per cent of pregnancies referred for amniocentesis are missed abortions and that the fetus is already dead. Sonography allows one to identify these gestations and to avoid an unnecessary procedure for the women.

The discovery of a twin gestation during sonography before a planned amniocentesis raises both counseling and technical problems. Before the amniocentesis is undertaken, the couple must be apprised of the changed situation and be allowed to determine whether or not to proceed. The basis for the discussion would be the theoretical risks for the diagnostic indication in the situation of twins. Assuming that one third of

Table 1. *Ultrasound Guidance of Genetic Amniocentesis**

	NO ULTRA-SOUND (%) (n = 75)	ULTRASOUND (%) (n = 75)
Failure to obtain fluid	5.3	4
More than one needle insertion	15.5	15.3
Absence of gross blood in fluid	60	56
Initially blood-tinged fluid	34	34
Persistently blood fluid	6	10
Tissue culture failure	1.3	4

* Adapted from Levine, S. C., Filly, R. A., and Golbus, M. S.: Ultrasonography for guidance of amniocentesis in genetic counseling. Clin. Genet., *14*:133, 1978.

twins are monozygotic and that two thirds are dizygotic, the probability of at least one fetus with a chromosomal abnormality related to advanced maternal age is 5/3 times the maternal age–specific risk.[15] The statistical alterations in the genetic risk of parents having twins has been derived for various situations, and this information should be given to the prospective parents so they can make an informed decision whether or not to proceed with the amniocentesis.[15]

The technical problems of obtaining amniotic fluid from each of twin gestational sacs can usually be overcome (Table 2). Sonography can identify the membrane between the two pregnancies and a pool of amniotic fluid in each gestational sac. We distinguish the two sacs by following the aspiration of the first fluid sample with an injection of 0.5 ml of indigo carmine dye. The abdomen is then manually manipulated to distribute the dye, and the second amniocentesis is performed. Aspiration of clear fluid indicates that the second sac was entered, whereas aspiration of dye-colored fluid indicates that the original sac was reentered.

The counseling and technical problems presented by discovering twins are overshadowed by the problems arising if the twins are found to be discordant for a genetic abnormality. The disease found in the affected fetus, including the possibilities of antepartum death or a short lifespan, must be discussed. Until recently, the family's choices included elective termination of both gestations, carrying the pregnancy and keeping both neonates, or carrying the pregnancy and putting the affected neonate up for adoptive or custodial care. The ethical and psychological issues involved in the abortion of a normal twin to prevent the birth of an abnormal twin are unresolved. A new approach, which averts these issues while raising a whole new set of problems, is to terminate selectively the life of the affected fetus while allowing the unaffected gestation to proceed. This option requires careful analysis of the ultrasonographic scan at the original amniocentesis. The positions of the fetuses when results are available must be compatible with the original description. Selective termination usually has been accomplished by intracardiac puncture of the affected fetus under sonographic guidance.[17] Use of a biopsy transducer with a slot through which the needle can be passed is advisable. Aspiration of cardiac blood may not be sufficient to cause fetal demise, and air embolization has been employed successfully.[24] Parents need a realistic discussion of the problems and techniques introduced by each new finding (for example, twins and a discordant abnormality) to decide how to proceed.

The last issue on the use of sonography for genetic amniocentesis concerns the avoidance of Rh isoimmunization in Rh-negative women. Some have suggested that Rh-negative women with Rh-positive husbands undergoing genetic amniocentesis face the potential hazard of isoimmunization. However, the actual incidence of isoimmunization after amniocentesis and the circumstances in which it may occur have not been established. We retrospectively examined a series of 8009 genetic amniocenteses and ascertained that 13 of 615 women estimated to be at risk (2.1 per cent) were sensitized after the procedure.[11]

Table 2. *Genetic Amniocentesis in Twins*

Undiagnosed		
Before routine ultrasound	22	
After routine ultrasound	4	
Diagnosed		
Before routine ultrasound (suspected by size)	5	
Both sacs sampled		4
One sac sampled		1
After routine ultrasound	61	
Both sacs sampled		59
One sac sampled		1
One sac sampled because of one twin's prior death		1

Eleven of the sensitizations occurred early in the programs, and a combination of ultrasound performed concurrently with the amniocentesis and experience appear to have reduced the risk of isoimmunization to that of control data from the literature.

FETOSCOPY

Several genetic loci are not expressed in amniotic fluid cells. Mendelian disorders caused by mutation at these loci and most multifactorially inherited congenital malformations occur without demonstrable chromosomal or biochemical abnormalities in amniotic fluid cells. The prenatal diagnosis of such disorders has been attempted by direct fetal visualization and by obtaining samples of fetal tissues other than amniotic fluid cells. These alternate tissues are chosen because they express a specific genetic attribute not expressed in amniotic fluid cells. The development of fetoscopy, using a small bore endoscope, has opened a new era in intrauterine diagnosis.

The first attempts at fetal visualization were made through a dilated cervix in the 1950s. Visualization was limited, but fetal parts and movements could be identified. Westin successfully performed transuterine visualization with a 10 mm hysteroscope in preabortal women.[33] In the early 1970s, the term "fetoscopy" was introduced to describe experience with a 2.2 mm fiberoptic endoscope used to search for neural tube defects.[28] Valenti used a modified 18 French pediatric cystoscope, which he called an endoamnioscope and reported the first aspiration of fetal blood.[32] Hobbins and Mahoney were the first to employ the most widely used instrument today, the Dyonics "needlescope," for fetal visualization and aspiration of fetal blood.[14] In the past several years, numerous investigators have reported the use of fetoscopy for fetal visualization and for obtaining fetal specimens in developing pregnancies.

Fetoscopy has proved useful in three main areas. The first is in the visualization of anatomic fetal defects. Although the field of vision is limited through the fetoscope, several fetal anomalies have been diagnosed or excluded. The second area of use is intrauterine fetal therapy. One example is early intrauterine transfusion for Rh isoimmunization, which has been described by Rodeck et al.[25] The third and most significant area of impact of the fetoscope has been in the biopsy of fetal tissues, to date blood, skin, and liver. The conditions already diagnosed are listed in Table 3.

Sonographic expertise is required to ensure that fetoscopy is carried out most safely. Both contact gray scale B scan and real-time ultrasound may be used, and the time spent on sonography often will exceed the time spent in the actual fetoscopy. Accurate information about placental localization, fetal lie, fetal age, fetal movement, any abnormalities of fetal configuration, the depth of the amniotic sac and placenta, and the site of umbilical cord insertion into the placenta is required. The ultrasound examination must immediately precede the fetoscopy because the configuration of the uterus and its contents may change in a period of minutes. Real-time sonography during the procedure provides constant surveillance of both fetal and fetoscope position, thereby supplying additional guidance to the fetoscopist. The transducer can be placed in a gas autoclave so it can be used in the operative field. We place the transducer in a position to observe the initial trocar entry into the amniotic sac. After the fetoscope is in place, the transducer is placed over the insertion site of the umbilical cord into the placenta, and the fetoscope is guided to the area. The sonographer then can verify that what the fetoscopist sees as umbilical cord really is

Table 3. *Conditions Diagnosed by Fetoscopy*

By visualization
  Amniotic bands
  Facial clefts
  Multiple malformation syndromes involving digital or limb anomalies
  Neural tube defects
  Sex determination

By skin biopsy
  Congenital bullous ichthyosiform erythroderma
  Epidermolysis bullosa
  Harlequin ichthyosis
  Lamellar ichthyosis

By fetal blood sampling
  α-1-antitrypsin deficiency
  β-thalassemia major
  Blood typing
  Chronic granulomatous disease
  Hemophilia A
  Hemophilia B
  Karyotyping
  Sickle cell anemia

that structure. We usually can see sonographically when the blood-drawing needle advances and touches the umbilical cord. After the fetal blood sample is obtained, the transducer is moved over the fetal chest, and a fetal heart rate is recorded. The procedure begins and ends with sonography.

ECHOCARDIOGRAPHY

A new role of ultrasound in prenatal diagnosis of genetic defects is the use of fetal echocardiography to detect congenital heart disease or cardiac arrhythmias.[19, 27] M-mode echocardiography may be performed as an isolated technique or may be processed from two-dimensional echocardiographic images. The addition of high resolution M-mode capabilities that are simultaneously recordable to either linear or sector scanners has been of great value for detecting and validating the findings on the two-dimensional studies. The use of simultaneous M-mode and two-dimensional echocardiography diminishes the time spent on the total study.

After a routine ultrasound examination, the fetal heart is considered. It is easier to obtain a good study by directing the ultrasound beams through the precordium or subcostal area rather than through the fetal back or rib cage. Because the transducer is some distance from the fetal heart, even slight transducer movements of a few degrees may cause the scan field to pass away from the heart. Maintaining the transducer position may require the ultrasonographer to use both hands.

Several echocardiographic views can be obtained for each fetus. In the four-chamber view, the two atrioventricular valves can be identified.[36] Cephalad manipulation of the transducer allows visualization of the inferior vena cava, the valve of the foramen ovale, and the aortic root.[30] The four-chamber view is useful for seeing ventricular septal defects, valve atresias, ventricular hypoplasia, univentricular hearts, endocardial cushion defects, the Ebstein anomaly, and pericardial effusions (Fig. 3).[30] A long axis view demonstrates the aortic valve, the ascending aorta, part of the aortic arch and descending aorta, and the pulmonary artery.[30] Aortic coarctation or atresia of hypoplastic left heart and of certain ventricular septal defects can be diagnosed from this view.[30] The short axis view, a series of tomographic planes from the base of the heart to the apex of the ventricles, visualizes the right ventricular outflow tract passing around the aorta, the bifurcation of the pulmonary artery, the ductus arteriosus, and the descending aorta.[30] These views potentially identify transposition of the great vessels, pulmonary atresia, aortic atresia, double outlet right ventricle, and truncus arteriosus.[30]

The indications for fetal echocardiography will change as the field develops. Because the incidence of cardiac abnormalities in utero is quite low, routine examinations would be time-consuming and have a very small yield. Additionally,

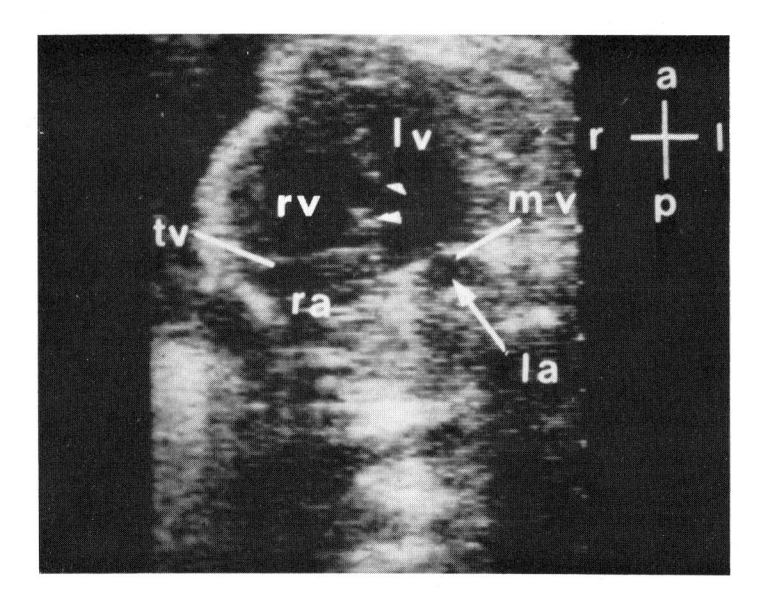

Figure 3. "Four-chamber" view from a fetal echocardiogram in which a ventricular septal defect (*arrows*) is demonstrated. RA, right atrium; LA, left atrium; LV, left ventricle; RV, right ventricle; TV, tricuspid valve; MV, mitral valve. (Courtesy of Norman H. Silverman, M.D., University of California, San Francisco, California.)

Figure 4. M-mode tracing obtained from a fetal echocardiogram in which complete heart block is demonstrated. Multiple atrial contractions (*small arrows*) are seen for every ventricular contraction (*large arrows*). (Courtesy of Norman H. Silverman, M.D., University of California, San Francisco, California.)

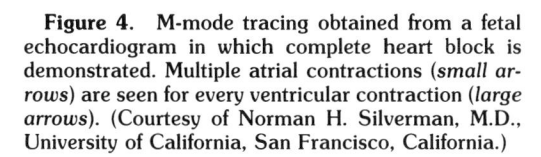

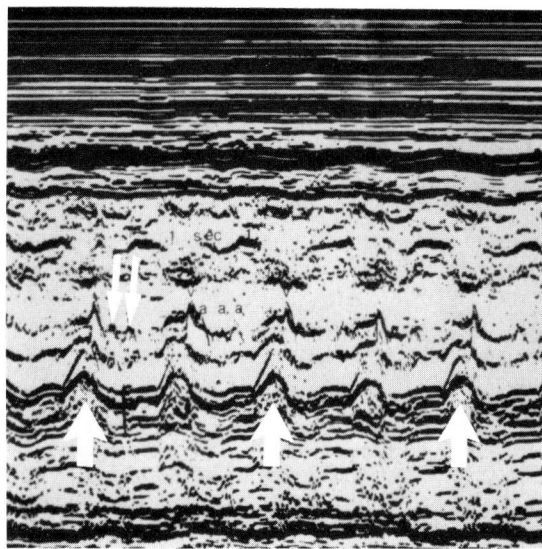

a low risk population accentuates the problem of false-positive and false-negative echocardiographic intepretations—a real concern in this area at its current stage of development. For these reasons, only situations in which there is a high prior probability of a fetal cardiac anomaly should be considered for echocardiography. These instances would include a chromosomally abnormal fetus, a fetus with multiple somatic anomalies seen by sonography, a fetus with cardiac arrhythmia, the presence of polyhydramnios, a family history of hereditary disease affecting the heart, or maternal exposure to drugs known to produce congenital heart disease.

Our pediatric cardiology group has studied seven fetuses with cardiac arrhythmias in utero.[30] One fetus had a heart block associated with maternal lupus erythematosus, one had a supraventricular tachycardia, one had premature ventricular beats, and four had premature atrial beats (Fig. 4). An additional five fetuses were seen with congenital heart defects: Three with ventricular septal defects and two with idiopathic cardiomyopathies. However, one of the fetuses with a ventricular septal defect also had undetected pulmonary atresia, and one fetus studied because of the presence of an omphalocele had a double outlet right ventricle which was not noted. There also were two false-positive diagnoses: one a tetralogy of Fallot and one a ventricular septal defect, both early in the experience. These errors in diagnosis must be eliminated by experience before the clinical application of this technique can become more widespread.

The accurate recognition of fetal cardiac lesions may allow better genetic counseling. Some cardiac anomalies incompatible with life may prompt couples to opt for selective termination of pregnancy. For a couple who is told their fetus has trisomy 21, the presence of a cardiac abnormality may influence their response to the situation. For the fetus with a correctable lesion (the vast majority), knowledge of the anomaly may influence the parents to have delivery at a center equipped for pediatric cardiac surgery. All of these situations should encourage us to continue developing this new area of ultrasound for diagnosing fetal abnormalities.

REFERENCES

1. Bebring, G. L., Dwyer, T. F., Huntington, D. S., et al.: A study of the psychological processes in pregnancy and of the earliest mother-child relationship. Psychoanal. Stud. Child., *16*:9, 1961.
2. Broome, D. L., Wilson, M. G., Weiss, B., et al.: Needle puncture of fetus: A complication of second-trimester amniocentesis. Am. J. Obstet. Gynecol., *126*:247, 1976.
3. Burnett, R. G., and Anderson, W. R.: The hazards of amniocentesis. J. Iowa Med. Soc., *58*:130, 1968.
4. Chandra, P., Nitowsky, H. M., Marion, R., et al.: Experience with sonography as an adjunct to amniocentesis for parental diagnosis of fetal genetic disorders. Am. J. Obstet. Gynecol., *133*:519, 1979.
5. Creasman, W. T., Lawrence, R. A., and Thiede, H. A.: Fetal complications of amniocentesis. J.A.M.A., *204*:91, 1968.

6. Fuchs, F.: Volume of amniotic fluid at various stages of pregnancy. Clin. Obstet. Gynecol., 9:449, 1966.
7. Galjaard, H.: European experience with prenatal diagnosis of congenital disease: A survey of 6121 cases. Cytogenet. Cell Genet., 16:453, 1976.
8. Gerbie, A. B., and Shkolnik, A. A.: Ultrasound prior to amniocentesis for genetic counseling, Obstet. Gynecol., 46:716, 1975.
9. Golbus, M. S. Conte, F. A., Schneider, E. L., et al.: Intrauterine diagnosis of genetic defects: Results, problems and follow-up of one hundred cases in a prenatal genetic detection center. Am. J. Obstet. Gynecol., 118:897, 1974.
10. Golbus, M. S., Loughman, W. D., Epstein, C. J., et al.: Prenatal genetic diagnosis in 3000 amniocenteses. N. Engl. J. Med., 300:157, 1979.
11. Golbus, M. S., Stephens, J. D., Cann, H. M., et al.: Rh isoimmunization following genetic amniocentesis. Prenatal Diagnosis, 2:149, 1982.
12. Goldstein, A., Dumars, K. W., and Kent, D. R.: Prenatal diagnosis of chromosomal and enzymatic defects. Obstet. Gynecol., 47:503, 1976.
13. Harrison, R., Campbell, S., and Craft, I.: Risks of fetomaternal hemorrhage resulting from amniocentesis with and without ultrasound placental localization. Obstet. Gynecol., 46:389, 1975.
14. Hobbins, J. C., and Mahoney, M. J.: In utero diagnosis of hemoglobinopathies: Technique for obtaining fetal blood. N. Engl. J. Med., 290:1065, 1974.
15. Hunter, A. G. W., and Cox, D. M.: Counseling problems when twins are discovered at genetic amniocentesis. Clin. Genet., 16:34, 1979.
16. Karp, L. E., Rothwell, R., Conrad, S. H., et al.: Ultrasonic placental localization and bloody taps in midtrimester amniocentesis for prenatal genetic diagnosis. Obstet. Gynecol., 50:589, 1977.
17. Kerenyi, T. D., and Chitkara, U.: Selective birth in twin pregnancy with discordancy for Down's syndrome. N. Engl. J. Med. 304:1525, 1981.
18. Kerenyi, T. D., and Walker, B.: The preventability of "bloody taps" in second trimester amniocentesis by ultrasound scanning. Obstet. Gynecol., 50:61, 1977.
19. Kleinman, C. S., Hobbins, J. C., Jaffe, C. C., et al.: Echocardiographic studies on the human fetus: Prenatal diagnosis of congenital heart disease and cardiac dysrhythmias. Pediatrics, 65:1059, 1980.
20. Lamb, M. P.: Gangrene of a fetal limb due to amniocentesis. Br. J. Obstet. Gynaecol., 82:829, 1975.
21. Levine, S. C., Filly, R. A., and Golbus, M. S.: Ultrasonography for guidance of amniocentesis in genetic counseling. Clin. Genet., 14:133, 1978.
22. Miskin, M., Doran, T. A., Rudd, N., et al.: Use of ultrasound for placental localization in genetic amniocentesis. Obstet. Gynecol., 43:872, 1974.
23. NICHD National Registry for Amniocentesis Study Group: Midtrimester amniocentesis for prenatal diagnosis. Safety and accuracy. J.A.M.A., 236:1471, 1976.
24. Petres, R. E., and Rewine, F.: Selective birth in twin pregnancy (letter). N. Engl. J. Med., 305:1218, 1981.
25. Rodeck, C. H., Kemp, J. R., Holman, C. R., et al.: Direct intravascular fetal blood transfusion by fetoscopy in severe Rhesus isoimmunization. Lancet, 1:625, 1981.
26. Ryan, G. T., Ivy, R., Jr., and Pearson, J. W.: Fetal bleeding as a major hazard of amniocentesis. Obstet. Gynecol., 40:702, 1972.
27. Sahn, D. J., Lange, L. W., Allen, H. D., et al.: Quantitative real-time cross-sectional echocardiography in the developing human fetus and newborn. Circulation, 62:588, 1980.
28. Scrimgeour, J. B.: Other techniques for antenatal diagnosis. In Emery, A. E. H. (ed.): Antenatal Diagnosis of Genetic Disease. New York, Churchill-Livingstone, 1973, p. 40–57.
29. Scrimgeour, J. B.: The diagnostic use of amniocentesis: Techniques and complications. Proc. R. Soc. Med., 64:1135, 1971.
30. Silverman, N. H., Snider, A. R., Golbus, M. S., et al.: Prospectives on fetal echocardiography. Proceedings of First Symposium on Fetal Echocardiography. France, Strasbourg, 1982.
31. Simpson, N. E., Dallaire, L., Miller, J. R., et al.: Prenatal diagnosis of genetic disease in Canada: Report of a collaborative study. Can. Med. Assoc. J., 115:739, 1976.
32. Valenti, C.: Antenatal detection of hemoglobinopathies. A preliminary report. Am. J. Obstet. Gynecol., 115:851, 1973.
33. Weston, B.: Hysteroscopy in early pregnancy. Lancet, 2:872, 1954.
34. Young, P. E., Matson, M. R., and Jones, O. W.: Amniocentesis antenatal diagnosis. Review of problems and outcomes in a large series, Am. J. Obstet. Gynecol., 125:495, 1976.

11

Perinatal Management of the Fetus with a Correctable Defect

Michael R. Harrison, M.D.

Fetal anatomy, normal and abnormal, can now be accurately delineated by ultrasonography and other imaging techniques. Although some fetal malformations with a known pattern of inheritance may be specifically sought, many are identified serendipitously during obstetric ultrasonography. Until recently, the only question raised by the prenatal diagnosis of a fetal malformation was whether the fetus should be aborted, but other therapeutic alternatives are becoming available. The detection of a fetal abnormality may now lead to a change in the timing of delivery, a change in the mode of delivery, and even treatment before birth. We have made a tenative outline of the diagnostic and therapeutic alternatives for the management of specific fetal malformations that can be recognized in utero.[10]

MALFORMATIONS BEST TREATED AFTER TERM DELIVERY

Most correctable malformations that can be diagnosed in utero are best managed by appropriate medical and surgical therapy after delivery at term. The term infant is a better anesthetic and surgical risk than the preterm infant. Examples of malformations that have been diagnosed in utero are given in the Table 1. Although this list is not exhaustive, the majority of neonatal surgical disorders fall into this category. Knowing that a fetus has one of these anomalies may improve perinatal management by allowing preparation for appropriate postnatal care. Therapy for polyhydramnios and preterm labor may be desirable to allow the fetus to remain in utero as long as possible. The delivery can be planned so that appropriate personnel (neonatologist, anesthesiologist, pediatric surgeon) are available. When the neonate will require highly specialized services, transporting the fetus in situ (maternal transport) may be preferable to postnatal transport of the fragile newborn infant.

MALFORMATIONS USUALLY MANAGED BY SELECTIVE ABORTION

When serious malformations incompatible with normal postnatal life are diagnosed early enough, the family has the option of terminating the pregnancy. When these malformations are recognized too late for safe termination, the family can be counseled and appropriate postnatal management arranged. Table 2 lists examples of severe anatomic malformations that are considered to be indications for selective abortion. These anatomic abnormalities join a long list of inherited chromosomal and metabolic disorders that can be diagnosed in utero and may lead to selective abortion.

PRENATAL DIAGNOSIS MAY LEAD TO EARLY DELIVERY

Early delivery may be indicated for certain fetal anomalies that require correction as soon as possible after diagnosis (Table 3.) In each of these cases, the risk of premature delivery must be weighed against the risk of continued gestation. This approach has already proved beneficial in managing the fetus with hydrops fetalis and intrauterine growth retardation. Recent advances in stimulating production of fetal surfactant with corticosteroids and in ventilating small babies have greatly improved the outcome for premature infants with respiratory distress syndrome.

Table 1. *Malformations Detectable In Utero but Best Corrected After Delivery at Term*

Esophageal, duodenal, jejunoileal and anorectal atresias
Meconium ileus (cystic fibrosis)
Enteric cysts and duplications
Small intact omphalocele
Small intact meningocele, myelomeningocele, and spina bifida
Unilateral multicystic dysplastic kidney
Craniofacial, extremity, and chest wall deformities
Cystic hygroma
Small sacrococcygeal teratoma
Ovarian cysts

The rationale for early correction is unique to each anomaly, but the principle remains the same: continued gestation would have a progressive ill effect on the fetus. In some cases, the function of a specific organ system is compromised by the lesion and will continue to deteriorate until the lesion is corrected. In congenital hydronephrosis, unrelieved urinary tract obstruction results in progressive deterioration of renal function. Preterm delivery for early decompression of the urinary tract should reverse the renal maldevelopment at the earliest possible time and thus maximize subsequent renal growth and development.[9] In obstructive hydrocephalus, high intraventricular pressure compresses the developing brain. Early delivery for ventricular decompression should maximize the opportunity for subsequent brain development and may avoid the difficult obstetric problem of delivering a baby with an abnormally large head.[19]

Anomalies associated with progressive organ ischemia should be corrected as soon as possible. Volvulus associated with intestinal malrotation or meconium ileus may lead to intestinal gangrene, perforation, and meconium peritonitis. Early delivery for correction of this type of bowel lesion would be aimed at minimizing the

Table 2. *Malformations Usually Managed by Selective Abortion*

Anencephaly, porencephaly, encephalocele, and giant hydrocephalus
Severe anomalies associated with chromosomal abnormalities (trisomy 13, trisomy 18, and others)
Renal agenesis or bilateral polycystic kidney disease
Inherited chromosomal, metabolic, and hematologic abnormalities (hemoglobinopathies, Tay-Sachs disease, and so on)

Table 3. *Malformations That May Require Induced Preterm Delivery for Early Correction Ex Utero*

Obstructive hydronephrosis
Obstructive hydrocephalus
Amniotic band malformation complex
Gastroschisis or ruptured omphalocele
Intestinal ischemia/necrosis secondary to volvulus, meconium ileus, and so on
Hydrops fetalis
Intrauterine growth retardation

amount of bowel lost to the ischemic process. In some malformations, the progressive ill effects on the fetus result directly from being in utero. In the amniotic band complex, a fetal part is compressed or strangulated by herniation through a defect in the fetal membranes, resulting in amputation or deformity. This simple mechanical restriction to growth and development should be relieved at the earliest possible time to prevent further deformity. In ruptured omphalocele or gastroschisis, the bowel exposed to amniotic fluid becomes coated with a thick, fibrous inflammatory peel that may hinder repair and delay resumption of function. Early delivery should minimize the damage by shortening the time the bowel is exposed to the amniotic fluid.

PRENATAL DIAGNOSIS MAY LEAD TO CESAREAN DELIVERY

Elective cesarean delivery rather than a trial at vaginal delivery may be indicated for the fetal malformations listed in Table 4. In most cases, this is because the malformation would cause dystocia. Another indication for elective cesarean delivery is a malformation requiring immediate surgical correction best performed in a sterile

Table 4. *Malformations That May Require Cesarean Delivery*

Conjoined twins
Giant omphalocele, ruptured omphalocele/gastroschisis
Large hydrocephalus
Large sacrococcygeal teratoma
Large cystic hygroma
Large or ruptured meningomyelocele
Malformations requiring preterm delivery in the presence of inadequate labor or fetal distress

environment. Examples are a ruptured omphalocele or an uncovered meningomyelocele. In this circumstance, the baby can be resuscitated in an adjacent sterile operating room and undergo immediate surgical correction. Finally, cesarean delivery may be required if preterm delivery of an affected fetus is elected but labor is inadequate or the fetus does not tolerate labor as determined by fetal monitoring.

PRENATAL DIAGNOSIS MAY LEAD TO INTERVENTION BEFORE BIRTH

Fetal Deficiencies

Some fetal deficiency states may be alleviated by treatment before birth (Table 5). In respiratory distress syndrome, glucocorticoids given to the mother increase deficient fetal pulmonary surfactant and alleviate the disease. Fetal anemia secondary to isoimmunization-induced hemolysis can be treated by transfusing red blood cells into the fetal peritoneal cavity. We have treated severe hydrops by administering digitalis and diuretics along with the blood. A fetus with vitamin B12–responsive methylmalonic acidemia has been treated in utero by giving massive doses of B12 to the mother, and a fetus with biotin-dependent multiple carboxylase deficiency has been treated by giving the mother pharmacologic doses of biotin during the last half of pregnancy.

Medications and nutrients injected into the amniotic fluid are swallowed and absorbed by the fetus. Intra-amniotic thyroid hormone can be used to treat congenital hypothyroidism and goiter and to help mature the fetal lung. The intrauterine growth-retarded fetus might be fed orally by instilling nutrients into the amniotic fluid.[6]

Anatomic Malformations

Correcting an anatomic malformation in utero is more difficult than providing a missing substrate, hormone, or medication to the fetus. The only anatomic malformations that warrant consideration are those that interfere with fetal organ development and that, if alleviated, would allow normal fetal development to proceed. At present, only three anatomic malformations deserve consideration, although others (for example, some rare cardiopulmonary lesions) may become candidates as their pathophysiology is unraveled.[20]

Congenital Hydronephrosis. Congenital hydronephrosis secondary to urethral obstruction is an excellent example of an anatomically simple lesion that has devastating consequences on the developing fetus which may be prevented by correction before birth. Fetal hydronephrosis is being recognized with increasing frequency because fluid-filled masses are particularly easy to detect by sonography and because associated oligohydramnios is a common obstetric indication for sonography. We have now managed more than 28 fetuses with urinary tract malformations. From this experience we have developed an approach based on the predictable pathophysiologic consequences of obstruction on renal and pulmonary development.[9, 12] The algorithm is presented in Figure 1.

If a renal cystic mass is suspected, it is important to distinguish multicystic dysplasia from hydronephrosis, because the renal functional damage associated with dysplasia is irreversible, whereas that secondary to obstruction is potentially reversible if the obstruction can be relieved. Although severe dysplasia associated with obstruction very early in fetal life may be difficult to distinguish from hydronephrosis, by the third trimester advanced dysplastic lesions can usually be distinguished by morphologic features and function from simple reversible hydronephrosis.

The most important clinical consideration is the effect of the malformation on

Table 5. *Malformations That May Require Treatment In Utero*

Deficiency States That May Be Alleviated
  Deficient pulmonary surfactant (pulmonary immaturity)
  Anemia–erythroblastosis and hydrops
  Hypothyroidism and goiter
  Methylmalonic acidemia (B12 dependent)
  Biotin-dependent multiple carboxylase deficiency
  Nutritional deficiency and intrauterine growth retardation

Anatomic Lesions That Interfere with Development
  Bilateral hydronephrosis (urethral obstruction)
  Diaphragmatic hernia
  Obstructive hydrocephalus

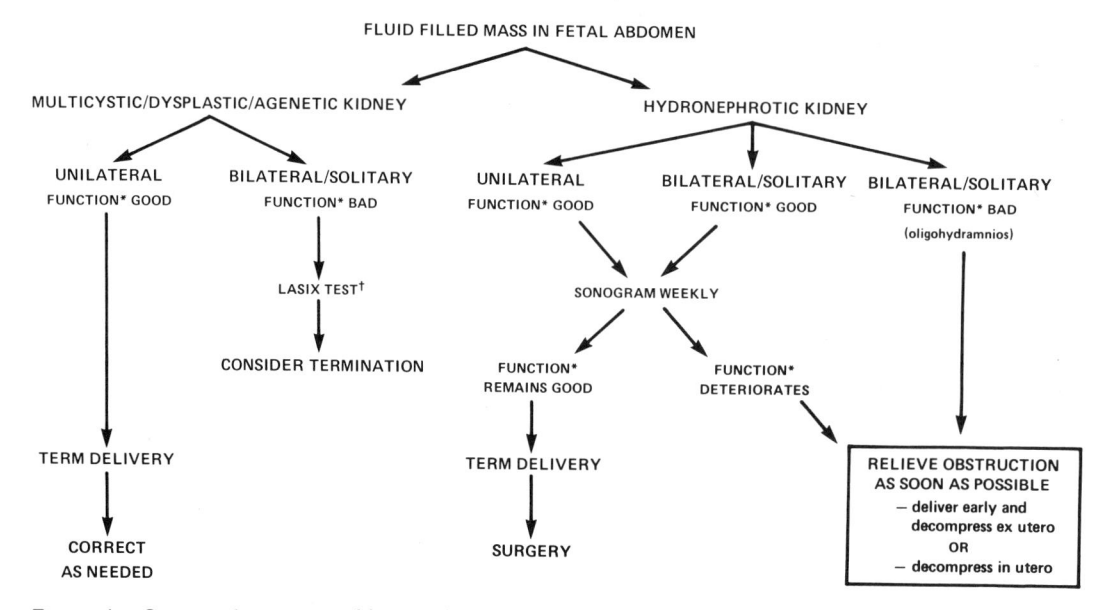

Figure 1. Suggested treatment of fetus with urinary tract malformation based on prenatal sonographic assessment of urinary tract anatomy and function. Asterisk, renal function inferred from volume of amniotic fluid and volume of urine in fetal bladder; dagger, sonographic assessment of fetal urine production (bladder filling, amniotic fluid volume) after giving furosemide to mother. (*From* Harrison, M.R., et al.: Management of the fetus with a urinary tract malformation. J.A.M.A., *246:* 635–639, 1981, with permission.)

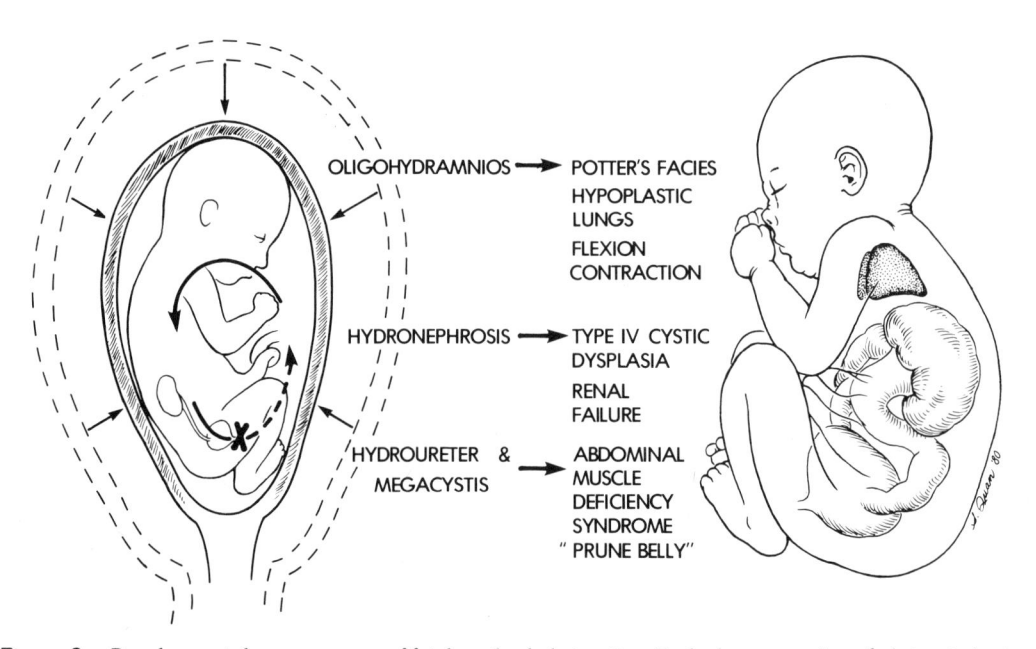

Figure 2. Developmental consequences of fetal urethral obstruction. Early decompression of obstructed urinary tract may abrogate these sequelae. (*From* Harrison, M.R., et al.: Management of the fetus with a urinary tract malformation. J.A.M.A., *246:* 635–639, 1981, with permission.)

renal function. We have found that fetal renal function can be inferred to some extent from the volume of amniotic fluid and the presence or absence of urine in the bladder. Oligohydramnios is probably the most important indicator of functional impairment. Since fetal urine is a major source of amniotic fluid in late pregnancy, it is not surprising that oligohydramnios accurately reflects decreased fetal urine excretion and that normal amniotic fluid volume accurately predicts the presence of at least one functioning kidney. Fetal urine output can also be estimated from real-time sonographic assessment of bladder filling and emptying. Inability to visualize the bladder on a routine sonogram does not in itself mean that fetal urine output is reduced, since the fetus may have recently voided. However, failure to visualize the bladder over a period of hours, especially after provoking fetal diuresis by giving furosemide to the mother, strongly suggests absence of adequate functioning renal tissue. More detailed functional and anatomic information can be obtained by aspiration of fetal urine under sonographic guidance. Urine production might then be measured directly, urine composition determined, and a fetal cystogram or pyelogram obtained.

When the findings suggest a unilateral multicystic kidney with adequate contralateral function, the fetus can be followed to term, for intervention even after birth is not urgent. When the prenatal findings suggest a severe bilateral dysgenetic or agenetic malformation that is incompatible with normal postnatal life, the family can be counseled and the pregnancy terminated or the neonate allowed to die without the emotionally and financially draining neonatal resuscitation and intensive care.

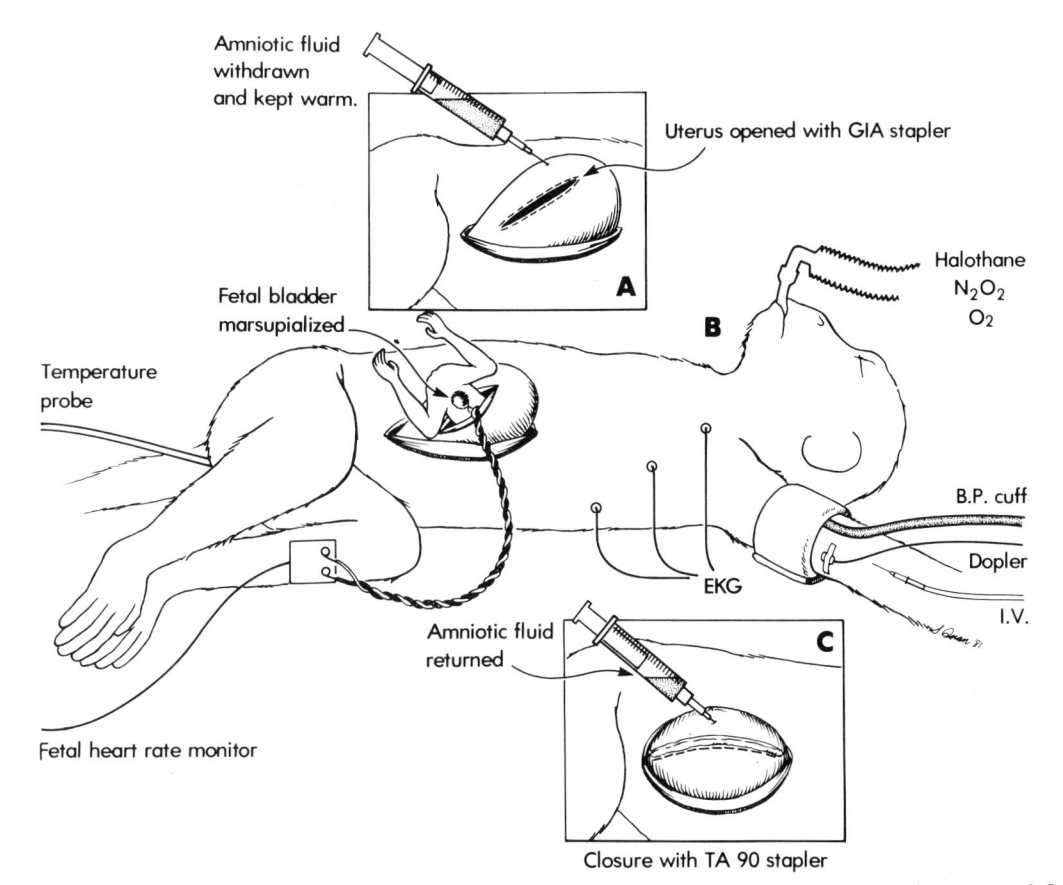

Figure 3. Technique for fetal surgery in the nonhuman primate. Mother and fetus are closely monitored. Indomethacin and antibiotics are given intravenously before surgery. Fluothane anesthesia provides uterine relaxation. The uterus is opened and closed with staples. (*From* Harrison, M.R., et al.: Fetal surgery in the primate. I. Anesthetic, surgical and tocolytic management to maximize fetal-neonatal survival. J. Pediatr. Surg., 17:115–122, 1982, with permission.)

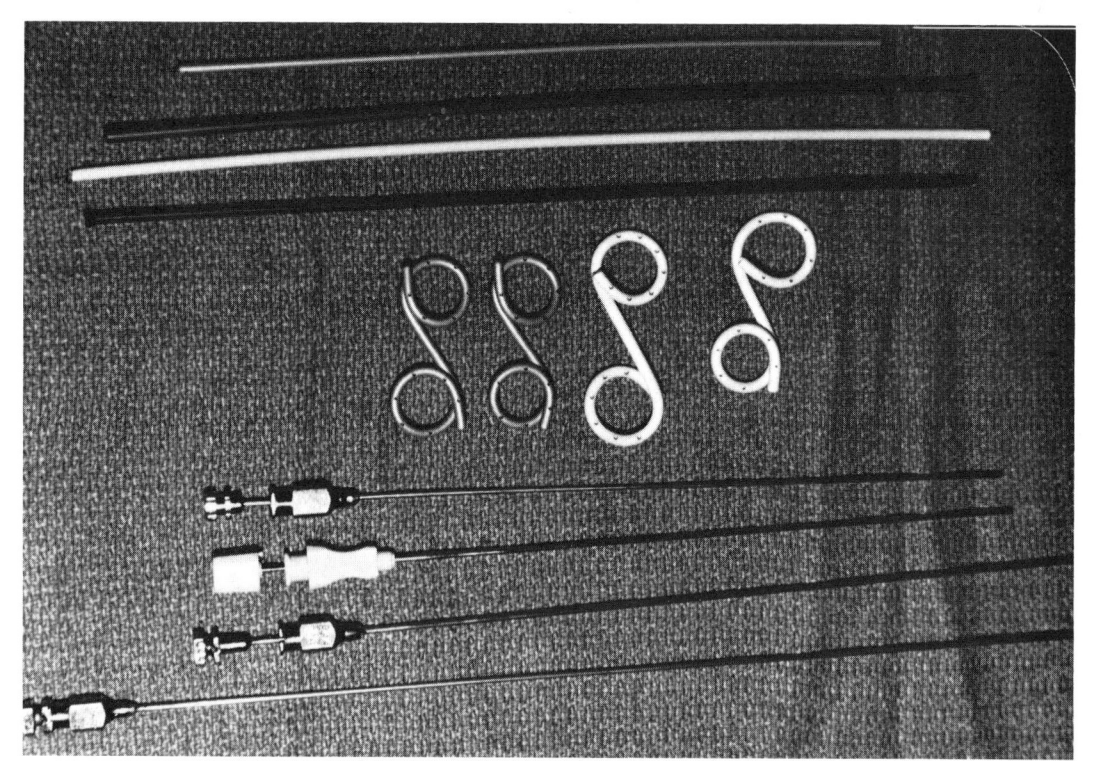

Figure 4. In selected cases an indwelling suprapubic catheter may be placed percutaneously under sonographic guidance. Photograph of the needles, catheters, and dilators used in percutaneous catheterization.

When the prenatal findings suggest urinary tract obstruction, intervention may be necessary because unrelieved urinary tract obstruction interferes with fetal development, and the severity of damage depends on the degree and duration of obstruction. Although infants born with partial obstruction may have only mild hydronephrosis, which is reversible with decompression after birth, infants born at term with high-grade obstruction may already have advanced hydronephrosis (type IV cystic disease) that is incompatible with life. In addition, oligohydramnios secondary to fetal urinary tract obstruction is associated with pulmonary hypoplasia as well as skeletal, facial, and abdominal wall deformities (Fig. 2). The pulmonary hypoplasia may be severe enough to prevent survival.[9, 12, 17]

In advanced cases with severe oligohydramnios, it may be necessary to relieve the obstruction at the earliest possible time to avert the progressive destructive consequences of obstruction and to allow normal development to proceed.[9, 12] There are several alternatives for decompressing the obstructed fetal urinary tract. The fetal bladder or renal pelvis can be aspirated percutaneously under sonographic guidance, but this offers only temporary relief, since the fetus makes a large amount of urine (greater than 5 ml per kg per hr) and will refill the bladder within hours. Early delivery can be electively induced so that the urinary tract can be decompressed ex utero. Preterm delivery for early decompression would maximize the opportunity for further renal development and minimize the adverse effects of oligohydramnios. The disadvantage of preterm delivery, fetal pulmonary immaturity, can be ameliorated by administration of corticosteroids to the mother before delivery. The efficacy of this approach has now been demonstrated in 10 of our cases.

Physiologically, the ideal management of fetal urinary tract obstruction is early decompression of the urinary tract and continued gestation. Transurethral or suprapubic drainage of urine from the bladder into the amniotic fluid would not only decompress the urinary tract and allow renal development to proceed, but would also restore normal amniotic fluid dynamics and thus prevent oligohydramnios and its severe sequelae.

Correction in utero is feasible. We have developed techniques for sonographically guided percutaneous placement of fetal shunt catheters and for surgical exteriorization of the fetal urinary tract. After we had studied the pathophysiology in a fetal lamb model,[14, 16] and established efficacy, feasibility, and safety in the more rigorous fetal monkey model (Fig. 3),[7] we began to apply these techniques clinically in a few highly selected cases (Figs. 4 to 7). In a male fetus (one of twins) with urethral obstruction, an indwelling suprapubic catheter was placed percutaneously under sonographic control.[3] This technique has been refined and used for diagnosis and treatment of a wide variety of fetal urinary tract obstructions at the Fetal Treatment Program at the University of California, San Francisco.[12] Open surgical decompression (bilateral fetal ureterostomies via hysterotomy) has also proved feasible (Fig. 8).[11] This more formidable technique requires extensive preparation in the non-human primate.

Congenital Diaphragmatic Hernia. Another fetal malformation that may require correction before birth is congenital diaphragmatic hernia. Although this simple defect is easily correctable in the neonatal period by removing the herniated viscera from the chest and closing the defect in the diaphragm, 50 to 90 per cent of these infants die of pulmonary insufficiency because the lung compressed by the herniated viscera is hypoplastic.[5] To allow the lung to grow and develop enough to support life at birth, the pulmonary compression must be relieved before birth. We have demonstrated in fetal lambs that

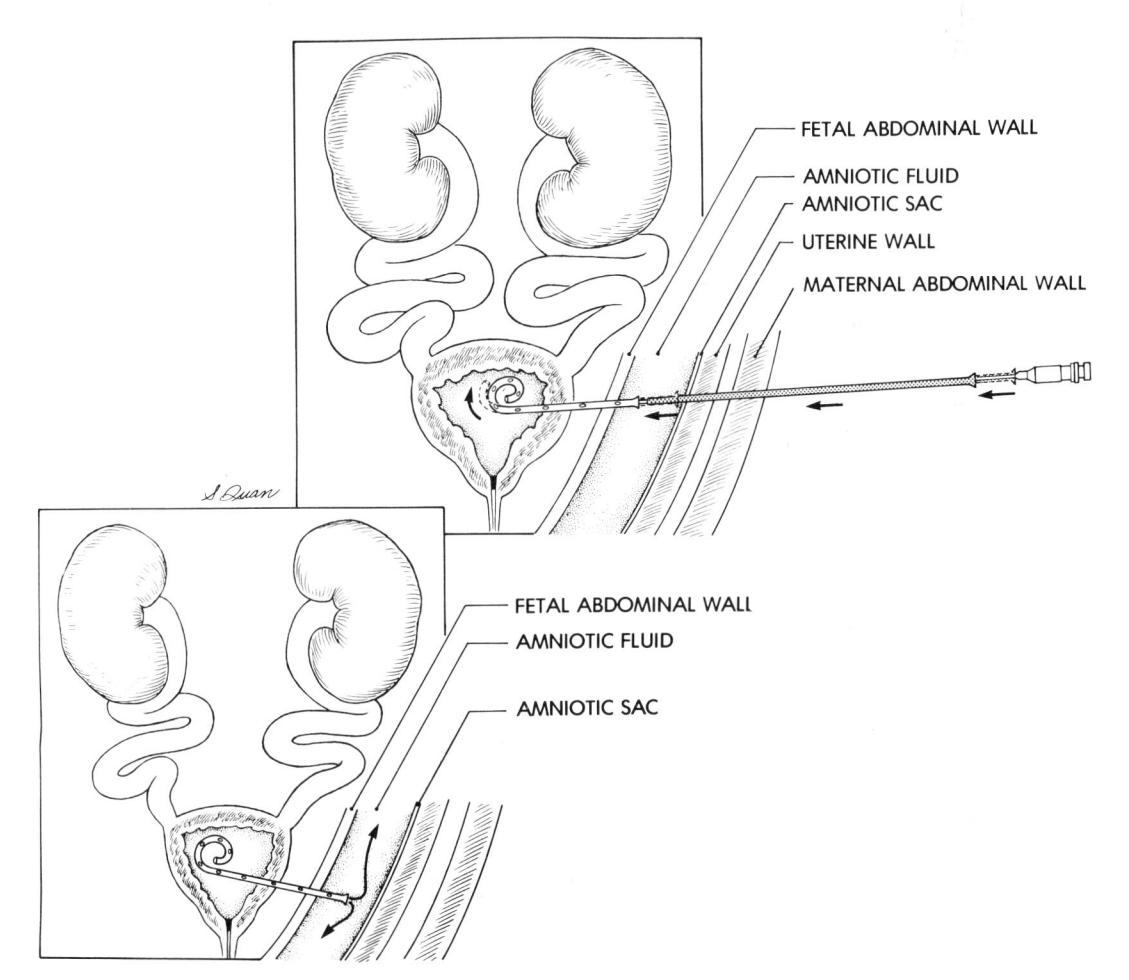

Figure 5. Artist's rendition of catheter placement technique. The catheter is pushed off the needle so that the curled end is in the fetal bladder and the flared end is in the amniotic cavity. (*From* Golbus, M.S., et al.: In utero treatment of urinary tract obstruction. Am. J. Obstet. Gynecol., *142*:383–388, 1982, with permission.)

compression of the fetal lung during the last trimester results in fatal pulmonary hypoplasia and that removal of the compressing lesion allows the lung to grow and develop sufficiently to reverse the fatal pulmonary hypoplasia and allow survival at birth.[8, 13] Congenital diaphragmatic hernia can be diagnosed in utero, and a technique for successful surgical correction in utero has been developed experimentally (Fig. 9).[15] In cases in which there is a suspicion of this abnormality after an ultrasonogram demonstrates an abnormal cystic structure within the thorax, a confirmatory amniogram demonstrating the abnormal location of the opacified fetal bowel within the thorax may be obtained. If the swallowed contrast material is not easily identified on a conventional pelvic radiograph, then one or two computed tomographic scans of the fetal thorax may be obtained (Fig. 10). Correction of diaphragmatic hernia is by far the most difficult of all procedures contemplated to date. It should not be attempted until the necessary skill is developed and success achieved in a rigorous animal model.

Congenital Obstructive Hydrocephalus. Another simple obstructive lesion with severe developmental consequences is obstructive hydrocephalus secondary to stenosis of the aqueduct of Sylvius. Obstruction to the flow of cerebrospinal fluid produces back pressure that dilates the ventricles, compresses the developing brain, and eventually destroys neurologic function. Decompressing the ventricles may reverse the adverse effects of high-pressure hydrocephalus and allow development to proceed normally.[19] The obstructed cerebrospinal fluid could be repeatedly aspirated or shunted into the amniotic fluid by means of a small one-way catheter placed by either surgical or sonographically guided percutaneous techniques.[1]

There are significant problems in managing the fetus with ventriculomegaly discovered by ultrasonogram. First, dilation of the ventricles may not result from simple obstruction to the flow of cerebrospinal fluid, but instead may be one part of a more extensive intrinsic central nervous system malformation. Ventricular drainage would not be expected to benefit the fetus with nonobstructive ventricular dilation. Second, even for true obstructive hydrocephalus, the pathophysiologic rationale that decompression will allow improved brain development, although reasonable, has not been tested in an appropriate animal model.

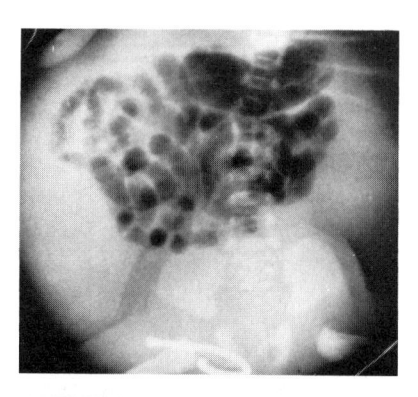

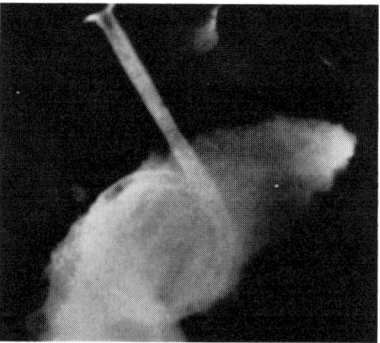

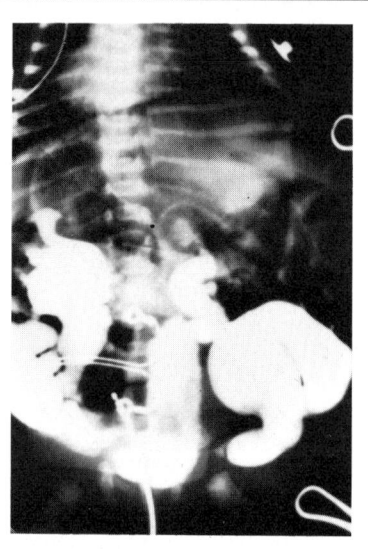

Figure 6. *Top,* Abdominal radiograph obtained shortly after birth of a baby with posterior urethral valves in which an indwelling catheter was placed in utero. *Middle,* Retrograde cystogram performed in the same baby demonstrating a markedly thickened bladder with the catheter still in place. *Bottom,* Markedly dilated upper collecting system, ureters, and thickened bladder wall in this infant with posterior urethral valves.

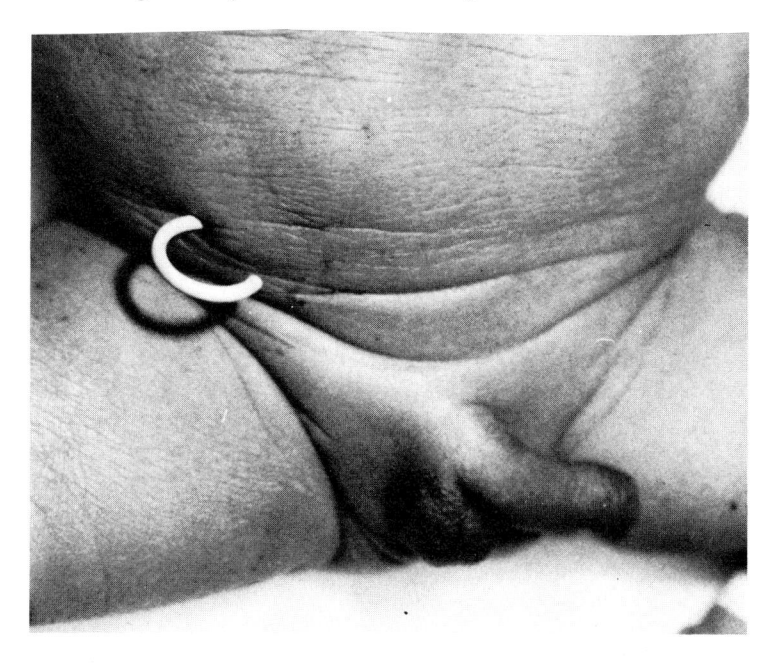

Figure 7. Photograph of an infant in whom a catheter was placed in utero leading from the bladder to the amniotic fluid.

For these reasons, we will continue to manage fetal hydrocephalus conservatively until we have sufficient clinical experience to be confident of the natural history of the disease and of our ability to distinguish obstructive hydrocephalus from other forms of ventriculomegaly, and until we can study the pathophysiology in an appropriate animal model. Fetal hydrocephalus continues to be an area of intense experimental and clinical investigation at our Fetal Treatment Program.[18, 19]

THE IMPACT OF FETAL THERAPY ON PRENATAL DIAGNOSIS

The potential for correction of some fetal malformations gives new importance to the rapidly developing field of prenatal diagnosis. Many fetal malformations are detectable in utero. In some cases, prenatal diagnosis will not alter management; some cannot be corrected, and most correctable lesions are best treated after normal term delivery. However, a few are amenable to treatment before term. Since their recognition will influence management of the pregnancy, prenatal diagnosis of these disorders assumes practical clinical importance.

Therapeutic decisions will require a thorough evaluation of the fetus beyond accurate anatomic definition of the malformation being considered for therapy.[10] Since it is known that malformations often occur as part of a syndrome, a search for associated abnormalities is necessary to avoid delivering a neonate with one corrected anomaly but other unrecognized disabling or lethal abnormalities. Real-time sonographic evaluation may yield important information on fetal breathing, fetal movements, and fetal vital functions. Amniocentesis allows culture of amniotic fluid cells for detection of chromosomal defects and inherited metabolic abnormalities, evaluation of fetal pulmonary maturity from lecithin-sphingomyelin analysis, and detection and quantitation of fetal hemolysis. Fetoscopy allows direct fetal visualization, fetal skin biopsy, and fetal blood sampling for diagnosis of hemoglobinopathies and other hematologic diseases. Amniography affords further definition of fetal anatomy, including the fetal gastrointestinal tract. Finally, fluid collections in the fetus (including blood, urine, ascites, cerebrospinal fluid) can be aspirated under real-time sonographic guidance for both diagnosis and therapy. The technique, in our experience, has proved safe and relatively simple.

In considering the ethical problems raised by fetal therapy, one clearly positive aspect is that prenatal diagnosis of a fetal malformation may now lead to treatment rather than abortion. However, the possibility of diagnosing and treating fetal disorders raises important questions about the

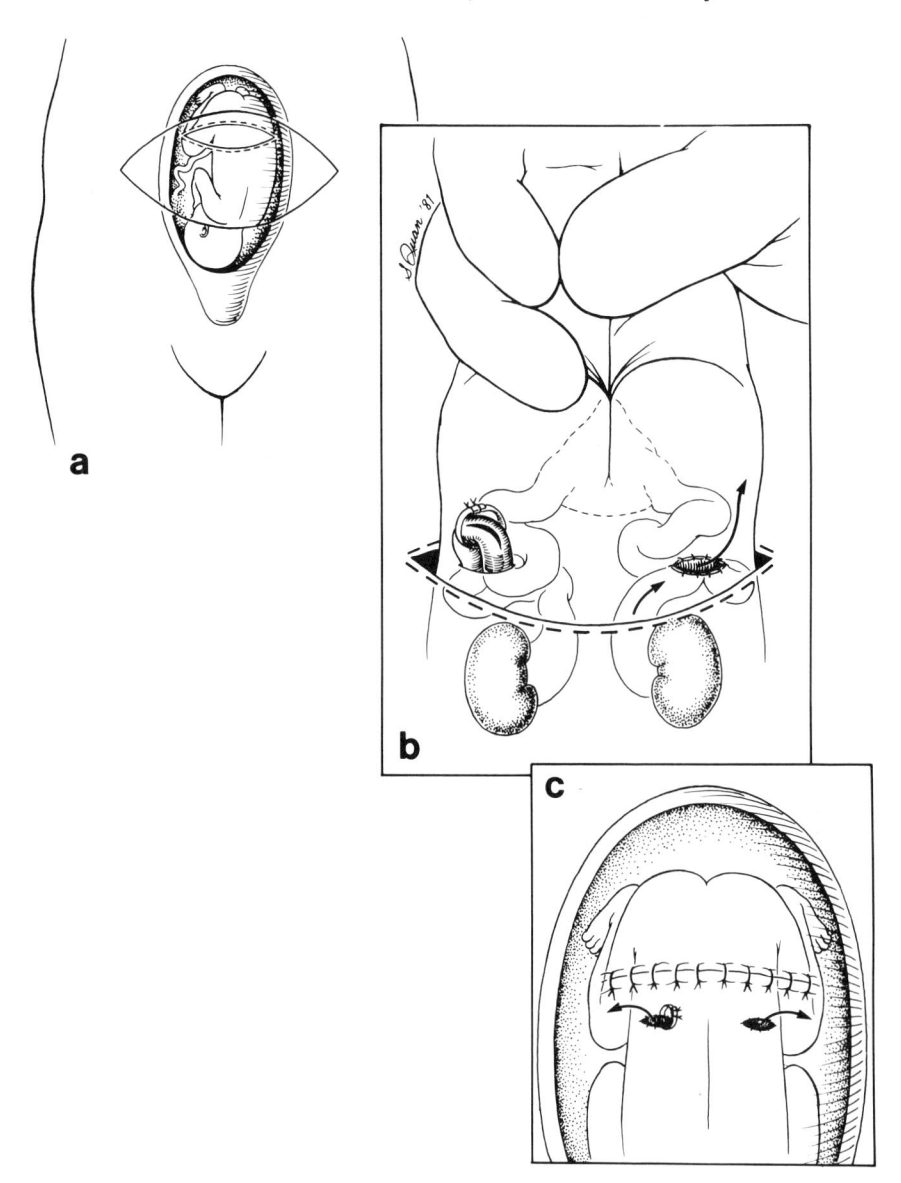

Figure 8. Ureterostomy in a fetus with hydronephrosis. Panel a shows the incisions in the maternal abdominal wall (*solid lines*) and in the uterus (*dashed lines*, which also represent staples). In panel b, the surgeon opens the obstructed ureters and sutures them to the skin while holding the legs of the fetus. A Silastic loop around the right ureter prevents retraction. Panel c shows the closed incisions of the fetus and uterus. The fetal urine is decompressed (*arrows*) into the amniotic fluid. (*From* Harrison, M.R., et al.: Fetal surgery for congenital hydronephrosis. N. Engl. J. Med., *306*:591–593, 1982, with permission.)

rights of the mother and fetus as patients.[2] Who makes decisions for the fetus? How can the risk of intervention be weighed against the burden of the malformation itself?

ASSESSING RISK AND BENEFIT

Fetal therapy raises complex medical and ethical issues. The first problem is defining the benefits and risks of fetal diagnosis and treatment. For the fetus, the risk of the procedure is weighed against the possibility of correction or amelioration of the malformation. The benefit to be derived from correction depends on the severity of the malformation and its predictable consequences on survival and quality of life, i.e., on the natural history of the disease. Assessing the risks and benefits for the mother is more difficult. Most fetal malformations do not directly threaten the mother's health, yet she must bear some risk from the procedure. She may choose to accept the risk to aid her unborn baby and increase his prospects for a normal life and to alleviate her own burden in carrying and preparing to raise a child with a severe malformation.

The risks involved in fetal diagnosis and treatment are generally greater for the fetus than for the mother and vary greatly according to the magnitude and invasiveness of the procedure.[10] Sonography carries no known risk. Amniography poses an increased risk of radiation exposure. Puncture of the amniotic cavity poses a small risk of fetal injury or loss. With appropriate equipment and expertise, fetoscopy, fetal blood sampling, and puncture of the fetal abdomen for intrauterine transfusion can be performed with acceptable risk. We have experience with sonographically guided aspiration of fetal ascites, pleural fluid, urine, and cerebrospinal fluid, but insufficient experience to judge risk adequately. The risk to fetus and mother of more extensive manipulation, such as placement of shunt catheters using sonographically guided percutaneous techniques or direct surgical exposure of the fetus by hysterotomy, is not known. Until recently, experience with surgical exposure of the human fetus was limited to catheterization of fetal vessels for exchange transfusion.[4] The greatest known risk of any fetal manipulation is induction of preterm labor and delivery. Although this remains the principal deterrent to fetal intervention, the pharmacologic control of uterine contractility with beta-mimetic drugs and prostaglandin synthetase inhibitors is improving. The electrophysiology of uterine muscle and the role of hormones, prostaglandins, and various tocolytic agents in preventing or controlling labor are areas of active investigation.[7]

THE FUTURE OF FETAL TREATMENT

The pathophysiologic arguments for fetal intervention are compelling, but extreme caution must be exercised in undertaking any new fetal manipulation. Extensive experience with fetal surgery in laboratory animals may not be readily translatable to the human. Survival after fetal surgery is easy to achieve in sheep but much more dif-

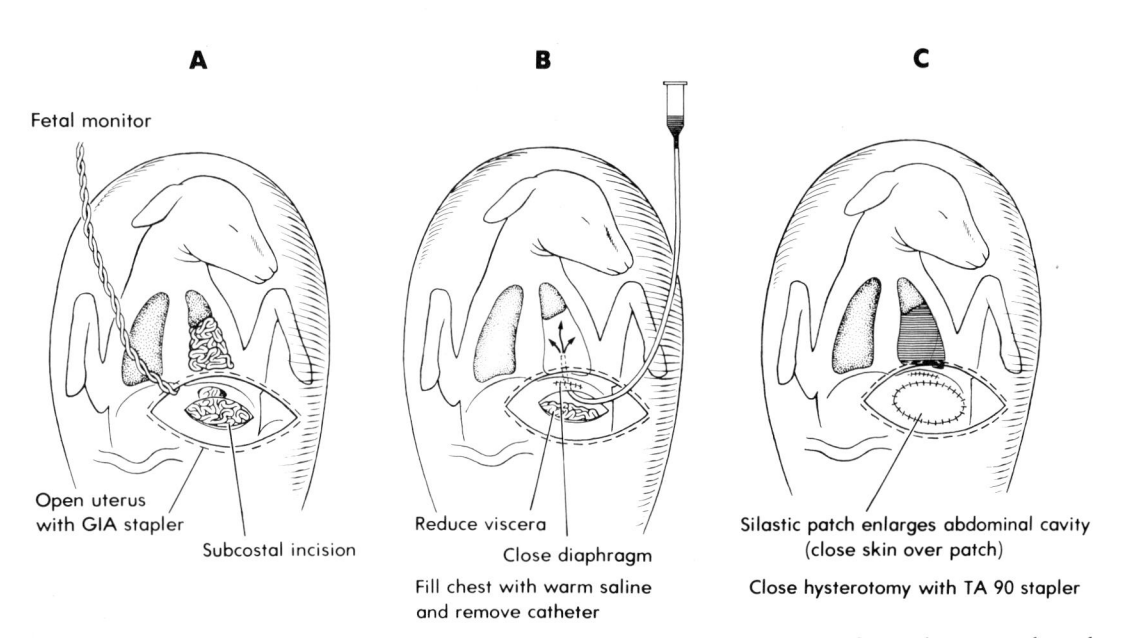

Figure 9. Technique for correction of congenital diaphragmatic hernia in utero. *A,* Surgical exposure through a stapled hysterotomy. A screw-in fetal scalp electrode monitors heart rate and variability during surgery. *B,* The herniated viscera are reduced, the air in the chest replaced with warm Ringer's lactate, and the diaphragm closed with a single layer of nonabsorbable sutures. *C,* The abdomen is enlarged by Silastic abdominoplasty, and the uterus closed with staples. Fetal operating time is less than 30 minutes. (*From* Harrison, M.R., et al.: Correction of congenital diaphragmatic hernia in utero. III. Development of a successful surgical technique using abdominoplasty to avoid compromise of umbilical blood flow. J. Pediatr. Surg., 16:934–942, 1981, with permission.)

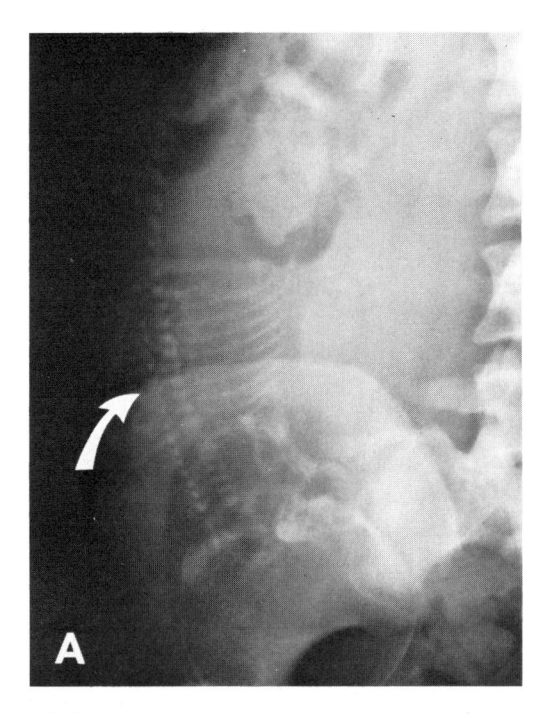

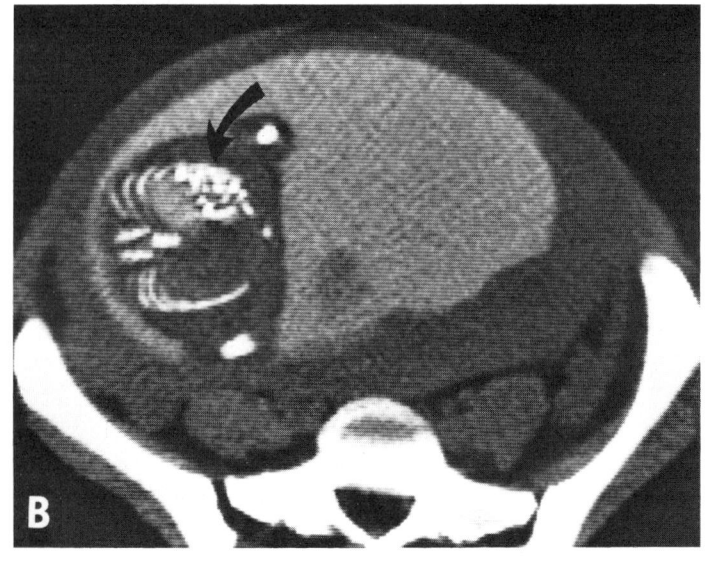

Figure 10. *A*, Amniogram in a fetus with congenital diaphragmatic hernia. The contrast-filled intestine can be seen only faintly (*arrow*) on a conventional radiograph. *B*, Computed tomographic section at the level of the fetal thorax from the same patient. The abnormally positioned contrast-filled intestine is well seen within the fetal chest (*arrow*).

ficult in primates, where preterm labor is often difficult to control. Certainly, repair of human fetal malformations should not be undertaken until competence and a high degree of success are achieved in a primate model. Recent advances in anesthetic and surgical technique and pharmacologic control of labor may soon make this feasible.[7]

Since the more invasive diagnostic and therapeutic procedures involve significant risks, a great deal of clinical and laboratory experience will be required to establish which are truly safe and feasible. In the meantime we should all maintain a healthy skepticism about fetal treatment. Because a procedure can be done does not mean that it should be done. A number of cases of obstructive hydronephrosis may be diagnosed in utero in which initially no therapy is performed and the fetus followed serially with "expectant management" (Fig. 11). At this very early stage, fetal intervention should be pursued only in centers committed to research and development as well as (and prior to) responsible clinical application. At

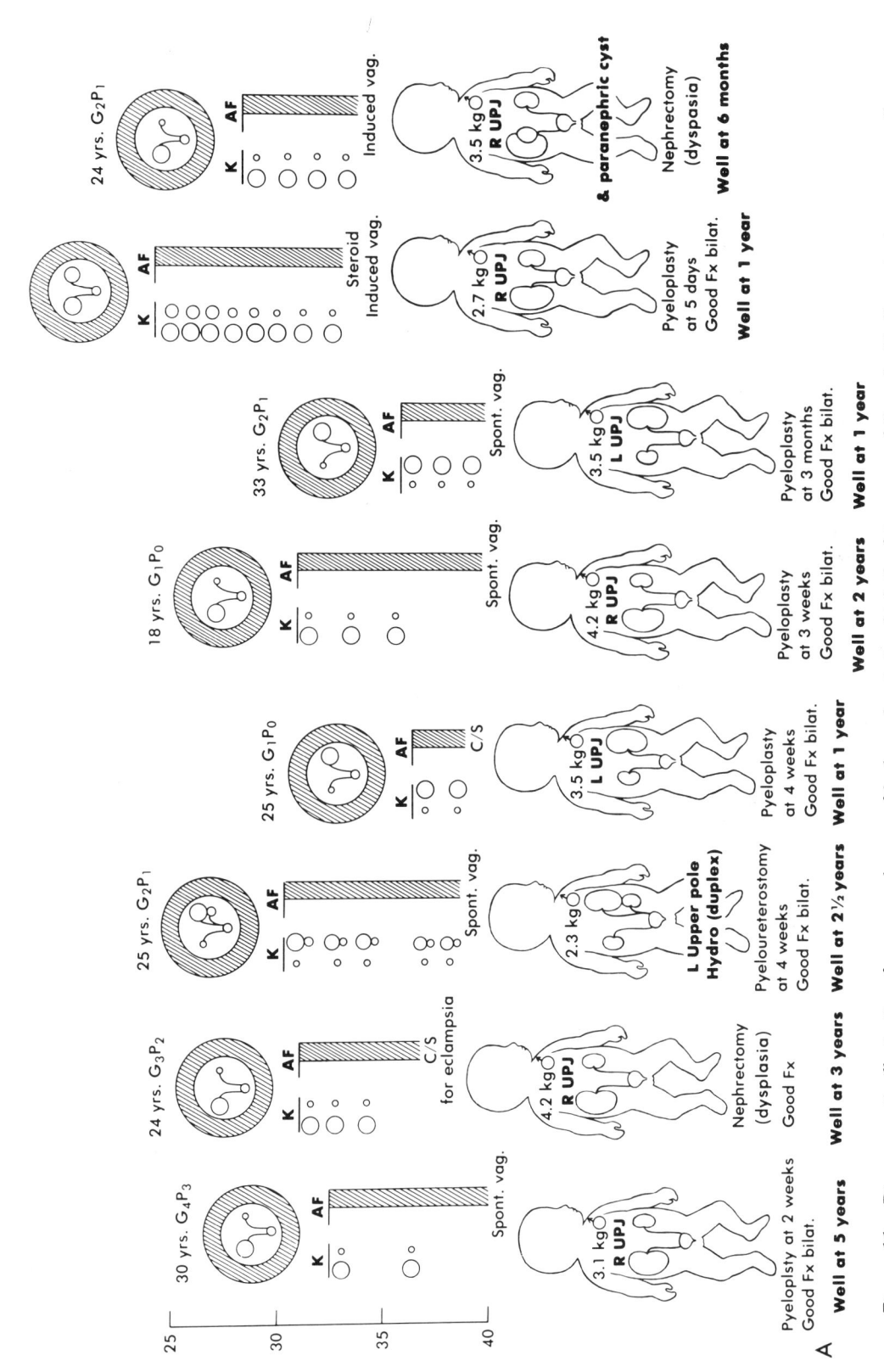

Figure 11. Diagrammatic illustrations from several cases of hydronephrosis in which the fetuses were followed with "expectant management" without in utero therapy. *A,* Eight cases of unilateral hydronephrosis followed serially by ultrasonography. K, kidney; AF, amniotic fluid; C/S, cesarean section. *B,* Three cases of bilateral hydronephrosis with good function and normal amounts of amniotic fluid. *C,* Three cases of bilateral hydronephrosis with poor function. (*From* Harrison, M.R., et al.: Management of the fetus with congenital hydronephrosis. J. Pediatr. Surg., in press, with permission.)

Illustration continued on following pages

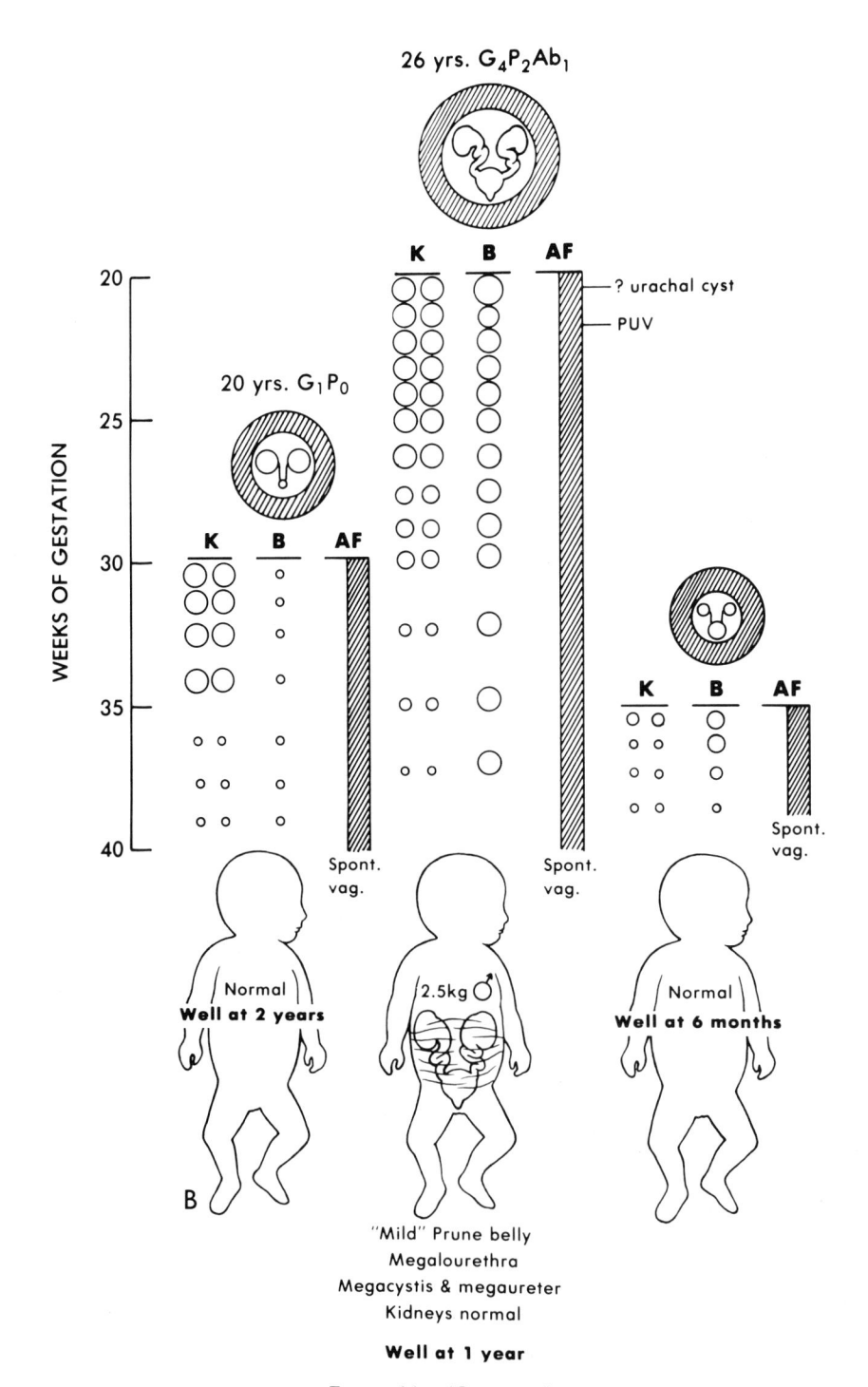

Figure 11. *(Continued)*

Figure 11. *(Continued)*

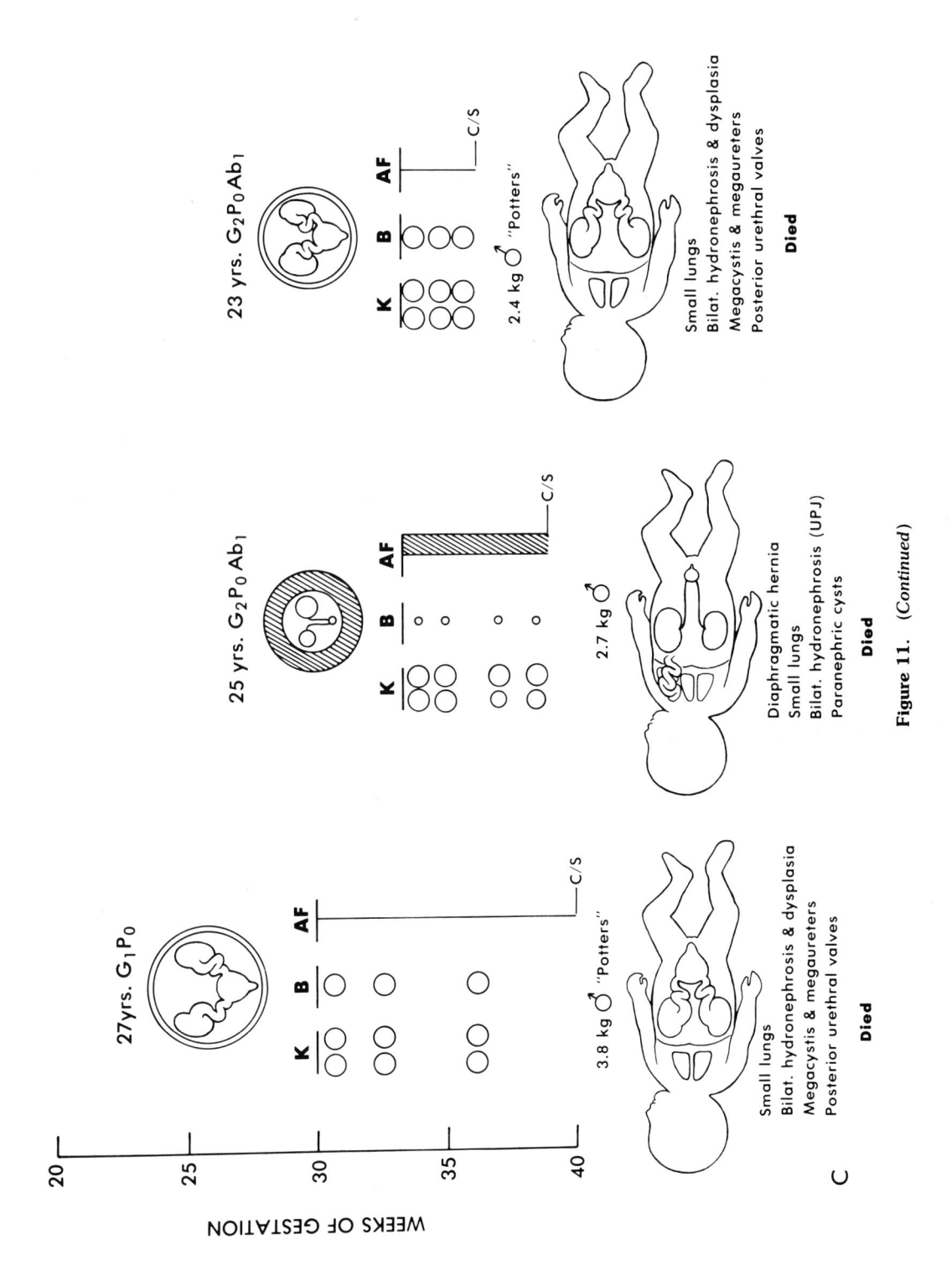

the present time the minimum requirements for fetal intervention include the cooperative efforts of an obstetrician experienced in prenatal intervention, a sonographer experienced and skilled in fetal diagnosis, a surgeon experienced in operating on tiny preterm infants and in performing fetal procedures in the laboratory, a perinatologist working in a high-risk obstetric unit associated with a tertiary intensive care nursery, a reasonable and compassionate bioethicist, and uninvolved professional . colleagues who will monitor such innovative therapy (a committee on human research). Since there is considerable potential for doing harm, a fetal abnormality of any type should never be treated simply "because it is there," and never by someone unprepared for this fearsome responsibility. The responsibility of those undertaking fetal therapy includes an obligation to report to the medical profession all results, good or bad, so that the merits and liabilities of fetal treatment can be established as soon as possible.

Our ability to diagnose fetal birth defects has achieved considerable sophistication. Treatment of several fetal disorders has proven feasible, and treatment of more complicated lesions will undoubtedly expand as techniques for fetal intervention improve.

REFERENCES

1. Clewell, W. H., Johnson, M. L., Meier, P. R., et al.: Placement of ventriculo-amniotic fluid shunt for hydrocephalus in a fetus (letter). N. Engl. J. Med., 305:955, 1981.
2. Fletcher, J. C.: The fetus as patient: Ethical issues. J.A.M.A., 246:772–773, 1981.
3. Golbus, M. S., Harrison, M. R., Filly, R. A., et al.: In utero treatment of urinary tract obstruction. Am. J. Obstet. Gynecol., 142:383–388, 1982.
4. Harrison, M. R.: Unborn: Historical perspective of the fetus as a patient. Pharos, 45:19–24, 1982.
5. Harrison, M. R., and de Lorimier, A. A.: Congenital diaphragmatic hernia. Surg. Clin. North Am., 61:1023–1035, 1981.
6. Harrison, M. R., and Villa, R.: Trans-amniotic fetal feeding. I. Development of an animal model: Continuous amniotic infusion in rabbits. J. Pediatr. Surg., 17:376–380, 1982.
7. Harrison, M. R., Anderson, J., Rosen, M. A., et al.: Fetal surgery in the primate. I. Anesthetic, surgical and tocolytic management of to maximize fetal-neonatal survival. J. Pediatr. Surg., 17:115–122, 1982.
8. Harrison, M. R., Bressack, M. A., Churg, A. M., et al.: Correction of congenital diaphragmatic hernia in utero. II. Simulated correction permits fetal lung growth with survival at birth. Surgery, 88:260–268, 1980.
9. Harrison, M. R., Filly, R. A., Parer, J. R. T., et al.: Management of the fetus with a urinary tract malformation. J.A.M.A., 246:635–639, 1981.
10. Harrison, M. R., Golbus, M. R., and Filly, R. A.: Management of the fetus with a correctable congenital defect. J.A.M.A., 246:774–777, 1981.
11. Harrison, M. R., Golbus, M. S., Filly, R. A., et al.: Fetal surgery for congenital hydronephrosis. N. Engl. J. Med., 306:591–593, 1982.
12. Harrison, M. R., Golbus, M. S., Filly, R. A., et al.: Management of the fetus with congenital hydronephrosis. J. Pediatr. Surg., in press.
13. Harrison, M. R., Jester, J. A., and Ross, N. A.: Correction of congenital diaphragmatic hernia in utero. I. The model: Intrathoracic balloon produces fatal pulmonary hypoplasia. Surgery, 88:174–182, 1980.
14. Harrison, M. R., Nakayama, D. K., Noall, R., et al.: Correction of congenital hydronephrosis in utero. II. Decompression permits renal and pulmonary development. J. Pediatr. Surg., in press.
15. Harrison, M. R., Ross, N. A., and de Lorimier, A. A.: Correction of congenital diaphragmatic hernia in utero. III. Development of a successful surgical technique using abdominoplasty to avoid compromise of umbilical blood flow. J. Pediatr. Surg., 16:934–942, 1981.
16. Harrison, M. R., Ross, N. A., Noall, R., et al.: Correction of congenital hydronephrosis in utero. I. The model: Fetal urethral obstruction produces hydronephrosis and pulmonary hypoplasia in fetal lambs. J. Pediatr. Surg., in press.
17. Harrison, M. R., Nakayama, D. K., Noall, R., et al.: Correction of congenital hydronephrosis in utero. II. Decompression reverses the effects of obstruction of the fetal lung and urinary tract. J. Pediatr. Surg., in press.
18. Nakayama, D. K., Harrison, M. R., and de Lorimier, A. A.: Morbidity and mortality of severe fetal urethral obstruction. J. Pediatr. Surg., in press.
19. Nakayama, D. K., Harrison, M. R., Berger, M. S., et al.: Correction of congenital hydrocephalus in utero. I. The model: Intracisternal Kaolin produces hydrocephalus in fetal lambs. J. Pediatr. Surg., submitted for publication.
20. Nakayama, D. K., Harrison, M. R., Edwards, M. S., et al.: Management of the fetus with a CNS malformation. Submitted for publication.
21. Turley, K., Vlahakes, G. J., Harrison, M. R., et al.: Intrauterine cardiothoracic surgery: The fetal lamb model. Ann. Thorac. Surg., in press.

12

Normal Anatomy of the Female Pelvis

Alfred B. Kurtz, M.D., and Matthew D. Rifkin, M.D.

The pelvis is a bony ring resembling a basin. Anatomically, it can be divided into the greater and lesser pelvis by an oblique line, termed the pelvic brim, which passes through the prominence of the sacrum, the arcuate and pectineal lines, and the superior margin of the pubic symphysis.[8] The greater or false pelvis is situated above this line and is bound posteriorly and laterally by the iliac crests. Anteriorly, the greater pelvis is incomplete and communicates cranially with the remainder of the abdomen and caudally with the lesser pelvis. The lesser or true pelvis is situated below the pelvic brim. Its bony walls are more complete and it resembles a bowl tilted back approximately 50 to 60 degrees from the vertical.[8] The cavity of the lesser pelvis is bound by the pubic symphysis and superior pubic rami anteriorly, by the pelvic surfaces of the sacrum and coccyx posteriorly, and by the ilium below the arcuate line and the inner surfaces of the body and superior ischial rami laterally. The lesser pelvis communicates with the greater pelvis cranially and is enclosed by a group of muscles caudally termed the pelvic diaphragm.

The accuracy of ultrasound in the analysis of disorders of the female pelvis has been shown to be between 82 and 91 per cent.[3, 5, 15, 19] This level of confidence can be approached only when the pelvic examination is performed with a distended urinary bladder. The filled bladder displaces loops of bowel out of the pelvis and serves as an acoustic "window" for evaluation of adjacent structures. Since the urinary bladder originates and distends within the lesser pelvis, the levator ani and obturator internus muscles, and the organs of reproduction (vagina, uterus, and adnexa) can be identified. In addition, when the rectosigmoid colon is concomitantly filled with fluid, almost complete evaluation of the lesser pelvic contents can be made.[4, 16]

Ultrasound examination of the greater pelvis is more difficult since the urinary bladder rarely distends sufficiently to aid in its imaging. The major structures within the greater pelvis are the iliopsoas muscles and loops of bowel filled with varying amounts of fluid and gas. The ascending and descending colons occupy the right and left flanks, while the midpelvis is filled with small bowel and mesentery. Although ultrasound is not able to adequately image bone directly, the anterior surfaces of the iliac bones can be seen as bright reflectors without distal acoustic transmission and thereby serve as specific landmarks. Visualization of the greater pelvis is inconsistent and only clearly imaged in thin patients with a paucity of bowel gas and prominent iliopsoas muscles.

It is the purpose of this chapter to define the role of ultrasound in the analysis of the true and false pelvis. The normal anatomy will be discussed in detail, comparing line drawings with ultrasonographic cross-sectional images. Because the osseous structures aside from their anterior surface cannot be imaged, they will not be discussed further. The major muscles, blood vessels, ureters, urinary bladder, vagina and uterus, adnexa, rectosigmoid colon, and potential spaces will be analyzed in order.

PELVIC MUSCULATURE

Three major groups of muscles are visualized on pelvic ultrasound examination. In the greater pelvis, the iliopsoas muscles can be seen, particularly in thin patients, while in the lesser pelvis, the obturator internus and the levator ani muscles are consistently identified (Figs. 1 to 3). The two other muscles of the lesser pelvis, the coccygeus and piriformis, are located deep, posteriorly and cranially (Fig. 2). They are not routinely visualized on ultrasound examination and, when imaged, cannot be accurately separated from the more inferiorly located levator ani muscle.

The iliopsoas muscle is a combination of the psoas major and the iliacus muscle.[6] The psoas major is a long thick muscle which originates bilaterally in the paralumbar vertebral regions and courses in a caudal direction, extending slightly anteriorly and laterally as it enters the greater pelvis over the iliac crest (Figs. 1 and 2). The iliacus muscle is a flat triangular structure arising posterior to the psoas major muscle from the superior two thirds of the iliac fossa (Fig. 2). These two muscles interdigitate to form the iliopsoas muscle which continues in an anterolateral direction as it moves caudally to its tendinous insertion on the femur. The muscle can vary greatly in size depending upon the patient's muscular development.

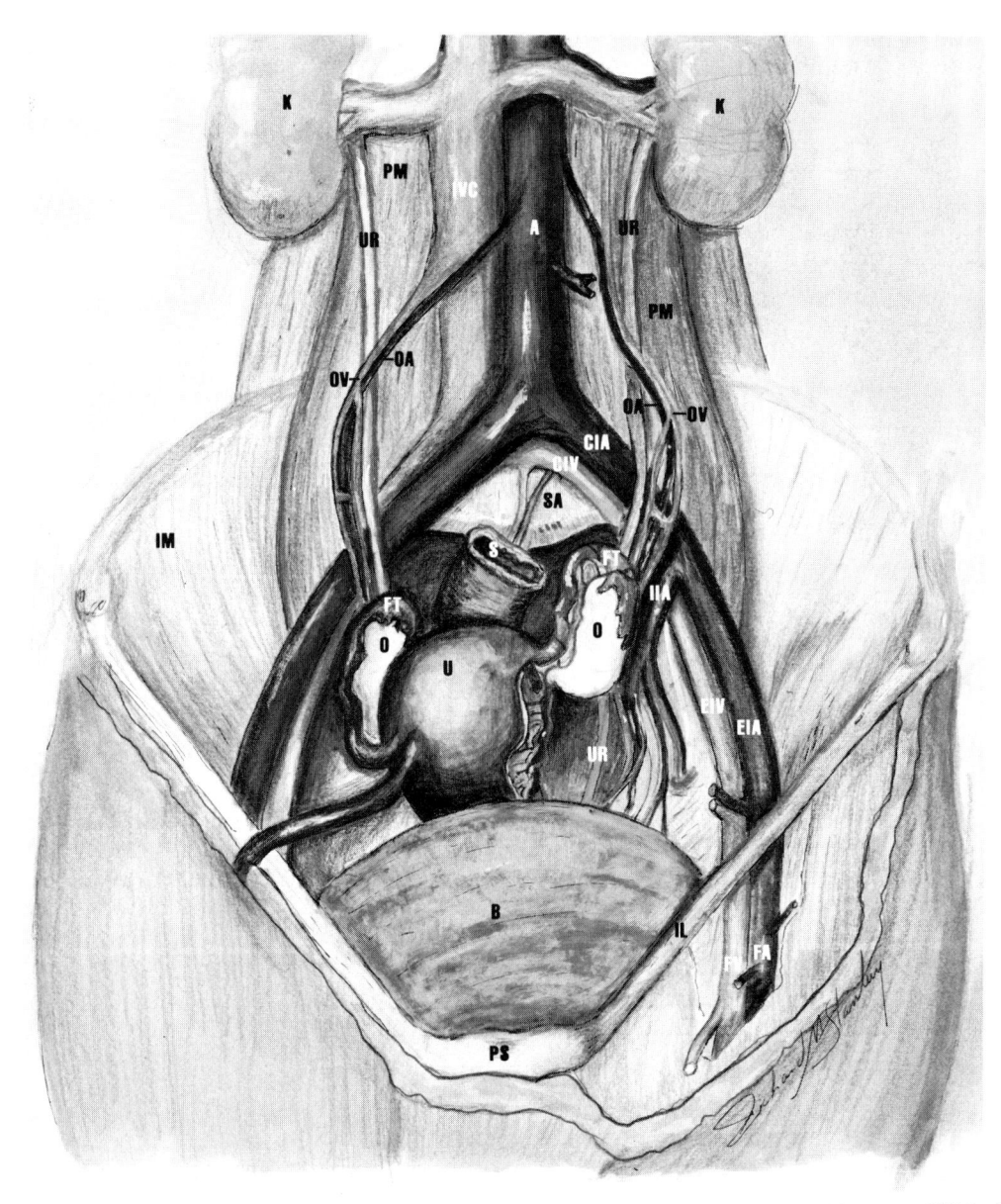

Figure 1. Anterior diagram of the lower abdominal and pelvic retroperitoneal structures. (See page 208 for key to abbreviations.)

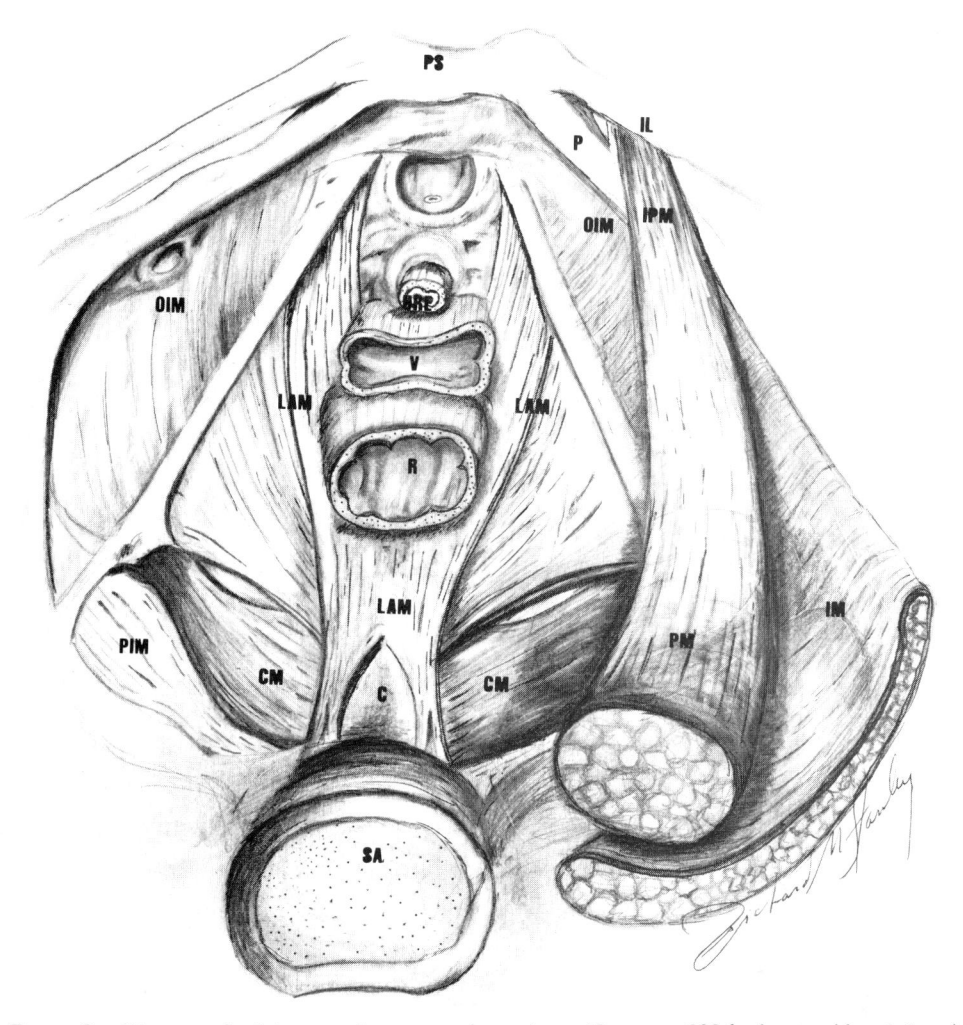

Figure 2. Diagram of pelvic musculature seen from above. (See page 208 for key to abbreviations.)

On ultrasound examination, the iliopsoas muscle is relatively hypoechoic and discretely marginated (Figs. 4 to 6).[17] The separation of the iliacus and psoas major muscles is frequently noted by a bright linear echo representing the interposed fascial sheath (Fig. 4). The superior aspect of the iliopsoas is often incompletely visualized because of varying amounts of overlying bowel gas. The more caudad portion is more completely imaged since it is more anteriorly located, has fewer interposed loops of bowel, and may be scanned obliquely through the distended urinary bladder. The long axis of the iliopsoas muscle is imaged in a longitudinal projection angled from the midline toward the hip (Fig. 4B). The muscle is also segmentally visualized in true transverse and longitudinal projection. In all of the described planes, the bright reflector seen immediately posterior to the iliopsoas muscle represents the anterior surface of the iliac bone (Fig. 4).

Within the lesser pelvis, the obturator internus muscle occupies a large part of the inner surface of the anterior and lateral pelvic walls (Fig. 2).[6] It is surrounded by the obturator fascia which serves as a tendinous attachment for the levator ani muscle.[6] On ultrasound examination, sections of this muscle are routinely imaged through the distended urinary bladder as elongated and relatively hypoechoic ovoid muscle surrounded by the bright reflector of the obturator fascia (Fig. 5, *B* and *C*).[12,17,18] The obturator internus muscle is most easily recognized in true transverse view and may be accentuated in transverse view by angling from the pubic symphysis superiorly (Fig. 6A). This cranially angled

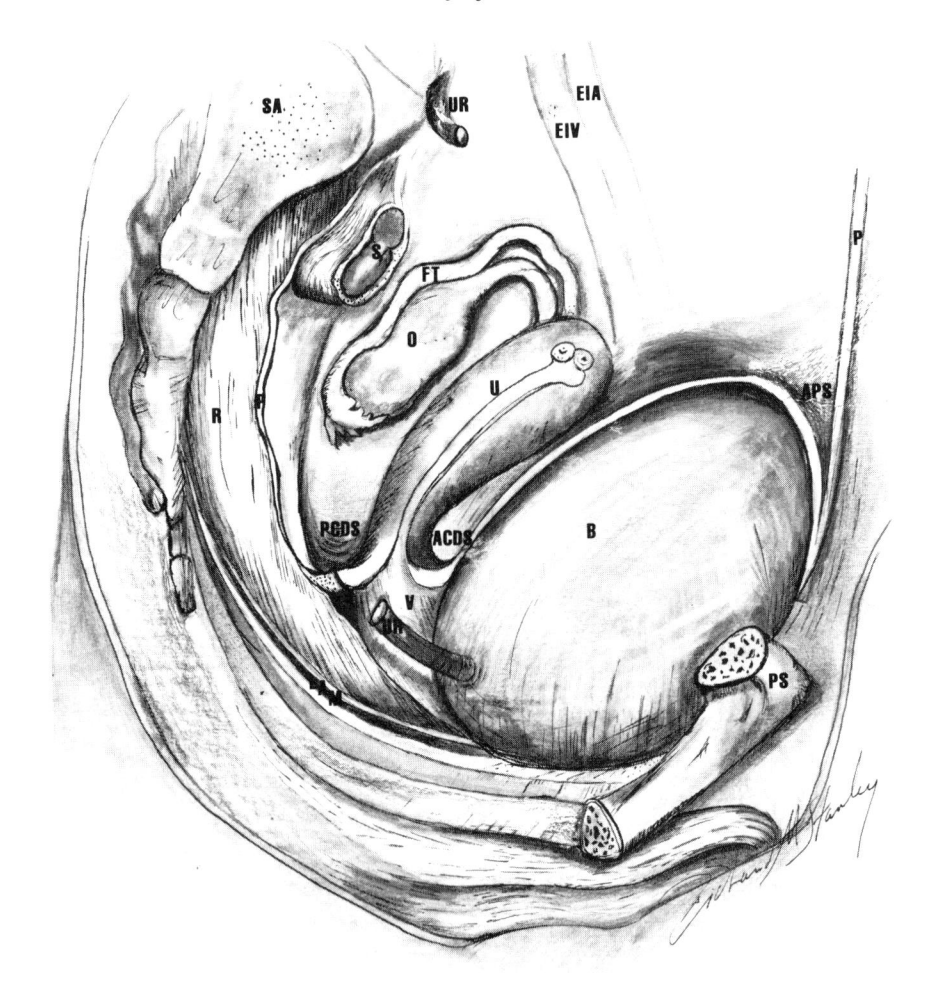

Figure 3. Sagittal diagram of pelvis, lateral to midline. (See page 208 for key to abbreviations.)

view will, at the same time, minimize the more caudally placed levator ani muscle. On occasion, the obturator internus muscle may also be seen on longitudinal scans angled toward the pelvic side walls (Fig. 7).

The levator ani muscle, together with the coccygeus muscle, form the pelvic diaphragm.[6] This muscle stretches across the pelvic floor like a hammock and is the most caudal structure defining the limits of the abdomino-pelvic cavity (Figs. 2 and 3). In lower animals, the levator ani muscle can be separated into two parts, the pubococcygeus and iliococcygeus muscles, but this separation cannot be made in man.[6] On ultrasound examination, the levator ani muscle is imaged as a relatively hypoechoic hammock-shaped area posterior, medial, and caudad to the obturator internus (Fig. 5, B to D). Because one of its major attachments is to the tendinous insertion from the obturator fascia, these two muscles are frequently inseparable laterally (Fig. 6B). The levator ani muscle is less commonly seen than the obturator internus muscle, even through a distended urinary bladder, owing to the interposition of loops of small bowel and rectosigmoid colon (Fig. 5D). While it is routinely imaged in true transverse plane (Fig. 5, B to D), the levator ani muscle may be accentuated by angling down in transverse projection from the superior aspect of the urinary bladder toward the feet since it is more prominent caudally (Fig. 6B). This same caudally angled transducer view will minimize the size of the obturator internus muscle, which is more superiorly located. On occasion, the levator ani muscle may be imaged on longitudinal scans angled toward the pelvic side walls (Fig. 7).

PELVIC BLOOD VESSELS

The common iliac arteries arise from the bifurcation of the abdominal aorta at approximately the fourth lumbar vertebral body and diverge laterally and caudally to enter the greater pelvis (Figs. 1 and 8).[7] The common iliac artery courses along the anteromedial aspect of the iliopsoas muscle and, in the superior aspect of the greater pelvis, divides into external and internal iliac arteries (Fig. 1). The external iliac artery remains within the greater pelvis, continuing along the anteromedial margin of the iliopsoas muscle through the inguinal canal to become the femoral artery in the thigh (Figs. 1, 3, and 8). The internal iliac artery, at its origin, immediately passes over the pelvic brim to descend into the lesser pelvis posterior and slightly lateral to the ureter and ovary (Fig. 1). The iliac veins (external, internal, and common) follow the same course as their companion arteries except they are slightly more posteriorly and medially placed.[12]

The ovarian artery and vein enter the greater pelvis anterior to the common iliac artery and vein and then descend into the lesser pelvis posterior to the ovaries (Figs. 1 and 8).[7] In general, the ovarian artery and vein are too small to be imaged routinely on ultrasound examination.

Ultrasound examination of the blood vessels shows them as tubular structures with bright walls and echo-free centers. Usually, the arteries can be seen to pulsate radially with each heartbeat. The common and external iliac vessels are incompletely visu-

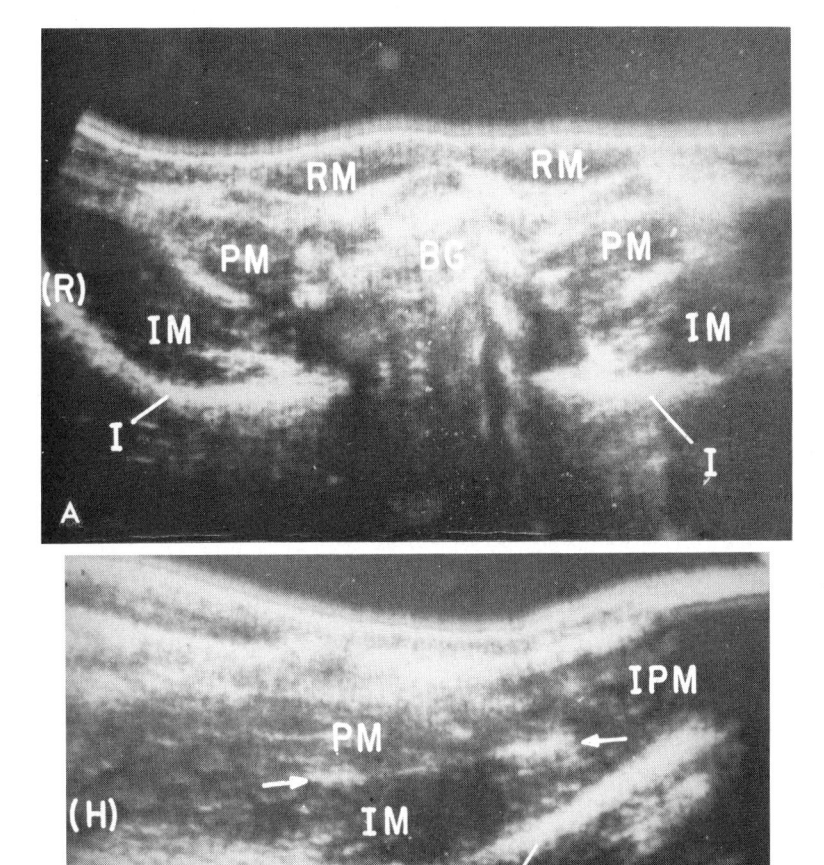

Figure 4. Greater pelvis. Transverse scan (*A*) and oblique longitudinal scan (*B*) imaged along the long axis of iliopsoas muscle (IPM) from midline toward hip. Arrow denotes fascia separating psoas muscle (PM) from iliacus muscle (IM). RM, rectus muscle; BG, bowel gas; I, iliac wing.

alized, particularly in the upper portion of the greater pelvis, because of the interposition of loops of gas-filled bowel. However, in the lower part of the greater pelvis, adjacent to the pelvic brim, the external iliac artery and vein can be imaged routinely, particularly through a very distended urinary bladder (Fig. 9).[12, 17] This distention, however, may occasionally compress the vein so that only the iliac artery is imaged (Fig. 6A). Optimal imaging of the common and external iliac vessels is obtained utilizing true transverse and angled longitudinal scans along the long axis of the blood vessels from the midline toward the hip (Fig. 9). Further evaluation of the blood vessels may be performed with pulsed range-gated Doppler.

The internal iliac artery and vein can usually be seen at their origins and followed for several centimeters distally.[12, 17] They can be imaged in the lesser pelvis in long axis posterior and slightly lateral to the ovary and ureter (Fig. 10). While it is necessary to have a very distended urinary bladder to image these vessels optimally,

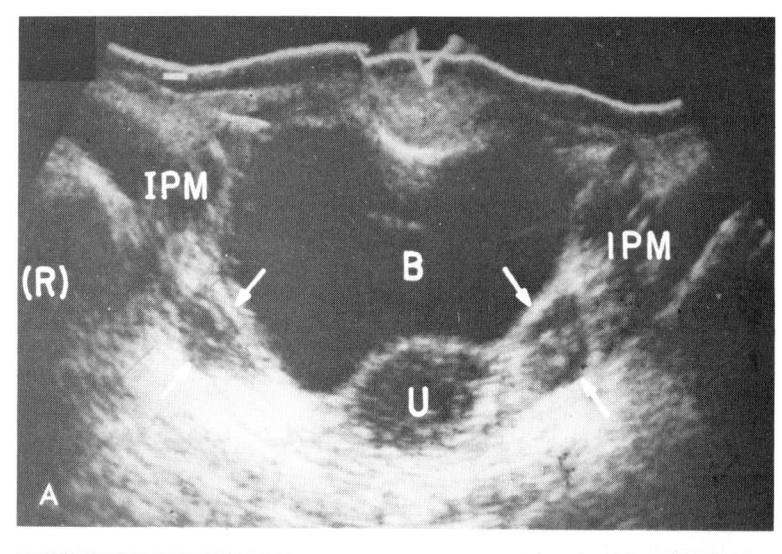

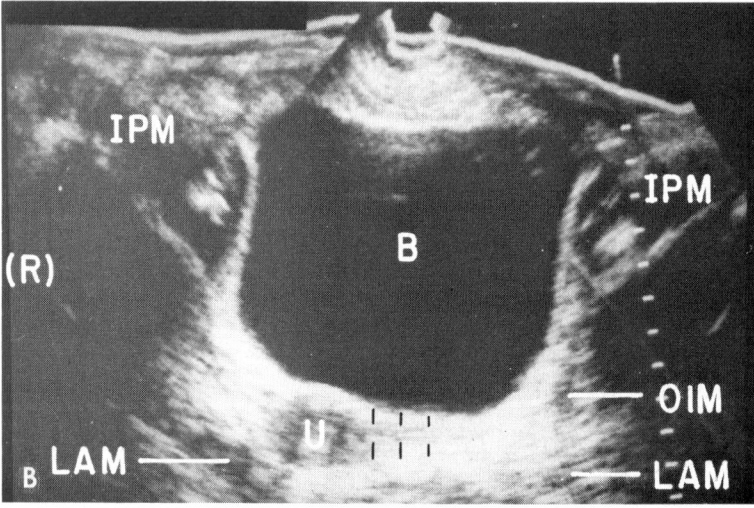

Figure 5. Transverse images of pelvis from cranial to caudal aspect of urinary bladder. Note slight bladder indentation by normal structures. A, Most superior scan. Arrows denote ovaries. The bladder is more rounded. IPM, iliopsoas muscle; U, uterus; B, bladder. B, Second-most superior scan. Lines denote left adnexal area. Note prominent iliopsoas muscles (IPM) causing "squaring" of bladder. LAM, levator ani muscle; OIM, obturator internus muscle; B, bladder; U, uterus.

Illustration continued on opposite page

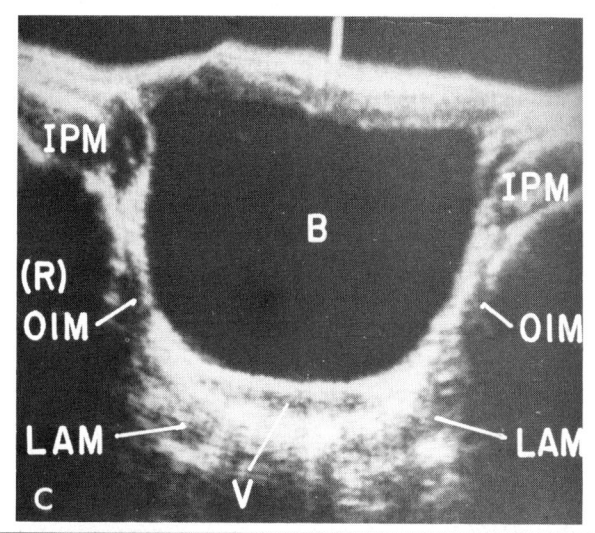

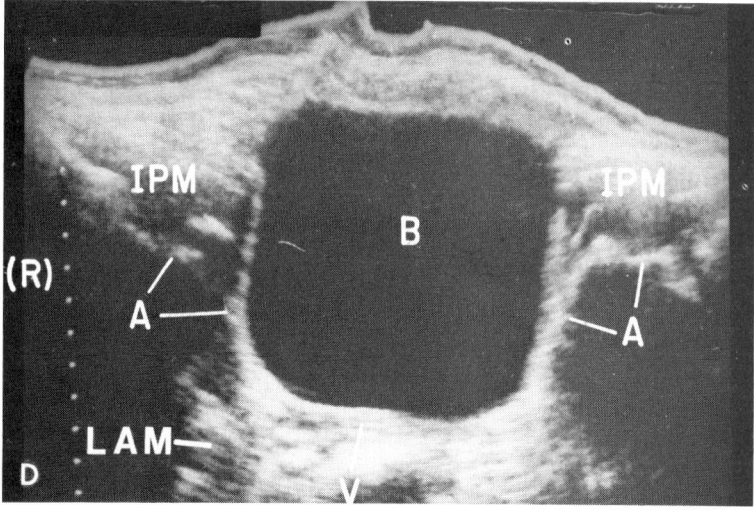

Figure 5 (*Continued*). *C*, Second-most inferior scan. V, vagina. *D*, Most inferior scan. Note "squaring" of bladder by effects of acetabulum (A). The levator ani muscle (LAM) is incompletely seen because of overlying bowel. IPM, iliopsoas muscle.

overdistention of the bladder may sometimes compress the internal iliac vein so that only the artery is imaged.

URETER

The ureters originate from the kidneys and extend longitudinally and caudally until they insert into the trigone at the posterolateral aspect of the urinary bladder (Figs. 1 and 8).[11] Initially, in the abdomen, the ureters lie anterior to the psoas muscles and upon entering the greater pelvis course anterior to the common iliac artery and vein. After passing over the pelvic brim, they descend into the lesser pelvis and pass posterior and slightly medial to the ovary.[11] The ureters then continue caudally to insert into the trigone on both sides of the cervix and upper vagina (Fig. 3).

On ultrasound examination, the ureter cannot be imaged within the greater pelvis owing to its small size and overlying bowel. While no measurements have been obtained for the upper limits of normal, the ureter can be routinely seen in the lesser pelvis through a very distended urinary bladder and traced until its insertion into the bladder trigone, at the upper level of the vaginal canal (Figs. 10 and 11).[12, 17] It is best imaged in long axis but can also be seen in transverse view as a bright-walled structure with a relatively echo-free center (Fig. 11). When posterior to the ovary, the

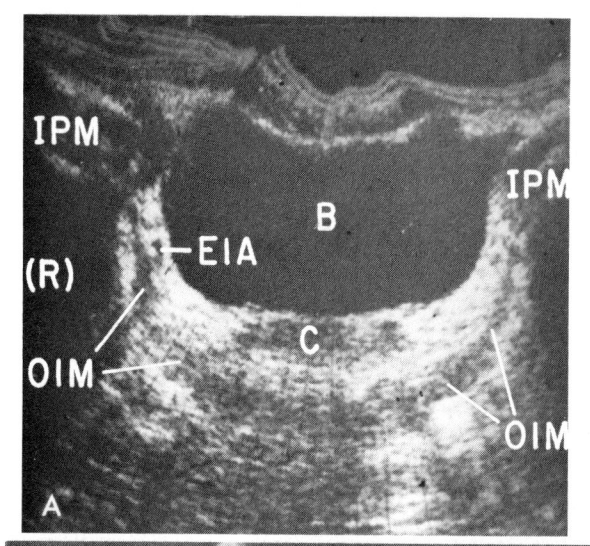

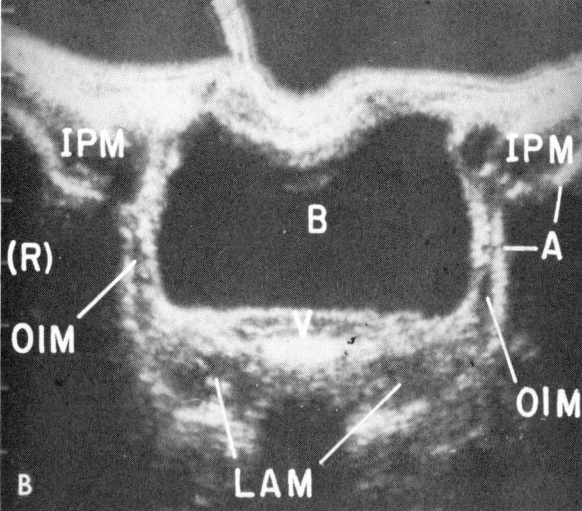

Figure 6. Angled transverse scans of pelvis showing levator ani muscle (LAM) and obturator internus muscle (OIM). Note difficulty in separating them laterally. *A,* Thirty degree cranial scan imaged from pubic symphysis upward showing more prominent obturator internus muscle. Because of distention of the urinary bladder, the external iliac vein has been compressed. IPM, iliopsoas muscle; C, cervix; EIA, external iliac artery. *B,* Thirty degree caudad scan imaged from superior aspect of bladder downward showing more prominent levator ani muscle. V, vagina.

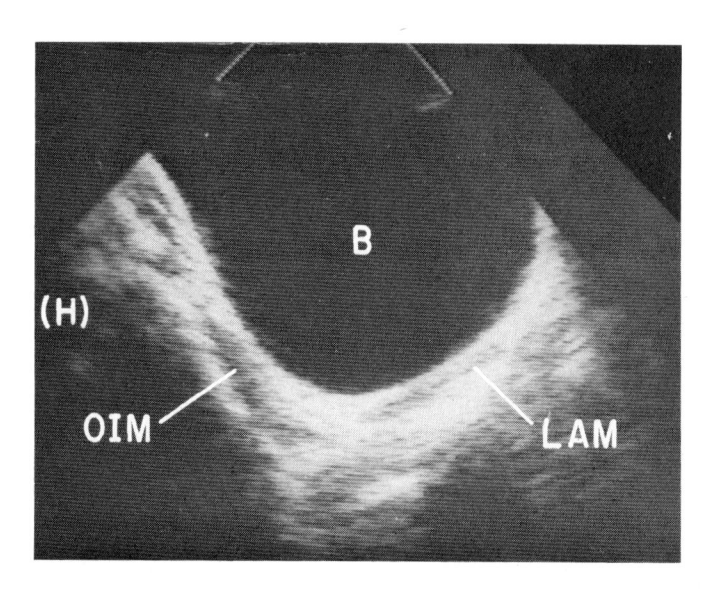

Figure 7. Longitudinal scan angled toward pelvic side wall. Note that the obturator internus muscle (OIM) is superior and posterior to the levator ani muscle (LAM). B, bladder.

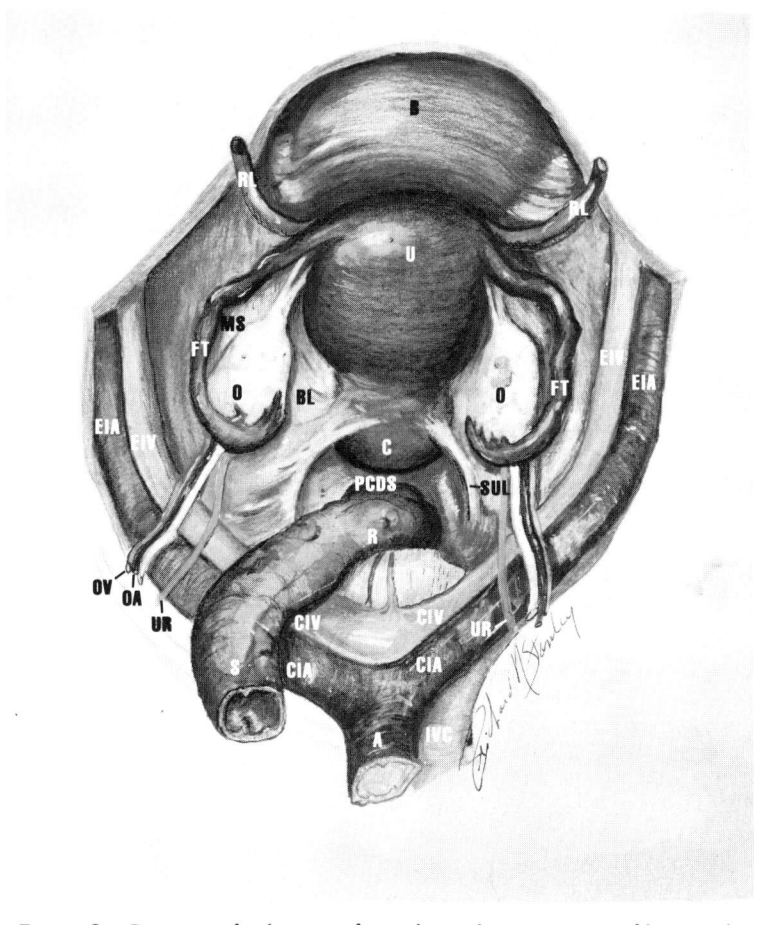

Figure 8. Diagram of pelvis seen from above showing organs of lesser pelvis.

ureter is anterior to the internal iliac vessels (Fig. 10). On real-time examination, normal peristalsis can be seen in the ureter as a sparkling pattern of intermittent echoes. Within the urinary bladder, intermittent showers of echoes can be imaged as the urine passes from the ureter into the bladder (Fig. 12).[4]

Because of their close proximity to the ovaries and cervix, any abnormality of these structures might involve the ureter and lead to ureterectasis and hydronephrosis. Therefore, on routine ultrasound examination, if an abnormality is seen in the ovary or cervix, the normal ureter should be evaluated. If the ureter cannot be visualized or if it is prominent without normal peristalsis, the ipsilateral kidney should be scanned for possible hydronephrosis. In addition, because of the position of the ureters as they pass over the pelvic brim, an enlarged uterus might also lead to ureteral obstruction.

URINARY BLADDER

The urinary bladder is the most anterior organ in the lesser pelvis, anchored inferiorly by the urethra and the trigone (Figs. 1, 2, 3, 8).[11] In its nondistended state, the bladder is collapsed against the trigone. When the bladder fills with urine, its posterior and superior aspects greatly distend, displacing a significant amount of small bowel and mesentery out of the pelvis. While the rectum and vagina are anchored in the pelvic diaphragm and therefore not displaced by the distention of the urinary bladder, bladder distention does affect the position of the uterus and sigmoid colon (Fig. 3).

On ultrasound examination, the distended urinary bladder is an echo-free structure with smooth thin walls. There are generalized shapes to the urinary bladder. In transverse view, the superior aspect of

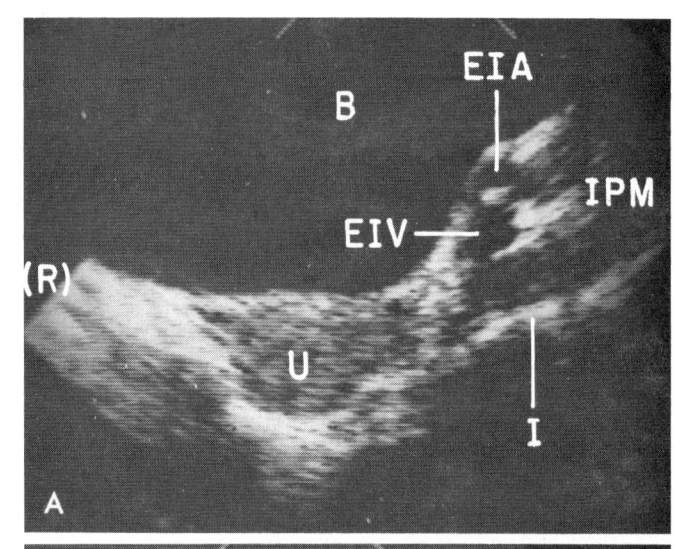

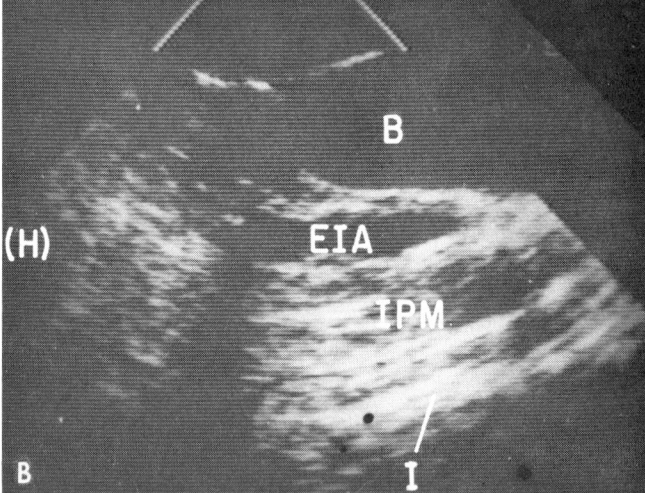

Figure 9. Scans of external iliac artery (EIA) and external iliac vein (EIV). Transverse scan (A) and oblique longitudinal scan (B) imaged from midline toward hip. Note position of vessels on medial aspect of iliopsoas muscle (IPM). U, uterus.

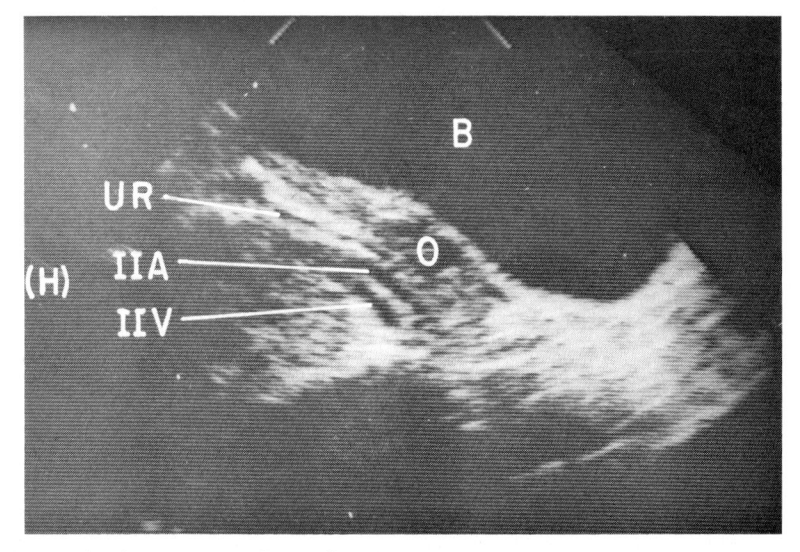

Figure 10. Longitudinal scan imaged 3 cm off midline showing internal iliac vessels (IIA, IIV) and ureter (UR) posterior to ovary (O).

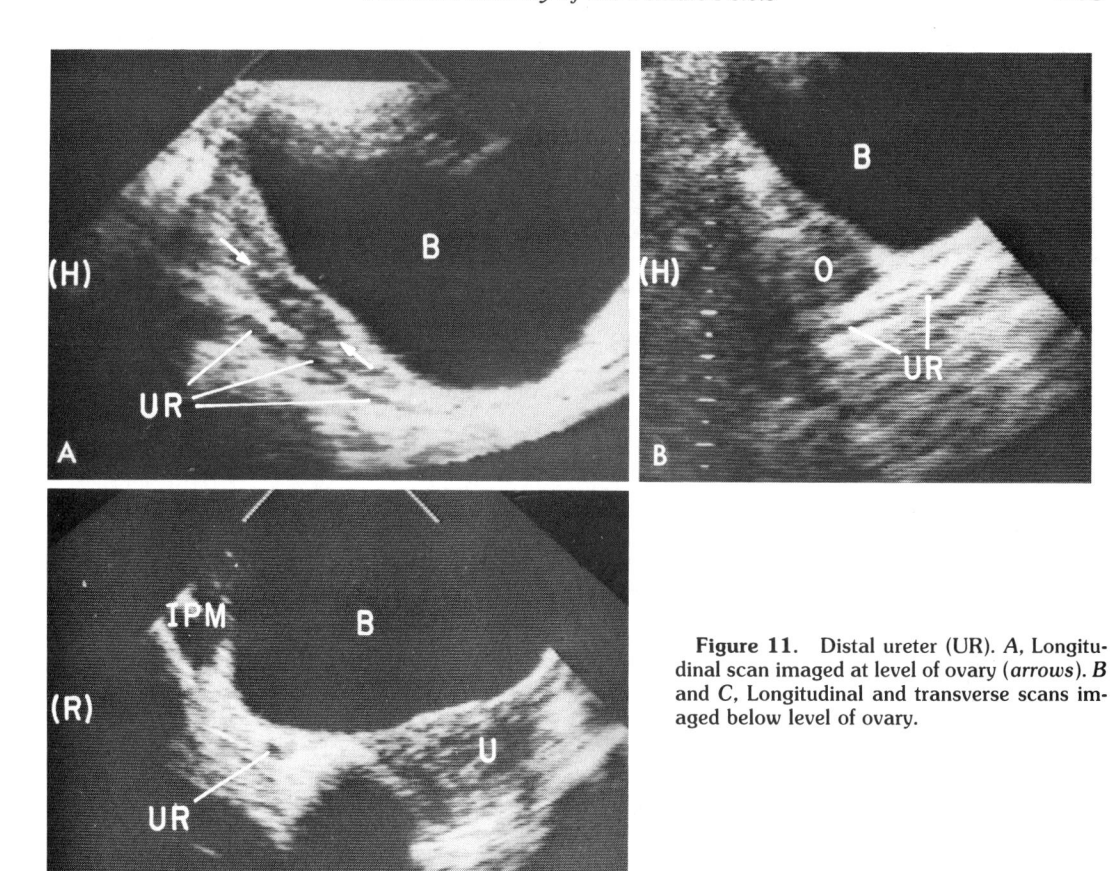

Figure 11. Distal ureter (UR). *A*, Longitudinal scan imaged at level of ovary (*arrows*). *B* and *C*, Longitudinal and transverse scans imaged below level of ovary.

the bladder is rounded except when the lateral walls are flattened by prominent iliopsoas muscles (Fig. 5, *A* to *C*). More caudally, the urinary bladder is squared owing to lateral indentation by the acetabula (Fig. 5*D*). In long axis, the urinary bladder is usually triangular in shape with the anterior side parallel to the anterior abdominal wall, the lowest or caudad side parallel to the vagina, and the third side extending obliquely from the superior aspect of the vagina toward the umbilicus (Figs. 11*A*, 13,

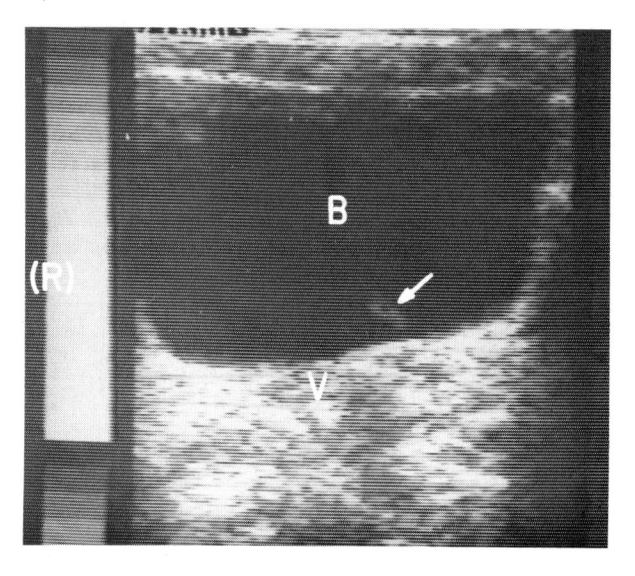

Figure 12. Transverse image of bladder showing "jet effect" of urine (*arrow*) entering urinary bladder from ureter.

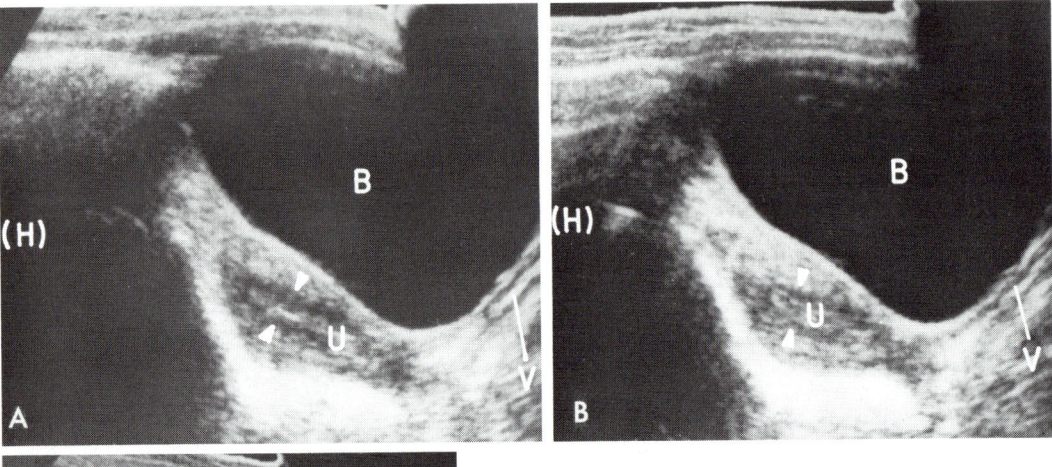

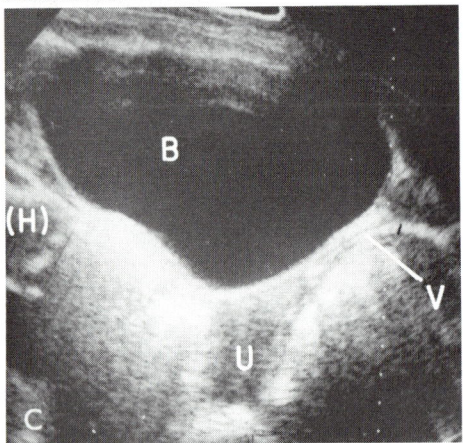

Figure 13. Longitudinal midline scans of uterus (U) and vagina (V). *A*, Uterus with bright endometrial canal surrounded by echo-free endometrium (*arrowheads*) of proliferative phase of menstrual cycle. *B*, Uterus in secretory phase of menstrual cycle in the same patient. Note more prominent and less bright endometrial echo (*arrowheads*). *C*, Retroverted uterus in a different patient. Note more globular uterine shape. Higher power was used to bring out normal uterine echo pattern but endometrial echo still not imaged.

14). At the area of the upper vagina, the ureteric orifices are occasionally imaged slightly to the right and left of the midline. While all normal structures cause slight indentation on the urinary bladder, it is unusual for normal bowel loops to indent the bladder, except when a fecal impaction is present.

VAGINA AND UTERUS

The vagina is anchored in the midline between the lower aspect of the urinary bladder anteriorly and rectum posteriorly (Figs. 2 and 3).[10] Although the position of the vagina is not affected by bladder distention, it may be elongated by a filled bladder. The uterus with its most caudad part, the cervix, is a thick-walled hollow muscular organ situated superior to the vagina.[10] While the most common uterine position is midline and anteverted, the uterus may extend to the right or left, be retroverted, or be additionally anteflexed or retroflexed.

Although the uterus is anchored at the superior aspect of the vagina, adjacent to the cervix, and loosely tethered by the round and broad ligaments, it is still movable and affected by bladder distention (Figs. 3 and 8).

On ultrasound examination, the vagina is imaged posterior to the lower part of the urinary bladder as a midline bright reflector, corresponding to the apposed mucosal linings, surrounded by the thin anterior and posterior hypoechoic vaginal walls (Figs. 13 and 14). If fluid is present within the vaginal canal, the bright reflector is lost and instead a relatively echo-free space is imaged,[17] and the anterior and posterior vaginal fornices surrounding the lower aspect of the cervix are visualized. The uterus is a pear-shaped organ with relatively low-level echoes, measuring less than 8 cm in long axis (from the base of the cervix to the top of the fundus), less than 5.5 cm in width, and less than 3 cm in anteroposterior dimension (Fig. 13, *A* and *B*).[12] The normal uterine canal, corresponding to the apposed endometrial linings, is usually thin and bright, extending up the midline of the uterus and surrounded by a relatively echo-free endometrium (Fig. 13, A and B).[12, 17] The endometrial echo can be imaged in almost 100 per cent of cases and is typically less bright than the midline vaginal echo (Fig. 13, A and B).[1] The thickness and brightness of the endometrial lining, however, are not constant but vary throughout the menstrual cycle, and during the secretory phase (post-ovulation) the lining is usually slightly thicker and less echogenic than during the proliferative stage (Fig. 13, A and B).[1] The appearance of the endometrial canal may also occasionally be affected by urinary bladder distention.

The vagina and uterus are usually imaged on true longitudinal and transverse scans (Figs. 5, 9A, 13). However, if the uterus extends to the right or left, scans should be performed in an oblique longitudinal direction to incorporate the vagina with the full length of the uterus. While the normal uterine shape, echogenicity, and endometrial echo are routinely imaged in the anteverted uterus, all of these may be distorted when the uterus is retroverted and/or retroflexed (Fig. 13C). Frequently the uterus then assumes a more globular shape with decrease in the normal echo pattern, occasionally mimicking a fibroid.[12] In addition, because of the change in angulation of the uterus, the endometrial echo is rarely seen.[1] With increased power or gain, however, the normal uterine echo pattern can be appreciated even in the most severe retroverted or retroflexed uteri but the endometrial echo is usually still not imaged.

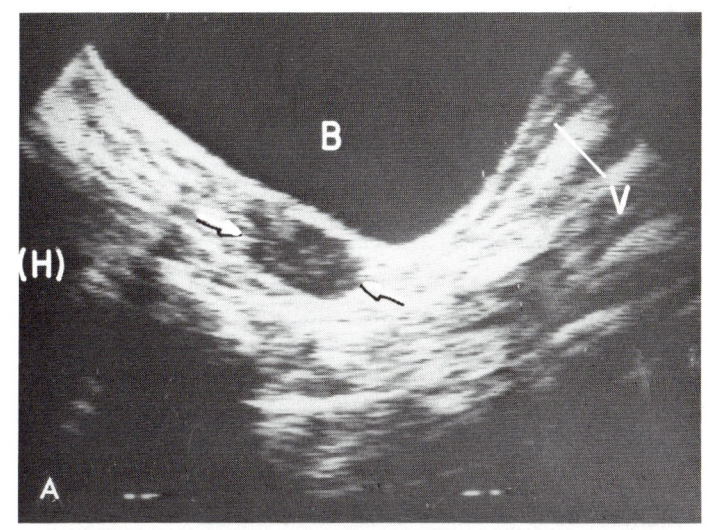

Figure 14. Longitudinal scans of ovaries (*arrows*) in the same patient. The ovaries are in their most common position lateral to uterus. *A*, Ovary without cysts at time of menstruation. *B*, Ovary with cysts just before ovulation.

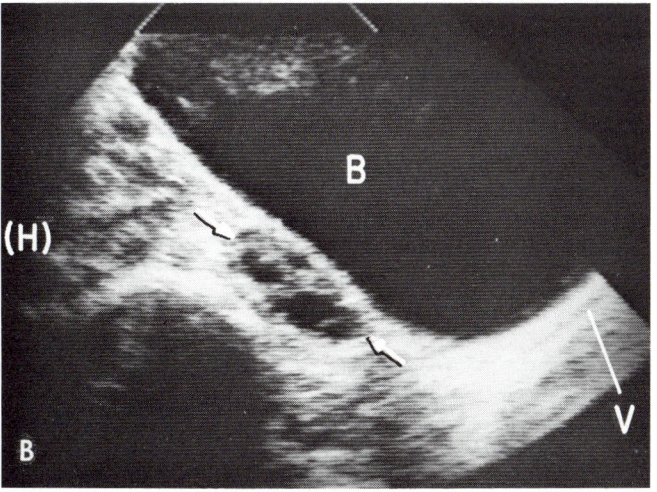

ADNEXA

The region of the adnexa consists of the fallopian tubes, broad ligaments, mesosalpinx, and ovaries (Figs. 1, 3, and 8).[10] Of these, only the ovaries are truly intraperitoneal. The fallopian tubes extend serpiginously off the fundal aspect of the uterus to finally terminate at the ovaries. The ovaries are usually lateral to the superior aspect of the body of the uterus but may be very variable in position. They may instead be posterolateral, directly posterior, or occasionally even superior to the uterus, and are frequently not seen at the same transverse level.[12,17] The ovarian position is frequently related to the uterine position. When the uterus is normally anteflexed and midline, the ovaries are usually lateral or posterolateral. When the uterus is deviated to one side, the ipsilateral ovary is frequently superior to the uterus, and when the uterus is midline and retroverted, both ovaries are commonly superior. When the ovary is in its normal position, the ureter and the internal iliac vessels can be commonly imaged posteriorly (Figs. 1 and 8).

On ultrasound examination, the ovaries are routinely imaged as ovoid structures with their longest axis cranial-caudal and with their echogenicity slightly greater than that of the uterus (Fig. 14). Assuming their shape to be a prolate ellipse, a simplified formula for their volume would be [length × width × height] ÷ 2.[2] Because of great variability in normal ovarian shape, however, all three dimensions should be obtained to determine if the ovary is enlarged. In the menstruating woman, the ovarian volume should be no greater than 6 cc and is much smaller in prepubescent and postmenopausal women.[17] In the menstruating woman, the ovary usually varies in size with each menstrual cycle.[13] It increases and is frequently filled with cysts during the first half of the cycle, peaking at the time of ovulation with regression following ovulation (Fig. 14). The ovaries are routinely imaged in true longitudinal and transverse projections (Figs. 5A and 14). When the ovary is at the lateral aspect of the urinary bladder, longitudinal scans obliqued from the opposite side toward the side of the ovary will frequently allow better imaging of the ovary since more of the urinary bladder is used as an "acoustical" window.

The remainder of the adnexa is only infrequently identified on ultrasound examination. When imaged, it is best seen in the transverse view as a thin, moderately echogenic area no greater than 5 mm in maximum thickness (Fig. 5B). Care must be taken that an edge of the urinary bladder is not incorrectly interpreted as part of the thickness of the adnexa. Abnormality of the fallopian tubes should be strongly suggested if the area is thicker than usual, if it is tubular with an echo-free center, or if rounded, particularly if the abnormality can be traced to the fundus of the uterus.

RECTOSIGMOID COLON

In the lesser pelvis, the caudad extent of the rectum is fixed in the retroperitoneum, posterior to the vagina (Figs. 2 and 3).[9] The sigmoid colon begins at the third sacral vertebral level, approximately one half the distance cranially within the lesser pelvis, is covered by peritoneum, and is attached to the pelvic wall by an extensive mesentery, the sigmoid mesocolon (Figs. 3 and 8).[9] As a result of this mesentery, the sigmoid colon may be quite redundant and may extend far to the right, far to the left, or remain in the midline. It finally courses anterior, superior, and to the left, to ascend into the left flank of the greater pelvis to become the descending colon (Fig. 8).

Only infrequently can the normal ultrasound evaluation identify the rectosigmoid colon since colonic feces and gas will appear as scattered intraluminal echoes and shadowing with poor bowel wall definition (Fig. 15A). With the introduction of water into the rectum, termed a water enema examination, the rectum can be clearly imaged in longitudinal, transverse, and oblique scans immediately posterior to the vagina and bladder (Fig. 15B).[4,16] The sigmoid colon can also be imaged but, owing to its variable position, is more difficult to find and, because of its mesocolon, may be displaced out of the pelvis by the distended bladder. Nevertheless, when water is introduced into the rectum, the sigmoid colon can be frequently imaged in transverse scans coursing obliquely from right to left at the superior aspect of the bladder (Fig. 15C). While the water enema technique has been described elsewhere, it is worth emphasizing that it is usually easier to

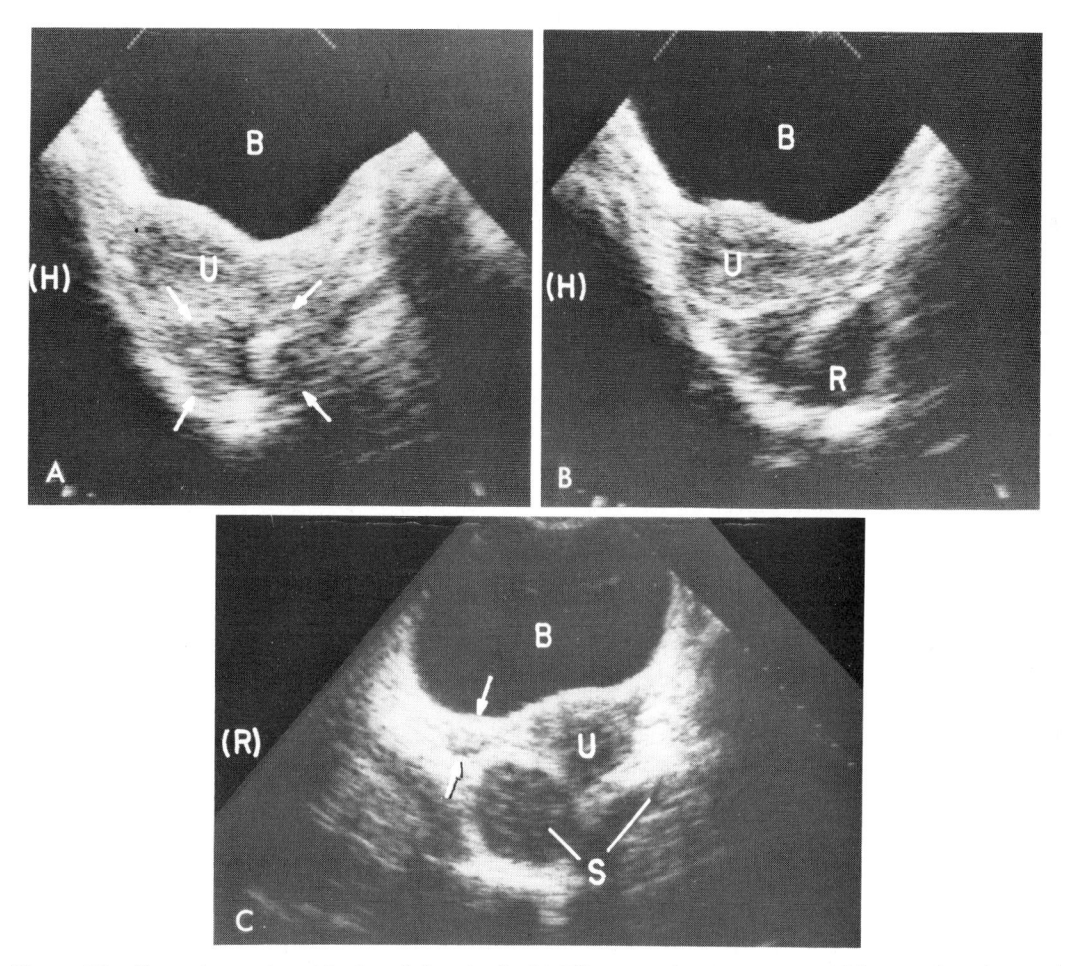

Figure 15. Normal rectosigmoid colon. *A,* Longitudinal midline scan showing rectum with feces and gas (*arrows*) posterior to uterus (U). *B,* Longitudinal midline scan in the same patient showing the water-filled rectum (R) after water enema. *C,* Transverse scan imaged at level of superior aspect of bladder showing water-filled sigmoid colon (S) after water enema. Note its redundancy to the right. Arrows denote right ovary.

image the rectosigmoid colon with real-time examination through a partially distended urinary bladder.[14, 16]

PERITONEAL REFLECTIONS

The peritoneal surface covers the superior aspect of the urinary bladder, uterus, and rectum. With distention of the urinary bladder, three potential peritoneal spaces are formed: the anterior peritoneal space between the anterior parietal peritoneum and the bladder, the anterior cul-de-sac between the bladder and anterior aspect of the uterus, and the posterior cul-de-sac between the uterus and rectum (Figs. 3 and 8). The posterior cul-de-sac extends caudally to at least the upper one-quarter of the vagina. It is potentially the largest of these spaces and frequently contains normal small bowel and mesentery. In addition, because of its posterior position, it is the most common pelvic area for intraperitoneal collections.

ACKNOWLEDGMENT

The authors would like to thank Mr. Larry Waldroup, B. S., R.D.M.S., for his technical assistance and Ms. Michele Fitzpatrick and Rosemarie Kayati for their editorial assistance.

REFERENCES

1. Callen, P. W., DeMartini, W. J., and Filly, R. A.: The central uterine cavity echo: A useful anatomic sign in the ultrasonographic evaluation of the female pelvis. Radiology, *131*:187–190, April 1979.

2. Campbell, S., Goessens, L., Goswamy, R., et al.: Real-time ultrasonography for determination of ovarian morphology and volume. Lancet, February 1982, pp. 425–426.
3. Cochrane, W. J., and Thomas, M. A.: Ultrasound diagnosis of gynecologic pelvic masses. Radiology, *110*:649–654, 1974.
4. Dubbins, P. A., Kurtz, A. B., Darby, J., et al.: Ureteric jet effect: The echographic appearance of urine entering the bladder. Radiology, *140*:513–515, 1981.
5. Fleischer, A. C., James, A. E., Millis, J. B., et al.: Differential diagnosis of pelvic masses by gray scale sonography. Am. J. Roentgenol., *131*:469–476, 1978.
6. Gray, H.: Muscles and fasciae. The muscles and fasciae of the lower limb. *In* Goss, C. M. (ed.): Anatomy of the Human Body. Edition 28. Philadelphia, Lea and Febiger, 1966, pp. 490–507.
7. Gray, H.: The arteries. The arteries of the trunk. *In* Goss, C. M. (ed.): Anatomy of the Human Body. Edition 28. Philadelphia, Lea and Febiger, 1966, pp. 628–656.
8. Gray, H.: Osteology. The bones of the lower limb (ossa membri inferioris). *In* Goss, C. M. (ed.): Anatomy of the Human Body. Edition 28. Philadelphia, Lea and Febiger, 1966, pp. 236–245.
9. Gray, H.: The digestive system. The sigmoid colon. The rectum. *In* Goss, C. M. (ed.): Anatomy of the Human Body. Edition 28. Philadelphia, Lea and Febiger, 1966, pp. 1238–1240.
10. Gray, H.: The urogenital system. The female genital organs. *In* Goss C. M. (ed.): Anatomy of the Human Body. Edition 28. Philadelphia, Lea and Febiger, 1966, pp. 1316–1334.
11. Gray, H.: The urogenital system. The ureters. The urinary bladder. *In* Goss, C. M. (ed.): Anatomy of the Human Body. Edition 28. Philadelphia, Lea and Febiger, 1966, pp. 1287–1296.
12. Green, B.: Pelvic ultrasonography. *In* Sarti, D. A., and Sample W. F. (eds.): Diagnostic Ultrasound Text and Cases. Boston, G. K. Hall and Co., 1980, pp. 502–589.
13. Hall, D. A., Hann, L. E., Ferrucci, J. T., et al.: Sonographic morphology of the normal menstrual cycle. Radiology, *133*:185–188, 1979.
14. Kurtz, A. B., Rubin, C. S., Kramer, F. L., et al.: Ultrasound evaluation of the posterior pelvic compartment. Radiology, *132*:677–682, 1979.
15. Lawson, T. L., and Albarelli, J. N.: Diagnosis of gynecologic pelvic masses by gray scale ultrasonography: Analysis of specificity and accuracy. Am. J. Roentgenol., *128*:1003–1006, 1977.
16. Rubin, C., Kurtz, A. B., and Goldberg, B. B.: Water Enema: A new ultrasound technique in defining pelvic anatomy. J. Clin. Ultrasound, *6*:28–33, 1978.
17. Sample, W. F.: Gray scale ultrasonography of the normal female pelvis. *In* Sanders, R. C., and James, A. E. (eds.): The Principles and Practice of Ultrasonography in Obstetrics and Gynecology. Edition 2. New York, Appleton-Century-Crofts, 1980, pp. 75–89.
18. Sample, W. F., Lippe, B. M., and Gyepes, M. T.: Gray-scale ultrasonography of the normal female pelvis. Radiology *125*:477–483, 1977.
19. Walsh, J. W., Taylor, K. J. W., Wasson, J. F. M., et al.: Gray-scale ultrasound in 204 proved gynecologic masses: Accuracy and specific diagnostic criteria. Radiology, *130*:391–397, 1979.

KEY TO ABBREVIATIONS in Figures 1, 2, and 3

APS	= Anterior peritoneal space		EIA	= External iliac artery
ACDS	= Anterior cul-de-sac		FA	= Femoral artery
PCDS	= Posterior cul-de-sac		FV	= Femoral vein
LAM	= Levator ani muscle		A	= Acetabulum
OIM	= Obturator internus muscles		I	= Iliac crest
PM	= Psoas muscle		PS	= Pubic symphysis
IM	= Iliacus muscle		P	= Pubic bone
IPM	= Iliopsoas muscle		SA	= Sacrum
CM	= Coccygeus muscle		B	= Urinary bladder
PIM	= Piriformis muscle		URE	= Urethra
RM	= Rectus muscle		P	= Peritoneum
IL	= Inguinal ligament		U	= Uterus
RL	= Round ligament		V	= Vagina
SUL	= Sacro-uterine ligament		C	= Cervix
BL	= Broad ligament		UR	= Ureter
OV	= Ovarian vein		MS	= Mesosalpinx
OA	= Ovarian artery		O	= Ovary
A	= Aorta		FT	= Fallopian tube
IVC	= Inferior vena cava		R	= Rectum
CIA	= Common iliac artery		S	= Sigmoid colon
CIV	= Common iliac vein		K	= Kidney
IIA	= Internal iliac artery		BG	= Bowel gas
IIV	= Internal iliac vein		(H)	= Toward patient's head
EIV	= External iliac vein		(R)	= Toward patient's right side

13

Ultrasound Evaluation of the Ovary

Arthur C. Fleischer, M.D., Anne Colston Wentz, M.D., Howard W. Jones, III, M.D., and A. Everette James, Jr., Sc.M., J.D., M.D.

Recent improvements in resolution capabilities of both static and real-time sonographic instrumentation have resulted in more consistent and detailed depiction of both normal and abnormally enlarged ovaries. After a discussion of normal anatomy and scanning techniques pertinent to sonographic imaging of the ovary, this chapter will present a variety of clinical applications of sonography for evaluation of the ovaries. The recent utilization of sonography as a means to monitor ovarian follicular development and the sonographic detection and evaluation of patients with ovarian masses will be emphasized.

NORMAL ANATOMY AND SCANNING TECHNIQUES

Although the depiction of the normal ovary by bistable sonography was described as early as 1972, the recent increased utilization and refinement of real-time scanning instrumentation has afforded more consistent and better detailed images of the normal and abnormal ovary.[17]

We prefer the use of mechanical sector real-time sonography for evaluation of the ovary because of the capability to dynamically and empirically alter the scan plane so that the region of interest is portrayed with greatest detail. A series of static scans can be helpful when a global depiction of the entire abdomen and pelvis is desired.

As in other examinations of the pelvic structures, a fully distended bladder is necessary for complete delineation of the ovary and surrounding structures. An exception to this preparation can be made when the patient has an extremely large pelvoabdominal mass which, by its compression of the urinary bladder, makes it uncomfortable for the patient to maintain a fully distended urinary bladder.

The size of the ovary correlates closely with the endocrinologic status of the patient.[29] Specifically, there is a significant difference between the size of the ovary in the prepubertal, postpubertal, and postmenopausal female (Table 1). Although the size and volume of the ovary may differ in patients of various ages, the shape of the ovary, in normal individuals, remains fusiform or almond-shaped (Fig. 1). Generally, the normal ovary measures approximately 3 cm in greatest transverse length, 2 cm in anteroposterior dimension, and 1 cm in the long axis. The ovary may become slightly rounded when it contains a preovulatory follicle or corpus luteum (Fig. 1A).

Since there is a difference in the linear dimensions of the ovary, we prefer calculation of an ovarian volume utilizing the geometric formula of a sphere or prolate ellipsoid. A nomogram for ovarian volume has been reported and is included as Figure 2.[29] The calculation of ovarian volume depends upon precisely obtaining all dimensions of the ovary.

The position of the ovaries within the pelvis is usually variable and depends upon the laxity of attachments of the ovaries to the peritoneum, meso-ovarium, and suspensory ligaments. For example, in a normal individual the ovary can be present in the cul-de-sac or superior to the uterine fundus. For this reason, it is unusual to delineate both ovaries on the same transverse image of a static sonogram since they are usually not oriented in a specific transverse plane. When static scanning is performed, the ovary of interest is best delineated on a longitudinal scan performed from the contralateral side directed through the dis-

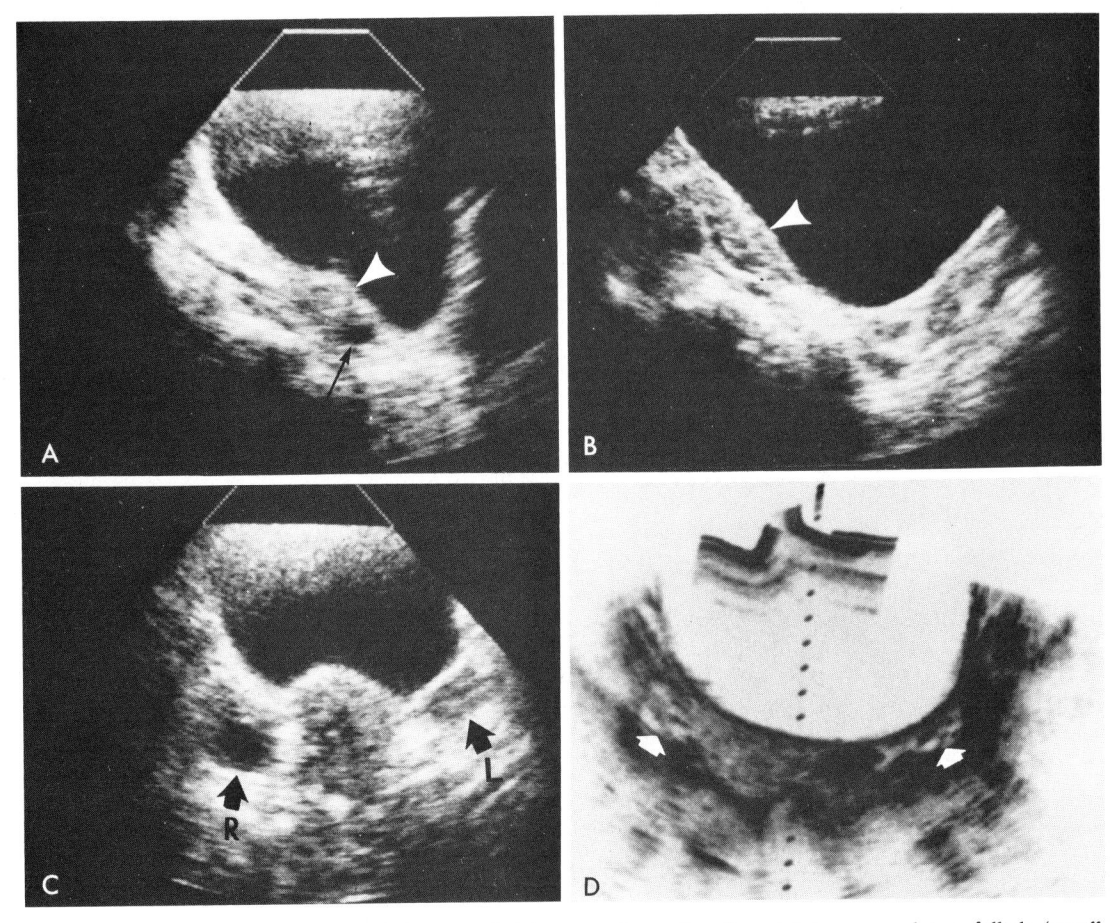

Figure 1. Normal ovary. *A,* Long axis view of right ovary (*arrowhead*) containing preovulatory follicle (*small arrow*). *B,* Long axis view of left ovary (*arrowhead*) in the same patient. *C,* Modified transverse real-time sonogram depicting both right (R) and left (L) ovaries. As depicted on the longitudinal sonogram, the right ovary contains a mature follicle. *D,* Normal ovaries. Although it is unusual to delineate both ovaries on the same transverse static sonogram, both ovaries (*arrows*) of this patient were clearly depicted.

tended bladder. For example, if the left ovary is being examined, the modified longitudinal static scans should be performed on the right side of the pelvis with the transducer directed toward the left side wall.

Several anatomic structures can be utilized as landmarks for delineation of the ovaries. One of the most constant relationships is the relationship of the ovary to the internal iliac vein, artery, and distal ureter.[29] Imaging with real-time scanning affords identification of some of the larger vascular structures by their pulsation and fluid-filled bowel loops by their characteristic changes in configuration and appearance with peristalsis.

The pubococcygeus, obturator internus, and iliopsoas muscles can simulate the texture and configuration of the ovary on scans obtained in the transverse plane.[29] However, the obturator internus muscle becomes larger as one angles caudad on transverse scans, whereas the pubococcygeus becomes more prominent on transverse scans angled cephalad. The inferior medial aspect of the iliopsoas muscle can be distinguished from the ovary by the echo-

Table 1. *Normal Ovarian Volume**

	AGE RANGE (YEARS)	NO. OF PATIENTS	VOLUME (cm³) Range	Mean
Prepuberty	1–2	4	0–0.7	—
	2–12	16	0.13–0.9	0.46
Postpuberty	13–20	25	1.8–5.7	4.0

* Adapted from Sample, W., et al.: *Radiology,* 125:477–483, 1977.

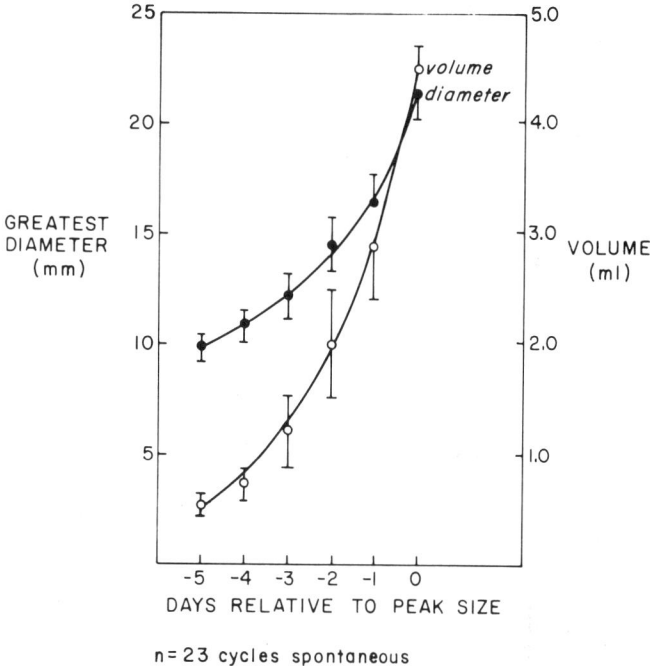

Figure 2. Nomogram for ovarian follicular volume and diameter. (*From* Queenan, J.: Fertil. Steril., *34*:99–105, 1981, with permission.)

n = 23 cycles spontaneous
Volume $4/3 \pi r^3$ if d ≈ 0.5 mm
$4/3 \pi r_1 r_2 r_3$ $1/2 L \times W \times AP$ if ellipsoid

genic borders, fusiform shape, and vessels typically contained within the iliopsoas. Other structures and non-ovarian masses that can mimic the sonographic features of the ovary are discussed in the section entitled "Sonographic Mimics of Ovarian Masses."

ANATOMIC ANOMALIES

One of the most frequently encountered anatomic anomalies is the polycystic ovary. The syndrome of polycystic ovaries, amenorrhea, and hirsutism is referred to as the Stein-Leventhal syndrome. However, in our experience and as reported by other groups, it is unusual for all of these features to be present in patients with polycystic ovaries.[32]

Sonographically, polycystic ovaries should be suspected when the ovaries are spherical and have abnormally large volume (Fig. 3A).[32] Occasionally, multiple immature follicles (less than 10 mm) can be identified along the periphery of the ovary (Fig. 3, A to C).

We have encountered enlarged ovaries in patients who do not have polycystic disease but were on ovulation suppression and/or ovulation hormonal induction therapy (Fig. 3D). The majority of the follicles in patients taking birth control pills will be small, irregular, and atretic. As will be discussed in greater detail in the section on ovarian follicular monitoring by sonography, patients who have polycystic ovary disease who are on ovulation induction therapy usually have one or two "dominant" follicles measuring twice the size of other follicles within the ovary.

Occasionally, an autonomously functioning follicle can be associated with precocious puberty (Fig. 3E). This condition is usually seen in premenarchal girls and has been associated with hypothyroidism.[27] It has been theorized that in hypothyroidism, a tropic hormone which may stimulate follicular maturation within the ovary is also elaborated.

Because of the small size and tubular configuration of streak ovaries, sonography is of little assistance in detecting their presence in patients with Turner's syndrome.

MONITORING OVARIAN FOLLICULAR MATURATION

Sonography has recently assumed an important role in evaluation of patients who are candidates for in vitro fertilization and

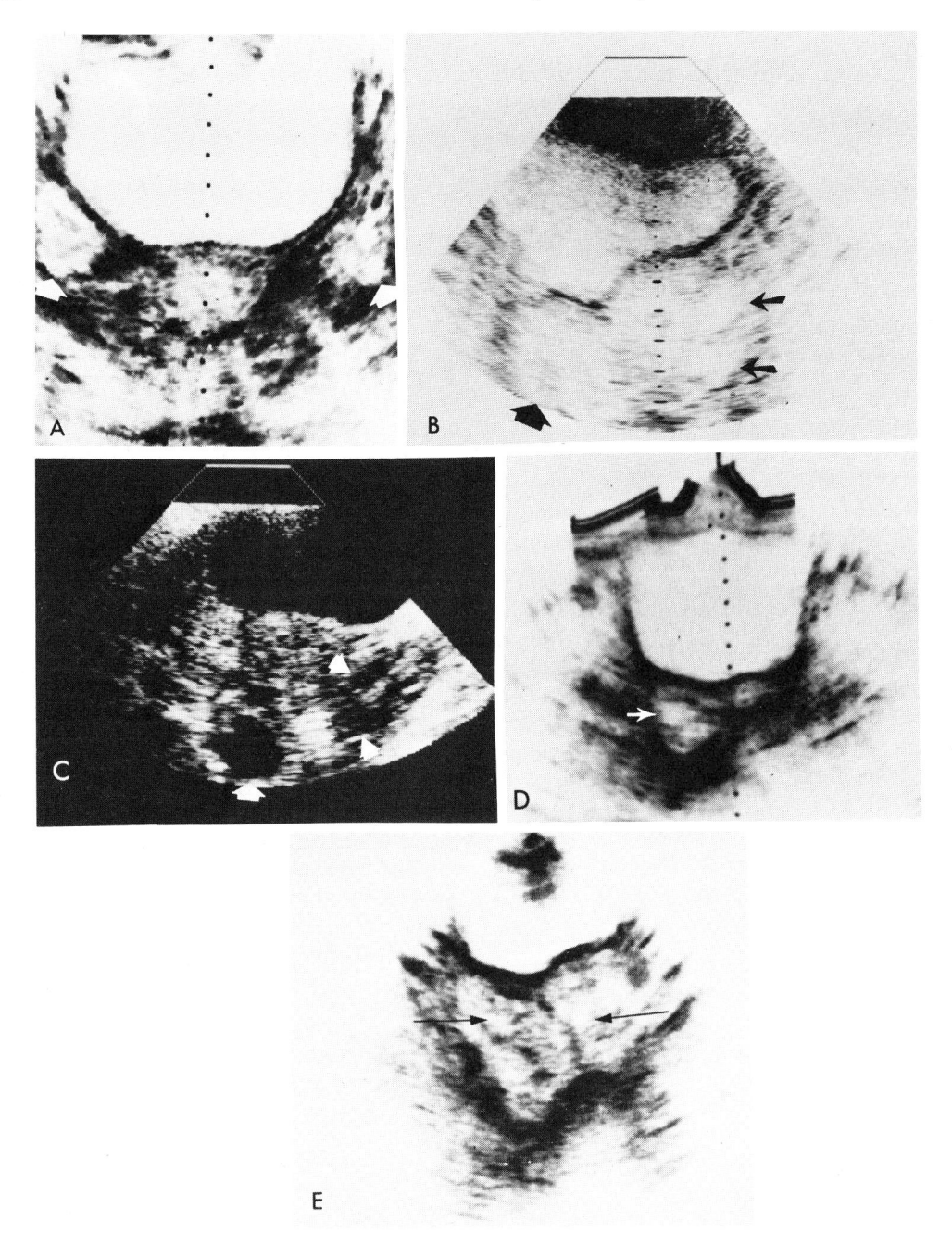

Figure 3. Anatomic anomalies. *A*, Polycystic ovaries (transverse static sonogram). Both ovaries (*arrows*) are enlarged and rounded and contain several follicles along their periphery. (*From* Fleischer, A., and James, A. E.: Introduction to Diagnostic Ultrasonography. New York, John Wiley and Sons, 1980, with permission.) *B*, Two developing follicles (*small arrows*) within a polycystic ovary in a patient receiving hormonal stimulation. The right ovary (*large arrow*) was also polycystic. *C*, Dominant follicle (*large arrow*) within the right polycystic ovary of patient undergoing hormonal stimulation. Although many follicles are present within both ovaries (*arrowheads*), only the follicle within the right ovary was of preovulatory size. (*From* Fleischer, A.: J. Clin. Ultrasound, 9:275–280, 1981, with permission.) *E*, Bilaterally enlarged ovaries with numerous irregularly outlined, atretic follicles (*arrows*) in a patient taking birth control pills. *D*, Premenarchal patient with precocious puberty. A preovulatory follicle (*arrow*) could be identified within the right ovary. This patient was later found to have hypothroidism. (*From* Fleischer, A., and James, A. E.: Introduction to Diagnostic Ultrasonography. New York, John Wiley and Sons, 1980, with permission.)

embryo transfer (IVF-ET).[6,9,15,21,24] Serial sonographic examinations can be used to determine: (1) the presence, number, size, and growth of pre-ovulatory follicles; (2) which ovary contains a mature follicle; and (3) whether ovulation has occurred. The sonographic data are coupled with estradiol and luteinizing hormone assays to determine the developmental status of the maturing follicle. For example, human chorionic gonadotropin is given to induce oocyte maturation if the follicle measures 17 mm or greater. Similarly, rapid assays of luteinizing hormone (LH) are performed only when sonography depicts adequate growth of the follicle. Sonography is also helpful in locating the exact position of the follicle within the ovary since, on occasion, it is difficult to locate the follicle by external inspection during laparoscopy. Sonography can also detect unsuspected hydrosalpinges or ovarian masses in a patient undergoing an evaluation for infertility.

Initial reports concerning serial sonographic monitoring of ovarian follicular maturation in spontaneous cycles have demonstrated a predictable enlargement of the ovarian follicle prior to the time of ovulation.[6,9,15,21,24] In general, the mature follicle at the time of ovulation in a patient undergoing spontaneous ovulation measures approximately 20 mm in average dimension (Fig. 2; Fig. 4, A to C). It has been shown that follicles that range between 18 and 25 mm in diameter have the greatest number of granulosa cells, an indication of follicular maturity.[19]

Several sonographic appearances of the corpus luteum have been described.[24] Some of the differences in the sonographic appearance can be attributed to the resolution of the scanner utilized. Most frequently, a corpus luteum can be distinguished from a developing follicle by its irregular wall and internal echoes (Fig 4, D to F). However, in some patients the corpus luteum can be indistinguishable from a mature follicle, whereas others become isoechogenic with respect to the ovary and therefore are difficult to identify after ovulation has occurred. This observation substantiates the necessity of serial rather than single observations of the ovary for follicular monitoring. In most patients, a small amount of fluid (10 to 15 ml) can be seen in the cul-de-sac immediately after ovulation occurs (Fig. 4D).[16] More importantly, however, if ovulation has occurred, the wall of the follicle becomes noticeably irregular, and low-level echoes can be identified within the developing corpus luteum.

Patients who are candidates for in vitro fertilization and embryo transfer are examined daily beginning approximately 5 days prior to the anticipated date of ovulation. The data concerning ovarian follicular size and hormonal levels are incorporated into a decision tree for management. At our institution, patients are examined daily utilizing a sector real-time scanner. The size of each ovarian follicle is noted on each examination. The average dimension of the follicle in transverse and anteroposterior or long axis is utilized. The volume of fluid contained within the follicle can also be estimated by utilizing the geometric formula of a sphere if the dimensions are within 0.5 mm of each other, or a prolate ellipsoid if the dimensions differ greater than 0.5 mm. The formula for the volume of a sphere is $4/3\pi r^3$ where r is the radius. For a prolate ellipsoid, the formula is $4/3\pi r_1 \times r_2 \times r_3$ where r_1, r_2, and r_3 are the different radii.[24]

As mentioned previously, another important use of sonography in the in vitro fertilization and embryo transfer program is the detection of ovulation in an examination immediately prior to laparoscopy. The sonographic signs that imply that ovulation has occurred include interval development of a collapsed follicle associated with blood and follicular fluid within the cul-de-sac. Once ovulation occurs, the previously well-defined follicle diminishes in size and has an irregular wall and usually low-level internal echoes. If there is conclusive sonographic proof of the ovulation, the laparoscopic procedure may be postponed, thus avoiding an inappropriate anesthetic risk when the chance of a successful oocyte collection is low. However, on some occasions, the oocyte has been recovered from within a cul-de-sac blood collection.

Serial sonographic examinations also have a very important role in the patient who is undergoing ovulation induction therapy.[31] Many of the patients who undergo ovulation induction have polycystic ovaries as their cause of infertility. In general, the follicles in patients with polycystic ovaries that undergo hormonal induction are larger than in patients with

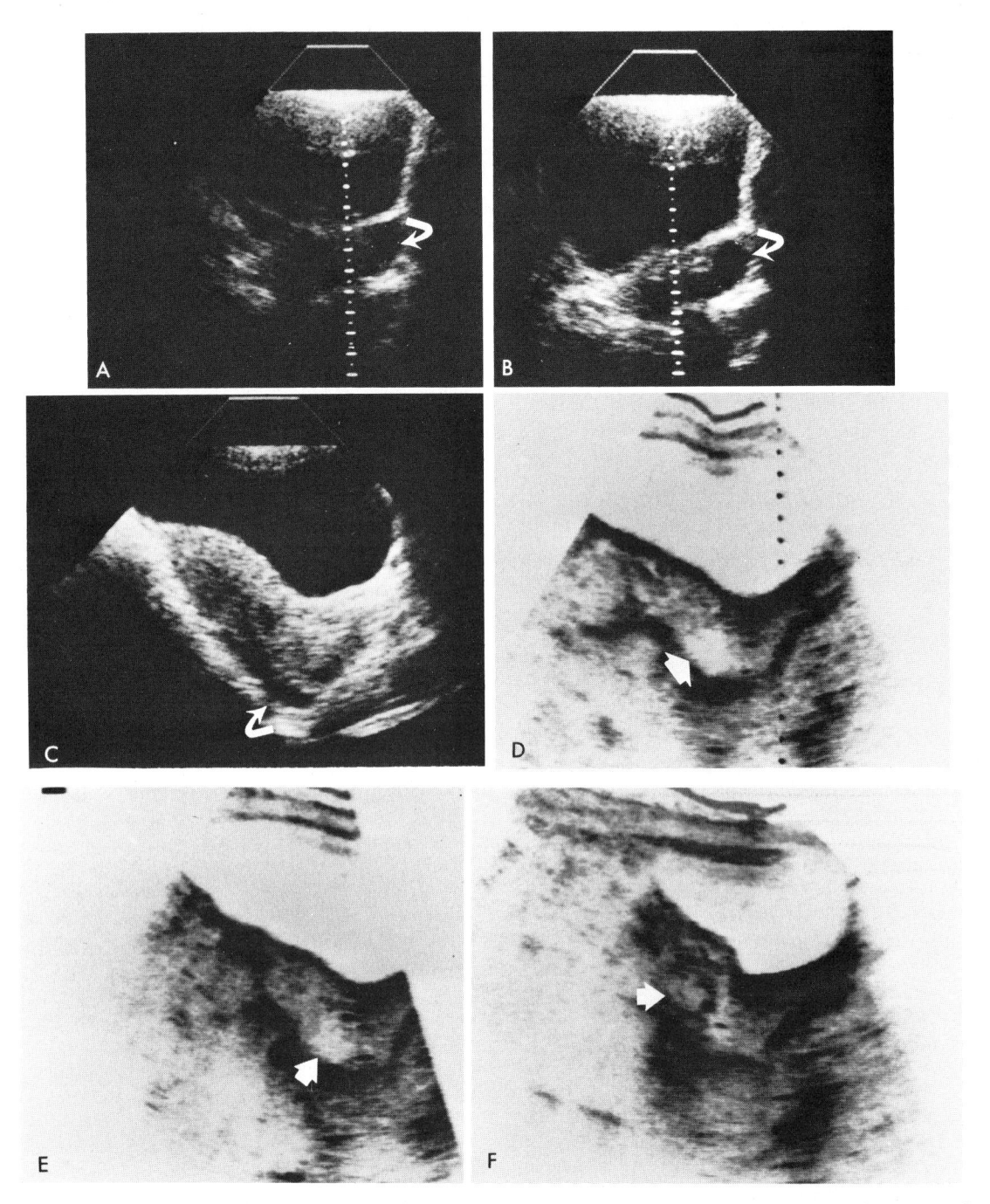

Figure 4. Sonographic monitoring of follicular development. *A,* Preovulatory follicle (*arrow*) is demonstrated on this modified transverse real-time sonogram on cycle day 10. The average dimension of the follicle was 14 mm. *B,* Same patient on cycle day 13. The follicle (*arrow*) has enlarged and has an average dimension of 18 mm. The shape of the follicle remains spherical and the walls are smooth. *C,* Real-time sonogram demonstrates a small amount of fluid (*arrow*) within the cul-de-sac associated with ovulation. *D,* A preovulatory follicle (*arrow*) is demonstrated on this longitudinal static sonogram one day prior to ovulation. The boundaries of the follicles are smooth and well-defined. *E,* Same patient one day after ovulation. The follicle (*arrow*) now contains low-level echoes and the wall of the follicle is irregular. *F,* Developing corpus luteum, three days after ovulation. The corpus luteum (*arrow*) has an echogenic internal texture and irregular wall. (*D, E, F from* Fleischer, A.: J. Clin. Ultrasound, 9:275–280, 1981.)

nonstimulated, spontaneous cycles. A mature follicle in a stimulated patient usually ranges from 25 to 35 mm in greatest dimension.[37] Usually, more than one preovulatory follicle can be identified in patients undergoing ovulation induction (Fig. 3B). Under optimal conditions, only one or two follicles exhibit growth. When more than four follicles attain a size of 25 to 30 mm, there may be a risk of a triplet or quintuplet pregnancy. However, even in the best of circumstances, mild to moderate hysterstimulation cannot always be prevented. It remains difficult to predict the multiplicity of gestation that may occur in these patients on the basis of sonography or hormonal assay.[4]

Sonography also has a role in evaluation of the patient with suspected ovarian hyperstimulation syndrome.[25] In these patients, the ovaries are massively enlarged, primarily because of edema of the stroma (Fig. 5A, B). This condition is usually associated with peritoneal effusions that appear as anechoic collections of fluid in the pericolic recesses.

In summary, sonography has an important role in monitoring ovarian follicular maturation since it can determine the number of follicles that appear to be maturing, the ovary which contains the most mature follicles, and whether or not ovulation has occurred. With further refinements in the in vitro fertilization and embryo transfer, such as the routine use of hormonal stimulation, it is envisioned that sonography will continue to play an important role in monitoring follicular maturation since responsiveness to hormonal stimulation seems to vary from individual to individual.

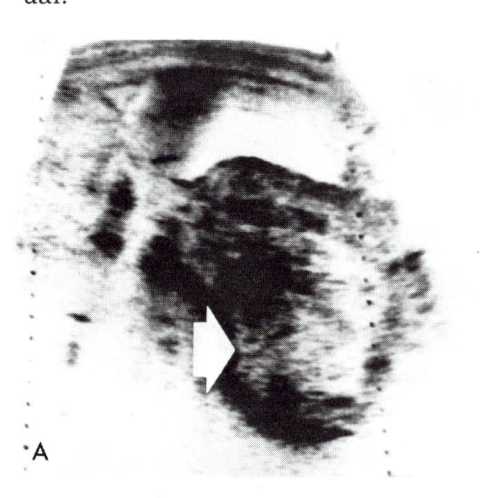

OVARIAN MASSES

Sonography has an important role in the evaluation of a patient with a pelvic mass since this determination has implications concerning management and surgical approach. This diagnostic technique is useful in determining the origin of a pelvic mass, its internal consistency, and the presence or absence of related disorders such as ascites, obstructive uropathy, and hepatic metastases. Cystic pelvic masses most often arise from the ovary whereas solid ones are of uterine origin.

This discussion of the sonographic evaluation of ovarian masses is subdivided according to the most typical sonographic appearance of a particular ovarian mass. This approach is utilized since it has practical relevance to daily practice of sonography. We will emphasize the relative specificity of a particular sonographic category of mass, realizing that some masses have more than one sonographic appearance (Table 2).

Completely Cystic Adnexal Masses

Cystic masses demonstrate no internal echoes, smooth and well-defined borders, and distal acoustic enhancement. Several types of adnexal masses exhibit a cystic texture, including physiologic ovarian cysts, cystadenomas, para-ovarian cysts, hydrosalpinges, and endometriomas to name a few (Fig. 6, A to C). Therefore, the specificity of the sonographic findings of a cystic adnexal mass is relatively low.[34]

The most common type of ovarian mass which is depicted as a cystic adnexal mass

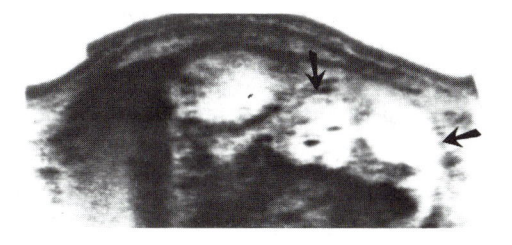

Figure 5. Sonographic features of hyperstimulation syndrome. A, Longitudinal static sonogram demonstrates a massively enlarged right ovary (arrow) posterior to the uterus. B, Transverse sonogram demonstrates several enlarged follicles (arrows) within the left ovary. A large intraperitoneal effusion (not shown) was also demonstrated.

Table 2. *Typical Sonographic Appearances of Ovarian Masses**

COMPLETELY CYSTIC	COMPLEX, PREDOMINANTLY CYSTIC	COMPLEX, PREDOMINANTLY SOLID	SOLID
Physiologic ovarian cyst Cystadenomas Cystic teratomas Ovarian abscess (Para-ovarian cyst) (Hydrosalpinx) (Endometrioma)	Cystadenoma (Ca) Dermoid cysts Tubo-ovarian abscess (Ectopic pregnancy) (Fluid-filled small bowel)	Cystadenoma (Ca) Dermoid cysts Granulosa cell tumor (Ectopic pregnancy)	Adenocarcinoma Solid teratoma (Ca) Arrhenoblastoma Fibroma Lymphomatous metastases to ovary Gastrointestinal metastases to ovary (Matted omentum) (Herniated fat)

* Non-ovarian masses that can mimic ovarian masses are denoted within parentheses.

is a physiologic ovarian cyst. Physiologic ovarian cysts are most common in the infant female and in women of childbearing age.[23] Physiologic cysts refer to masses such as corpus luteum cysts which occur after continued hemorrhage or lack of resolution of corpus luteum.

Physiologic ovarian cysts appear as rounded anechoic adnexal masses (Fig. 6A). In some patients, the contiguity of the cyst within the ovary can be delineated. Serial evaluation of such unilocular cysts by sonography may be quite helpful since physiologic cysts tend to regress sponta-

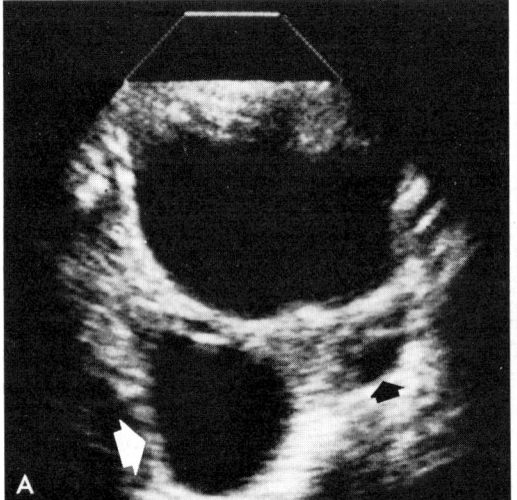

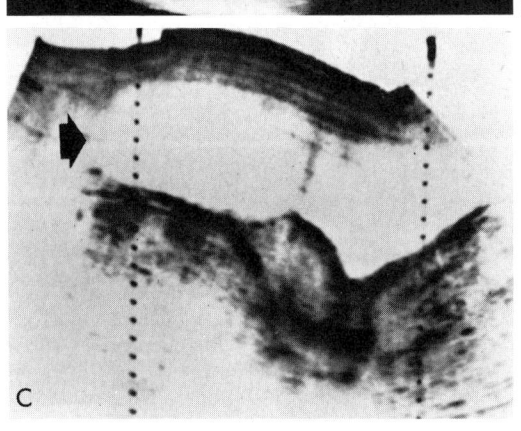

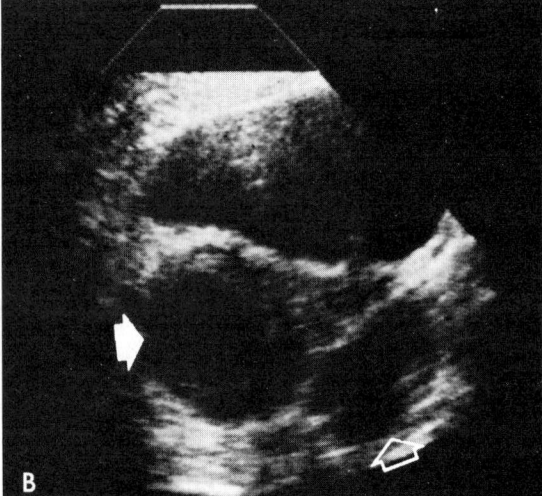

Figure 6. Cystic ovarian masses. *A,* Physiologic ovarian cysts (transverse real-time sonogram). As compared with the normal developing follicle within the left ovary (*small arrow*), the right ovary contains a large physiologic ovarian cyst (*large arrow*). This mass underwent regression on reexamination one month after this sonogram. *B,* Intra-ovarian abscess in a patient with an intrauterine contraceptive device (IUCD). An abscess (*arrow*) developed within a corpus luteum hematoma of the right ovary in this patient who had an IUCD in place. Note the rim of ovarian tissue around the cystic mass within the ovary. A left hydrosalpinx (*open arrow*) was also present. *C,* Serous cystadenoma (longitudinal static sonogram). This cystic mass (*arrow*) was encountered in an asymptomatic girl. Because of its completely cystic character, this mass was correctly diagnosed as a benign ovarian tumor.

neously over several cycles whereas endometriomas and neoplastic ovarian cysts do not.

Besides physiologic ovarian cysts and neoplasms, tubo-ovarian abscesses, para-ovarian cysts, and hydrosalpinges can appear as cystic adnexal masses. Hydrosalpinges tend to be fusiform in shape whereas ovarian cysts are usually spherical. Tubo-ovarian abscesses result from chronic pelvic inflammatory disease. As opposed to a simple hydrosalpinx that contains serous fluid and does not include an ovary, a tubo-ovarian abscess involves the ovary as a portion of an abscess cavity. Occasionally, hydrosalpinges can be differentiated from tubo-ovarian abscesses when a rim of ovarian tissue bordering a tubo-ovarian abscess is identified. These masses tend to have a layer of low-level echoes which represent pus within the tubo-ovarian abscess (Fig. 7C). A similar appearance can be encountered in endometriomas that contain clotted blood or cysts that have undergone torsion and internal hemorrhage.

Patients with a hydrosalpinx or tubo-ovarian abscess may present with right upper quadrant pain as the result of infected fluid tracking up the right paracolic recess to localize in the subhepatic and perihepatic spaces. This phenomenon has been termed the Fitz-Hugh-Curtis syndrome and explains why some patients with pelvic inflammatory disease can first present with right upper quadrant pain.

Abscesses confined to the ovary have been associated with intrauterine contraceptive devices. These abscesses are thought to be the result of an ascending infection localizing within a corpus luteum arising from the low grade endometritis produced by an intrauterine contraceptive device. Ovarian abscesses can also appear as anechoic adnexal masses (Fig. 6B).

Para-ovarian cysts arise from the remnants of wolffian duct system (Gartner's duct) which courses within the mesovarium. These masses range from 2 to 3 cm to pelvo-abdominal in dimensions (Figs. 10, B and C). Like ovarian epithelial tumors and endometriomas, para-ovarian cysts do not demonstrate cyclical regression and growth associated with physiologic ovarian cysts.

Rarely, cystic masses can be encountered in patients who have undergone an oophorectomy. The cystic mass arises from a retained remnant of the ovary. The "ovarian remnant syndrome" usually occurs when a portion of the ovary is incompletely resected. The ovarian remnant can contain corpus luteum hematoma and can occasionally be so large as to be associated with ureteric obstruction.[23]

Complex, Predominantly Cystic Masses

This category of masses includes those predominantly cystic masses that contain septa, internal contents, or solid material. The most common type of complex, predominantly cystic mass is the ovarian epithelial tumor, specifically cystadenoma (Figs. 7, A and B). Dermoid cysts and tubo-ovarian abscesses are also included in this sonographic category. An ectopic pregnancy should be considered when a complex, predominantly cystic adnexal mass is encountered in a patient of childbearing age.

The sonographic appearance of ovarian epithelial tumors such as cystadenomas is highly specific. Typically, these tumors appear as large cystic masses with internal septa (Fig. 7A).[12, 34] Usually, patients with this type of tumor are postmenopausal and present with progressive abdominal enlargement over several months.

The number and arrangement of the internal septa within ovarian epithelial tumors do not appear to correlate with whether the mass is benign or malignant. However, the more solid and irregular areas within the mass, the more likely is the tumor malignant (Fig. 7, D and E).[20] Malignancy can also be inferred when ascites is associated with the mass. However, the absence of ascites is not a totally reliable indicator that the mass is benign.

Once a mass of this variety is encountered, one should examine the pericolic recesses, subhepatic space, and cul-de-sac for the presence of ascites, the kidneys for presence of obstructive uropathy, the liver for the presence of hepatic metastases, and the peritoneal surfaces for the presence of peritoneal and/or omental metastases (Fig. 8, D to F).[13] Peritoneal metastases greater than 2 cm in size can be delineated when surrounded by ascites. However, smaller metastases (less than 2 cm) near the subdiaphragmatic areas may be difficult to delineate on sonography.[5] Although rare, in

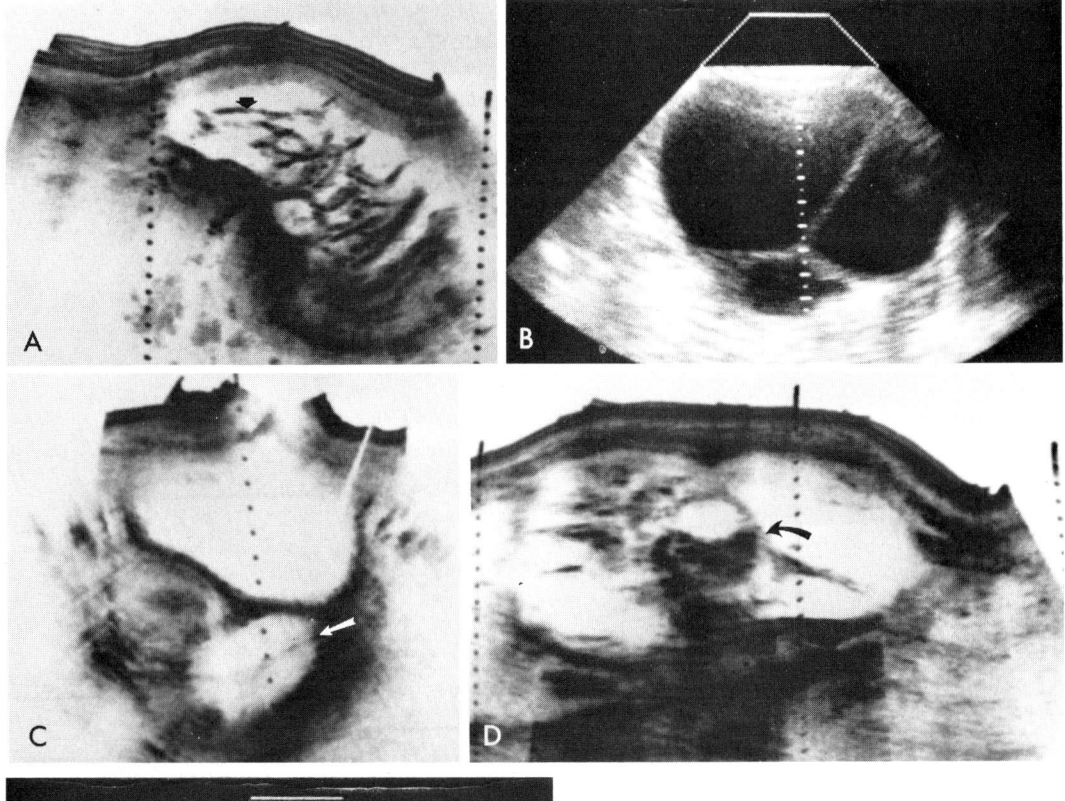

Figure 7. Complex, predominantly cystic ovarian masses. *A*, Mucinous cystadenoma (longitudinal static sonogram). This mass contained several thin and well-defined septations (*arrow*) characteristic of a mucinous cystadenoma. *B*, Real-time sonogram of a mucinous cystadenoma with typical thin internal septae. *C*, Tubo-ovarian abscess (transverse static sonogram). This predominantly cystic mass had two components that seemed to be separated by a well-defined layer (*arrow*). Pus was located in the more dependent portion of the mass. *D*, Malignant teratoma encountered in young child (longitudinal static sonogram). Although this mass is predominantly cystic and has several well-defined and thin internal septations, the solid irregular areas within the mass (*arrow*) suggested the possibility of a malignant tumor. (*From* Fleischer, A., and James, A. E.: Introduction to Diagnostic Ultrasonography. New York, John Wiley and Sons, 1980, with permission.) *E*, The possibility of malignancy of this complex, predominantly cystic mass was correctly postulated by the presence of an irregular solid internal component (*arrow*).

some patients with advanced ovarian carcinoma, intrahepatic metastases will be present (Fig. 8, *E* and *F*).[22] Hepatic metastases associated with ovarian carcinoma usually appear as either relatively hypoechoic masses within the liver or as anechoic masses with irregular borders (Fig. 8, *F* and *G*). Exophytic metastases which enlarge from the surface of the liver are also encountered in some patients with advanced ovarian carcinoma (Fig. 8*E*).

Complex, Predominantly Solid Masses

A complex, predominantly solid mass consists primarily of soft tissue components or contains echogenic internal material such as sebum within a dermoid cyst, or numerous floating cells contained within the mass (Fig. 8, *A* and *B*). This type of mass can also result from cystic degeneration within a solid mass such as that characteristically found in granulosa cell tumors. The most common types of complex, predominantly solid ovarian masses are a germ cell tumor or an ovarian neoplasm (Fig. 9, A to C).

Tumors arising from the germ cells of the ovary are most common in patients from approximately 5 to 25 years of age.[33] Germ cell tumors include benign cystic teratomas or dermoid cysts as well as malignant teratomas. In the adolescent group, 30 per cent of teratomas will be malignant. As when any complex adnexal mass is encountered, an ectopic pregnancy should be considered if the clinical presentation and laboratory findings indicate that the patient is pregnant.

The most common type of germ cell tumor is the dermoid cyst. As their name implies, these masses consist of skin, hair, teeth, and fatty elements which typically arise from ectoderm. Dermoid cysts frequently tend to be located superior to the uterine fundus (Fig. 9D). Since they are usually pedunculated, they may undergo torsion and produce exquisite abdominal pain. Their sonographic appearance varies from completely cystic to solid masses.[30] However, the most common appearance of dermoid cyst is that of a complex, predominantly solid mass containing high level echoes arising from hair and/or calcification within the dermoid cyst (Fig. 7A). The

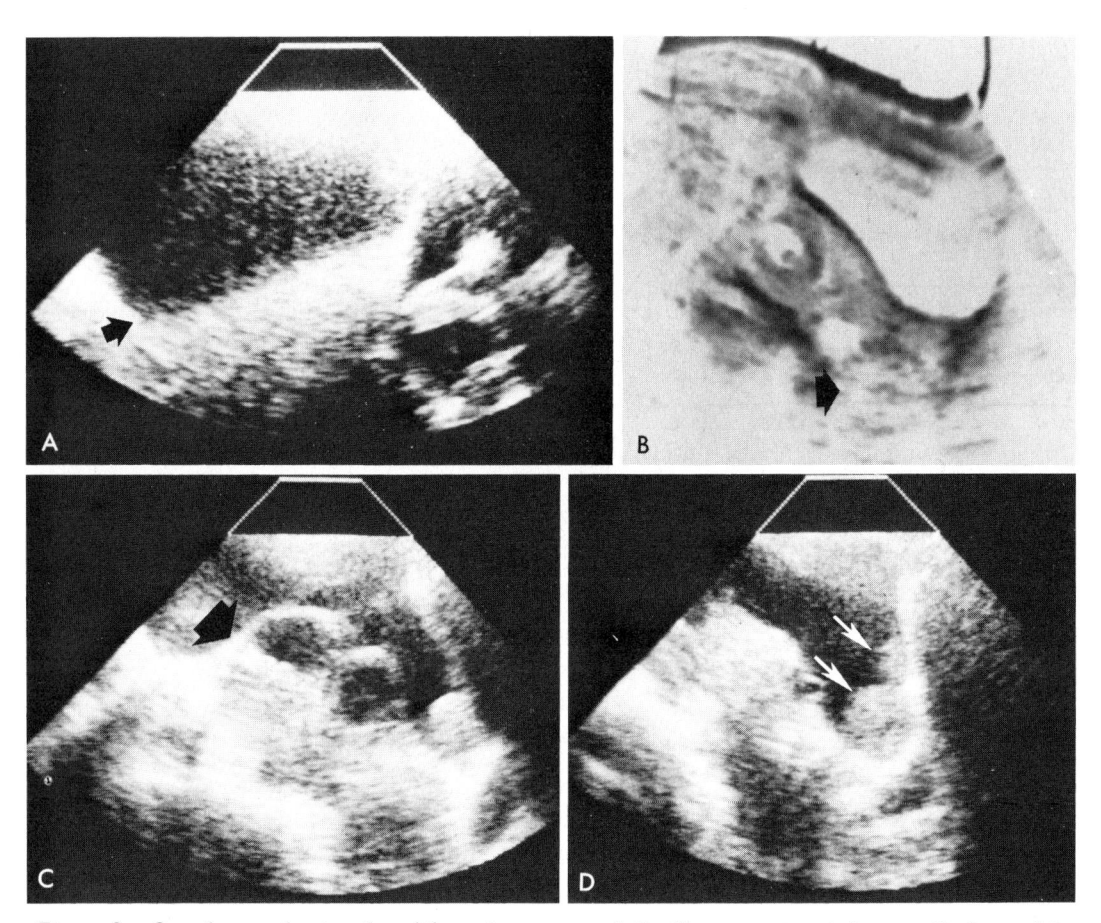

Figure 8. Complex, predominantly solid ovarian masses. *A,* Papillary serous cystadenoma. During real-time examination, the internal contents of this mass could be demonstrated to be gravity dependent. A gravity-dependent layer (*arrow*) of solid material was present within this mass with the more echogenic components corresponding to cellular debris within the cystadenoma. *B,* Dermoid cyst and seven weeks intrauterine pregnancy (longitudinal static sonogram). Posterior to the lower uterine segment is a complex, predominantly solid mass (*arrow*) representing a dermoid cyst. *C,* Mucinous cystadenocarcinoma. This mass (*arrow*) had some cystic components but was predominantly solid and was associated with ascites. *D,* Serosal implants associated with the ovarian tumor depicted in A. Several serosal implants along the bladder dome could be identified (*arrows*).

Illustration continued on following page

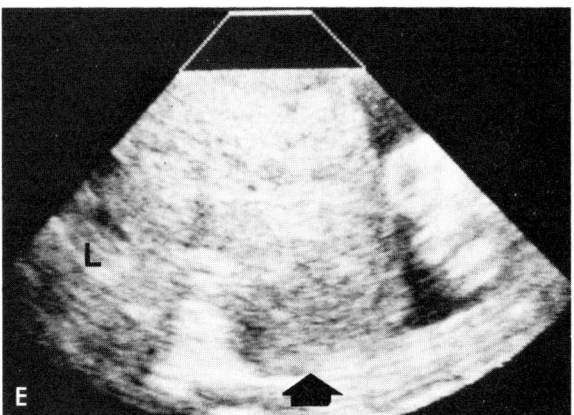

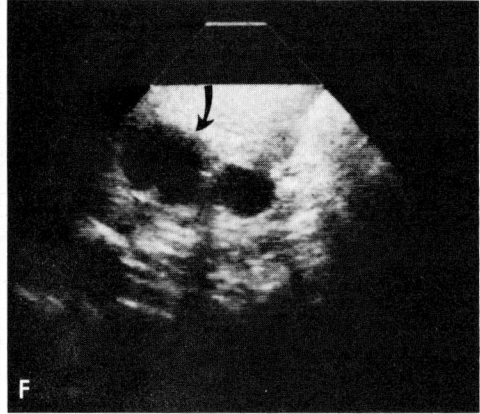

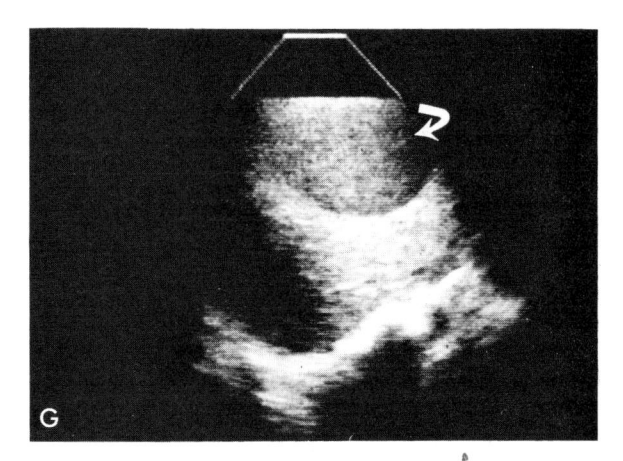

Figure 8 (*Continued*). *E*, Exophytic liver mass in patient with cystadenocarcinoma (longitudinal real-time sonogram). A large mass (*arrow*) could be identified arising from the inferior surface of the liver (L) in this patient with advanced ovarian carcinoma. Several small bowel loops were suspended within ascites. *F*, Cystic intrahepatic metastases (*arrow*). These were associated with advanced ovarian carcinoma. *G*, Hypoechoic intrahepatic metastasis (*arrow*) associated with advanced ovarian carcinoma (transverse real-time sonogram).

highly echogenic nature of these masses may make it difficult to completely delineate the mass or distinguish it from surrounding gas-containing loops of bowel.[14,36] Typically, this situation may be encountered when the gynecologist is confident that a pelvic mass of 5 to 6 cm in size is present on palpation and the sonographer cannot definitely delineate a mass. If this situation occurs, a pelvic radiograph may be helpful to identify areas of calcification and/or fat within these masses. One should also recognize that fully distended urinary bladder can displace a pelvic mass out of the pelvis and into the lower to mid-abdomen.[18]

As in other ovarian tumors, the more irregular and solid the internal components of an ovarian mass, the more likely is it malignant (Fig. 7*E*).[20] A solid teratoma is an unusual germ cell tumor. Because of its solid texture, it may blend in with the outline of the uterus, giving rise to the "indefinite uterus" sign described when a mass of similar echogenicity is adjacent to the uterus (Fig. 9*E*).[3]

Solid Ovarian Tumors

Solid tumors of the ovary are rare compared to cystic ovarian neoplasms. Adenocarcinomas, fibromas, and arrhenoblastomas are some of the most common types of solid ovarian masses (Fig. 9, *A* to *C*). Ovarian fibromas can be associated with ascites and pleural effusions in Meig's syndrome. Since the solid type of ovarian masses is so rare, one should consider non-ovarian causes of solid adnexal masses such as subserous or intraligamentous leiomyoma, fat, conglomerated omentum, or thickened

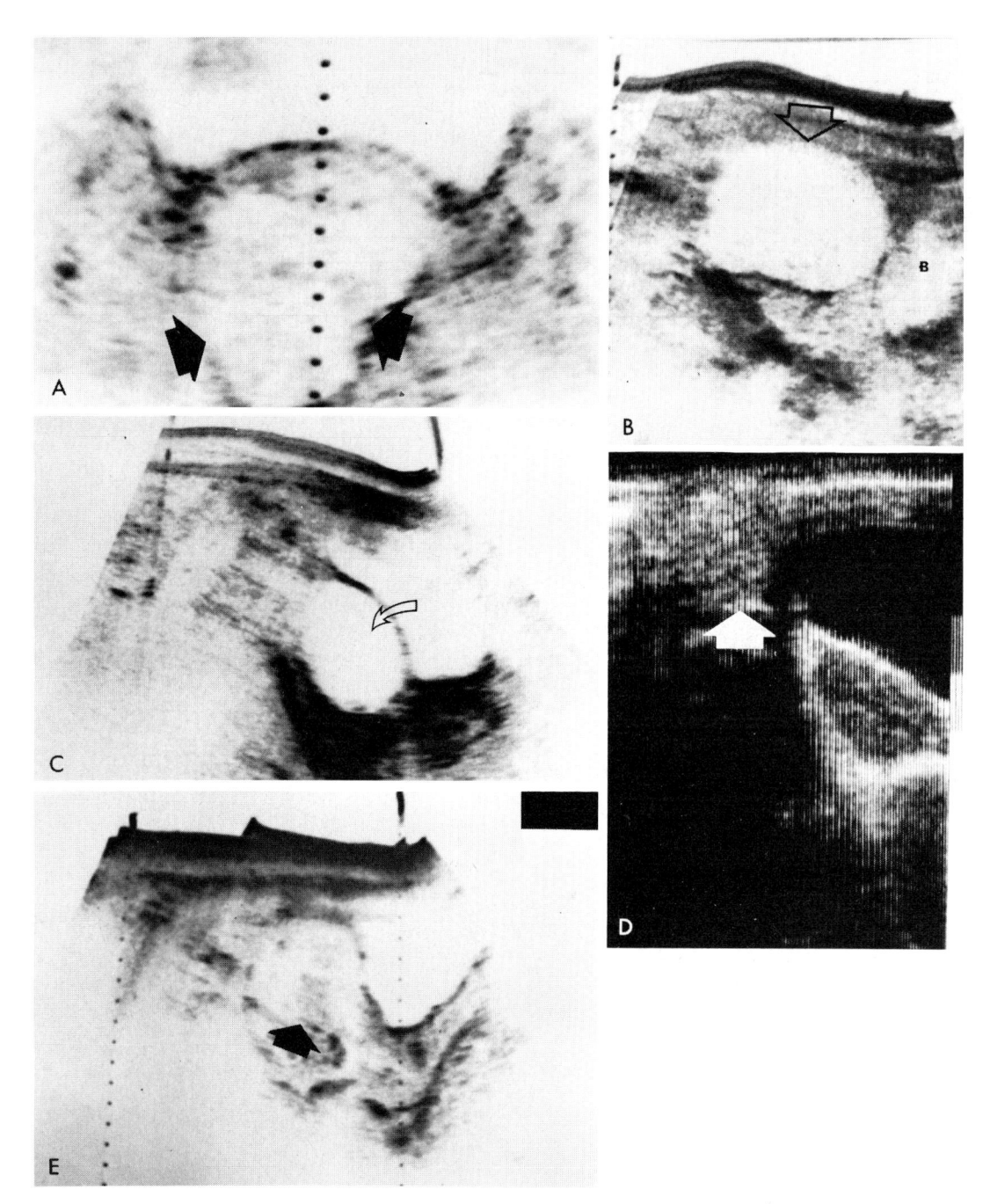

Figure 9. Solid ovarian masses. *A*, Adenocarcinoma of the ovary depicted as a solid ovarian mass (*arrow*) on this transverse static sonogram. *B*, Lymphomatous involvement of the ovary in a patient with a B-cell lymphoma (longitudinal static sonogram; B = urinary bladder). Although lymphatomous involvement of the ovary produces a solid mass (open arrow), there is typically very little stromal component and thus the mass is usually typically anechoic. (*A* and *B* from Fleischer, A., and James, A. E.: Introduction to Diagnostic Ultrasonography. New York, John Wiley and Sons, 1980, with permission.) *C*, Lymphomatous involvement of the ovary. Similar to that depicted in Figure 8B, this mass (*curved open arrow*) was produced by lymphomatous involvement of the ovary. Because of its anechoic appearance and enhanced through transmission, it would be mistaken for a cystic ovarian mass. *D*, Dermoid cyst presenting as ill-defined mass (*arrow*) superior to the uterine fundus. This mass contained a large amount of sebum; thus it demonstrated a very echogenic appearance. *E*, Solid teratoma (*arrow*) adjacent to the uterus producing the "indefinite uterus sign."

mesentery or hematoma (Fig. 10, *E* to *G*).[8, 10, 35] A rare cause of solid adnexal mass is a hematoma associated with a chronic ectopic pregnancy. As with any solid mass that is adjacent to the uterus, one may get the sonographic impression of an enlarged uterus ("indefinite uterus sign") (Fig. 10*G*).

Although rare, several types of primary neoplasms can metastasize to the ovary. Most frequently these include metastases from primary lesions of the gastrointestinal tract (Krukenberg tumor), lymphoma, and leukemia (Figs. 9, *B* and *C*).[2, 28] All these processes result in overall enlargement of the ovary with a mass of hypoechoic texture.

Sonographic Mimics of Ovarian Masses

One should be aware of the variety of structures and masses not of ovarian origin that can sonographically mimic an ovarian mass. For example, fluid-filled loops of small bowel produced by ingestion of water can mimic the sonographic appearance of a cystic ovarian mass. However, fluid-filled loops of bowel demonstrate a characteristic change of configuration with peristalsis as

Figure 10. Sonographic mimics of ovarian masses. *A*, Fluid-filled loops of ileum (*large arrow*) appearing as a predominantly cystic adnexal mass. The mucosal folds (*small arrows*) of the small bowel could be delineated, thereby identifying this mass as created by a loop of small bowel. (*From* Fleischer, A., et al.: Radiology, *133*:681–685, 1979, with permission.) *B*, Large para-ovarian cyst (*arrow*) in pregnant patient mimicking a cystadenoma (longitudinal static sonogram). *C*, Para-ovarian cyst appearing as fusiform cystic adnexal mass (*arrow*) (transverse static sonogram).

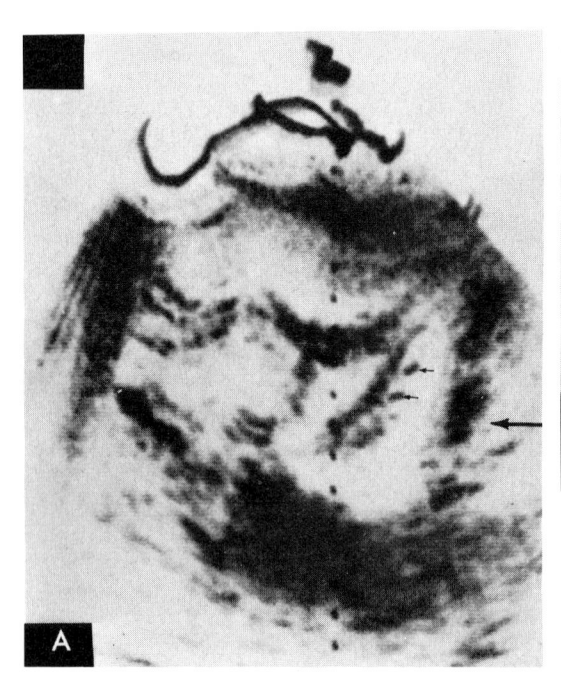

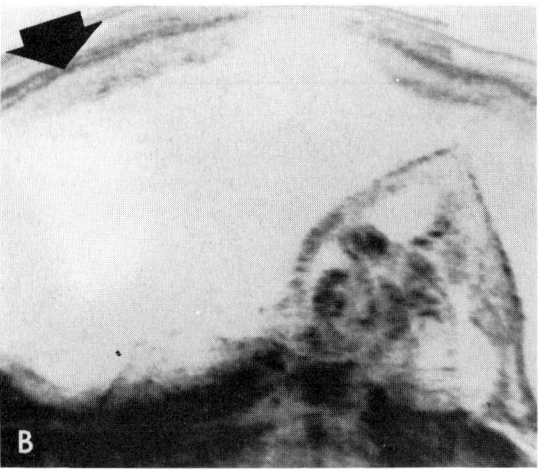

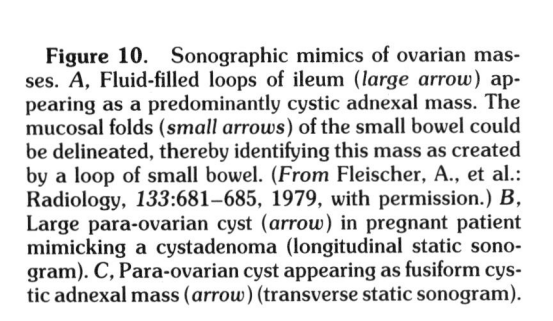

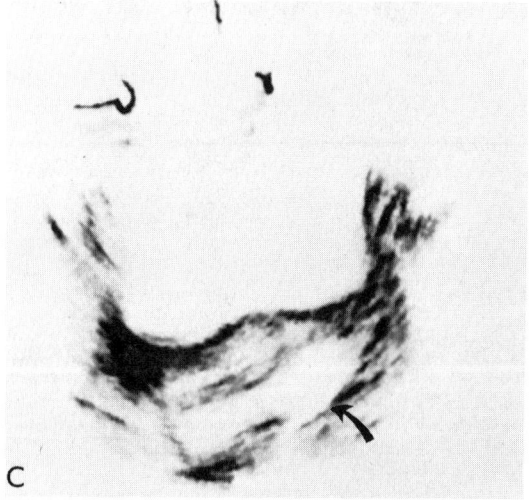

Illustration continued on opposite page

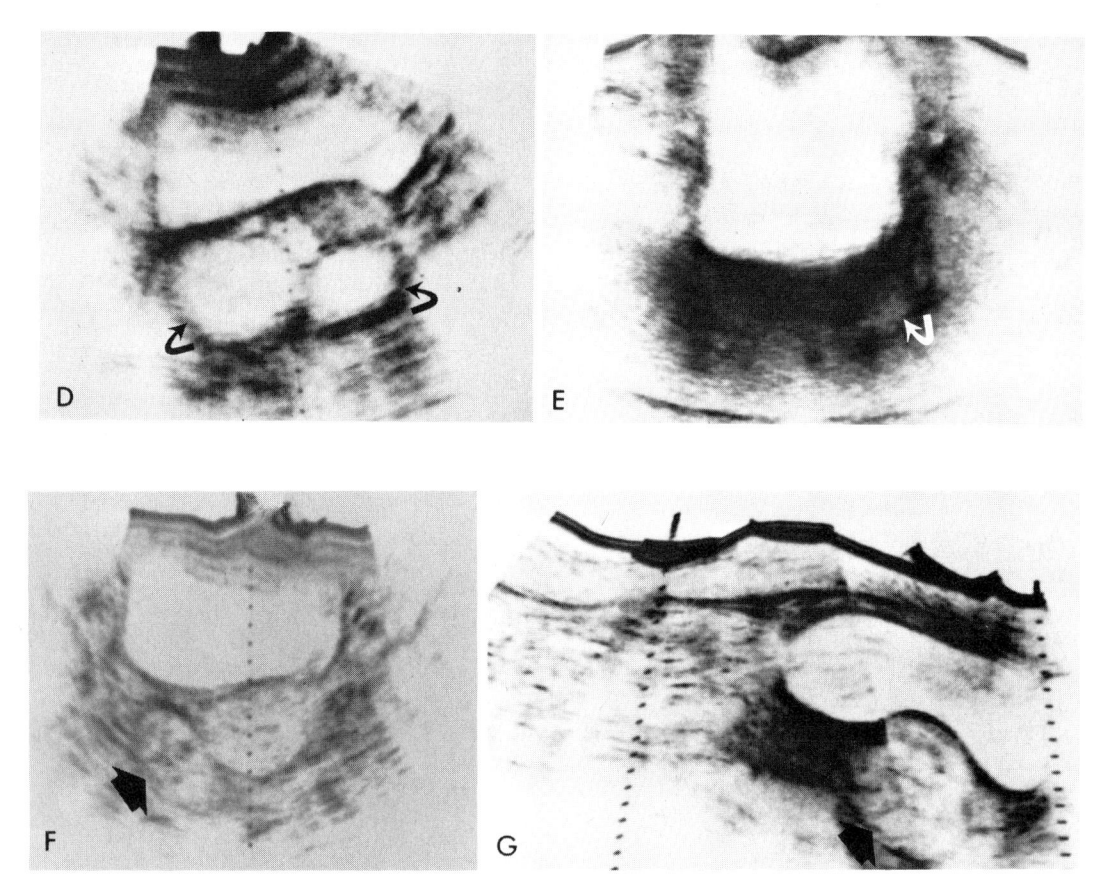

Figure 10. (*Continued*) *D*, Multiple endometriomas (*arrows*) which might be confused for multiple follicular cysts arising from the ovary. (*From* Fleischer, A., and James, A. E.: Introduction to Diagnostic Ultrasonography. New York, John Wiley and Sons, with permission.) *E*, Ill-defined solid left adnexal mass (*arrow*) in this patient who has undergone hysterectomy. The mass was mistaken for an enlarged ovary preoperatively. A matted portion of omentum was identified at surgery. *F*, Herniated fat through the broad ligament producing an apparently solid adnexal mass (*arrow*). Herniation of the ovary and/or fat through a rent in the broad ligament has been termed the Allen-Masters syndrome. (*From* Weinstein, M., et al.: J. Tenn. Med. Assoc. J., 72:121–122, 1979, with permission.) *G*, Chronic ectopic pregnancy (longitudinal static sonogram). A solid mass (*arrow*) posterior to the uterus corresponding to a hematoma from a ruptured ectopic pregnancy blends into the outline of the uterus. This condition might mimic the sonographic appearance of a solid ovarian mass.

depicted best by real-time scanning. Occasionally, a fluid-filled segment of small bowel that is affected by a mechanical obstruction (closed loop obstruction) will mimic the sonographic appearance of a cystic ovarian mass. In most cases of closed loop obstruction, however, linear echogenic interfaces that arise from mucosal folds can be recognized sonographically (Fig. 10*D*).

Masses that arise from the surrounding structures of the ovary can be difficult to distinguish sonographically from those masses that arise directly from the ovary. For instance, para-ovarian cysts that arise from the mesoovarium can appear as masses that arise from the ovaries (Figs. 10, *B* and *C*). Similarly, multiple endometriomas may demonstrate the same sonographic features as multiple follicular cysts (Fig. 10*D*).

Several types of solid structures can mimic a solid ovarian mass. These include masses consisting of a hematoma, fat, or conglomerated omentum (Figs. 10, *D* to *G*).

SUMMARY

The resolution capabilities of sonography afford excellent depiction of both normal and abnormal ovaries. As discussed in this chapter, the major applications of sonography include follicular maturation monitoring and evaluation of the presence or absence of masses within the ovary. Since the long-term prognosis of patients with ovarian carcinoma has been correlated with the completeness of tumor resection, sonographic evaluation of ovarian neoplasms has attained an important status in the clinical presurgical and postsurgical evaluation of the patient with an ovarian mass.[29] Sonography should be utilized with additional radiologic procedures such as excretory urography and barium enema for the most complete preoperative assessment of tumor extent and associated disorders.[26]

REFERENCES

1. Bendon, J., Poleynard, G., and Bordin, G.: Fibrosing mesenteritis simulating pelvis carcinomatosis. Gastro. Rad., 4:195–197, 1979.
2. Bickers, G., Siebert, J., Anderson, J., et al.: Sonography of ovarian involvement in childhood acute lymphocytic leukemia. Am. J. Roentgenol., 137:399–401, 1981.
3. Bowie, J.: Ultrasound of gynecologic pelvic masses: The indefinite uterus sign and other patterns associated with diagnostic error. J. Clin. Ultrasound, 5:323–328, 1977.
4. Caball, A., and Bessis, R.: Monitoring of ovulation induction with human menopausal gonadotropin and human chorionic gonadotropin by ultrasound. Fertil. Steril., 36:178–182, 1981.
5. Coulam, C., Julian, C., and Fleischer, A.: Clinical efficacy of sonography and computed tomography of gynecologic neoplasms. Appl. Rad., 11:78–88, 1982.
6. Dabelstein, S., Hackeloer, B., and Sturm, G.: Ovulation and corpus luteum formation observed by ultrasonography. Ultrasound in Med, 7:33–39, 1981.
7. DeLand, M., Fried, A., Van Nagell, J., et al.: Ultrasonography in the diagnosis of tumors of the ovary. Surg. Gynecol. Obstet., 148:346–348, 1979.
8. Engel, J., and Deitsch, E.: Omentum mimicking cystic masses in the pelvis. J. Clin. Ultrasound, 8:31–33, 1980.
9. Fleischer, A., Daniel, J., Rodier, J., et al.: Sonographic monitoring of ovarian follicular development. J. Clin. Ultrasound, 9:275–280, 1981.
10. Fleischer, A., Dowling, A., Weinstein, M., et al.: Sonographic features of distended, fluid-filled bowel. Radiology, 133:681–685, 1979.
11. Fleischer, A., and James, A. E.: Introduction to Diagnostic Sonography. New York, John Wiley and Sons, 1980.
12. Fleischer, A., James, A. E., Millis, J., et al.: Differential diagnosis of pelvic masses by gray scale sonography. Am. J. Roentgenol., 131:469–476, 1978.
13. Fleischer, A., Walsh, J., Jones, H., et al.: Sonographic evaluation of pelvic masses: Method of examination and role of sonography relative to other imaging modalities. Radiol. Clin. North Am., 20:397–412, 1982.
14. Guttman, P.: In search of the elusive benign cystic teratoma: "Tip of the iceberg" syndrome. J. Clin. Ultrasound, 5:83–87, 1977.
15. Hackeloer, B., Fleming, R., Robinson, H., et al.: Correlation of ultrasonic and endocrinologic assessment of human follicular development. Am. J. Obstet. Gynecol., 135:122–126, 1979.
16. Hall, D., Hann, L., Ferrucci, J., et al.: Sonographic morphology of the normal menstrual cycle. Radiology, 133:185, 1979.
17. Kratochwil, A., Urban, G., and Friedrich, F.: Ultrasonic tomography of the ovaries. Ann. Chir. Gynecol. Fenn., 61:211–214, 1972.
18. Kurtz, A., Ashman, F., Dubbins, P., et al.: Ultrasound evaluation of palpable ovarian masses: Comparison of filled and partially emptied urinary bladder techniques. Appl. Radiol., 11:101–105, 1982.
19. McNatty, K., Smith, D., and Mahvis, A.: The microenvironment of the human antral follicle: Interrelationships among the steroid levels in antral fluid, the population of granulosa cells and the status of the oocyte in vivo and in vitro. J. Clin. Endocrinol Metab., 49:859–863, 1980.
20. Meire, H., Farrant, P., and Guha, T.: Distinction of benign from malignant ovarian cysts by ultrasound. Br. J. Obstet. Gynaecol., 85:893–899, 1978.
21. O'Herlihy, L., deCrespigny, L., Copata, A., et al.: Preovulatory follicular size: A comparison of ultrasound and laparoscopic measurements. Fertil. Steril., 34:24, 1980.
22. Paling, M., and Shawker, T.: Abdominal ultrasound in advanced ovarian carcinoma. J. Clin. Ultrasound, 9:435–441, 1981.
23. Phillips, H., and McGohan, J.: Ovarian remnant syndrome: A case report. Radiology, 142:487–488, 1982.
24. Queenan, J., O'Brien, G., Baris, L., et al.: Ultrasonic scanning of ovaries to detect ovulation in women. Fertil. Steril., 34:99–105, 1980.
25. Rankin, R., and Hutton, L.: Ultrasound in the ovarian hyperstimulation syndrome. J. Clin. Ultrasound, 9:473–476, 1981.
26. Requard, C., Mettler, F., and Wicks, J.: Preoperative sonography of malignant ovarian neoplasms. Am. J. Roentgenol., 137:79–82, 1981.
27. Riddlesberger, M., Kuhn, J., and Muncshauer, R.: The association of juvenile hypothyroidism and cystic ovaries. Radiology, 139:77–80, 1981.
28. Rochester, D., Levin, B., Bowie, J., et al.: Ultrasonic appearance of the Krukenberg tumor, a case report. Am. J. Roentgenol., 129:919–920, 1977.
29. Sample, W., Lippe, B., and Gyepes, M.: Gray-scale ultrasonography of the normal female pelvis. Radiology, 125:477–483, 1977.
30. Sandler, M., Silver, T., and Karo, J.: Gray-scale ultrasonic features of ovarian teratomas. Radiology, 131:705–709, 1979.
31. Smith, D., Picker, R., and Simosich, P.: Assessment of ovulation by ultrasound and estradiol levels during spontaneous and induced cycles. Fertil. Steril., 33:387–390, 1980.

32. Swanson, M., Sauerbrei, E., and Cooperberg, P.: Medical implication of ultrasonically detected polycystic ovaries. J. Clin. Ultrasound, 9:219–222, 1981.
33. Towne, B., Haholar, H., Wooley, M., et al.: Ovarian cysts and tumors in infancy and childhood. J. Pediatr. Surg., 10:311–320, 1975.
34. Walsh, J., Taylor, K., Wasson, J., et al.: Gray-scale ultrasound in 204 proved gynecologic masses: Accuracy and specific diagnosis criteria. Radiology, 130:391–397, 1979.
35. Weinstein, M., Fleischer, A., Daniell, J., et al.: Sonographic detection of Allen-Masters syndrome. J. Tenn. Med. Assoc., 72:121–122, 1979.
36. White, E., and Filly, R.: Cholesterol crystals as the source of both diffuse and layered echoes in a cystic ovarian tumor: A case report. J. Clin. Ultrasound, 8:241–243, 1980.
37. Ylostalo, P., Ronnberg, L., and Jouppila, P.: Measurement of the ovarian follicle by ultrasound in ovulation induction. Fertil. Steril., 31:651–655, 1981.

14

Ultrasound of the Uterus

Barry H. Gross, M.D., and Peter W. Callen, M.D.

Ultrasound is a technique uniquely suited to the structure of the uterus. The uterus is readily evaluated by ultrasound because of its location posterior to the urinary bladder, which in the distended state acts as an acoustic window. Ultrasound is ideal for evaluating the uterus because images are obtained without radiating a clinically undetected intrauterine pregnancy. Since the initial report in 1958 describing ultrasonographic detection of gynecologic masses,[8] the accuracy of ultrasound in diagnosing uterine abnormalities has been well established.[7, 10, 24, 25, 45]

In this chapter, ultrasonographic examination of the uterus is reviewed. Ultrasonography of developmental anomalies and of benign and malignant disease processes of the uterus is discussed. Pregnancy and its complications are discussed elsewhere in this text, as are gestational trophoblastic disease and intrauterine contraceptive devices.

THE NORMAL UTERUS AND ITS ULTRASONOGRAPHIC APPEARANCE

Position. The uterus is typically located in the midline between the bladder and the rectum (Fig. 1). However, the uterus can have various right-to-left and anterior-to-posterior positions in the absence of pelvic disease, depending on the degree of bladder and rectal distention and on normal anatomic variation.[35] Nevertheless, when the uterus is away from the midline, displacement by a pelvic mass should be excluded. Pelvic relaxation may result in a lower than normal uterine position.

Size. The size of a normal uterus depends on the developmental status of the patient. The normal prepubertal uterus measures 2.0 to 3.3 cm long and 0.5 to 1.0 cm wide (Fig. 2).[26, 35] The most common cause of enlarged uterus in children is hormonal stimulation (Fig. 3). Uterine rhabdomyosarcoma and hydrometrocolpos are less common causes.[19]

Various measurements have been given for the normal postpubertal uterine size.[5, 26, 31, 35] The maximum postpubertal size is approximately 4 by 7 by 4 cm,[5] but multiparity increases the normal size by 1.2 cm in all directions.[31] The postmenopausal uterus atrophies, with a reported range of 1.2 to 1.8 cm thick and 3.5 to 6.5 cm long in postmenopausal women (Fig. 4).[31]

The uterus remains small with delayed menarche (see Fig. 2) and primary ovarian failure.[19] The most common postpubertal causes of an enlarged uterus are pregnancy and uterine leiomyomata.[13] Causes of uterine enlargement are listed in Table 1.

Shape. Uterine shape varies with the maturation of the patient. The prepubertal cervix makes up 2/3 to 5/6 of total uterine length, and its anteroposterior diameter is twice that of the uterine corpus (see Fig. 2).[35] This contrasts with the postpubertal uterus, in which the fundus is larger and longer than the cervix (see Fig. 1). Precocious puberty results in a postpubertal uterine shape (see Fig. 3).

In most patients, the uterus is anteverted or tilted forward so that the fundus is more anterior than the cervix (see Fig. 1). Strictly speaking, there are two types of uterine retroposition. In retroversion, the entire uterus is tilted backward, whereas in retroflexion, the body of the uterus bends backward with respect to the cervix.[18] The two are usually indistinguishable sonographically (Fig. 5). Retrodisplaced gravid uteri typically become anteverted during the third month of pregnancy (Fig. 6). Adhesions may prevent spontaneous reduction, and if manual repositioning is not performed, abortion or even uterine rupture may result.[21]

Table 1. *Causes of Uterine Enlargement*

Adenomyosis
Congenital uterine anomalies
Endometrial polyps
Gestational trophoblastic disease
Hemato-, hydro-, or pyometra
Multiparity
Neoplasms, benign or malignant
Postpartum state
Precocious puberty
Pregnancy
Recent abortion

Uterine tumors, particularly pedunculated ones, may distort normal uterine shape. Alterations in shape also occur with various congenital uterine anomalies (Table 2).

Contour. The uterus is normally smooth in contour and distinctly outlined (see Fig. 1). Subtle irregularity of contour may be the only diagnostic feature in some patients with uterine leiomyomata (Fig. 7). Similar changes may be detected after cesarean section (Fig. 8). These changes may be accentuated by postoperative hematoma or abscess (Fig. 9). Retrodisplaced uteri tend to be somewhat lobulated (see Fig. 5), so that in these patients the diagnosis of myomas based on changes in contour alone is difficult.

Loss of the normally distinct uterine outline is an ultrasonographic pattern associated with diagnostic error.[2] In a study of 99 suspected pelvic masses, ultrasound detected the abnormality in 85 per cent, and most errors occurred with homogeneous pelvic masses hiding the uterine borders. In that study, the uterus with an indefinite outline most often resulted from myomas or pelvic inflammatory disease (Fig. 10). Recurrent pelvic bleeding, as in endometriosis, and malignant pelvic tumors also obscure the uterine outline.[22] Abnormalities of uterine contour are listed in Table 3.

Texture. With proper ultrasound technique, the uterus shows homogeneous, low

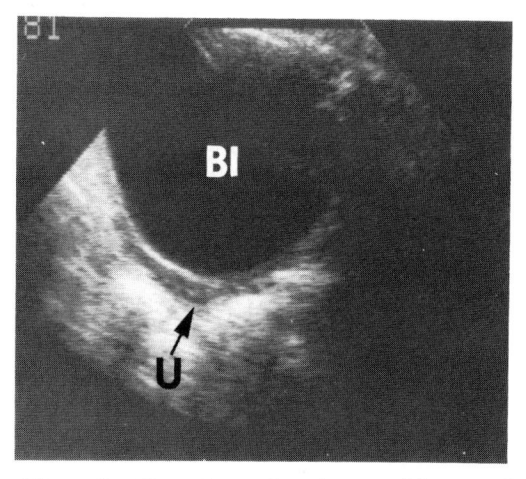

Figure 2. Normal prepubertal uterus (U) in an 18-year-old with delayed menarche. Longitudinal scan demonstrates the predominance of the cervix, which is larger and longer than the fundus. Overall uterine size is significantly smaller than in the postpubertal female. Bl, bladder.

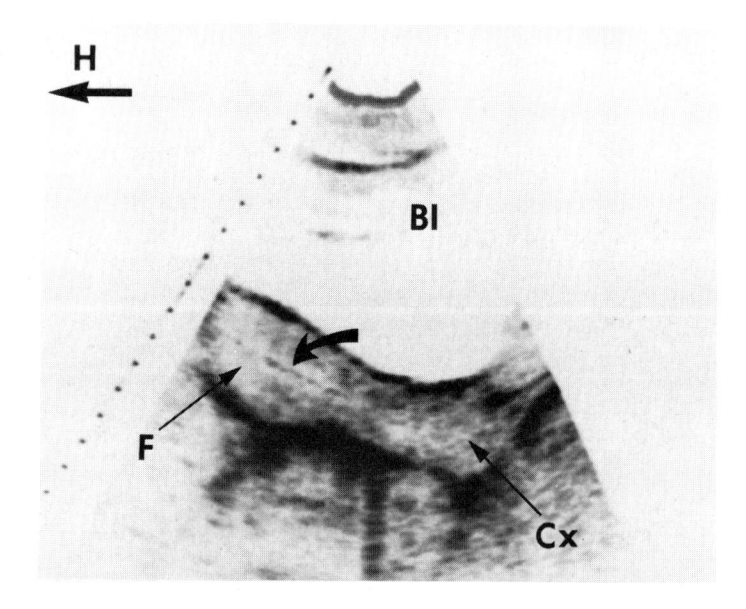

Figure 1. Normal longitudinal ultrasonogram of the uterus. In the postpubertal uterus, the fundus (F) is larger and longer than the cervix (Cx) and is also more anterior. The uterus is smooth in contour and sharply outlined. The central uterine cavity echo (*curved arrow*) is surrounded by the hypoechoic endometrium. The myometrium demonstrates homogeneous, low to moderate echogenicity. Bl, bladder; H, head.

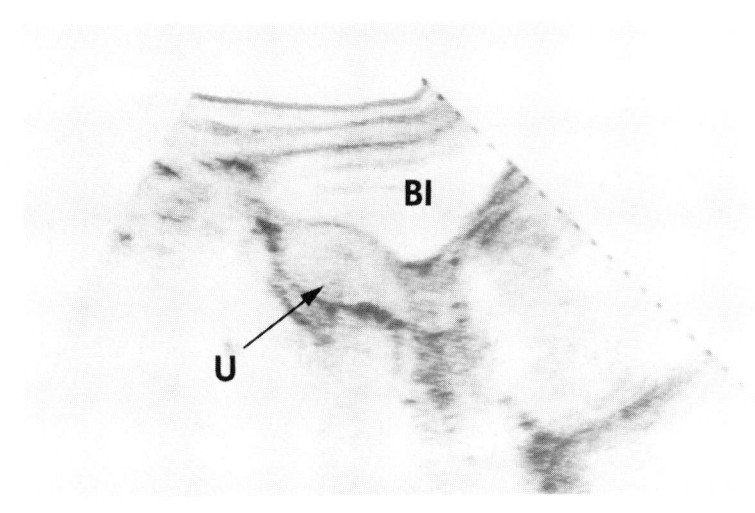

Figure 3. Precocious puberty. Longitudinal scan of the uterus (U) of a 12-year-old girl shows postpubertal uterine size and shape (see Figures 1 and 2).

to moderate echogenicity (see Fig. 1). Benign and malignant neoplasms may disrupt uterine homogeneity. There may be associated increased echogenicity, sometimes because of calcification within the neoplasm. Areas of decreased echogenicity occur in adenomyosis,[44] nabothian cysts (Fig. 11), and pyo-, hydro-, or hematometra. Alterations in uterine texture are listed in Table 4.

Central Uterine Cavity Echo. Within the uterus in most normal patients, there is a centrally located linear echo of moderate to high amplitude (see Fig. 1). In one study, this echo was seen in 90 per cent of examinations retrospectively reviewed, and in 20 of 20 prospective examinations.[6] The central uterine echo is thought to be a specular reflection from the uterine cavity, resulting from a smooth interface that is larger than the sound beam width and is relatively perpendicular to the beam direction. This echo may not be shown in retroverted uteri, in which the uterine cavity is not perpendicular to the sound beam. The central uterine cavity echo is seen in all phases of the menstrual cycle as well as in postmenopausal patients (see Fig. 4).

Often, a 2 to 3 mm zone of low amplitude echoes surrounds the central cavity echo (see Fig. 1) and is believed to represent the endometrium. A sonographic study of the normal menstrual cycle showed a characteristic hypoechoic transformation of this zone of low amplitude echoes during the midluteal stage.[15] The transformation probably reflects vascular engorgement and glandular fluid in the thickened secretory endometrium.

Identification of the central uterine cavity echo is useful in the evaluation of pa-

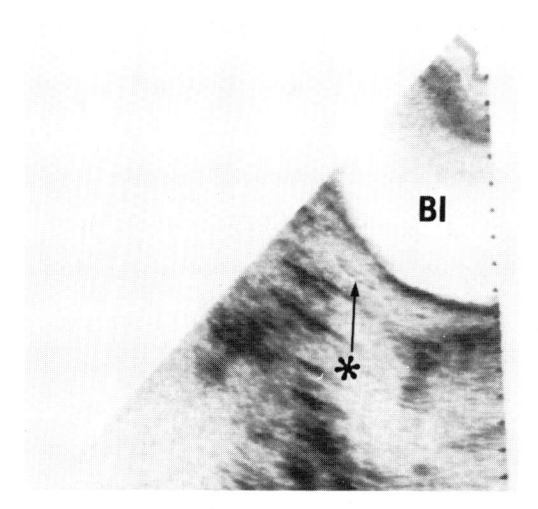

Figure 4. Normal postmenopausal uterus. Longitudinal sonogram reveals diminished uterine size in comparison with the postpubertal premenopausal uterus. The central uterine cavity echo (*asterisk*) is demonstrated, confirming that it is not related to menstruation.

Table 2. *Abnormalities of Uterine Shape*

Congenital uterine anomalies
Delayed menarche
Neoplasms, benign or malignant
Precocious puberty
Pregnancy
Primary ovarian failure
Retroposition

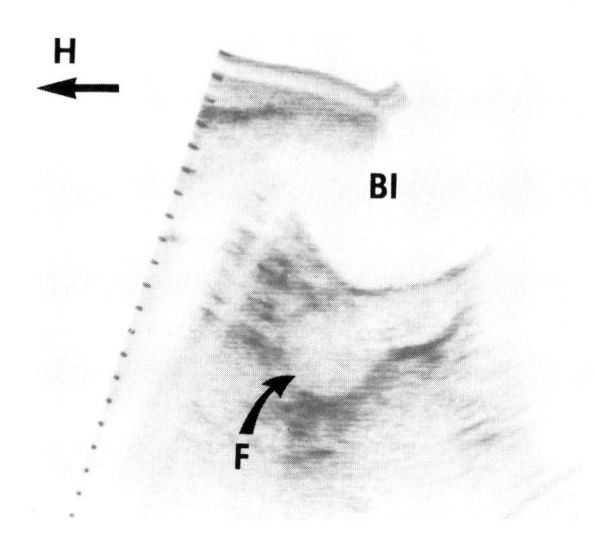

Figure 5. Uterine retroposition. Longitudinal sonogram demonstrates posterior orientation of the uterine fundus (F), which shows the lobular contour typical of uterine retrodisplacement.

tients with pelvic masses. When there is extensive pelvic disease, it may be difficult to differentiate adnexal masses from the uterus. Identifying the central uterine cavity echo establishes conclusively which structure represents the uterus and which structure represents an extrauterine adnexal mass. Furthermore, a pelvic mass that touches the central uterine cavity echo must be uterine in origin (Fig. 12).[6]

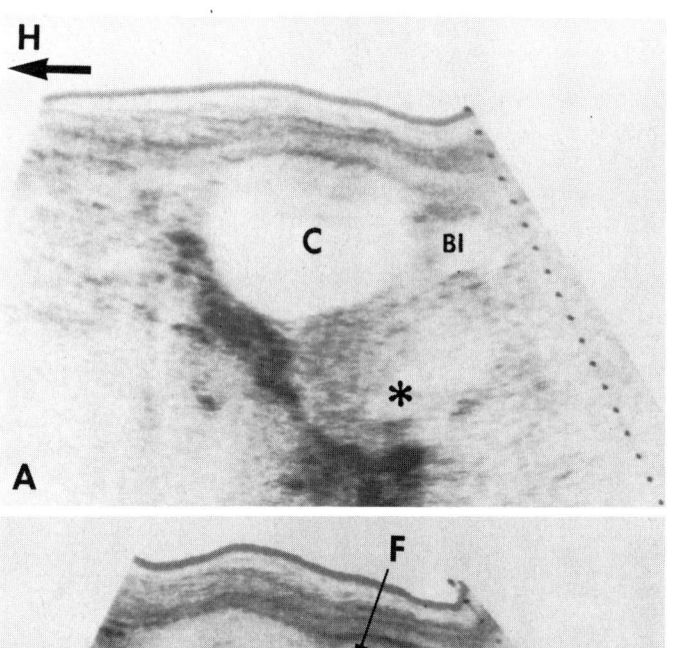

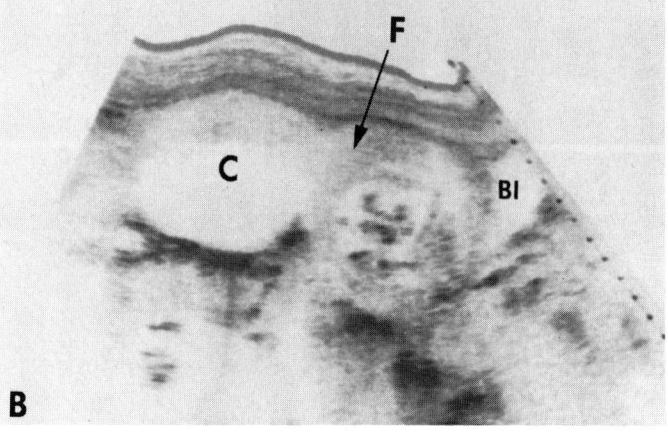

Figure 6. Spontaneous reduction of uterine retroposition during pregnancy. *A*, Longitudinal scan displays an early gestational sac (*asterisk*) in the fundus of a retrodisplaced uterus. There is a large corpus luteum cyst (C) anterior and cephalad to the uterus. *B*, Two weeks later, the fundus (F) has become anteverted, and contains fetal parts. The corpus luteum cyst (C) persists. Bl, bladder.

Table 3. *Abnormalities of Uterine Contour*

Endometriosis
Neoplasms, benign or malignant
Pelvic inflammatory disease
Post-surgery
Retroposition

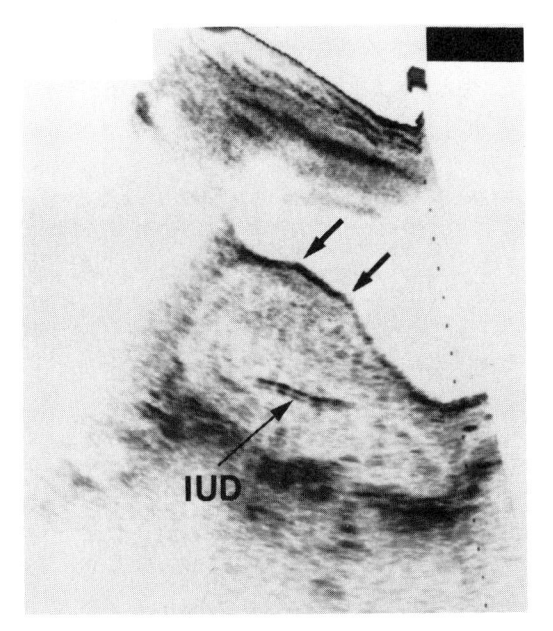

Figure 7. Uterine leiomyomata. Subtle irregularity of contour anteriorly (*arrows*) is demonstrated on this longitudinal scan from a woman with leiomyomata and an intrauterine contraceptive device (IUD).

Other features may help distinguish a uterine mass from an extrauterine one. Although occasionally one may see a cleavage plane separating an adnexal mass from the uterus,[22, 39] in many cases such a distinction will not be clearly seen. In such patients, evaluating the ultrasonographic character of the pelvic lesion will help separate uterine and adnexal lesions. Predominantly solid lesions will usually be uterine in origin, generally secondary to myomas. Predominantly cystic lesions will generally be adnexal in origin, usually secondary to an ovarian mass.[5] Though these guidelines are not absolute, they are helpful in evaluating pelvic masses.

The presence of a normal central uterine cavity echo may also help show that the uterus is nongravid and empty. A normal central cavity echo on the ultrasonogram assures one that the appropriate tomographic plane of section has been obtained where a gestational sac would be present, and thus the uterus can be stated to be nongravid and empty. The central echo may be replaced by various collections of fluid. Most commonly, this occurs with early intrauterine pregnancy. However, in one study, eight of 39 ectopic pregnancies had collections of fluid indistinguishable from early intrauterine pregnancies.[27] Similar collections of fluid have been associated with vaginal bleeding (Fig. 13) and inflammation of the endometrium or adnexae (Fig. 14).[23] The causes of the collection of intrauterine fluid are listed in Table 5.[23]

The central cavity echo may be increased in thickness or echogenicity with various endometrial alterations. Endometrial hyperplasia and polyps typically produce this ultrasound pattern (Fig. 15). Many diseases that sometimes produce a collection of intrauterine fluid (Table 5) can instead cause a prominent central uterine cavity echo. In patients with pelvic inflammatory disease, associated intrauterine fluid or prominence of the central echo (Fig. 16)

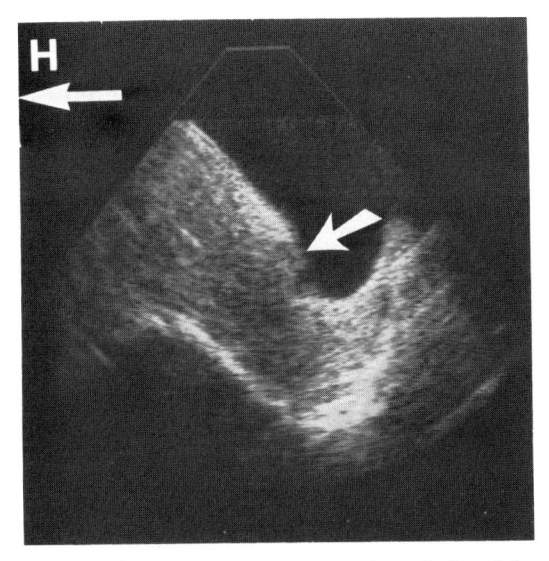

Figure 8. Postcesarean section. Irregularity of the uterus (*arrow*) is similar to that seen in Figure 7 at the site of a cesarean section performed one week prior to this longitudinal sonogram.

Table 4. *Alterations in Uterine Texture*

Adenomyosis
Gestational trophoblastic disease
Hemato-, hydro-, or pyometra
Nabothian cysts
Neoplasms, benign or malignant
Pregnancy

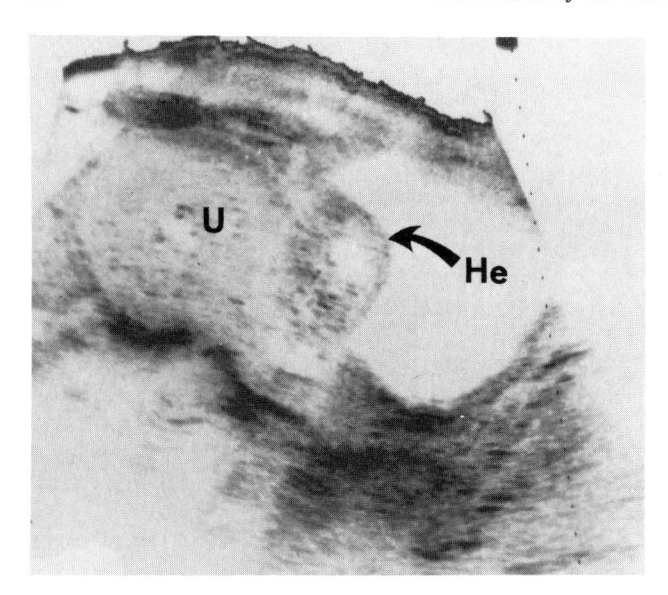

Figure 9. Longitudinal scan of a hematoma after cesarean section. There is a mass (He) along the anterior margin of the uterus (U) instead of the subtle contour irregularity demonstrated in Figure 8. The uterus is enlarged, consistent with the early postpartum state.

probably reflects concomitant endometritis.[5] The differential diagnosis for a prominent central uterine echo is listed in Table 6.

The central cavity echo will rarely cause acoustic shadowing, even when prominent.[22] Acoustic shadowing usually indicates the presence of an intrauterine contraceptive device. Intrauterine gas may also result in acoustic shadowing and may occur during uterine surgery (Fig. 17) or in association with severe infections. Contents of the uterus associated with acoustic shadowing are listed in Table 7.

DEVELOPMENTAL VARIANTS

The uterus is derived from the paired müllerian ducts. The cranial ends of the ducts form the ostia of the fallopian tubes; the caudal ends fuse to form the uterus.[18] The overall incidence of congenital uterine abnormalities is estimated to be 0.1 to 0.5 per cent,[17] although a higher incidence is detected in women undergoing hysterosalpingography.[29, 49]

Uterine malformations can be classified according to the development of the müllerian ducts:[49]

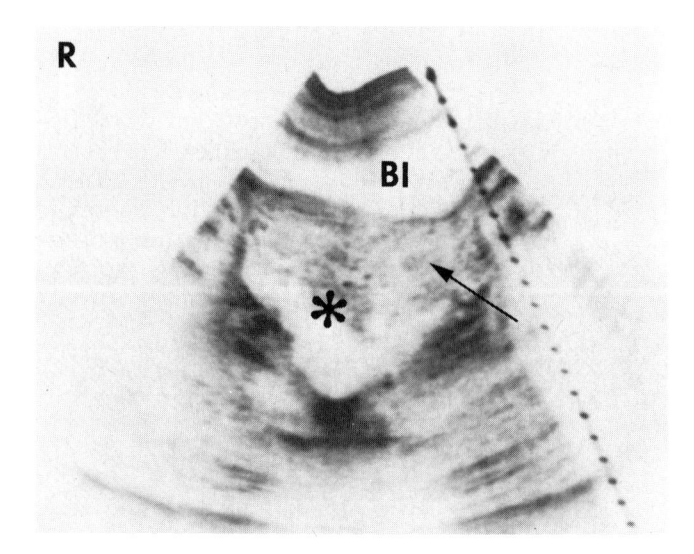

Figure 10. The indefinite uterus, transverse scan. Pelvic inflammatory disease (*asterisk*) obscures the uterus, which is identified only by the presence of the central cavity echo (*arrow*). R, right.

Figure 11. Nabothian cyst. Longitudinal scan demonstrates a rounded, echo-free area in the cervix showing increased through transmission of sound, typical for a nabothian cyst (C).

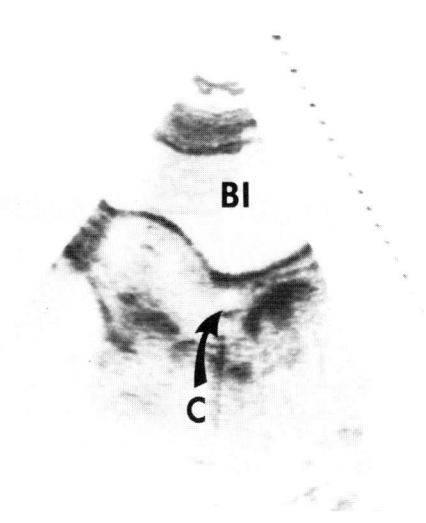

I. Arrested development of the müllerian ducts
   1. Uterine aplasia — bilateral arrested development
   2. Uterus unicornis unicollis — unilateral arrested development
II. Failure of fusion of the müllerian ducts
   1. Uterus didelphys — total failure of fusion (two vaginas, two cervices, two uterine bodies)
   2. Uterus bicornis bicollis — partial fusion (one vagina, two cervices, two uterine bodies)
   3. Uterus bicornis unicollis — partial fusion (one vagina, one cervix, two uterine horns)
   4. Uterus arcuatus — near complete fusion

III. Incomplete resorption of the sagittal septum
   1. Uterus septus — nonresorption of the septum
   2. Uterus subseptus — partial resorption of the septum
IV. Miscellaneous defects, including various anomalies of shape

Some of these malformations are illustrated in Figure 18.

From 1160 malformations detected in 13,470 hysterosalpingograms, the most common anomaly is uterus arcuatus. Uterine hypoplasia, uterus bicornis unicollis, and uterus unicornis unicollis are other rel-

Figure 12. Use of the central cavity echo to identify the origin of a pelvic mass. Transverse scan reveals a large echogenic mass (M) adjacent to the uterus. The mass touches the central cavity echo (*arrow*), establishing conclusively that it is uterine in origin. The mass proved to be a leiomyoma.

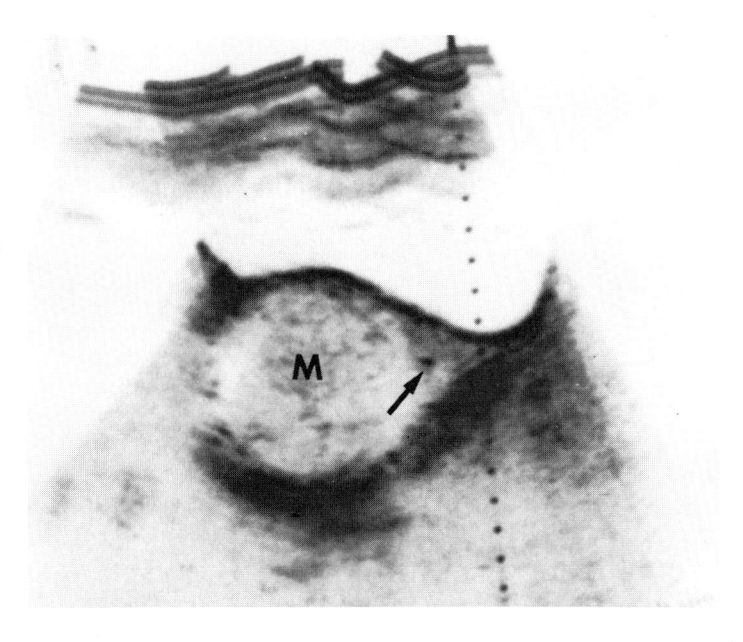

234   *Ultrasound of the Uterus*

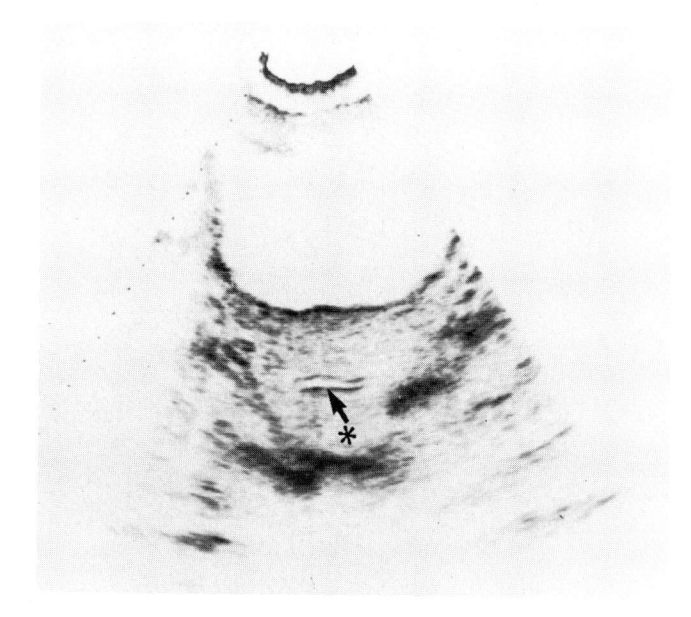

Figure 13. Menstrual blood. There is a fluid collection (*asterisk*) replacing the central cavity echo on this transverse scan of a menstruating woman.

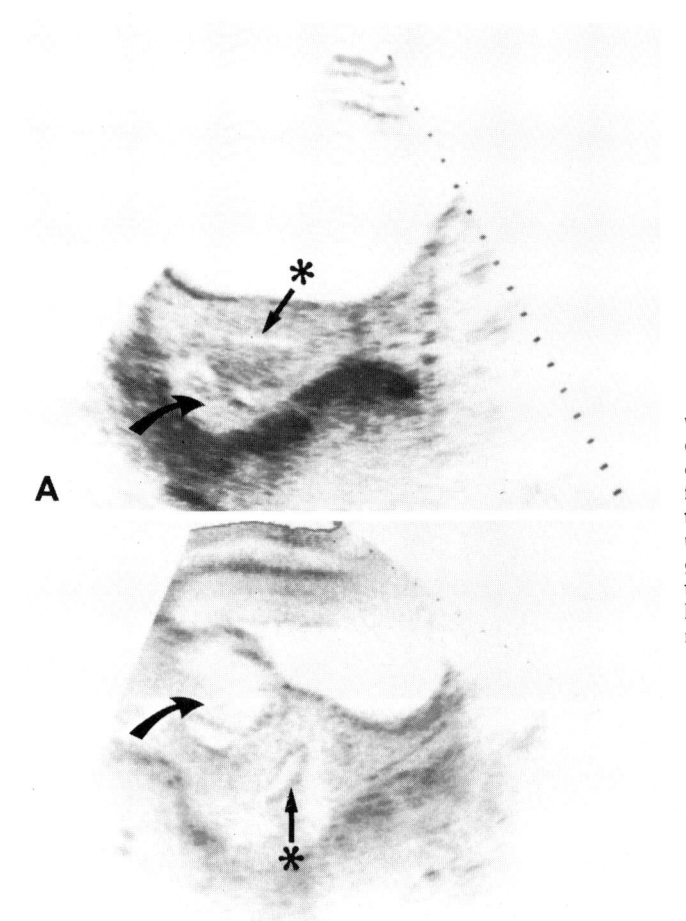

Figure 14. Pelvic inflammatory disease with intrauterine fluid, probably as a result of coexisting endometritis. *A,* There is a fluid collection (*asterisk*) in the uterus and an inflammatory mass (*curved arrow*) posterior to it on this transverse scan. *B,* This intrauterine fluid collection displays an echogenic rind (*asterisk*), simulating a gestational sac of early intrauterine pregnancy. Longitudinal scan also shows an inflammatory mass (*curved arrow*).

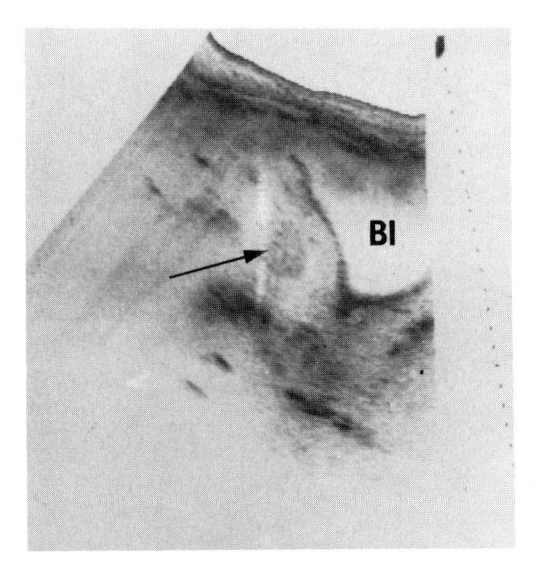

Figure 15. Endometrial adenomatous hyperplasia. Longitudinal sonogram reveals increased thickness and echogenicity of the central uterine cavity echo (*arrow*).

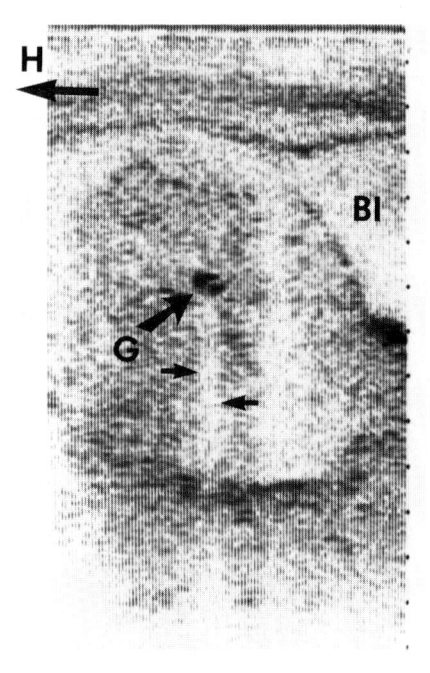

Figure 17. Intrauterine gas. Intraoperative longitudinal sonogram during fetal extraction shows a high amplitude echo (G) producing acoustic shadowing (*arrows*) in an enlarged uterus. There were no retained fetal parts.

atively common malformations. Uterine anomalies may be associated with sterility or early loss of the fetus.[17] There is also a frequent association with unilateral renal agenesis,[11, 17, 38] usually on the side of the genital anomaly.[17] Renal agenesis occurs throughout the range of uterine malformations.[17] In light of this association, all patients with uterine anomalies should undergo sonographic examination of the kidneys, and all patients with renal agenesis should have pelvic sonography.

The ability of ultrasound to detect anomalies of the nongravid uterus depends on deformity of the external uterine contour.

With a bicornuate uterus, the transverse uterine diameter is typically bilobed and increased. Ultrasound may also detect hydrometra or hydrometrocolpos when one of the uterine horns is occluded.[17]

Most anomalies are more easily detected during pregnancy because morphologic changes from the nongravid state are accentuated.[29] Uterus septus and subseptus, in which the external uterine morphology

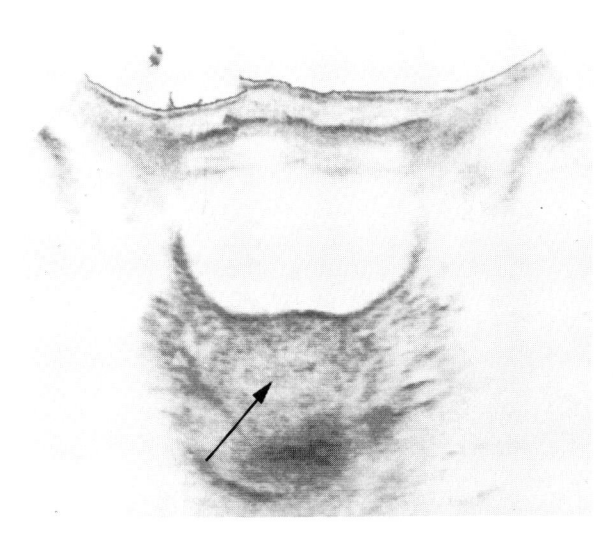

Figure 16. Pelvic inflammatory disease with concomitant endometritis. There is thickening of the central cavity echo (*arrow*) on this transverse scan.

Uterus didelphys   Uterus bicornis bicollis

Uterus bicornis unicollis   Uterus unicornis

Uterus subseptus   Uterus septus   Uterus arcuatus

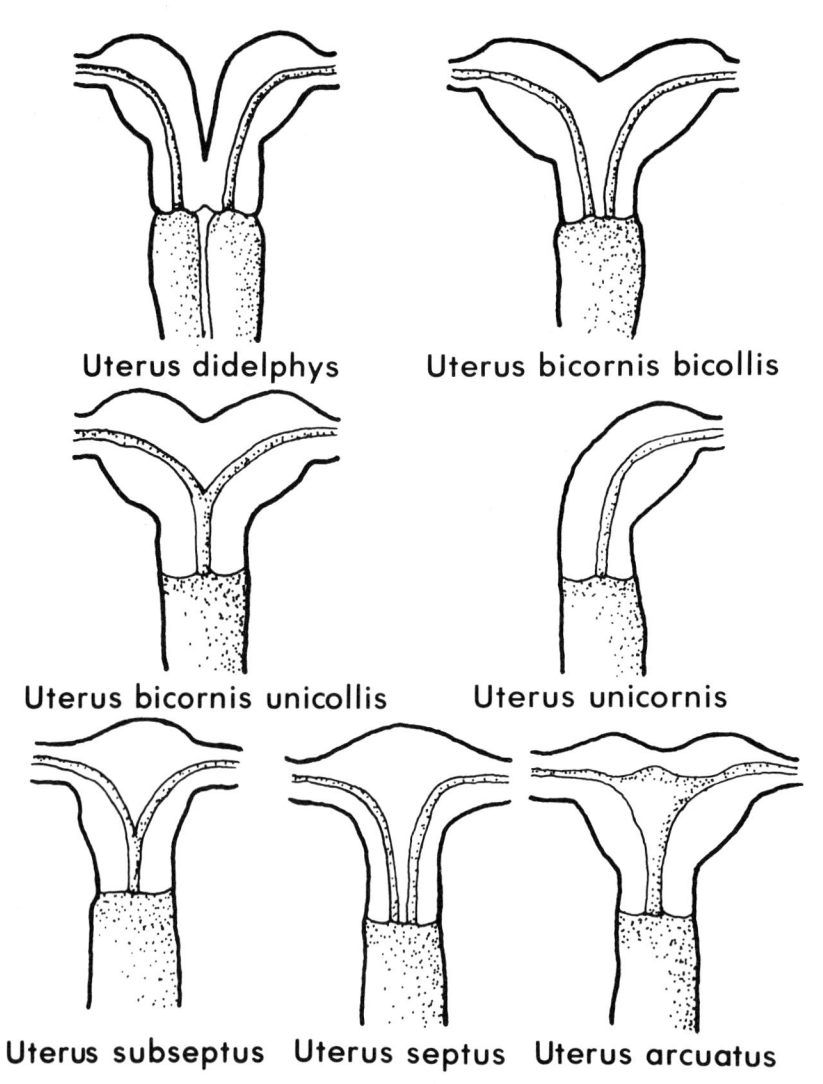

Figure 18. Diagrammatic representation of developmental anomalies of the uterus. Uterus arcuatus, the most common anomaly, produces only minimal external contour deformity. Most anomalies produce more marked morphologic alterations. However, uterus septus and subseptus result in normal external morphology, and are detected only when intrauterine fluid outlines the persistent sagittal septum.

Table 5. *Intrauterine Fluid Collections*

Decidual cast of ectopic pregnancy
Degenerated leiomyoma
Early intrauterine pregnancy
Endometritis with or without pelvic inflammatory disease
Gestational trophoblastic disease
Hemato-, hydro-, or pyometra
Menstruation
Retained products of conception
Vaginal bleeding

is normal, are also more easily detected during pregnancy. This occurs because fluid in the amniotic sac may outline the septum. A bicornuate uterus may show decidual reaction in one horn when there is a pregnancy in the other horn (Fig. 19). There may even be one fetus in each horn.[14]

A myoma adjacent to a pregnancy may simulate the nongravid horn of a bicornuate uterus, but the myoma is usually hypoechoic and inhomogeneous and does not show decidual reaction (see Fig. 19). Later in pregnancy, the nongravid horn becomes difficult to detect. Uterine anomalies may

Table 6. Prominence of the Central Uterine Cavity Echo
Early intrauterine pregnancy
Ectopic pregnancy
Endometrial hyperplasia
Endometrial polyps
Endometritis, with or without pelvic inflammatory disease
Retained products of conception

Table 7. Uterine Contents Causing Acoustic Shadowing
Calcification
Cerclage tape
Gas
Implant for radiation therapy
Intrauterine contraceptive device
Pregnancy
Retained fetal parts following uterine evacuation
Suture material
Tampon

result in delayed involution of the postpartum uterus.[29]

Diethylstilbestrol is associated with various abnormalities of the genital tract in women who were exposed to the drug in utero. By 1977, there had been 330 reported cases of vaginal adenocarcinoma attributed to diethylstilbestrol, and benign disorders such as vaginal adenosis and cervical ectropion are common. Diethylstilbestrol also causes morphologic changes in the uterus.

Hysterosalpingography of 60 women exposed in utero to diethylstilbestrol showed 28 patients with a T-shaped uterus, lacking the characteristic bulbous fundus. There were five hypoplastic uteri, one unicornuate uterus, and six miscellaneous morphologic abnormalities.[20] The T-shaped uterus can be detected by ultrasound, and ultrasound has also shown the size of the

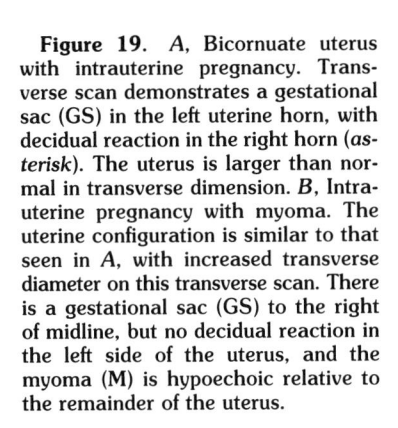

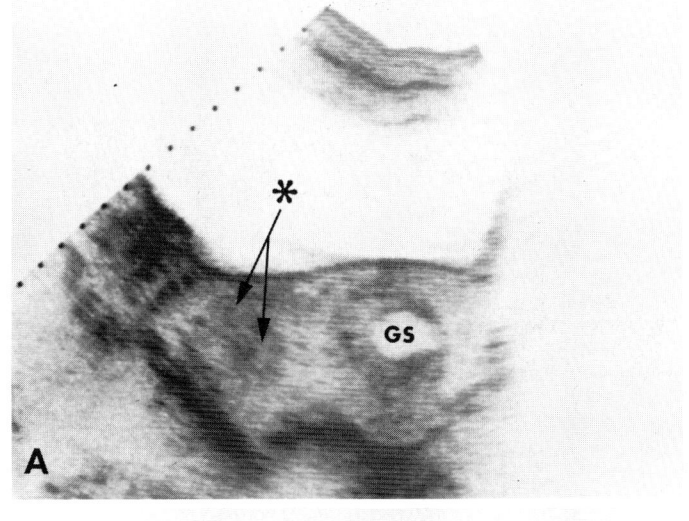

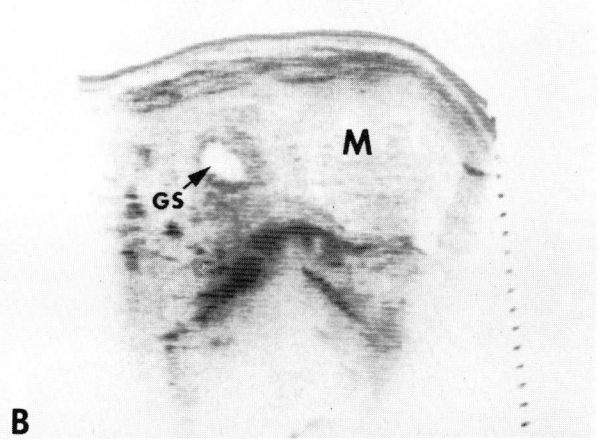

Figure 19. A, Bicornuate uterus with intrauterine pregnancy. Transverse scan demonstrates a gestational sac (GS) in the left uterine horn, with decidual reaction in the right horn (asterisk). The uterus is larger than normal in transverse dimension. B, Intrauterine pregnancy with myoma. The uterine configuration is similar to that seen in A, with increased transverse diameter on this transverse scan. There is a gestational sac (GS) to the right of midline, but no decidual reaction in the left side of the uterus, and the myoma (M) is hypoechoic relative to the remainder of the uterus.

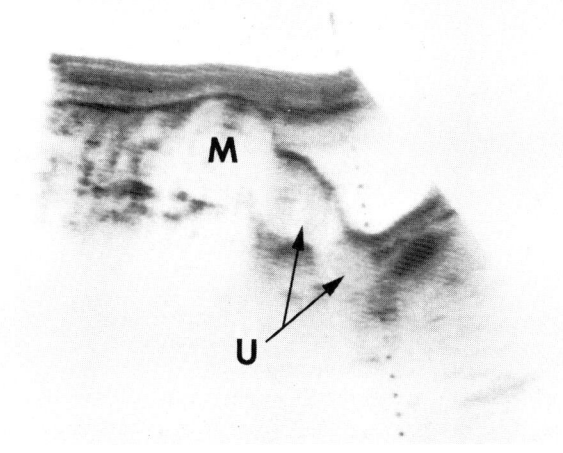

Figure 20. Pedunculated leiomyoma, longitudital sonogram. There is a hypoechoic mass (**M**) projecting from the fundus of the uterus (**U**). Decreased sound transmission through the mass indicates its solid nature.

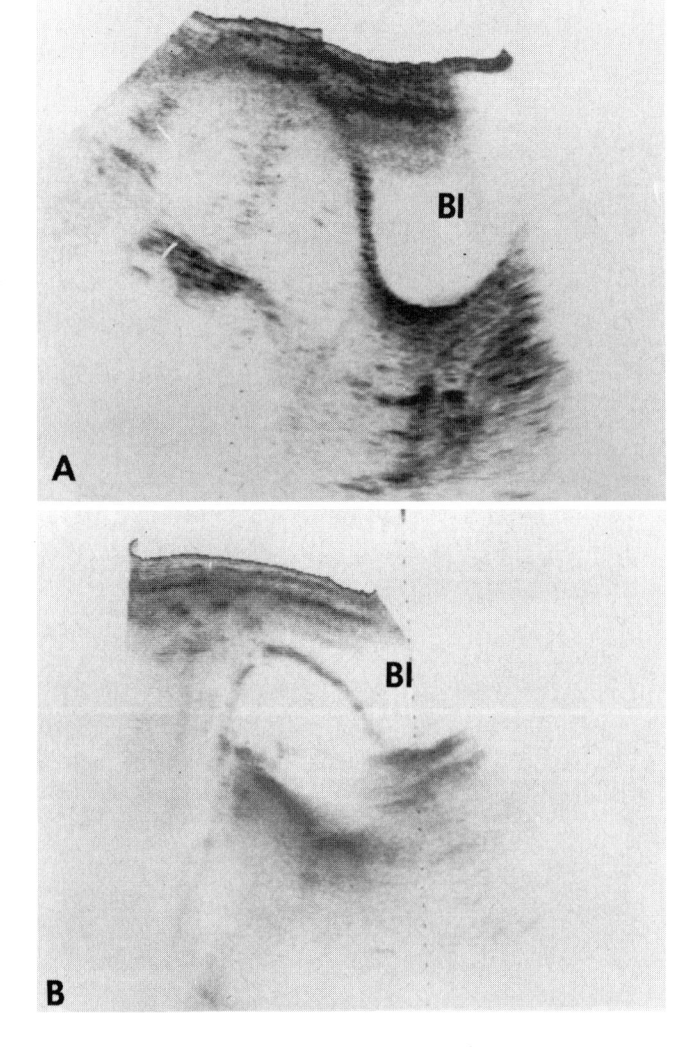

Figure 21. *A*, Multiple leiomyomata, longitudinal scan. The uterus is enlarged and inhomogeneous, with a bulbous contour. There is decreased echogenicity and poor through transmission of sound. *B*, Longitudinal scan of a benign serous cyst of the pelvic peritoneum following hysterectomy. The mass arising at the vaginal apex also has a bulbous, irregular contour with inhomogeneity and decreased internal echogenicity, simulating a myomatous uterus. However, increased through transmission of sound and an internal septation reveal its cystic nature.

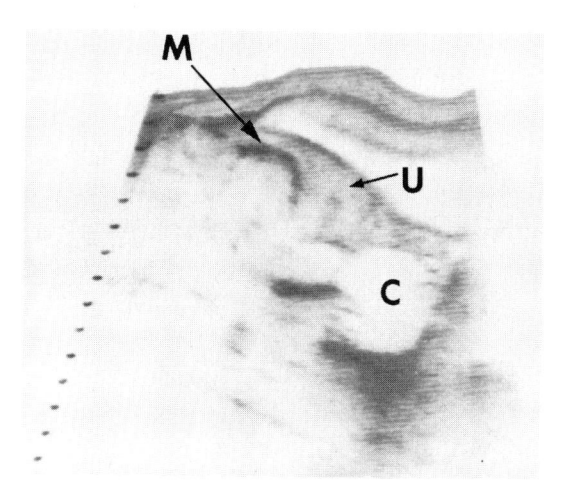

Figure 22. Calcified leiomyoma. Longitudinal sonogram reveals a high amplitude echo (M) within the uterus (U) with resultant acoustic shadowing. Incidentally noted is a cystic adnexal mass (C).

uterus to be significantly reduced in women exposed to diethylstilbestrol.[41]

ACQUIRED UTERINE DISORDERS

Neoplasms

Leiomyoma. The leiomyoma is a common benign neoplasm of the uterus, occurring in up to 40 per cent of women beyond the age of 35 years.[12] Leiomyomata are usually multiple,[28] and many are asymptomatic. The most frequent symptoms are pain and uterine bleeding. Myomas also impair fertility.[18]

Myomas are classified as submucous, intramural, and subserous. Submucous fibroids are the least common but are the most likely to produce symptoms,[42] to become infected,[28] and to undergo sarcomatous change.[18] Intramural fibroids are the most common. Subserous fibroids are frequently pedunculated (Fig. 20) and may simulate adnexal masses. Broad ligament myomas may also simulate adnexal pathology.[12] Cervical myomas are rare.

Myomas undergo a spectrum of secondary changes that includes hyaline degeneration, fatty degeneration, calcification, hemorrhage, and necrosis. The sonographic appearance of a myoma depends on its location and the presence or absence of secondary change and also on the relative amounts of its stromal and muscular constituents.[42] The classic ultrasound appearance of a myoma is a hypoechoic, solid, contour-deforming mass in an enlarged, inhomogeneous uterus (Fig. 21). However, any one of these changes may constitute the only sonographic evidence of myomas (see Fig. 7). Focal increased echogenicity occurs with fatty degeneration and calcification, and the latter may result in acoustic shadowing (Fig. 22). Alternatively, degeneration or necrosis may result in decreased echogenicity and increased through transmission,[16] sometimes appearing cystic (Fig. 23).[42] The fundus of a retroverted uterus typically appears hypoechoic, and a lobular contour is common, so that myomas are more difficult to diagnose in these patients.

Figure 23. Hemorrhagic pedunculated leiomyoma with necrosis. Transverse scan of a gravid uterus (U) shows a hypoechoic mass (M) projecting from the right side of the uterus. There is relatively good transmission of sound, so that a cystic adnexal mass was suspected. At surgery, a necrotic pedunculated myoma was found.

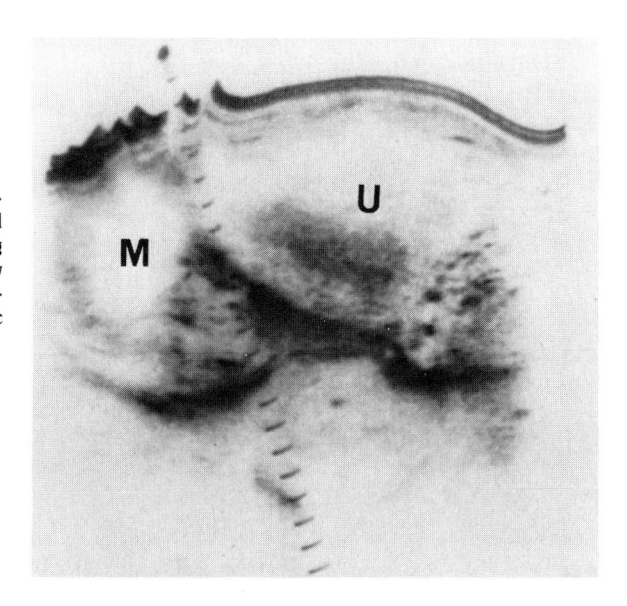

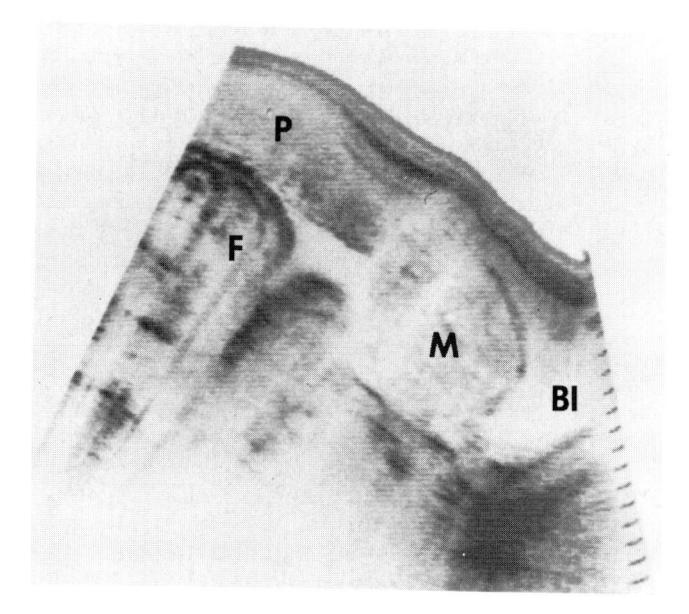

Figure 24. Large cervical myoma, which might interfere with vaginal delivery. Longitudinal sonogram reveals an echogenic mass (M) at the cervical os, with the fetus (F) more cephalad. P, placenta; Bl, bladder.

Although the etiology of myomas is not established, they are clearly stimulated by estrogens.[12] Myomas may grow rapidly during anovulatory menstrual cycles,[40] and the majority of myomas increase in size during pregnancy.[16] Myomas also tend to become more hypoechoic during pregnancy.[40] In the gravid uterus, myometrial contractions should not be mistaken for myomas.[4, 34, 48] Unlike myomas, myometrial contractions tend to bulge into the amniotic cavity without deforming the external uterine contour. Furthermore, myometrial contractions are usually more echogenic than myomas. Most important of all, contractions only last for minutes or hours, conclusively distinguishing them from myomas. Myomas may cause uterine inertia, and large cervical myomas may mechanically block vaginal delivery (Fig. 24).[18] Nevertheless, even very large myomas are compatible with uncomplicated pregnancy and normal vaginal delivery.

Myomas rarely develop in postmenopausal patients, and most tumors typically stabilize or diminish in size after menopause.[18] Postmenopausal increase in size of the uterus may result from the aforementioned secondary changes but should always cause one to suspect sarcomatous change. However, sarcomatous change is rare, occurring in less than 0.3 per cent of patients.[28]

Endometrial Polyps. The common endometrial polyp is composed of an immature type of endometrium that is unresponsive to progesterone. The incidence is difficult to assess, because polyps may go unrecognized at curettage. Although most polyps are asymptomatic, the usual symptom is uterine bleeding. In rare cases, a polyp will have a pedicle long enough to allow it to protrude beyond the cervix or even the vagina. In premenopausal women, polyps have very little premalignant potential. Although this is also true of postmenopausal polyps, there is a 10 to 15 per cent association with malignant disease in the postmenopausal group.[18]

Sonographically, polyps cause a prominent central uterine cavity echo. Polyps are also a cause of uterine enlargement.[37]

Endometrial Carcinoma. Carcinoma of the endometrium constitutes 90 per cent of malignant neoplasms of the uterine corpus[18] and is the most common invasive gynecologic neoplasm.[12, 18] In contrast to myomas, the onset of endometrial carcinoma typically occurs after age 50.[12] The etiology is unknown, but the tumor seems to be associated with estrogen stimulation, as in nulliparity, failure of ovulation, late menopause, and obesity.[12] Postmenopausal bleeding is an important symptom that should raise the possibility of endometrial carcinoma. Overall, one third of women with postmenopausal bleeding have underlying malignant neoplasms, and one half of these malignant neoplasms are endometrial carcinomas.[32]

The typical ultrasound appearance of endometrial carcinoma is an enlarged uterus with irregular areas of low-level echoes and bizarre clusters of high-intensity echoes (Fig. 25). Occasionally, local invasion can be demonstrated.[45] In a study of 21 patients with endometrial carcinoma, 71 per cent had uterine enlargement, 62 per cent had a bulbous or lobular uterine contour, and 48 per cent had hypoechoic or inhomogeneous texture.[32] The findings on an ultrasonographic scan of endometrial carcinoma, other than local invasion, are those of leiomyomata.[32, 42, 45] Worse yet, 35 per cent of patients with endometrial carcinoma also have myomas.[42]

Nevertheless, ultrasound has a role in the treatment of endometrial carcinoma by helping to separate carcinoma limited to the uterus (Stages I and II) from carcinoma extending beyond the uterus (Stages III and IV). A lobular uterine contour was associated with advanced disease in four of five patients; a normal or bulbous contour was noted in 15 of 16 patients with local disease. Furthermore, all four patients with inhomogeneous echogenicity had advanced disease, and 16 of 17 patients with homogeneous texture had local disease. Seven of 21 patients had a normal pelvic sonogram.[32]

Ultrasound may also aid in the planning of intracavitary radiotherapy. In the pretreatment phase, ultrasound assessment of uterine size and shape allows the selection of an appropriate applicator. Postinsertion scans allow calculation of critical doses and localization of incorrectly placed applicators.[3]

Endometrial carcinoma may obstruct the endometrial cavity, resulting in hydrometra, pyometra, or hematometra.[32, 37] There is also a reported case of hematometra secondary to radiation-induced cervical stenosis with an endometrial carcinoma in the wall of the distended uterus.[33]

Leiomyosarcoma. Leiomyosarcoma is the most frequent uterine sarcoma,[12] but sarcomas account for only 3 per cent of uterine tumors.[42] As a group, sarcomas are the most lethal of uterine tumors. Uterine bleeding is the usual symptom, but symptoms may be absent. Most leiomyosarcomas are believed to arise in preexisting leiomyomata.[28]

Sonographically, these tumors typically show large areas of degeneration, bizarre patches of high intensity echoes, invasion of surrounding structures, and even distant metastases.[42] In the absence of the latter two findings, they are indistinguishable from myomas. Leiomyosarcoma is rarely diagnosed preoperatively.[18]

Cervical Carcinoma. Once the most common invasive gynecologic neoplasm, carcinoma of the cervix is now second only to endometrial carcinoma in incidence.[12] This tumor typically occurs in women between 45 and 55 years of age. The etiology is unknown but among the factors that appear to be related to the development of cervical carcinoma are multiparity, early onset of sexual relations, and intercourse with uncircumcised males.[12]

The ultrasound scan usually shows a solid retrovesical mass (Fig. 26),[43] and is indistinguishable from a cervical myoma. Ultrasound may also detect parametrial or paracervical thickening of soft tissue, involvement of the pelvic sidewalls, extension into the bladder, and pelvic adenopathy.[42] Ultrasound is thus useful not for histologic diagnosis but for staging of cervical carcinoma.[13] However, computed tomography is preferable for staging.[42] Cervical carcinoma also causes hydrometra, pyometra, or hematometra.[32, 37]

Differentiation of Benign and Malignant Neoplasms. Simply put, ultrasound usually cannot distinguish myomas from malignant uterine lesions. The pres-

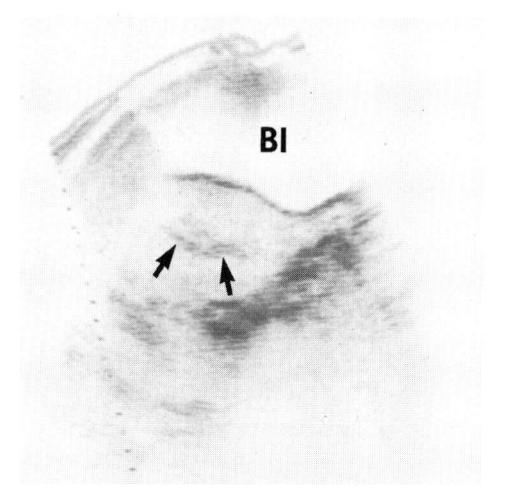

Figure 25. Endometrial carcinoma. The uterus is enlarged and bulbous on this longitudinal scan. There are clusters of high amplitude echoes (arrows) in the region of the central cavity echo. This appearance is difficult to differentiate from other causes of a prominent central echo. See Figures 15 and 16.

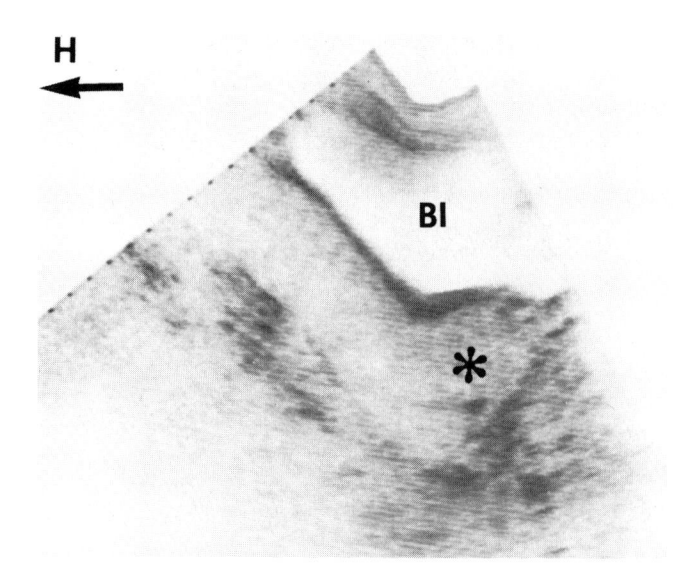

Figure 26. Carcinoma of the cervix. There is an echogenic cervical mass (*asterisk*), reversing the normal predominance of the postpubertal uterine fundus.

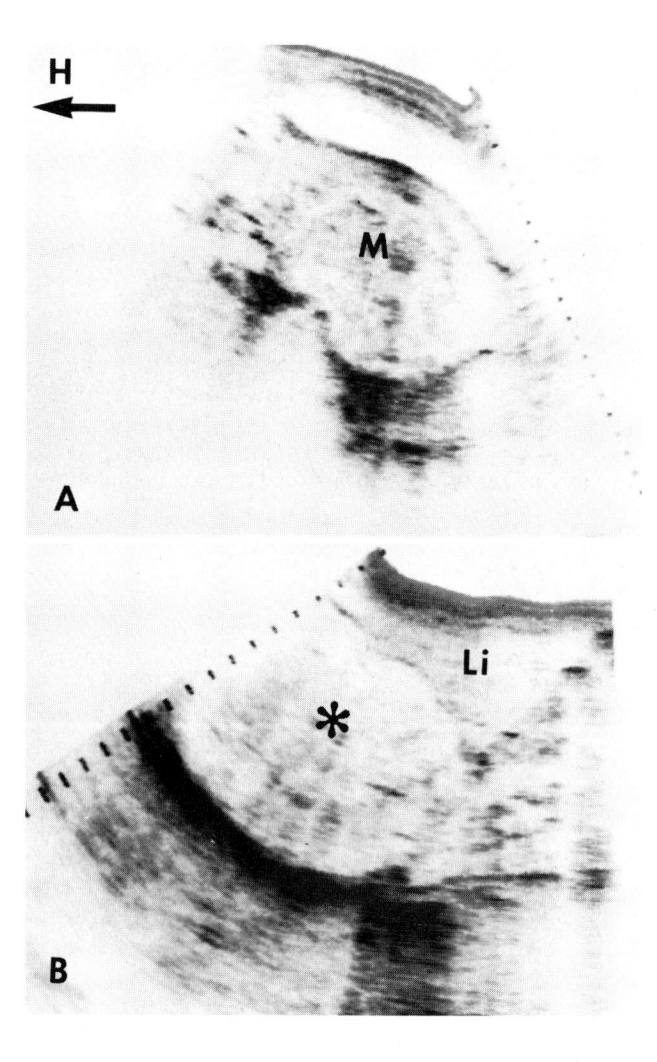

Figure 27. Difficulty in differentiating benign from malignant uterine masses. *A*, There is a large, inhomogeneous mass (M) deforming the uterine contour on this longitudinal scan. *B*, Longitudinal scan of the liver (Li) demonstrates a large mass (*asterisk*) posterosuperiorly. Because of this liver lesion, a malignant uterine neoplasm with hepatic metastasis was suspected. The patient underwent total abdominal hysterectomy, and was found to have multiple leiomyomata. At angiography, the liver mass proved to be a cavernous hemangioma.

ence of patchy, high-amplitude echoes in malignant neoplasms is often emphasized, but similar echoes occur with fatty degeneration or calcification of myomas. The overwhelmingly greater incidence of myomas means that most patients with patchy, high-amplitude intrauterine echoes will have myomas, not malignant neoplasms. Similarly, invasion of surrounding structures is said to be diagnostic of malignant disease. However, myomas are a common cause of the indefinite uterus, in which a homogeneous pelvic mass obscures the borders between pelvic organs,[2] simulating invasion of adjacent structures.

Nevertheless, some sonographic guidelines can be formulated. Applied with caution, these findings raise the possibility of malignant disease: (1) rapid increase in size of a uterine mass (though myomas also behave this way in pregnancy[16] and anovulatory menstrual cycles[40]), (2) postmenopausal increase in size of a uterine mass (though most such patients will have degenerating myomas[18]), (3) extrauterine extension (see preceding), and (4) distant metastases with a uterine mass. The latter criterion is the best indicator of uterine malignant disease but is not foolproof (Fig. 27).

Nonneoplastic Disorders

Endometrial Hyperplasia. Endometrial hyperplasia is a spectrum of histologic changes of the endometrium produced by unopposed estrogen stimulation. Endometrial hyperplasia is the most common cause of uterine bleeding. It occurs during the menstrual years as well as in postmenopausal women. In the majority of patients, the microscopic pattern is frankly benign. Adenomatous hyperplasia, characterized by glandular proliferation into the surrounding stroma, occurs in a small proportion of patients. When there is associated cellular atypia, the histologic appearance may be difficult to separate from endometrial carcinoma.[18]

As with endometrial polyps, ultrasound may demonstrate a prominent central uterine cavity echo (see Fig. 15).

Adenomyosis. Adenomyosis is characterized by ingrowths of endometrium into the myometrium, with glandular and stromal tissue among the uterine muscle fibers.[44] It occurs mainly in parous women beyond the age of 40. Adenomyosis is usually asymptomatic, but there may be uterine bleeding and pain. Adenomyosis has an overall incidence of 8 to 27 per cent,[46] and is found in 25 to 40 per cent of hysterectomy specimens.[42] Although also called internal endometriosis, adenomyosis appears to be a separate disease.[46] Nevertheless, there is associated endometriosis in 13 per cent of patients with adenomyosis.[44]

Adenomyosis occurs in two distinct forms; it may be diffuse or encapsulated. In the latter circumstance, it is called an adenomyoma. It is generally accepted that adenomyosis results from ingrowth of endometrial tissue rather than from embryonic cell rests.[46]

In an ultrasound study of 25 patients with endometriosis, nine had intrauterine changes of adenomyosis. Characteristically, irregular cystic spaces disrupt the homogeneity of the uterine texture (Fig. 28). Pathologic confirmation in four patients revealed blood-containing cavities.[44] Adenomyosis may also cause uterine enlargement.[37] The differentiation of adenomyosis, either diffuse or encapsulated, from myomas may be difficult.[10]

Hydrometra, Pyometra, and Hematometra. Hydrometrocolpos is the accumulation of secretions in the vagina and uterus caused by obstruction of the genital tract. Hydrometra is an accumulation of fluid limited to the uterus; hydrocolpos is an accumulation of fluid limited to the vagina.[47] Superimposed infection is called pyometra. At puberty, menstruation results in hematometra.

The causes of accumulation of uterine fluid fall into two distinct categories, depending on the patient's age. In the young patient, the usual cause is a congenital abnormality of the genital tract. If there is hydrometrocolpos, the abnormality may be an intact hymen, vaginal membrane, or vaginal atresia.[47] Hydrometra may result from a duplication anomaly of the uterus with obstruction of one uterine horn. In this age group, accumulation of uterine fluid may be associated with renal agenesis.[19]

In the older age group, hydrometra, pyometra, or hematometra usually results from uterine or cervical malignant disease[32, 37] or from radiation-induced cervical stenosis.[33] Delayed onset of hydrometra after treatment of cervical carcinoma is

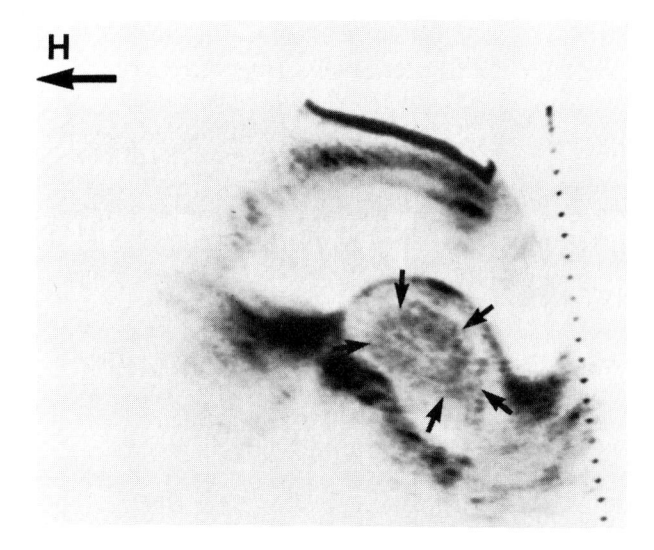

Figure 28. Adenomyosis. Longitudinal sonogram shows inhomogeneous increased echogenicity (*arrows*) surrounding the echolucent endometrium. There are small hypoechoic areas within the zone of increased echogenicity, probably resulting from blood-filled cavities within the myometrium.

usually *not* associated with recurrent tumor.[37] Adhesions after surgery may also cause uterine distention.[9]

Typically, ultrasound demonstrates cystic enlargement of the uterine cavity. There may be layering of echogenic material.[33] Hydrometra and pyometra are not usually distinguishable by ultrasound.[37]

Incompetent Cervix. Incompetent cervix is defined as premature dilatation of the endocervical canal in the absence of labor.[22] This occurs in 0.2 to 2 per 1000 pregnancies. The causes include previous obstetrical trauma, previous dilatation and curettage or cone biopsy, and anatomic variations leading to defective structure of the cervical ring.[36] Patients with incompetent cervix may carry their pregnancies to term, but, more often, midtrimester abortion occurs.[30] If the diagnosis can be established early in pregnancy, placing tape or a purse-string suture at the cervical os saves 58 to 77 per cent of the fetuses (Fig. 29).[36]

Detection of the incompetent cervix by ultrasound is based on the demonstration of a shortened cervix,[1] sometimes with fluid or fetal parts in the endocervical canal.[22] The lower limit of normal for cervical length is 3 cm (Fig. 30).[1] The method of scanning is crucial, because a full bladder may compress the opposing cervical walls, obscuring the diagnosis of incompetency. When incompetent cervix is a clinical consideration, scans after partial emptying of the bladder must be obtained (Fig. 31).

A sonolucency is frequently demonstrated within the cervical canal in pa-

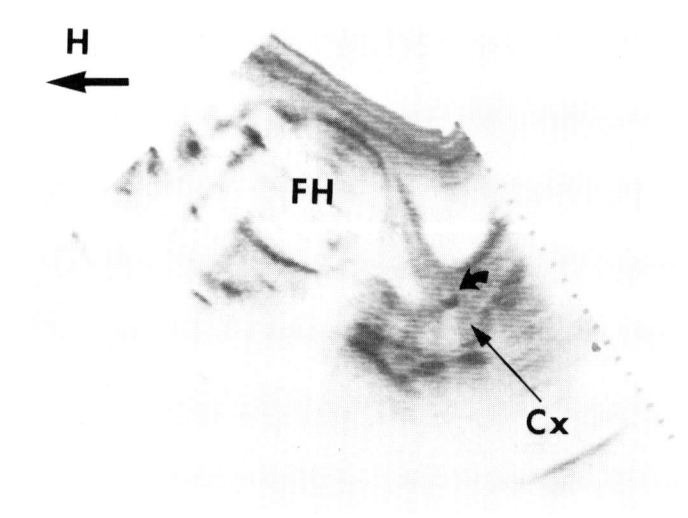

Figure 29. Cerclage suture. Longitudinal scan of a patient with incompetent cervix following cerclage demonstrates the echogenic suture (*curved arrow*) maintaining closure of the cervix (Cx). FH, fetal head.

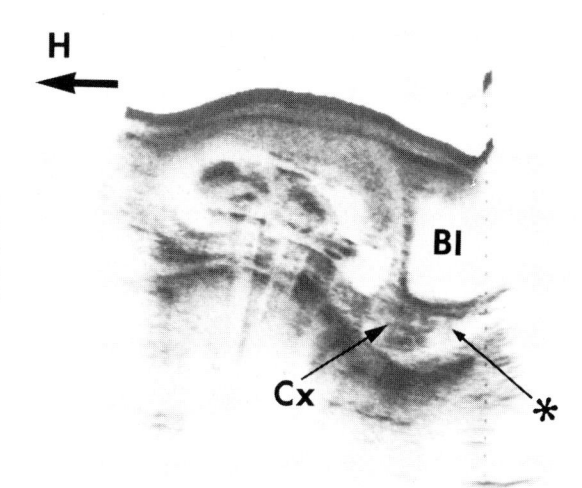

Figure 30. Normal cervical length. On a longitudinal postvoid sonogram of a gravid uterus, there has been reflux of urine into the vagina (*asterisk*), so that the cervix (Cx) is outlined by fluid at both the internal and external os. The normal cervix exceeds 3 cm in length.

tients with normal cervical length. This probably represents the mucous plug, and these patients generally deliver at term. The normal length of the cervix distinguishes this entity from incompetent cervix.[1]

At the far end of the spectrum of cervical shortening is prolapse of the amniotic sac ("hourglass membranes") (Fig. 32). This is probably a separate entity representing the sonographic picture of abortion in progress.[30] In one study, none of five patients

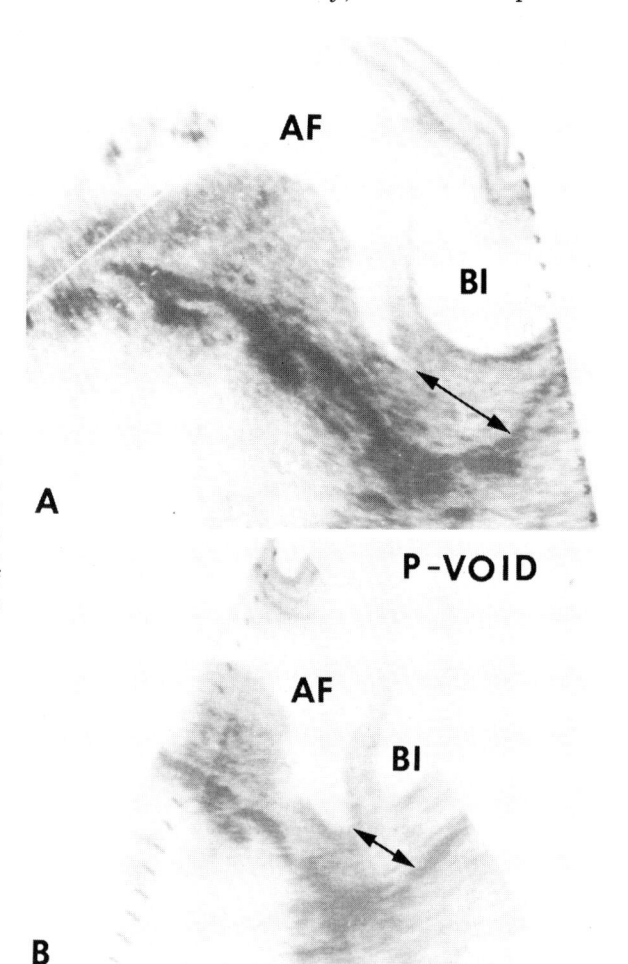

Figure 31. Importance of a postvoid scan for incompetent cervix. *A*, With the bladder (Bl) relatively full, the opposing cervical walls are compressed and the cervix appears to be normal in length (*arrow*). *B*, Following emptying of the bladder, the true cervical length (*arrow*) is considerably shorter, establishing the diagnosis of incompetent cervix. (Same patient as in Figure 29, prior to cerclage.) AF, amniotic fluid.

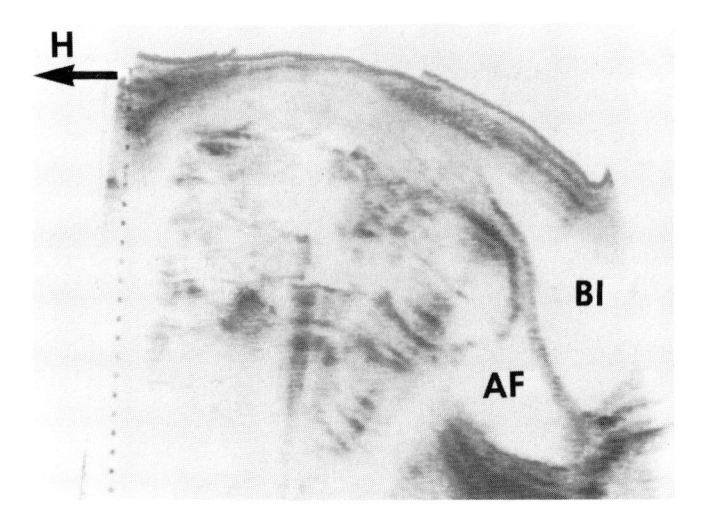

Figure 32. Hourglass membranes. There is prolapse of the amniotic sac (AF) through the effaced and dilated cervix, with virtually no closed cervix demonstrated. The so-called hourglass appearance results from the prolapsed amniotic sac below and the intrauterine cavity above, with the internal cervical os serving as the "waist" of the hourglass. This patient had a spontaneous abortion shortly after the sonogram was obtained.

with hourglass membranes had a history of incompetent cervix, and all were spontaneously delivered of an infant shortly after being scanned. A similar hourglass appearance can result from a lower uterine contraction or myoma. As with incompetent cervix, cervical length is the key to differentiating hourglass membranes from its simulators.

CONCLUSION

Ultrasound has some limitations in diagnosing uterine abnormalities. It fails to detect some uterine conditions (such as Asherman's syndrome) and is of limited value in others (such as differentiating benign and malignant uterine neoplasms). Nevertheless, ultrasound is an important tool in diagnosing and managing various uterine disorders.

REFERENCES

1. Bernstine, R. L., Lee, S. H., Crawford, W. L., et al.: Sonographic evaluation of the incompetent cervix. J. Clin. Ultrasound, 9:417–420, 1981.
2. Bowie, J. D.: Ultrasound of gynecologic pelvic masses: The indefinite uterus and other patterns associated with diagnostic error. J. Clin. Ultrasound, 5:323–328, 1977.
3. Brascho, D. J., Kim, R. Y., and Wilson, E. E.: Use of ultrasonography in planning intracavitary radiotherapy of endometrial carcinoma. Radiology, 129:163–167, 1978.
4. Buttery, B., and Davison, G.: The dynamic uterus revealed by time-lapse echography. J. Clin. Ultrasound, 6:19–22, 1978.
5. Callen, P. W.: Ultrasonographic evaluation of pelvic disease. In Goldberg, H. I. (ed.): Interventional Radiology and Diagnostic Imaging Modalities. Department of Radiology, University of California, San Francisco, 1982, p. 209–214.
6. Callen, P. W., DeMartini, W. J., and Filly, R. A.: The central uterine cavity echo: A useful anatomic sign in the ultrasonographic evaluation of the female pelvis. Radiology, 131:187–190, 1979.
7. Cochrane, W. J., and Thomas, M. A.: Ultrasound diagnosis of gynecologic pelvic masses. Radiology, 110:649–654, 1974.
8. Donald, I., MacVicar, J., and Brown, T. G.: Investigation of abdominal masses by pulsed ultrasound. Lancet, 1:1188–1194, 1958.
9. Fisch, A. E., and Jacobson, J. B.: Ultrasound findings in segmental uterine distension. J. Clin. Ultrasound, 4:209–211, 1976.
10. Fleischer, A. C., James, A. E., Jr., Millis, J. B., et al.: Differential diagnosis of pelvic masses by gray scale sonography. Am. J. Roentgenol., 131:469–476, 1978.
11. Fried, A. M., Oliff, M., Wilson, E. A., et al.: Uterine anomalies associated with renal agenesis: Role of gray scale ultrasonography. Am. J. Roentgenol., 131:973–975, 1978.
12. Gompel, C., and Silverberg, S. G.: Pathology in Gynecology and Obstetrics. Philadelphia, J. B. Lippincott Co., 1977.
13. Gottesfeld, K. R.: The role of ultrasound in gynecologic diagnosis. Clin. Diagn. Ultrasound, 2:207–227, 1979.
14. Green, W. M., Berry, S., and Wilkinson, G.: Twin pregnancy in a bicornuate uterus. J. Clin. Ultrasound, 7:303–304, 1979.
15. Hall, D. A., Hann, L. E., Ferrucci, J. T., Jr., et al.: Sonographic morphology of the normal menstrual cycle. Radiology, 133:185–188, 1979.
16. Hassani, S., and Bard, R.: Ultrasonic changes of uterine fibroids in pregnancy. Abstract presented at the annual meeting of the American Institute of Ultrasound in Medicine, San Francisco, California, 1979.
17. Jones, T. B., Fleischer, A. C., Daniell, J. F., et al.: Sonographic characteristics of congenital uterine abnormalities and associated pregnancy. J. Clin. Ultrasound, 8:435–437, 1980.

18. Jones, H. W., Jr., and Jones, G. S.: Novak's Textbook of Gynecology. Baltimore, Williams and Wilkins, 1981.
19. Kangarloo, H., Sarti, D. A., and Sample, W. F.: Ultrasound of the pediatric pelvis. Semin. Ultrasound, *1*:51–60, 1980.
20. Kaufman, R. H., Binder, G. L., Gray, P. M., Jr., et al.: Upper genital tract changes associated with exposure in utero to diethylstilbestrol. Am. J. Obstet. Gynecol., *128*:51–59, 1977.
21. Laing, F. C.,: Sonography of a persistently retroverted gravid uterus. Am. J. Roentgenol., *136*:413–414, 1981.
22. Laing, F. C.: Diagnostic dilemmas in obstetrical and gynecologic ultrasound. Syllabus for the Categorical Course in Ultrasonography, Presented at the annual meeting of the American Roentgen Ray Society, San Francisco, California, March 22–27, 1981, p. 229–251.
23. Laing, F. C., Filly, R. A., Marks, W. M., et al.: Ultrasonic demonstration of endometrial fluid collections unassociated with pregnancy. Radiology, *137*:471–474, 1980.
24. Lawson, T. L., and Albarelli, J. N.: Diagnosis of gynecologic pelvic masses by gray scale ultrasonography: Analysis of specificity and accuracy. Am. J. Roentgenol., *128*:1003–1006, 1977.
25. Levi, S., and Delval, R.: Value of ultrasonic diagnosis of gynecological tumors in 370 surgical cases. Acta Obstet. Gynecol. Scand., *55*:261–266, 1976.
26. Lippe, B. M., and Sample, W. F.: Pelvic ultrasonography in pediatric and adolescent endocrine disorders. J. Pediatr., *92*:897–902, 1978.
27. Marks, W. M., Filly, R. A., Callen, P. W., et al.: The decidual cast of ectopic pregnancy: A confusing ultrasonographic appearance. Radiology, *133*:451–454, 1979.
28. Mattingly, R. F.: TeLinde's Operative Gynecology. Philadelphia, J. B. Lippincott Co., 1977.
29. McArdle, C. R., and Berezin, A. F.: Ultrasound demonstration of uterus subseptus. J. Clin. Ultrasound, *8*:139–141, 1980.
30. McGahan, J. P., Phillips, H. E., and Bowen, M. S.: Prolapse of the amniotic sac ("hourglass membranes"): Ultrasound appearance. Radiology, *140*:463–466, 1981.
31. Miller, E. I., Thomas, R. H., and Lines, P.: The atrophic postmenopausal uterus. J. Clin. Ultrasound, *5*:261–263, 1977.
32. Requard, C. K., Wicks, J. D., and Mettler, F. A., Jr.: Ultrasonography in the staging of endometrial adenocarcinoma. Radiology, *140*:781–785, 1981.
33. Ruhe, A. H., and Mulder, B. D.: Gravity-dependent layering in primary endometrial carcinoma of the uterus. J. Clin. Ultrasound, *6*:193–194, 1978.
34. Sample, W. F.: The unsoftened portion of the uterus: A pitfall in gray-scale ultrasound studies during mid-trimester pregnancy. Radiology, *126*:227–230, 1978.
35. Sample, W. F., Lippe, B. M., and Gyepes, M. T.: Gray-scale ultrasonography of the normal female pelvis. Radiology, *125*:477–483, 1977.
36. Sarti, D. A., Sample, W. F., Hobel, C. J., et al.: Ultrasonic visualization of a dilated cervix during pregnancy. Radiology, *130*:417–420, 1979.
37. Scott, W. W., Jr., Rosenshein, N. B., Siegelman, S. S., et al.: The obstructed uterus. Radiology, *141*:767–770, 1981.
38. Shenker, L., and Brickman, F. E.: Bicornuate uterus with incomplete vaginal septum and unilateral renal agenesis. Radiology, *133*:455–457, 1979.
39. Simonds, B. D.: An approach to pelvic diagnosis. Semin. Ultrasound, *1*:61–68, 1980.
40. Smith, J. P., Weiser, E. B., Karnei, R. F., Jr., et al.: Ultrasonography of rapidly growing uterine leiomyomata associated with anovulatory cycles. Radiology, *134*:713–716, 1980.
41. Viscomi, G. N., Gonzalez, R., and Taylor, K. J. W.,: Ultrasound detection of uterine abnormalities after diethylstilbestrol (DES) exposure. Radiology, *136*:733–735, 1980.
42. Walsh, J. W., Brewer, W. H., and Schneider, V.: Ultrasound diagnosis in diseases of the uterine corpus and cervix. Semin. Ultrasound, *1*:30–40, 1980.
43. Walsh, J. W., Rosenfield, A. T., Jaffe, C. C., et al.: Prospective comparison of ultrasound and computed tomography in the evaluation of gynecologic pelvic masses. Am. J. Roentgenol., *131*:955–960, 1978.
44. Walsh, J. W., Taylor, K. J. W., and Rosenfield, A. T.: Gray scale ultrasonography in the diagnosis of endometriosis and adenomyosis. Am. J. Roentgenol., *132*:87–90, 1979.
45. Walsh, J. W., Taylor, K. J. W., Wasson, J. F. M., et al.: Gray-scale ultrasound in 204 proved gynecologic masses: Accuracy and specific diagnostic criteria. Radiology, *130*:391–397, 1979.
46. Wharton, L. R., Jr.: Endometriosis. In Mattingly, R. F. (ed.): TeLinde's Operative Gynecology. Philadelphia, J. B. Lippincott Co., 1977.
47. Wilson, D. A., Stacy, T. M., and Smith, E. I.: Ultrasound diagnosis of hydrocolpos and hydrometrocolpos. Radiology, *128*:451–454, 1978.
48. Wilson, R. L., and Worthen, N. J.: Ultrasonic demonstration of myometrial contractions in intrauterine pregnancy. Am. J. Roentgenol., *132*:243–247, 1979.
49. Zanetti, E., Ferrari, L. R., and Rossi, G.: Classification and radiographic features of uterine malformations: Hysterosalpingographic study. Br. J. Radiol., *51*:161–170, 1978.

15

Ultrasonography in the Detection of Intrauterine Contraceptive Devices

Barry H. Gross, M.D., and Peter W. Callen, M.D.

Intrauterine contraceptive devices (IUD's) constitute an important method of preventing pregnancy. It is estimated that worldwide, more than 50 million are in use, with up to 3 million women using IUD's in the United States.[18]

To be effective at preventing pregnancy, an IUD must be appropriately positioned within the uterus. Most IUD's have a vaginal marker thread to verify intrauterine position. When the thread is no longer present on physical examination, the IUD is presumed to be "misplaced." Disappearance of the thread has four possible explanations:[3, 9] (1) expulsion of the IUD, often not noticed by the patient;[3] (2) perforation of the IUD into or through the uterine wall, also often asymptomatic;[3] (3) detachment of the thread; (4) intrauterine migration of the thread. Expulsion and perforation account for less than 25 per cent of missing threads,[3, 8, 9, 13] but their detection is essential to prevent unwanted pregnancy.

Verification of the position of the IUD may be performed by "invasively" attempting to retrieve the IUD when no thread is seen, or by attempting to image the IUD by non-invasive radiologic means. Among the radiographic techniques that have been used to locate missing IUD's are obtaining: radiographs of the pelvis, radiographs after insertion of a metal probe into the uterine cavity, and hysterosalpingography.[9]

Ultrasonography was first used to identify IUD's in 1966.[26] Using a finger probe to apply pulsed high frequency sound waves transvaginally, Winter correctly identified the presence or absence of an IUD in 45 of 47 patients.[26] A major advantage of ultrasound imaging of IUD's is that the uterus can be scanned without radiating a possible early intrauterine pregnancy. Technical advances since 1966 have made ultrasound the most optimal method of choice for evaluating IUD's.

BACKGROUND

Currently marketed IUD's have a net pregnancy rate of 1 to 6 per 100 women by the end of the first year of use.[14] The mortality rate associated with the use of IUD's in the United States is 1 to 10 per million woman-years of use, with complications requiring hospitalization in 0.3 to 1 per 100 woman-years.[14] IUD's have a higher morbidity rate and a lower mortality rate than oral contraceptives, but pregnancy exceeds both in terms of morbidity and mortality.[14]

IUD's now in use include the Lippes Loop, double coil, Copper-7, Copper-T, and Progestasert (Fig. 1). The copper and hormonal IUD's have lower expulsion rates and produce less menstrual bleeding without significantly altered pregnancy rates. The disadvantage of these IUD's is their limited time of activity. The Copper-7 is currently approved for only 3 years of use, and the Progestasert for 1 year. Other types of IUD's have been removed from the market for various reasons. These include closed devices such as the Birnberg bow (risk of bowel obstruction following uterine perforation), spirals (trauma to male partner during intercourse), the Majzlin spring (embedment and difficult removal), and the Dalkon shield (mid-trimester septic abortion).[14]

IDENTIFICATION OF IUD'S

Early studies on sonographic identification of IUD's achieved high sensitivity[3, 8, 9, 13, 15, 16, 25] by relying on the dem-

249

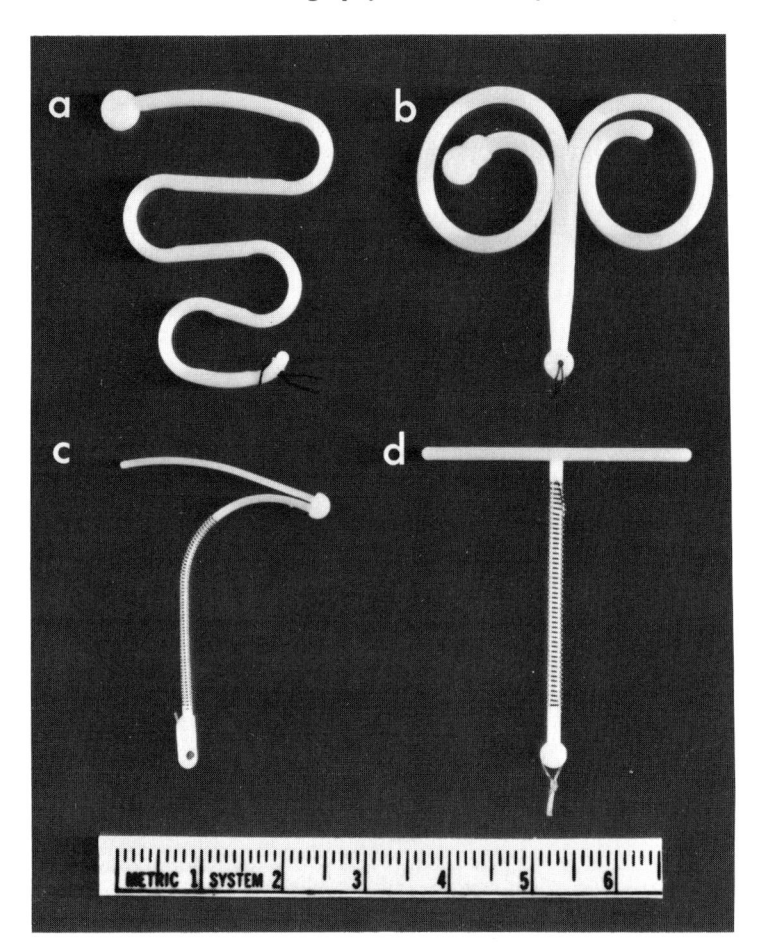

Figure 1. Commonly used intrauterine devices (IUD's). *A*, Lippes Loop. *B*, Double coil. *C*, Copper-7. *D*, Copper-T. (*Note:* Progestasert, not pictured, is a T-shaped device.)

onstration of high amplitude intrauterine echoes[9, 25] or characteristic type-specific echo patterns.[3, 8] With the advent of gray-scale ultrasound, more sophisticated criteria have been developed.[2] They are *type-specific morphology, acoustic shadowing, entrance-exit reflections, and high amplitude echoes.*

Type-specific morphology is the most specific finding.[10] With a Lippes Loop, one should see five interrupted moderate-to-high amplitude echoes on a longitudinal scan of the uterus (Fig. 2). These echoes represent the transected rungs of the Lippes Loop. With a Copper-7, longitudinal scans reveal a moderate amplitude echo from the short limb and a longer, higher amplitude echo from the long copper-wrapped limb (Fig. 2). In a retrospective review of 50 consecutive patients referred for localization of IUD's, type-specific morphology could be demonstrated in 32 of 34 Lippes Loops (94 per cent) and 13 of 16 Copper-7's (81 per cent).[2] The five patients in whom morphology was not visible all had retroverted uteri.

All commonly used IUD's produce *acoustic shadowing* when scanned in vitro (Fig. 3).[2] However, as with gallstones[7] and renal calculi,[20] the ability of ultrasound to demonstrate the shadow depends on the relationship of the IUD to the acoustic beam (Fig. 4). If the peripheral edge of the beam encounters the IUD, there will be no acoustic shadow. This results from averaging of the shadow with adjacent soft tissue. Beam width versus IUD diameter is also important in the demonstration of shadowing. Narrowing beam width by using a higher frequency or a focused transducer may aid in the detection of an acoustic shadow.[7] If the IUD falls within this narrow portion of the beam the sound will be absorbed and reflected, resulting in an acoustic shadow. Finally, high gain setting may obscure an acoustic shadow, whereas low overall gain or disproportionately low far gain may bring out a subtle shadow.[20]

The importance of acoustic shadowing lies in the fact that it can be demonstrated in a high percentage of patients with an IUD in place (Fig. 5). Acoustic shadowing is not seen emanating from the normal uterus. In a recent study, a shadow was demonstrated in 46 of 50 patients with IUD's, while there was no shadowing in 200 patients without IUD's.[2] Therefore, when a shadow is not visible in a patient thought to have an intrauterine contraceptive device, one should rescan with transducers of higher frequency and varying focal zones (narrowest portion of the ultrasound beam) and with lower overall gain setting.

Entrance-exit reflections have been noted in 65 per cent of patients with IUD's (Fig. 6).[10] This finding may also be helpful in identifying an IUD and in differentiating it from the normal central uterine cavity echo. The source of this echo pattern is not proved, but it is felt to result from reflection of sound at both the anterior and posterior interfaces of the IUD. As with acoustic shadowing, entrance-exit reflections are better seen and are more discretely demonstrated using higher frequency transducers.[2]

High amplitude echoes alone constitute the least reliable criterion for identifying an IUD. Prominence of the central uterine cavity echo from any cause may simulate an IUD and this prominence at times may be related solely to technical factors. Much less often, acoustic shadowing and entrance-exit reflections can occur in patients without IUD's (Fig. 7). Even apparent type-specific morphology will on rare occasions be seen in the absence of an IUD.[2] However, the four criteria as a whole provide

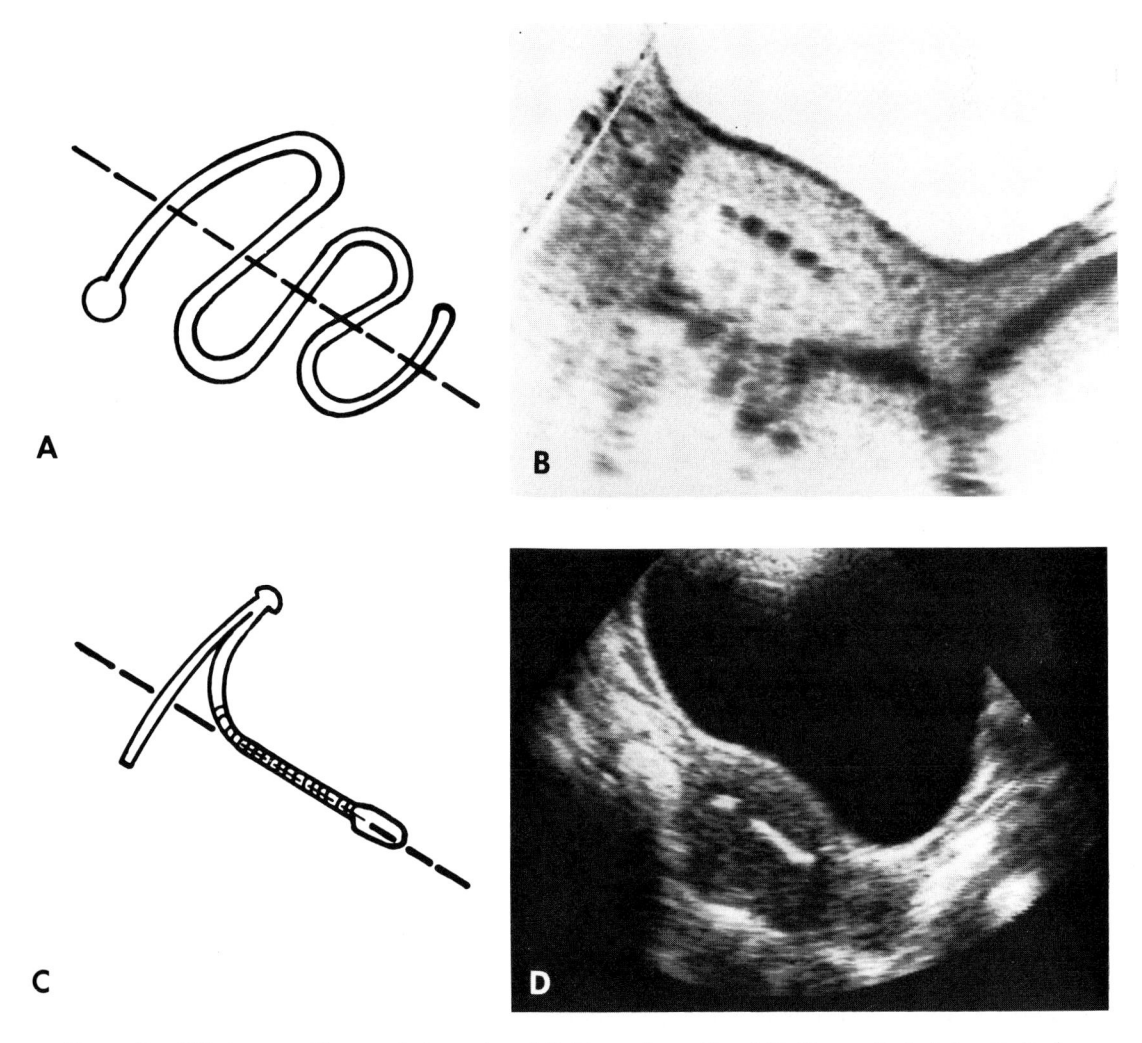

Figure 2. IUD type-specific morphology. *A* and *B*, Lippes loop. *C* and *D*, Copper-7. *A*, A longitudinal scan intersects the loop five times. *B*, Resultant characteristic morphology. *C*, A longitudinal scan intersects the short limb and then traverses the long, copper-wrapped limb. *D*, Characteristic sonographic morphology.

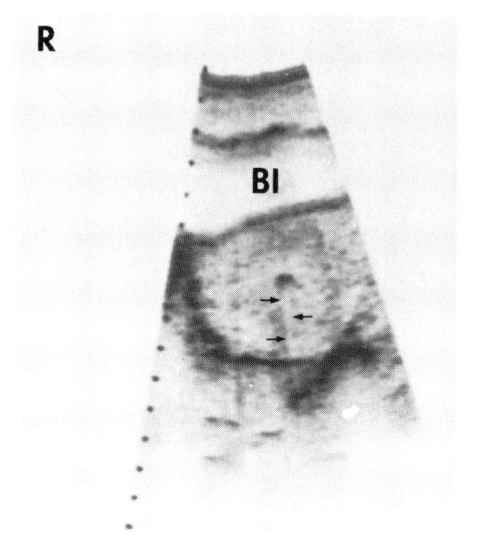

Figure 3. Transverse sonogram of a Copper-7 IUD demonstrating acoustic shadowing (*arrows*). Bl, bladder.

an accurate means of identifying the presence and, in most patients, the specific type of an IUD.

LOCALIZATION OF IUD'S

As previously noted, if an IUD is to be used for contraception it should be positioned appropriately within the uterus. More specifically, it should be in the endometrial cavity of the uterine fundus.[14, 24]

Attention should be directed to the location of an IUD once its presence is established by ultrasound.

In patients without IUD's, the normal central uterine cavity echo is often surrounded by a 2 to 3 mm zone of low amplitude echoes. This is felt to represent the endometrium.[1] Demonstration of this hypoechoic halo around an IUD verifies its endometrial position (Fig. 8). Such a halo was demonstrated in 36 of 50 consecutive patients referred for IUD localization.[2] It was more frequently seen with Copper-7's (14 of 16) than with Lippes Loops (22 of 34).

COMPLICATIONS OF IUD'S

Expulsion

The expulsion rate for IUD's varies from 4 to 18 of every 100 users by the end of the first year. Expulsion is most likely to occur during the first month after insertion, especially during the first menstruation after insertion.[14] As previously stated, expulsion may go unnoticed.[3]

Incomplete expulsion (IUD in the lower uterine segment) or perforation (IUD embedded in the myometrium) places the user at risk for pregnancy.[14] Displacement into the lower uterine segment is readily diagnosed by ultrasound.[24] Gray-scale sonography allows a better appreciation of the

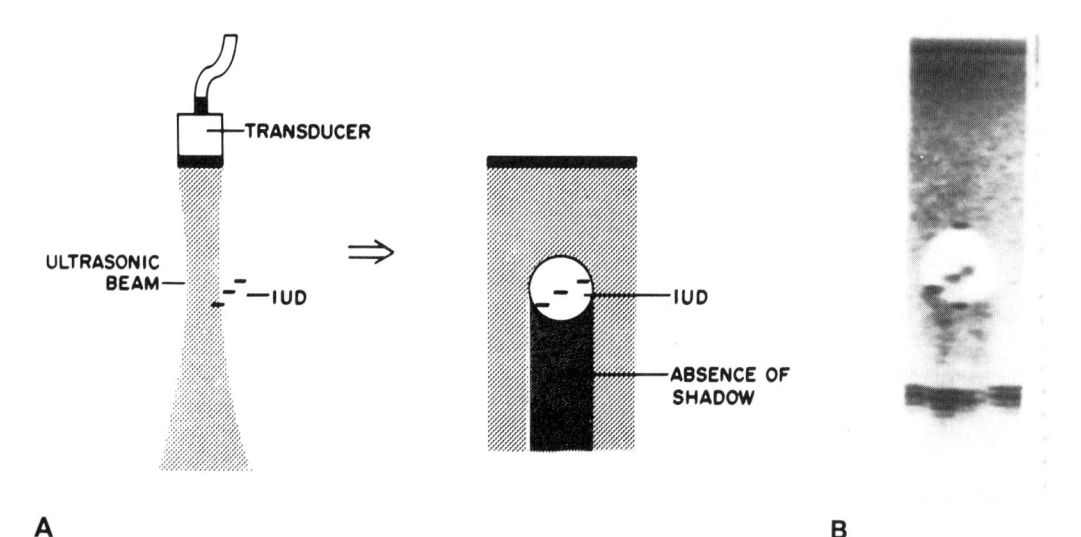

Figure 4. Importance of relationship between IUD and acoustic beam. Scans of an IUD within a gelatin-containing phantom. *A* and *B*, With the IUD at the edge of the acoustic beam, there is no acoustic shadow. *C* and *D*, With the ultrasound transducer repositioned slightly so that the same IUD lies within the "focal zone," acoustic shadows are demonstrated (*arrows*).

C

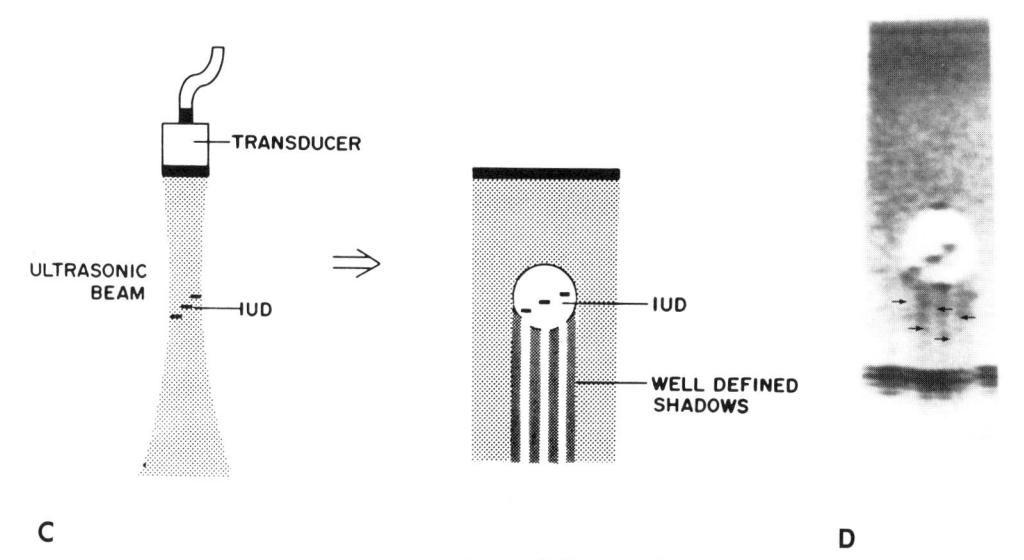

D

Figure 4 (*Continued*)

relationship between IUD and myometrium,[4] so that embedment can also be detected in some instances (Fig. 9).

Perforation

Perforation occurs in up to 8.7 of every 1000 insertions,[14] and is usually asymptomatic.[3, 5, 23] The rate depends mainly on the skill and experience of the person inserting the device and on the design of the IUD and its mechanical inserter. Most perforations probably occur during insertion,[23] and the softer consistency of the early postpartum uterine wall has been implicated as a causative factor.[11] Sharply anteflexed or retroverted uteri, severe cervical stenosis, and congenital uterine anomalies also increase the risk of perforation.[14] Partial perforations are less common. Occasionally, perforation occurs through the wall of the cervix into the upper vagina, particularly with T-shaped and 7-shaped devices.[14]

The most common complication of uterine perforation by an IUD is a normal pregnancy.[3] Closed loop IUD's outside the uterus may cause bowel obstruction,[5, 14, 22] whereas copper IUD's produce an intense reaction in the peritoneal cavity, resulting in dense adhesions.[14, 22] Otherwise, perforated IUD's are typically asymptomatic. Nevertheless, current opinion recommends removal of all extrauterine IUD's.[14]

Using ultrasound, it is very difficult to locate an IUD that has penetrated outside the uterine confines.[6] The difficulty in identification of a perforated IUD lies in the similarity of its echogenicity to that of periuterine soft tissue. At times, shadowing may be seen from echogenic structures outside of the uterus. Caution is advised to avoid the erroneous conclusion that this is due to an IUD (Fig. 10). Nevertheless, in some patients an IUD has been correctly identified in an extrauterine position using

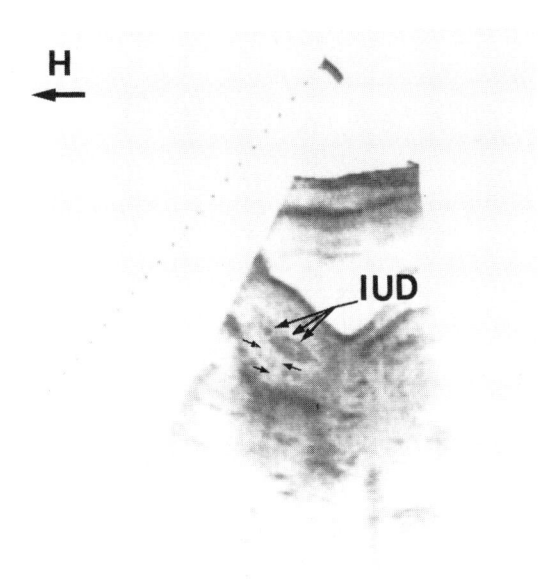

Figure 5. Type-specific morphology is obscured by blood in the endometrial canal, but acoustic shadowing (*short arrows*) confirms the presence of an IUD (*long arrows*). H, head.

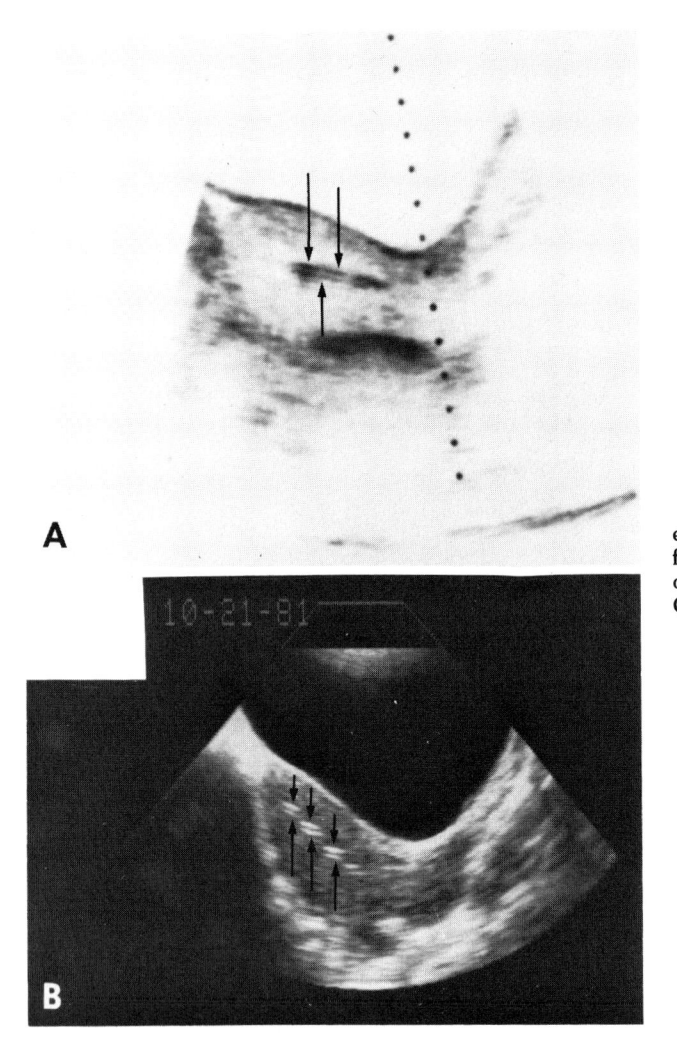

Figure 6. Entrance-exit reflections. This echo pattern probably results from sound reflection at the anterior and posterior inferfaces of the IUD (*arrows*). *A*, Longitudinal scan of Copper-7. *B*, Longitudinal scan of Lippes loop.

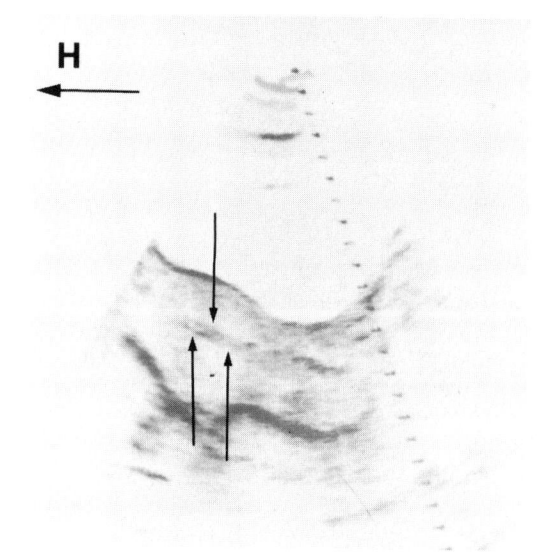

Figure 7. Longitudinal sonogram of the uterus in a patient with retained products of conception simulating entrance-exit reflections (*arrows*). H, head.

ultrasound. In nearly all such patients fluid has surrounded the IUD, making it more apparent.

If a lost IUD cannot be located after careful scanning of the uterus, a plain film of the abdomen and pelvis is recommended. Absence of the IUD confirms unnoticed expulsion, while its presence on the plain film verifies asymptomatic perforation. In equivocal cases, computed tomography (CT) has been suggested for further localization.[19] A digital scout view is obtained, and is used to position the patient for an axial CT scan through the IUD. In one such case, CT clearly showed the IUD outside the uterine wall, just anterior to the rectum.[19]

Pelvic Inflammatory Disease

The occurrence of pelvic inflammatory disease in patients with IUD's was initially

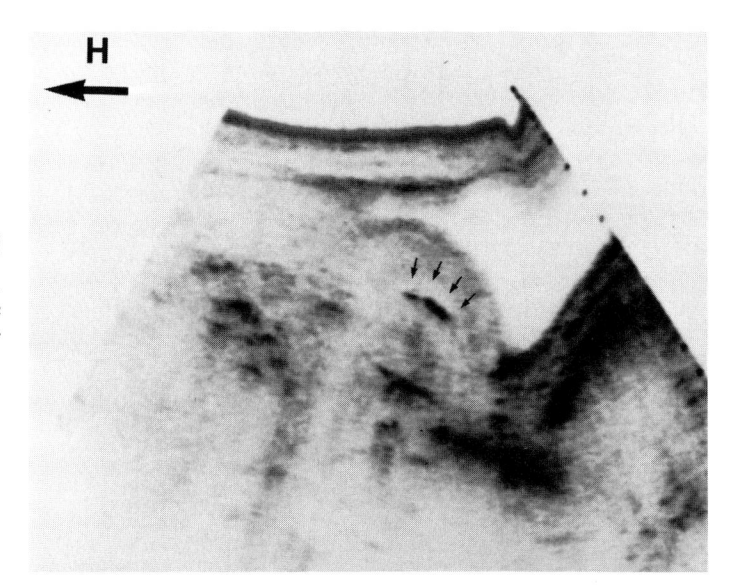

Figure 8. Longitudinal scan of the uterus reveals a sonolucent "halo" (*arrows*) surrounding a Copper-7 IUD. This lucency probably represents the endometrium, and thus verifies appropriate central position of the IUD.

noted by Tietze in 1966.[23] In a cooperative study based on the work of 33 investigators, pelvic inflammatory disease was reported in 606 of 22,403 women with IUD's. In many patients, this represented recurrence of previous pelvic inflammatory disease, so that IUD's were not clearly implicated as a cause of pelvic inflammatory disease.

More recent information suggests an increased risk of pelvic inflammatory disease secondary to IUD's, and this includes a risk of nongonorrheal infections.[14] In one study, young nulliparous women with IUD's had three to five times more infections compared to women in the same age group without IUD's. Most workers feel that there is no added risk from a transcervical appendage. To minimize the risk of pelvic inflammatory disease, IUD's must be sterile and should be inserted properly. Furthermore, insertion is not advised in patients with acute pelvic inflammatory disease or with a history of repeated attacks of pelvic inflammatory disease.

When pelvic inflammatory disease is diagnosed in a woman with an IUD, antibiotic therapy is indicated. The current opinion is to leave the IUD in place, removing it only if striking improvement does not occur promptly.[14] Ultrasound is useful, as in patients with pelvic inflammatory disease unrelated to IUD's, for the demonstration of tubo-ovarian abscesses (Fig. 11).[21]

Miscellaneous

IUD's may be associated with an increased risk of ectopic pregnancy.[14] A woman who becomes pregnant with an IUD in place is said to have a 5 per cent chance of an ectopic pregnancy.[14] The risk of an ectopic pregnancy may persist for some time after removal of the IUD. Women who have had ectopic pregnancies prior to insertion of an IUD may be at even greater risk. However, a recent cooperative study disputes the existence of any association between IUD's and ectopic pregnancies.[17]

There may be an increased incidence of infertility in women who have used IUD's.[14] This has not been well studied, particularly in women who had IUD's removed because of side effects. In light of this potential risk, nulligravid patients in

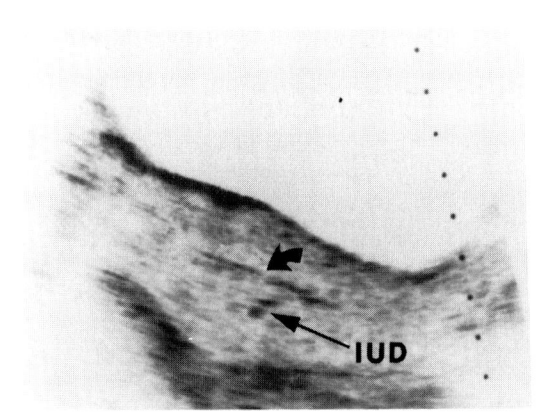

Figure 9. Longitudinal scan of the uterus demonstrating an IUD with several rungs (IUD) penetrating into the myometrium, away from the central cavity echo region (*curved arrow*).

particular should be carefully counseled prior to placement of an IUD.

Removal of IUD's for medical reasons total 12 to 16 per 100 women at the end of the first year of use. More than half of all removals are performed because of cramping and uterine bleeding. Typically, bleeding manifests as increased menstrual flow. Copper devices produce less menstrual bleeding than in women without IUD's, but there may be moderate intermenstrual spotting.[14]

There is as yet no known risk of gynecologic malignant disease in women who have used IUD's.[14]

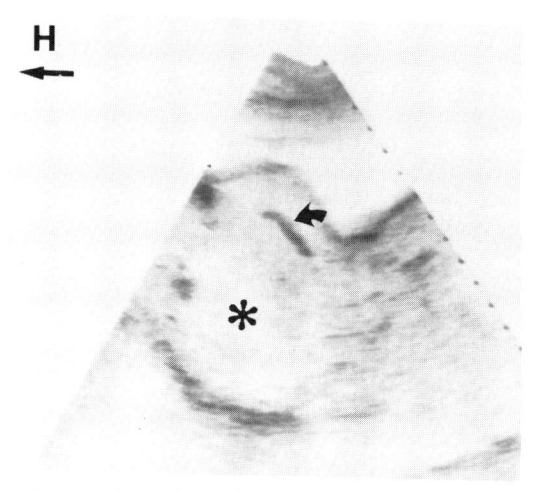

Figure 11. Pelvic inflammatory disease in a patient with an IUD. Longitudinal scan of the uterus reveals a tubo-ovarian abscess (*asterisk*) posterior to the uterus, which contains a Copper-7 IUD (*arrow*). H, head.

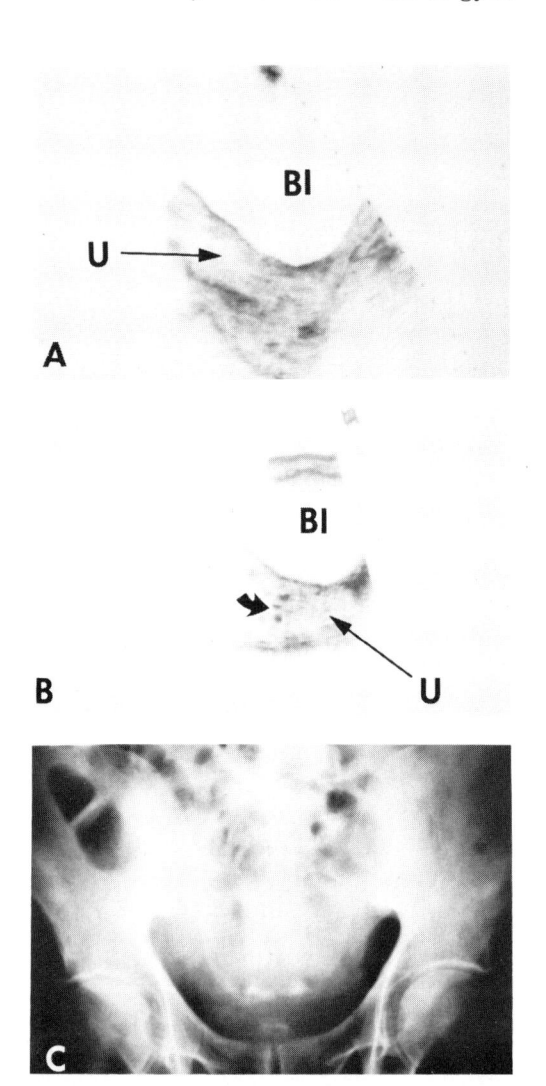

Figure 10. A, Longitudinal sonogram in a patient with a lost IUD reveals no evidence of an IUD within the uterus (U). Bl, bladder. B, Transverse scan shows several high amplitude echoes (*arrow*) in the right adnexa, giving the appearance of an extrauterine IUD. U, uterus; Bl, bladder. C, Pelvic radiograph demonstrates no IUD. This proves that the echoes in B were not caused by an IUD.

IUD'S AND INTRAUTERINE PREGNANCY

Use of an IUD is associated with a small but definite risk of pregnancy. In some women, this results from unnoticed expulsion or perforation of the IUD, but intrauterine pregnancies do occur with intrauterine IUD's. In 11 such patients studied by Tsai et al.,[24] four had IUD's very low in the uterus near the cervix, six had IUD's lower than the preferred position in the uterine fundus, and only one had an IUD adjacent to the gestational sac of pregnancy. They postulated that a downwardly displaced IUD leaves exposed endometrium in the upper uterine cavity as a site for implantation. In our experience, IUD's are more often found immediately adjacent to coexisting pregnancies (Fig. 12). In virtually all instances, the IUD remains extraovular.[14] An IUD is readily detected in the first trimester of pregnancy,[24] but localization is difficult in the second trimester (Fig. 13).[15, 24]

Pregnancy associated with an IUD carries a high risk of spontaneous abortion.[12] The abortion rate is 53.9 per cent for tailed IUD's and 42.6 per cent for tail-less IUD's. It is currently recommended that an IUD be removed, if the marker thread is visible, as soon as pregnancy is diagnosed.[14] This reduces the abortion rate to approximately 25 per cent, and also decreases the risk of bleeding, midtrimester septic abortion, premature delivery, stillbirth, amnionitis, and amniotic fluid embolus. If the marker thread is not visible, removal requires insertion into the uterus of an instrument with which the IUD can be hooked, and this further increases the already high rate of abortion.[12] There is no evidence of congenital anomalies referable to the continued presence of an IUD during pregnancy.[14]

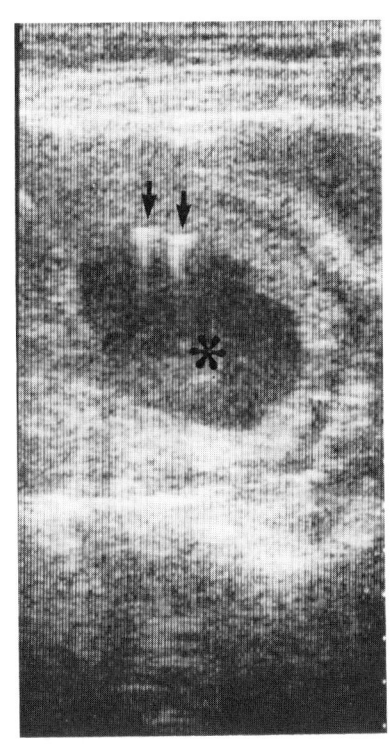

Figure 13. Second trimester pregnancy in a patient with an IUD. Longitudinal scan of the uterus demonstrates an IUD (*arrows*) in a patient whose fetus was 25 weeks of menstrual age. Asterisk, amniotic cavity.

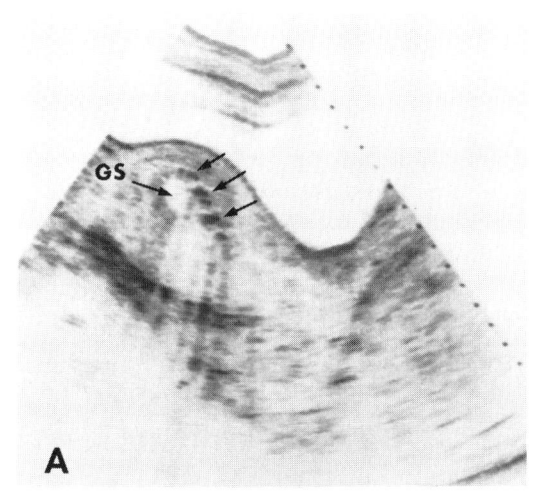

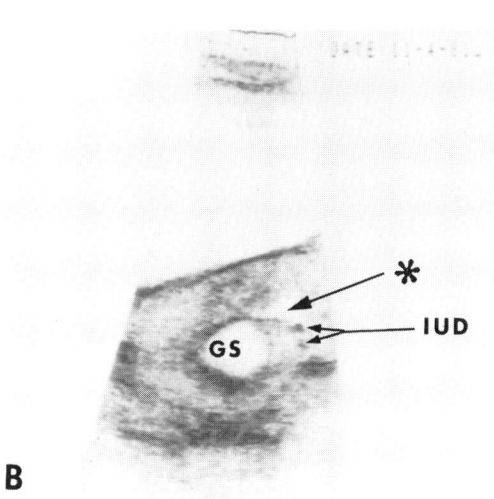

Figure 12. Early intrauterine pregnancy in a patient with an IUD. *A,* Longitudinal sonogram of the uterus shows a Lippes Loop (*arrows*) immediately adjacent to a gestational sac (GS). *B,* Transverse scan demonstrates fluid in the endometrial canal (*asterisk*) surrounding the Lippes Loop (IUD), which again abuts the gestational sac (GS).

CONCLUSION

Ultrasonography is the established method of choice for evaluating IUD's. Sonography can identify the presence, type, and location of an IUD, and is the indicated diagnostic examination when the vaginal marker thread is missing. Associated conditions, including pelvic inflammatory disease, ectopic pregnancy, and intrauterine pregnancy, are also well delineated.

REFERENCES

1. Callen, P. W., DeMartini, W. J., and Filly, R. A.: The central uterine cavity echo: A useful anatomic sign in the ultrasonographic evaluation of the female pelvis. Radiology, *131*:187–190, 1979.
2. Callen, P. W., Filly, R. A., and Munyer, T. P.: Intrauterine contraceptive devices: Evaluation by sonography. Am. J. Roentgenol., *135*:797–800, 1980.
3. Cochrane, W. J., and Thomas, M. A.: The use of ultrasound B-mode scanning in the localization of intrauterine contraceptive devices. Radiology, *104*:623–627, 1972.

4. Defoort, P., and Thiery, M.: IUD typing by ultrasound—an *in vitro* study. Contraception, 9:609–614, 1974.
5. Esposito, J. M.: Perforation of the uterus, secondary to insertion of IUCD. Obstet. Gynecol., 28:799–805, 1966.
6. Filly, R. A., and Callen, P. W.: Ultrasonography in the evaluation of nontraumatic abdominopelvic emergencies. Radiol. Clin. North Am., 16:159–173, 1978.
7. Filly, R. A., Moss, A. A., and Way, L. W.: *In vitro* investigation of gallstone shadowing with ultrasound tomography. J. Clin. Ultrasound, 7:255–262, 1979.
8. Ianniruberto, A., and Mastroberardino, A.: Ultrasound localization of the Lippes Loop. Am. J. Obstet. Gynecol., 114:78–82, 1972.
9. Jouppila, P.: Location of the missing intrauterine contraceptive device. Acta Obstet. Gynecol. Scand., 54:71–75, 1975.
10. Laing, F. C.: Diagnostic dilemmas in obstetrical and gynecologic ultrasound. Syllabus for the Categorical Course in Ultrasonography. Presented at the annual meeting of the American Roentgen Ray Society, San Francisco, March 22–27, 1981, pp. 239–241.
11. Ledger, W. J., and Willson, J. R.: Intrauterine contraceptive devices: The recognition and management of uterine perforations. Obstet. Gynecol., 28:806–811, 1966.
12. Lewit, S.: Outcome of pregnancy with intrauterine devices. Contraception, 2:47–57, 1970.
13. McArdle, C. R.: Ultrasonic localization of missing intrauterine contraceptive devices. Obstet. Gynecol., 51:330–333, 1978.
14. The Medical Device and Drug Advisory Committees on Obstetrics and Gynecology. Second Report on Intrauterine Contraceptive Devices. Washington, D. C., U.S. Department of Health, Education, and Welfare—Food and Drug Administration, 1978.
15. Nelson, L. H., and Miller, J. B.: Real-time ultrasound in locating intrauterine contraceptive devices. Obstet. Gynecol., 54:711–714, 1979.
16. Nemes, G., and Kerenyi, T. D.: Ultrasonic localization of the IUCD: A new technique. Am. J. Obstet. Gynecol., 109:1219–1220, 1971.
17. Ory, H. W.: Ectopic pregnancy and intrauterine contraceptive devices: New perspectives. Obstet. Gynecol., 57:137–144, 1981.
18. Piotrow, P.T., Rinehart, W., and Schmidt, J.C.: Intrauterine devices. Popul. Rep. (B), 7:49–98, 1979.
19. Richardson, M. L., Kinard, R. E., and Watters, D. H.: Location of intrauterine devices: Evaluation by computed tomography. Radiology, 142:690, 1982.
20. Rosenfield, A. T., Taylor, K. J. W., Dembner, A. G., et al.: Ultrasound of renal sinus: New observations. Am. J. Roentgenol., 133:441–448, 1979.
21. Sample, W. F.: Pelvic inflammatory disease and endometriosis. *In* Sanders, R. C., and James, A. E., Jr. (eds.): The Principles and Practice of Ultrasonography in Obstetrics and Gynecology. New York, Appleton-Century-Crofts, 1980, pp. 321–334.
22. Seymour, E. O., and Williamson H. O.: A review of commonly used intrauterine contraceptive devices. Radiology, 115:359–360, 1975.
23. Tietze, C.: Contraception with intrauterine devices: 1959–1966. Am. J. Obstet. Gynecol., 96:1043–1054, 1966.
24. Tsai, W. S., Chen, H. Y., Chen, Y. P., et al.: Sonographic visualization of coexisting gestation sac and IUD in the uterus and a consideration of a causative factor of accidental pregnancy. Int. J. Fertil., 18:85–92, 1973.
25. Watt, I., Watt, E., Halliwell, M., et al.: Sonographic demonstration of intrauterine contraceptive devices. J. Clin. Ultrasound, 5:378–382, 1977.
26. Winters, H. S.: Ultrasound detection of intrauterine contraceptive devices. Am. J. Obstet. Gynecol., 95:880–882, 1966.

16

Ultrasonography in Evaluation of Gestational Trophoblastic Disease

Peter W. Callen, M.D.

During the past several years, the ultrasonographer has played an increasing role in evaluating both the patient with complications related to pregnancy and those patients with gynecologic malignancies. Trophoblastic disease, a pregnancy-related malignancy, is certainly no exception. The role of ultrasound in evaluating patients with gestational trophoblastic disease as well as the clinical and pathologic features of this disease will be discussed.

The term "gestational trophoblastic disease" describes a spectrum of proliferative diseases of the trophoblast, from the benign hydatidiform mole to the more malignant and frequently metastatic choriocarcinoma. In considering this disease process, one must remember that these tumors are derived from the trophoblastic elements of the developing blastocyst and, as such, retain certain properties of the normal placenta such as invasive tendencies and the ability to secrete the polypeptide hormone human chorionic gonadotropin. In addition, these tumors are always related to pregnancy and as such differ specifically from germ cell tumors of the ovaries and testes.

CLASSIFICATION

In a standard text on gynecology or pathology, one may frequently find trophoblastic disease divided into three major categories: hydatidiform mole, invasive mole (chorioadenoma destruens), and choriocarcinoma.[5, 6] Though in one sense the division of this disease entity into these three categories is useful for understanding the various manifestations and progession of this disease, one should realize that since the advent of an accurate immunologic, biologic marker for this disease, specifically the beta subunit of human chorionic gonadotropin (β-HCG), the division of trophoblastic disease into these categories is less significant for therapy.

DIAGNOSIS

Trophoblastic disease has been detected more accurately the past several years with the advent of β-HCG. The earlier assays of human chorionic gonadotropin were less sensitive and specific because there was marked overlap with the three other polypeptide hormones with similar alpha subunits, specifically luteinizing hormone, follicle-stimulating hormone, and thyroid-stimulating hormone. Although measuring the level of β-HCG is useful for detecting patients with a suspected molar pregnancy, one must remember that the measured level of β-HCG from patients with trophoblastic disease may overlap that of patients with a normal pregnancy. In situations in which a molar pregnancy is suspected and the serum β-HCG level is elevated, the ultrasound examination will be extremely valuable in isolating patients with trophoblastic disease.

HYDATIDIFORM MOLE

This form of trophoblastic disease is the most benign and the most common. The incidence of hydatidiform mole varies geographically. In the United States, the incidence is approximately 1 in 1200 to 2000; in France, the incidence is said to be 1 in 500; and in Japan and Hong Kong, the incidence is as high as 1 in 250 patients. The explanation for this geographic variability is not yet known; however it is hypothe-

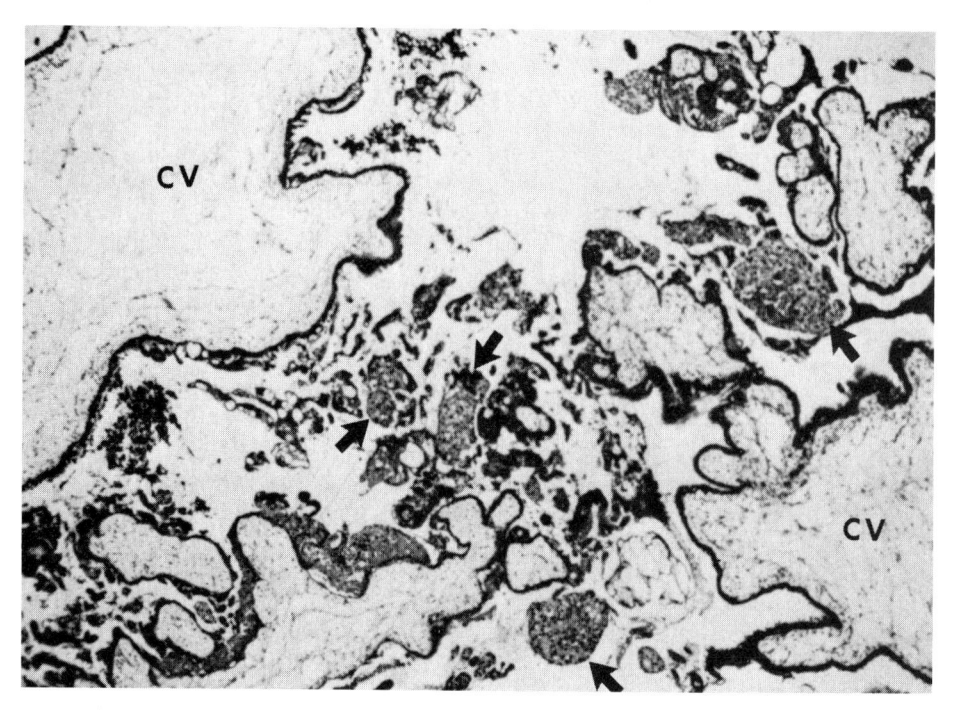

Figure 1. Photomicrograph from a patient with hydatidiform mole. Abnormal nest of trophoblastic cells (*arrows*) are seen scattered among markedly swollen chorionic villi (CV). The degree of hydropic changes of the chorionic villus in addition to the presence of trophoblastic proliferation separates this from hydropic degeneration occurring in otherwise normal pregnancies.

sized that this may be secondary to dietary factors and to a genetic predisposition.

The standard explanation for the pathophysiology of hydatidiform mole is that the chorionic villi of a blighted ovum in a missed abortion persist and continue to undergo increasing hydatid swelling. This explanation accounts for the characteristic vesicular appearance of the swollen chorionic villi, but not for the primary pathologic feature of this disease, which is trophoblastic proliferation. Thus, some investigators have postulated that the primary event may well be abnormal proliferation of the trophoblastic elements, with the hydropic change of the chorionic villi being a secondary phenomenon.

The pathologic characteristics of hydatiform mole are (1) marked edema and enlargement of the chorionic villi, (2) disappearance of the villus blood vessels, (3) proliferation of the lining trophoblast of the chorionic villi, and (4) absence of fetal tissue. As stated earlier, perhaps the most important characteristic that separates hydatidiform mole from other nontrophoblastic diseases is the proliferation of the lining trophoblast of the chorionic villi.

Normally, one sees small islands of the chorionic villus in the normal placenta, and the trophoblastic elements form a thin "limiting border." With hydatidiform mole, the chorionic villus becomes markedly swollen with proliferating nests of trophoblastic cells seen scattered throughout (Fig. 1).

The clinical features of hydatidiform mole can be divided into two categories: those features related to the tumor mass itself including abnormal vaginal bleeding and a uterus that appears large for dates; and those features related to the abnormally high levels of human chorionic gonadotropin including hyperemesis gravidarum and, in some patients, thyrotoxicosis.

Ultrasonographic Appearance. Normally, a hydatidiform mole appears as a large, soft-tissue mass filling the uterine cavity containing low to moderate amplitude echoes with numerous small cystic fluid-containing spaces scattered throughout (Fig. 2). When the tumor volume is small, the myometrium may be perceived as less echogenic soft tissue surrounding the more echogenic mass filling the uterine

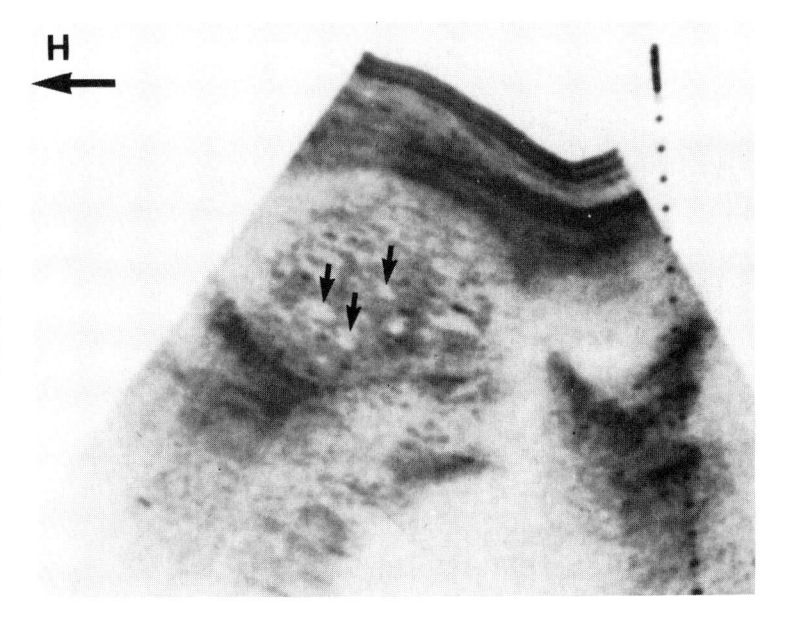

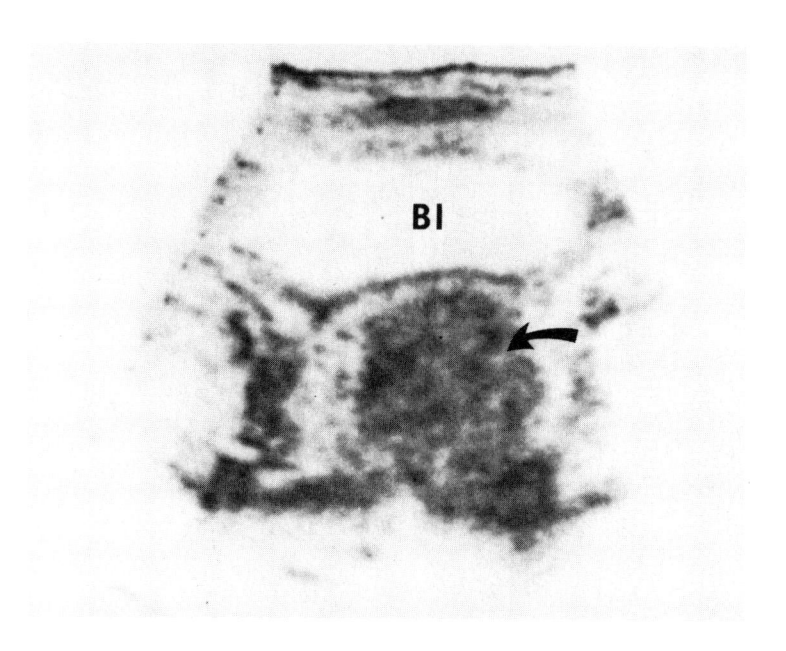

Figure 2. Longitudinal ultrasonogram in a patient with a second trimester hydatidiform mole. A large moderately echogenic mass with numerous small cystic spaces (arrows) is seen filling the central uterine cavity. The cystic spaces undoubtedly represent the markedly hydropic chorionic villi.

cavity. Though these features have come to be recognized as typical of a hydatidiform mole, this appearance is only specific for a second trimester hydatidiform mole.[7] Cases of first trimester molar pregnancies have been reported in the literature widely and have a variable appearance. First trimester moles in some cases may have an appearance simulating a blighted ovum or a threatened abortion; others may show a small echogenic mass filling the uterine cavity without the characteristic vesicular appearance (Fig. 3).[11] In these cases, only a high index of suspicion will allow the ultrasonographer to suggest the diagnosis.

COMPLICATIONS OF TROPHOBLASTIC DISEASE

Hemorrhage. Perhaps, one of the most common complications of trophoblastic disease, which can be readily identified on the ultrasonogram, is a hemorrhage internally within this lesion or within the adjacent tissues. The areas of hemorrhage

Figure 3. Transverse ultrasonogram from a patient with a first trimester hydatidiform mole. In this case an echogenic mass (arrow) is seen filling the central uterine cavity. Noticeably absent are the multiple small cystic spaces which are characteristically seen in more advanced molar pregnancies. BL, urinary bladder. (*From* Munyer, T.P., Callen, P.W., Filly, R.A., et al: Further observations on the ultrasonographic spectrum of gestational trophoblastic disease. J. Clin. Ultrasound, 9:349–358, 1981, with permission.)

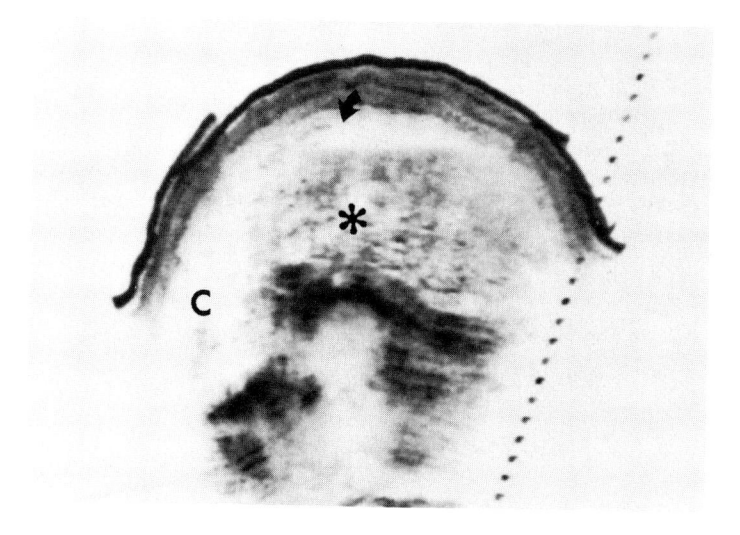

Figure 4. Transverse ultrasonogram from a patient with a second trimester hydatidiform mole. A moderately echogenic mass (*asterisk*) is filling the uterine cavity. In addition a crescentic anechoic region (*arrow*) is seen anteriorly adjacent to the anterior abdominal wall probably representing hemorrhage. In addition evidence of a theca-lutein cyst (C) is seen on the right side.

usually appear as crescentic anechoic regions surrounding the tumor (Fig. 4).

Theca-Lutein Cysts. The other feature frequently associated with hydatidiform mole and trophoblastic disease is theca-lutein cysts. The incidence of theca-lutein cysts in patients with trophoblastic disease is approximately 20 to 50 per cent. The number detected using ultrasonography is usually higher than that with the use of clinical examination. The explanation for this difference is probably secondary to the fact that with excessive uterine enlargement the ovaries may be difficult to palpate since they are displaced in a cephalic direction out of the true pelvis. Theca-lutein cysts are thought to occur secondary to a markedly elevated circulating level of human chorionic gonadotropin. Analysis of the cysts shows them to be multilocular, containing amber-colored or serosanguineous fluid.[6] The ultrasonogram ac-

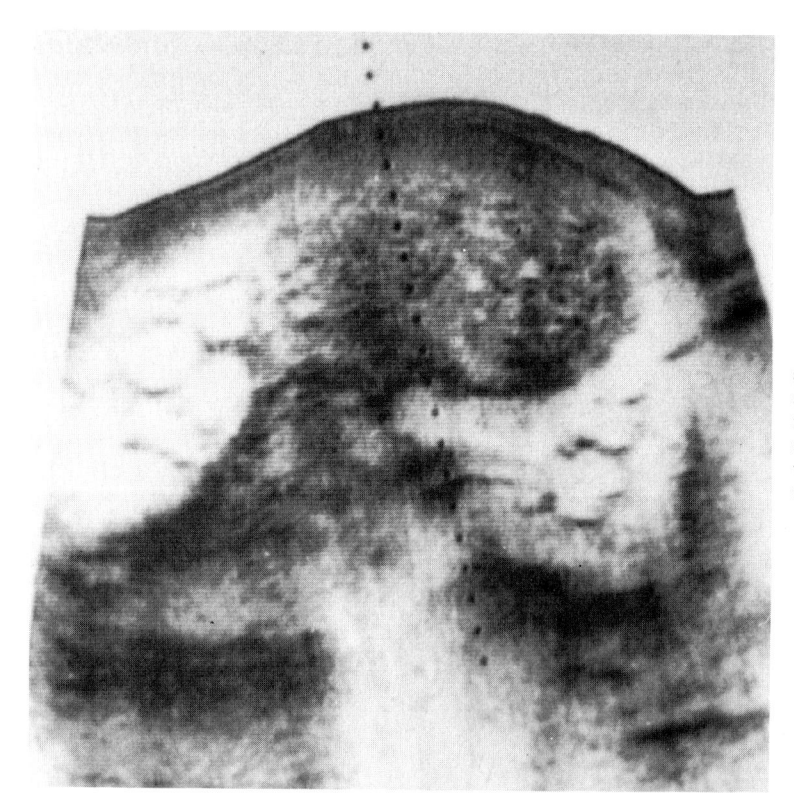

Figure 5. Transverse ultrasonogram from a patient with a second trimester hydatidiform mole. Large theca-lutein cysts are seen bilaterally. The characteristic multiseptated appearance is readily demonstrated.

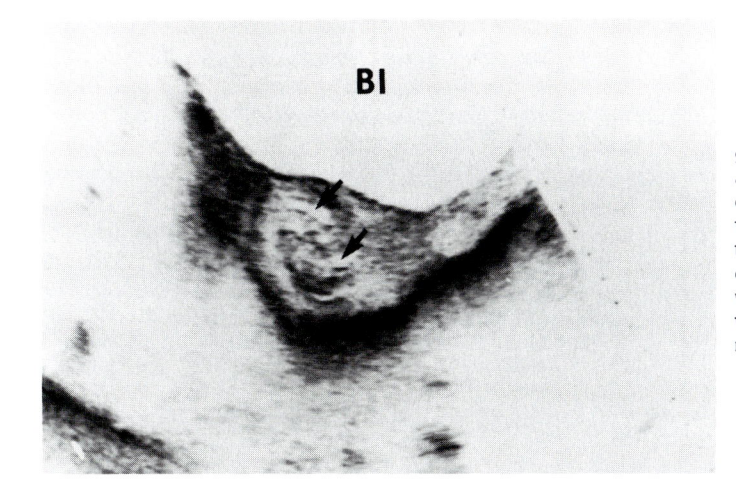

Figure 6. Longitudinal ultrasonogram of a patient with vaginal bleeding and a positive pregnancy test. Irregular cystic spaces (*arrows*) can be seen within the uterus. While the appearance is certainly not specific, this case of hydropic degeneration with fetal demise may be very difficult to differentiate from a first trimester molar pregnancy. BL, maternal urinary bladder.

curately depicts this pathologic description: multiseptated cysts are the most common presentation (Fig. 5). The ultrasonographer should remember that it may take approximately two to four months for these cysts to regress after molar evacuation; thus, they cannot be used as evidence of persistent or recurrent disease.[3]

DISEASES SIMULATING HYDATIDIFORM MOLE

The older literature about trophoblastic disease tended to be confusing since several diseases that were not truly hydatidiform moles such as hydropic degeneration or partial moles were included in this classification. If one adheres strictly to the pathologic criterion stated earlier for hydatidiform mole, one will be less prone to overestimate the prevalence of this disease. One entity that has been frequently included with hydatidiform mole should remain separate: hydropic degeneration of the placenta.

Hydropic changes of the placenta may occur in approximately 1 to 3 per cent of normal pregnancies.[4] Although the chorionic villi may be engorged, a specific feature of trophoblastic disease — proliferation of the lining trophoblast of the chorionic villi — is not seen. The ultrasonographer may find it extemely difficult to distinguish between a missed abortion — in which there is hydropic degeneration — and a molar pregnancy (Fig. 6). In these cases, the levels of serum human chorionic gonadotropin as well as pathologic evaluation of the specimen will be needed to make this distinction.

Although leiomyomas involving the uterus do not usually present a diagnostic dilemma, occasionally a leiomyoma with cystic degeneration may simulate the appearance of a mole (Fig. 7). In these cases, carefully evaluating the highly attenuating nature of this disease may help distinguish the diseases.

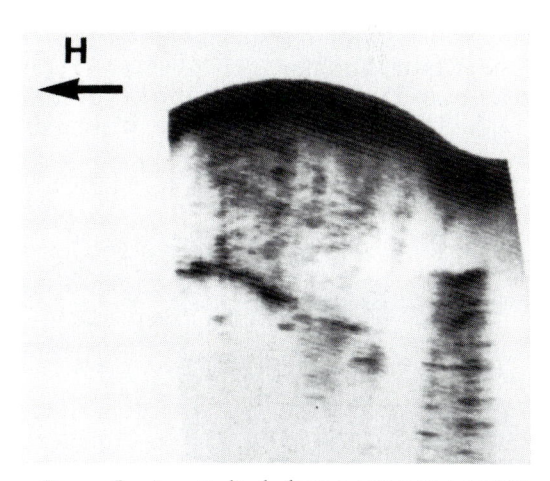

Figure 7. Longitudinal ultrasonogram in a patient with vaginal bleeding and a large pelvic mass. While at first glance the enlarged moderately echogenic uterus with lucent spaces may simulate a molar pregnancy, attenuation of sound and absence of numerous well defined cystic spaces would make this atypical for a second trimester mole. The serum beta HCG was negative and may be useful in making the distinction between leiomyomata with cystic degeneration and a molar pregnancy.

FOLLOW-UP EVALUATION AND TREATMENT

The treatment and follow-up of trophoblastic disease are beyond the scope of this discussion, but some general points will be mentioned. Once hydatidiform mole has been diagnosed, suction evacuation of the uterus is usually performed, followed by curettage of the endometrium to examine for evidence of myometrial invasion. A baseline chest radiograph is used to examine for evidence of metastatic disease. Serum levels of β-HCG may then be followed until the level is normal. Normally, the serum β-HCG level falls into the normal range approximately 10 to 12 weeks after evacuation of the molar pregnancy.[3]

VARIATIONS OF MOLAR PREGNANCY

Coexistent Mole and Fetus

Several reports in the literature have noted that a living fetus was associated with a molar pregnancy.[1, 2, 8] Unfortunately, many patients were included in this category in whom there was hydropic degeneration or an incomplete mole rather than a true hydatidiform mole. Nevertheless, several well-documented cases of coexistent fetus and mole have been seen. Because absence of fetal structure is one of the pathologic requirements for a true hydatidiform mole, the presumed mechanism for coexistence of a true mole and normal fetus is molar transformation of one of binovular twin placenta (Fig. 8). Although the diagnosis may be suggested and made with a high degree of certainty on the ultrasonogram, it should be confirmed pathologically since these lesions must be considered as having the same malignant potential as a more classically appearing molar pregnancy.

INCOMPLETE OR PARTIAL MOLE

Several entities, including hydropic degeneration, have been placed in this category. The following pathologic findings for incomplete or partial moles are well presented in a review by Szulman and Surti: (1) identifiable fetal tissues, (2) edematous chorionic villi with little to no trophoblastic proliferation, and (3) multiple congenital anomalies in which a chromosomal analysis usually reveals a triploid chromosomal complement (Fig. 9).[9]

Invasive Mole

Approximately 80 per cent of patients initially diagnosed as having hydatidiform mole will follow a benign course with resolution after evacuation.[1] However, in approximately 12 to 15 per cent of patients, invasive mole will develop, and in 5 to 8

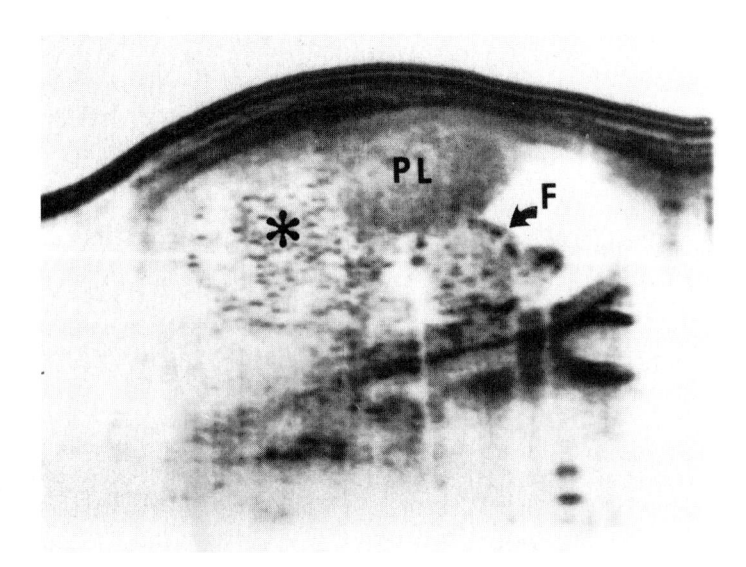

Figure 8. Longitudinal ultrasonogram from a patient with coexistence of a true hydatidiform mole and a normal fetus. The fetus (*arrow*) was living at the time of the examination and the placenta (PL) was normal in appearance. The more characteristically appearing molar pregnancy can be seen (*asterisk*) superior and adjacent to the normal pregnancy.

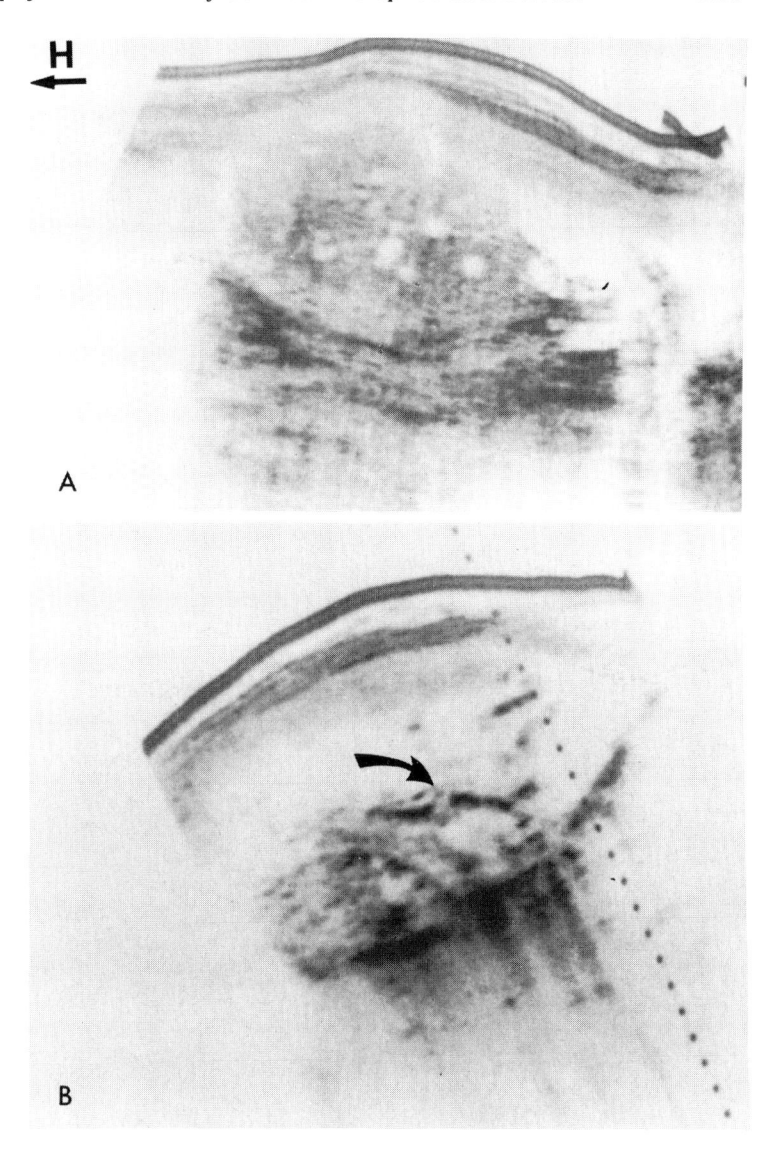

Figure 9. Partial molar pregnancy. *A*, Longitudinal scan shows enlarged uterus filled with vesicular tissue. No identifiable normal placenta. *B*, A transverse scan through the lower uterine segment shows a portion of the fetal extremity (*arrow*). No fetal motion was detected. (*From* Munyer, T.P., Callen, P.W., Filly, R.A., et al.: Further observations on the ultrasonographic spectrum of gestational trophoblastic disease. J. Clin. Ultrasound, 9: 349–358, 1981, with permission.)

per cent metastatic choriocarcinoma will develop.

The pathologic features of invasive mole are extensive local invasion, excessive trophoblastic proliferation, and preservation of the villous pattern. The differentiating feature between invasive mole and the more malignant form of trophoblastic disease—choriocarcinoma—is preservation of the villous pattern in invasive molar disease. Examination of a specimen from a patient with an invasive mole reveals that the characteristic elements seen with hydatidiform mole — nests of trophoblastic cells as well as swollen chorionic villi — rather than being within the central cavity of the uterus are found within the myometrium.

Invasive mole is infrequently diagnosed without hysterectomy, since it is uncommon to obtain myometrium during curettage. And since hysterectomies are not commonly being performed for any form of trophoblastic disease, the diagnosis may not be suggested by the clinician. The morbidity and mortality of invasive mole result from the penetration of the tumor through the myometrium and then through the pelvic vessels; this results in hemorrhage.[5, 6] Although the ultrasonographer may have a difficult time diagnosing this more aggressive form of the disease, hemorrhagic necrosis involving the myometrium extending into the parametrial areas should make one suspect this entity (Fig. 10).

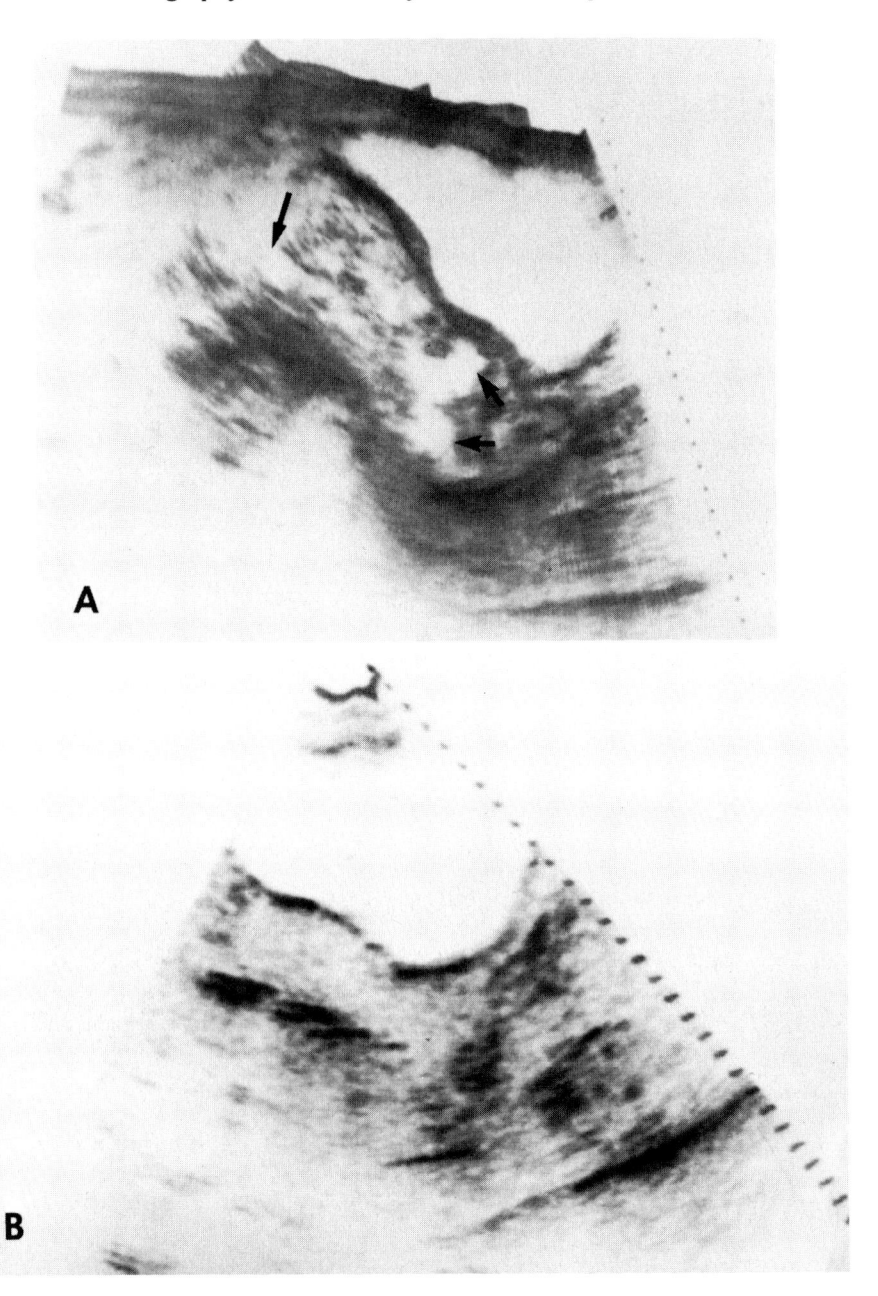

Figure 10. *A*, Longitudinal ultrasonogram from patient with invasive trophoblastic disease. A large complex mass in the expected position of the uterus is identified in which highly echogenic tissue is seen interspersed with multiple cystic areas (*arrows*) probably representing hemorrhage. Surgery confirmed evidence of extension of trophoblastic disease beyond the uterine cavity into the parametrium. *B*, Longitudinal ultrasonogram from the same patient after chemotherapy. Dramatic response is seen with return of the uterus to a more normal size and echogenicity.

Choriocarcinoma

This most malignant form of trophoblastic disease has an incidence of approximately 1 in 40,000 pregnancies in the United States. Approximately 50 per cent of the cases of choriocarcinoma are preceded by a molar pregnancy; however, only 3 to 5 per cent of all molar pregnancies will result in choriocarcinoma. Approximately one half of cases of choriocarcinoma occur in association with a molar pregnancy, 25 per cent occur after an abortion, 22 per cent occur after normal pregnancy, and approx-

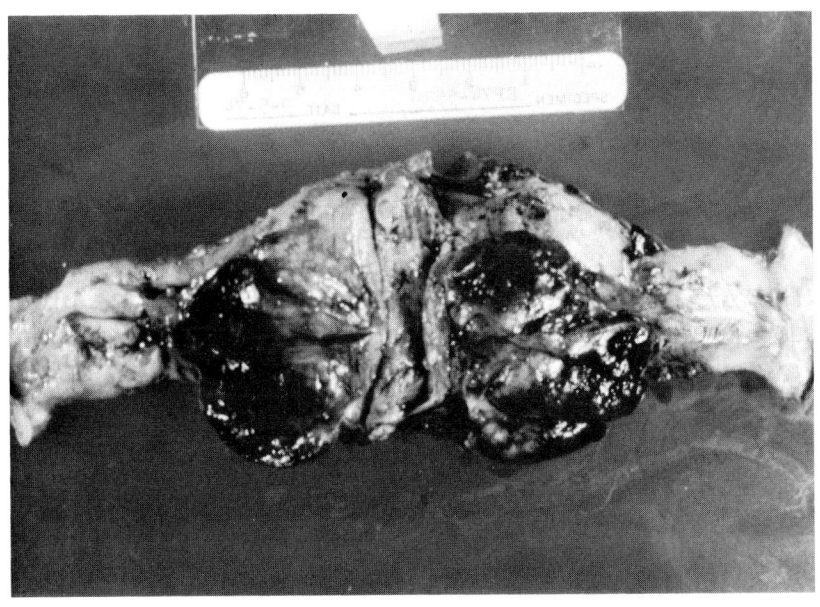

Figure 11. Pathologic specimen from a patient with choriocarcinoma. The bivalved uterus demonstrates a large hemorrhagic necrotic mass involving the body of the uterus.

imately 3 per cent may occur after an ectopic pregnancy.

Pathology. Gross examination of the uterus in a patient with choriocarcinoma will reveal a dark, hemorrhagic mass on the uterine wall, cervix, or vagina, which may show extensive ulceration and penetration of the tumor into the musculature (Fig. 11). Microscopically, the villous pattern is completely blotted out by the proliferating trophoblast (Fig. 12). This feature separates this disease entity from the

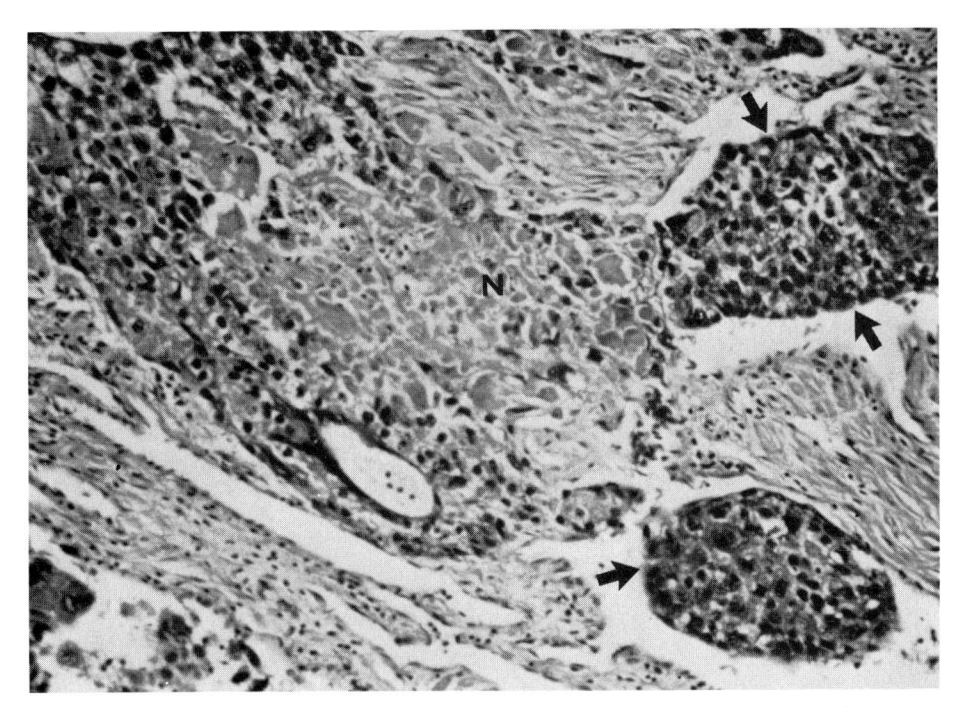

Figure 12. Photomicrograph from a patient with choriocarcinoma. Multiple cords (*arrows*) of malignant trophoblastic tissue infiltrate the uterine stroma. The absence of villi and necrosis (N) of tumor differentiate this process from invasive trophoblastic disease.

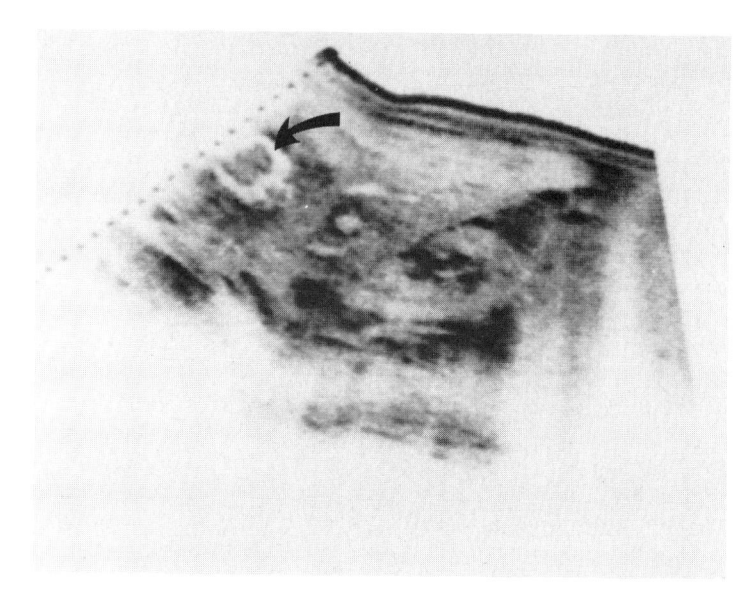

Figure 13. Longitudinal ultrasonogram in a patient with metastatic choriocarcinoma. Evidence of metastatic disease involving the liver in which a necrotic metastasis with hemorrhage (*arrow*) is seen. The patient died of massive hemoperitoneum from bleeding hepatic metastases.

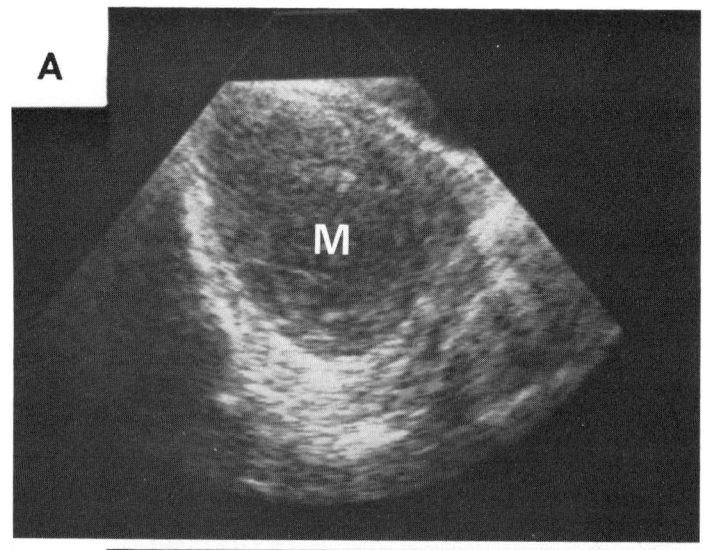

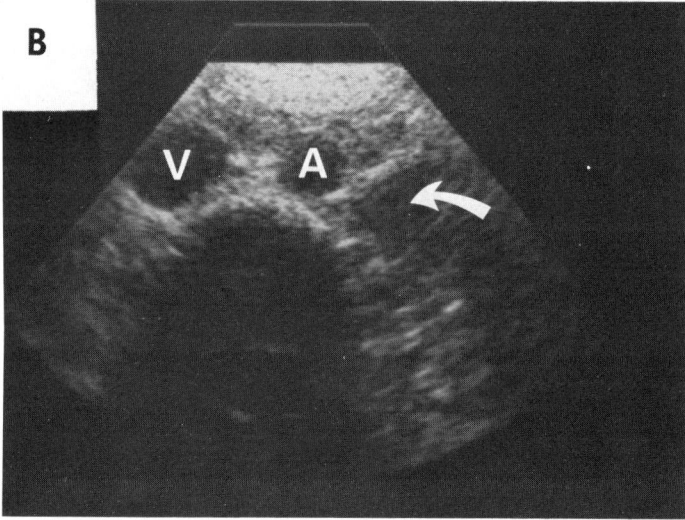

Figure 14. *A,* Longitudinal sector scan in a patient with choriocarcinoma. A large tumor mass that is uncharacteristically poorly echogenic (M) is seen expanding the uterine cavity and extending posteriorly. The only normal appearing myometrium was seen anteriorly. This was confirmed at surgery. *B,* Limited transverse ultrasonogram from the same patient in which evidence of adenopathy (*arrow*) is seen adjacent to the aorta (A). V, inferior vena cava.

less benign forms of trophoblastic disease.[5,6] Choriocarcinoma is known to metastasize to the lung, brain, liver, bone, gastrointestinal tract, and skin. As such, the ultrasonographer may help in evaluating the extent of the disease particularly in the liver (Fig. 13).

PROGRESSION OF DISEASE

The appearance of persistent trophoblastic disease is not specific on the ultrasonogram; however, the ultrasonographer still has an important role in the follow-up of these patients. When serial examinations of the serum β-HCG level reveal a plateau or a respiking of the level of the hormone, it becomes important to differentiate the cause of this elevation as being from persistent disease or a normal pregnancy. The ultrasonographer can obviously help distinguish the causes. In patients with malignant forms of trophoblastic disease, the extent of disease, specifically the parametrium and liver, can be assessed by the ultrasonographer and is important in determination of the appropriate therapy.

Although pathologic confirmation of the appearance of choriocarcinoma is difficult because hysterectomies are now infrequently performed for this disease, correlation of the appearance of the uterus with an evaluation of known metastatic survey as well as the level of serum β-HCG has proved interesting in assessing local involvement (Fig. 14).[7] Patients with persistent trophoblastic disease may have focal areas of increased echogenicity within the myometrium as the only imaged evidence of disease (Fig. 15).

CHARACTERIZATION OF TROPHOBLASTIC DISEASE BY ULTRASONOGRAPHY

The major pathologic feature of trophoblastic disease is abnormal proliferation of trophoblastic tissue after a gestational event. We hypothesize that trophoblastic disease appears on the ultrasonogram as highly echogenic tissue within the uterus in which visualization depends upon the amount of tissue present as well as secondary changes (see Figs. 3 and 15).[7,11] If molar pregnancy is detected early, that is, first trimester mole or in cases of early detection of persistent or locally invasive disease, the vesicles that give hydatidiform mole its characteristic and easily recognizable appearance either may not be present or may be too small to be seen. Therefore, first trimester molar pregnancies may often be misdiagnosed as a missed abortion, or persistent disease may not be readily apparent on the ultrasonogram. As the molar pregnancy progresses into the second trimester, the pathognomonic vesicles and

Figure 15. Longitudinal ultrasonogram from a patient with persistent trophoblastic disease. Despite a markedly elevated serum beta HCG, the results of a metastatic workup were negative. There was, however, a focus of increased echogenic tissue (arrow) adjacent to the central uterine cavity which most likely represents persistent trophoblastic tissue.

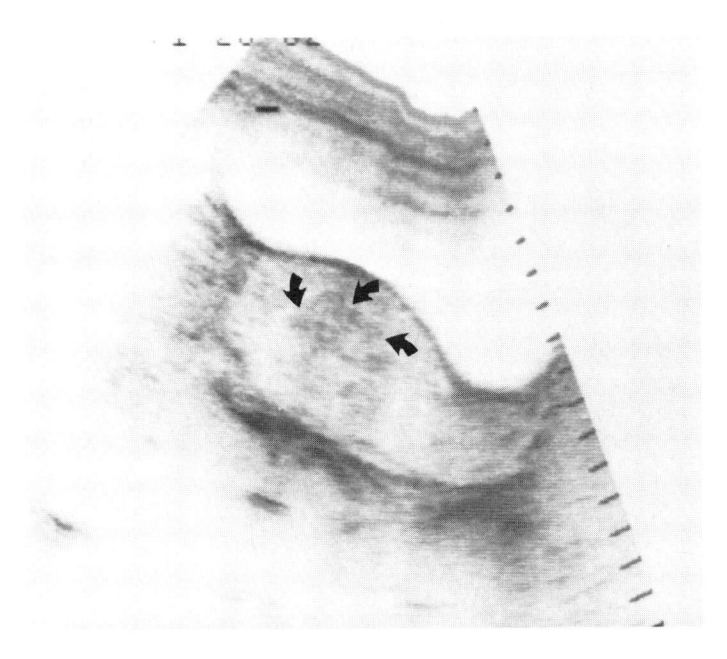

theca-lutein cysts become evident. This concept is supported by studies of Szulman and Surti who have established a roughly linear relationship between gestational age of the molar pregnancy and the microscopic size of the swollen chorionic villi.[10] For example, their earliest hydatidiform mole with a gestational age of 8½ gestational weeks yielded vesicles with a maximum diameter of 2 mm. This result contrasts with their most advanced case of 18½ gestational weeks yielding vesicles with a maximum diameter of 10 mm. As stated previously, in cases of first trimester molar pregnancy or in cases of persistent or locally invasive disease when recurrence is detected by serial determinations of human chorionic gonadotropin levels, the characteristic vesicles may be too small to be imaged by ultrasound.

Knowledge of the various manifestations of trophoblastic disease as well as the complications that can be seen on the ultrasonogram will aid the clinician in managing the disease. Differentiation between trophoblastic disease and a normal intrauterine pregnancy as well as extent of spread of disease or response to therapy in advanced cases may all be followed up using ultrasonography.

REFERENCES

1. Bree, R. L., Silver, T. M., Wicks, J. D., et al.: Trophoblastic disease with coexistent fetus: A sonographic and clinical spectrum. J. Clin. Ultrasound, 6:310, 1978.
2. Fleisher, A. C., James, A. E., Krause, D. A., et al.: Sonographic patterns in trophoblastic diseases. Radiology, 126:215, 1978.
3. Goldstein, D. P., Berkowitz, R. J., and Cohen, S. M.: The current management of molar pregnancy. Curr. Probl. Obstet. Gynecol., 3:1–40, 1979.
4. Hertig, A. T.: Human Trophoblast. Springfield, Ill., Charles C Thomas, 1968, pp. 228–237.
5. Jones, H. W., III.: Gestational trophoblastic disease. In Jones, H., and Jones, G. S. (eds.): Novak's Textbook of Gynecology. Edition 10. Baltimore, Williams and Wilkins, 1981.
6. Kraus, F. T.: Female genitalia. In Anderson, W. A. D., and Kissane, J. M. (eds.): Pathology. Edition 7. St. Louis, C. V. Mosby, 1977.
7. Munyer, T. P., Callen, P. W., Filley, R. A., et al.: Further observations on the sonographic spectrum of gestational trophoblastic disease. J. Clin. Ultrasound, 9:349–358, 1981.
8. Sauerbrei, E. E., Salem, S., and Fayle, B.: Coexistent hydatidiform mole and live fetus in the second trimester. Radiology, 135:415, 1980.
9. Szulman, A. E., and Surti, U.: The syndromes of hydatidiform mole. I. Cytogenic and morphologic correlations. Am. J. Obstet. Gynecol., 13:655, 1978.
10. Szulman, A. E., and Surti, U.: The syndromes of hydatidiform mole. II. Morphologic evolution of the complete and partial mole. Am. J. Obstet. Gynecol., 132:20, 1978.

17

Sonographic Evaluation of Pelvic Infections

Lincoln L. Berland, M.D., Thomas L. Lawson, M.D., and W. Dennis Foley, M.D.

Numerous reports have indicated that sonography is highly accurate in diagnosing gynecologic pelvic masses,[6, 7, 9, 18, 31, 32, 36, 41] but inflammatory disease accounted for only 10 to 20 per cent of the cases reviewed in these reports. Furthermore, the 1981 edition of *Novak's Textbook of Gynecology*[12] fails to even acknowledge the use of ultrasound in diagnosing pelvic inflammatory diseases. Nevertheless, in some patients with inflammatory diseases of the pelvis, sonography may contribute significantly to diagnosis and treatment. The sonogram is most valuable when there is a dialogue between the clinician and sonographer, leading to a full appreciation of the accuracy, indications, and failings of ultrasonography. The following discussion will focus on the various clinical presentations of inflammatory pelvic diseases, will highlight areas in which sonography contributes most, and will enumerate factors that lead to false interpretations. Sonography will be evaluated in the perspective of other often complementary diagnostic modalities, and the technical aspects of the sonographic examination will be considered. We will also speculate on possible future uses of sonography in patients with pelvic infections.

ACUTE PELVIC INFLAMMATORY DISEASE

Pathology

The term "pelvic inflammatory disease" has been used to designate several conditions with different causes, but in this chapter we use pelvic inflammatory disease to refer only to the spectrum of entities arising from venereal diseases in women of childbearing age. Pelvic inflammatory disease results from ascending infection traveling through the endometrium, salpinges, and into the pelvic peritoneum,[12] and *Neisseria gonorrhoeae* is isolated from about 50 per cent of patients.[25] The "nongonococcal" form probably begins most often as a Neisseria infection which provides a favorable environment for growth of other native bacterial flora.[25] These superinfecting bacteria are usually anaerobes or are polymicrobial, and they compete with and eradicate the gonococcus.

If pelvic inflammatory disease is not promptly and adequately treated, adhesions may obstruct the fallopian tube and lead to a pyosalpinx. If the ovary is also involved in the infection, a tubo-ovarian abscess may form, usually bilaterally. The ovary itself is relatively resistant to infection, and therefore infection commonly causes a perioophoritis, but rarely destroys the ovary.[26]

Pelvic peritonitis and pelvic abscess may also develop when purulent material spills from the fallopian tubes. Rupture of a pyosalpinx, a tubo-ovarian abscess, or a pelvic abscess may lead to more extensive peritoneal abscess formation, often presenting in the right subphrenic or subhepatic spaces. Uncommonly, the peritonitis is localized to the right upper quadrant, causing fever and abdominal pain. This gonococcal perihepatitis is termed the Fitz-Hugh-Curtis syndrome. Pelvic or tubo-ovarian abscesses are usually treated with antibiotics first, but may require surgical drainage.[12]

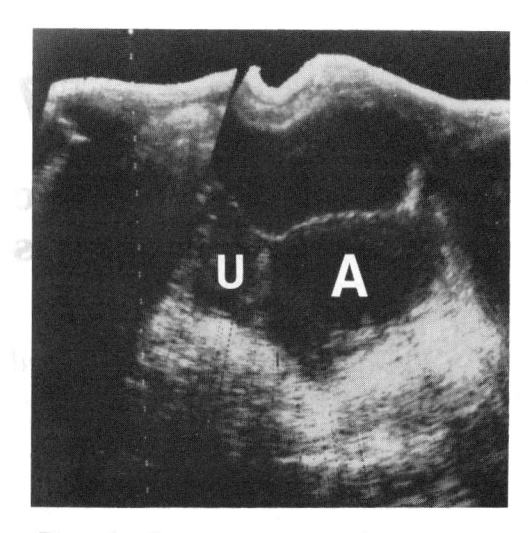

Figure 1. Transverse sonogram shows an irregular, thick-walled, tubo-ovarian abscess (A) to the left of the uterus (U).

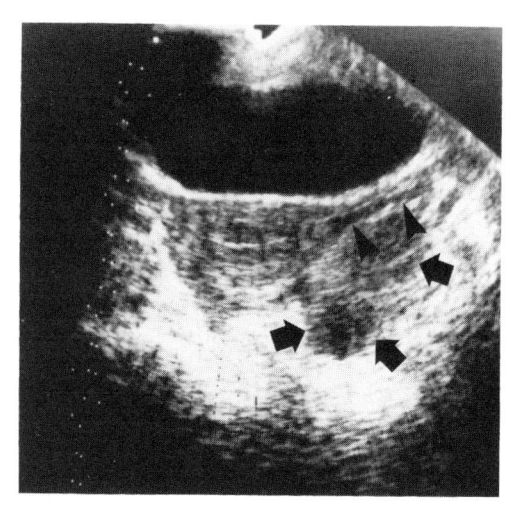

Figure 2. Transverse sonogram of an inhomogeneous, hyperechoic, left pelvic abscess (*arrows*). Note the tubular structure anterior to the abscess, probably representing a thickened fallopian tube (*arrowheads*).

Sonography

If discovered early, a first episode of acute pelvic inflammatory disease is likely to produce no abnormalities on the pelvic sonogram. Uterine borders may become indistinct, and this finding has been called the "indefinite uterus."[2] However, like decreased uterine echogenicity, the indefinite uterus is a subtle sign that is not easily appreciated, and thus is of limited usefulness.

Pyosalpinx and tubo-ovarian abscesses are characteristically tubular adnexal masses because the fallopian tubes tend to elongate and may appear serpentine. These abscesses usually have the typical sonographic features of fluid collections. However, abscesses may also have thick and irregular or "shaggy" walls (Fig. 1), or may contain echoes (Fig. 2) or fluid levels representing the layering of purulent debris (Fig. 3).[40, 41] Free pelvic fluid may indicate peritonitis. If the free fluid becomes loculated, an abscess may form, which is usually ovoid and often acts aggressively,

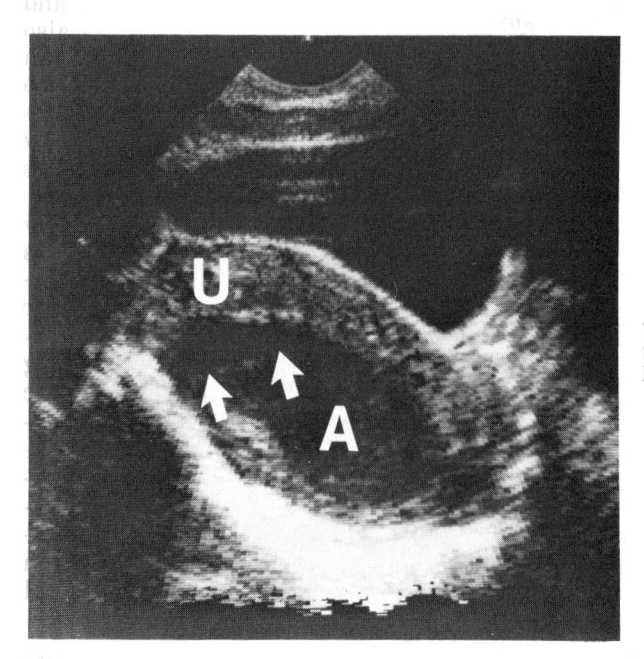

Figure 3. Longitudinal sonogram in a patient with a tubo-ovarian abscess (A) posterior to the uterus (U). A fluid-fluid level (*arrows*) represents layering of purulent debris.

displacing and distorting adjacent organs.[8] A peritoneal abscess usually becomes established within the cul-de-sac because this is the most dependent point of the peritoneal space in the supine patient,[24] whereas a tubo-ovarian abscess is commonly higher in the adnexa.[40] However, the larger an abscess, the more difficult the task of determining whether it is tubal or pelvic because the tubo-ovarian abscess may enlarge to occupy the pouch of Douglas which is the usual position of a pelvic abscess (Fig. 4). Some abscesses may have a very echogenic appearance from small gas bubbles created by gas-forming organisms, and such bubbles may even be too small to discern by radiography.[15]

Because the clinical diagnosis of acute pelvic inflammatory disease is usually straightforward, the sonogram is ordinarily reserved for patients with equivocal pelvic examinations because of obesity or tenderness, for detecting complications including abscess, or for localizing such an abscess and indicating whether it is amenable to transvaginal drainage.[33, 40] Another use of the ultrasound examination in acute pelvic inflammatory disease is to con-

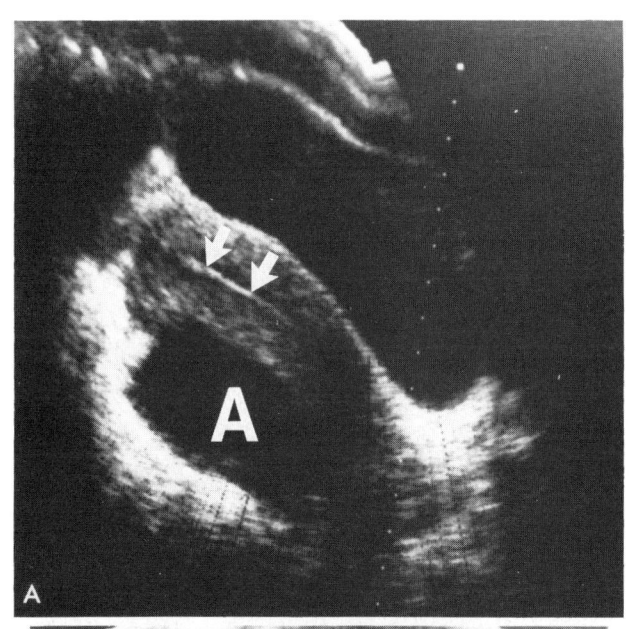

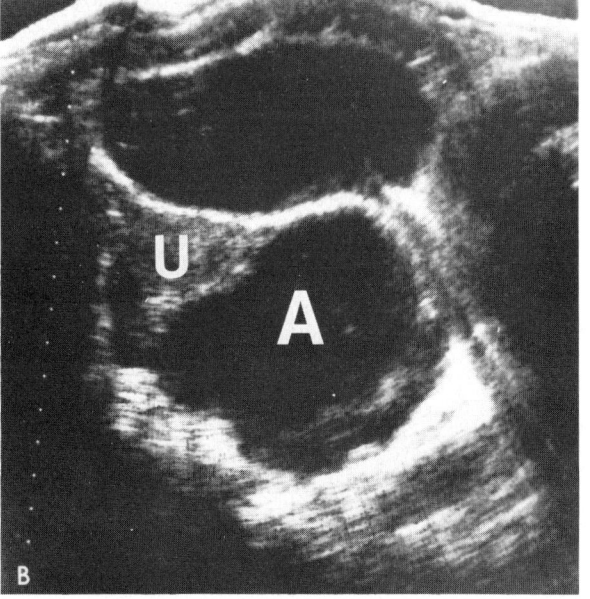

Figure 4. *A*, Longitudinal sonogram of a patient with a large tubo-ovarian abscess (A) in the pouch of Douglas. Arrows indicate central cavity echo. *B*, Transverse sonogram in the same patient shows the complete extent of the left tubo-ovarian abscess (A) which has enlarged sufficiently to occupy the cul-de-sac. U, uterus.

firm the diagnosis of pelvic abscess and thus avoid laparoscopy prior to surgical drainage.[31] Follow-up studies help assess the efficacy of medical or surgical therapy and provide a baseline for future evaluations. Imaging studies other than ultrasonography presently have no significant role in acute pelvic inflammatory disease.

Differential Diagnosis

There is a wide spectrum of sonographic findings in acute pelvic inflammatory disease. Abnormalities may be absent or difficult to demonstrate, or the variable appearance may mimic other conditions. The uterine borders may be poorly marginated with pelvic inflammatory disease, endometriosis, ovarian neoplasm, and uterine leiomyoma.[2, 9, 18] Endometriomas may be confused with abscesses because both commonly have thick walls and internal echoes, and both diseases cause pain and infertility (Fig. 5).[9] Both ectopic pregnancy and abscess may appear as complex adnexal masses, and while the prominent central uterine echoes of a decidual reaction of a normal or ectopic pregnancy are usually characteristic, they occasionally resemble

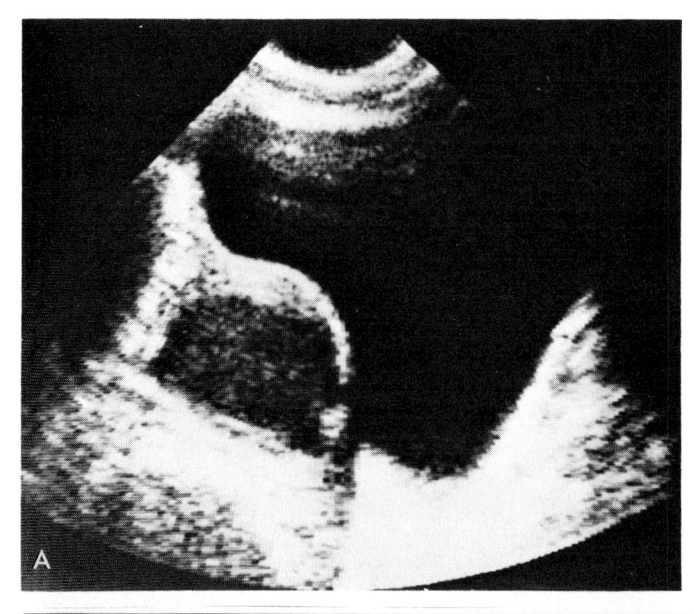

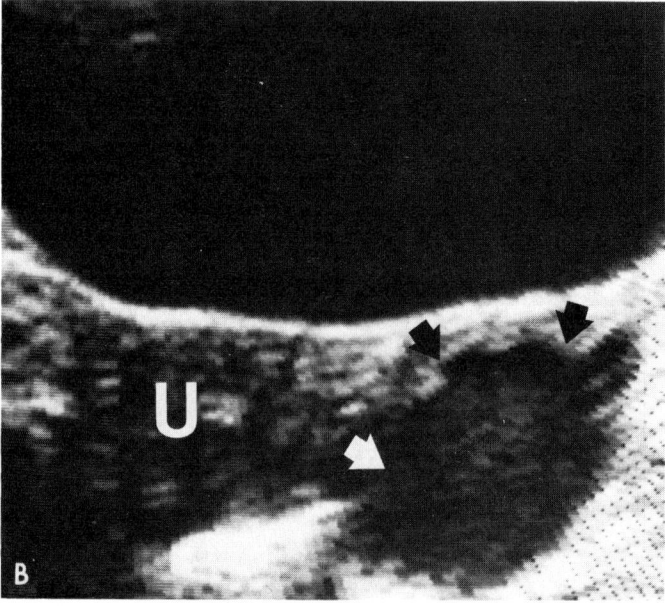

Figure 5. A, Longitudinal sonogram demonstrates a tubo-ovarian abscess with low-level echoes. The uterus is not seen in this image. B, Oblique transverse sonogram in another patient with a very similar appearing endometrioma (arrows) to the left of the uterus (U). Both tubo-ovarian abscesses and endometriomas may also have complex internal textures.

findings of endometritis. A corpus luteum cyst in a pregnant woman can sonographically mimic a pelvic abscess. However, recently developed serum pregnancy tests are very sensitive and values elevated early in pregnancy may help discriminate pelvic inflammatory disease from a cyst related to pregnancy.

Functional ovarian retention cysts may undergo hemorrhage, torsion, or rupture, causing pain and creating a complex sonographic appearance. If an inflamed appendix is located within the pelvis because it or the cecum is low lying, then a periappendiceal abscess may develop within the pelvis. Also, inflammatory masses from Crohn's disease commonly occur within the pelvis. A cystic teratoma complicated by torsion or rupture may look both sonographically and clinically like a pelvic or tubo-ovarian abscess, and both conditions most commonly affect young adult women.

The frequency of simultaneous abnormalities of different etiologies further limits the specificity of ultrasound.[2] Functional cysts, ectopic pregnancy, and pelvic inflammatory disease are common conditions that may coexist and indeed are etiologically related. Pelvic inflammatory disease may lead to tubal adhesions, predisposing to ectopic pregnancy. Corpus luteum cysts appear normally during ectopic and normal pregnancies and therefore further complicate the sonographic diagnosis. Thus, because of the nonspecificity of pelvic sonography, a detailed knowledge of the clinical findings is crucial to narrowing the differential diagnosis.

CHRONIC PELVIC INFLAMMATORY DISEASE

Pathology

The term "chronic pelvic inflammatory disease" refers to the residua of acute infection and to subacute reinfection of previous acute pelvic inflammatory disease. Several kinds of chronic pelvic changes may occur even after one episode of acute pelvic inflammatory disease. Pelvic adhesions develop first, fixing pelvic structures to each other and to adjacent bowel and omentum.[26] If a pyosalpinx occurs it may evolve into a hydrosalpinx in which purulent exudate is replaced by serous fluid. The hydrosalpinx may then further expand by osmotic pressure to become a rounded cystic adnexal mass which is potentially subject to torsion,[26] as are other large adnexal cysts. Alternatively, subacute inflammation limited to the fallopian tube may produce chronic interstitial salpingitis in which the tube becomes large, but thick-walled, rather than thin-walled as with a hydrosalpinx.[26]

Another variety of chronic pelvic inflammatory disease is the inflammatory cyst of the pelvic peritoneum, which has been recently described by Lees et al. and is of obscure cause.[20] These lesions are large, multiloculated, serous or serosanguinous cysts adherent to inflamed fallopian tubes.

Sonography

Pelvic sonograms may be confusing in the presence of chronic pelvic inflammatory disease and adhesions. While the adhesions themselves are invisible, they may lead to fixation of bowel loops and omentum in the pelvis which may be mistaken for pelvic cysts or masses.[9, 18] The chronic residua of tubo-ovarian and pelvic abscesses such as a hydrosalpinx, inflammatory cysts, or adhesions may produce complex patterns of pelvic fluid loculations often markedly expanding the pouch of Douglas and encompassing the uterus (Fig. 6).[40] Adhesions may prevent free peritoneal fluid from occupying the usual most dependent position within the cul-de-sac, and

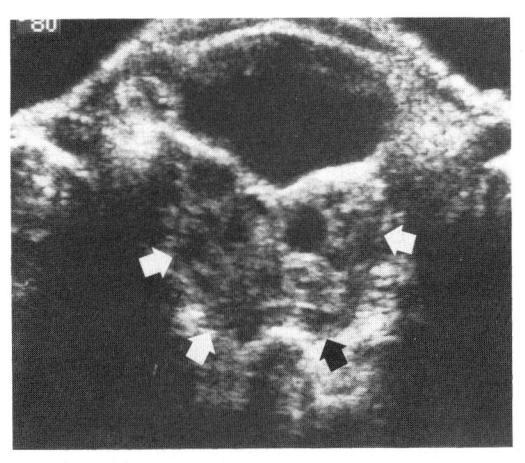

Figure 6. Transverse sonogram of a patient with severe chronic pelvic inflammatory disease shows large complex cystic and echogenic masses (*arrows*).

thus the fluid may not be identified. Despite adhesions, in chronic pelvic inflammatory disease without active infection the "indefinite uterus" of acute pelvic inflammatory disease regains its sharp borders, and the echogenicity of the uterus and endometrial cavity return to normal. A hydrosalpinx may retain a tubular appearance, leading to its identification as a fallopian tube (Fig. 7), but when markedly distended it appears similar to other large simple adnexal cysts. A large hydrosalpinx may occasionally be recognized because it may have a small fluid-filled tail at the junction of the tube with the uterus.[26] An acute abscess with echogenic debris and a shaggy irregular wall may resolve into a collection that is more sharply defined (Fig. 8). Inflammatory pelvic peritoneal cysts are large, multiseptated, and thin-walled and thus mimic serous or mucinous cystadenomas or cystadenocarcinomas.

Without classic clinical findings or serial sonographic changes, the ultrasound examination is not specific. For example, an echo-free tubular pelvic structure may not represent the expected hydrosalpinx, but rather a dilated distal ureter (Fig. 9). Complex residua of abscesses and inflammatory cysts may be indistinguishable from cystic neoplasms, endometriosis, or chronic ruptured ectopic pregnancy. Functional cysts frequently coexist with chronic pelvic inflammatory disease; however, cysts usually resolve, whereas chronic pelvic inflammatory disease does not. Normal fluid-filled bowel loops may even masquerade as abscesses (Fig. 10).

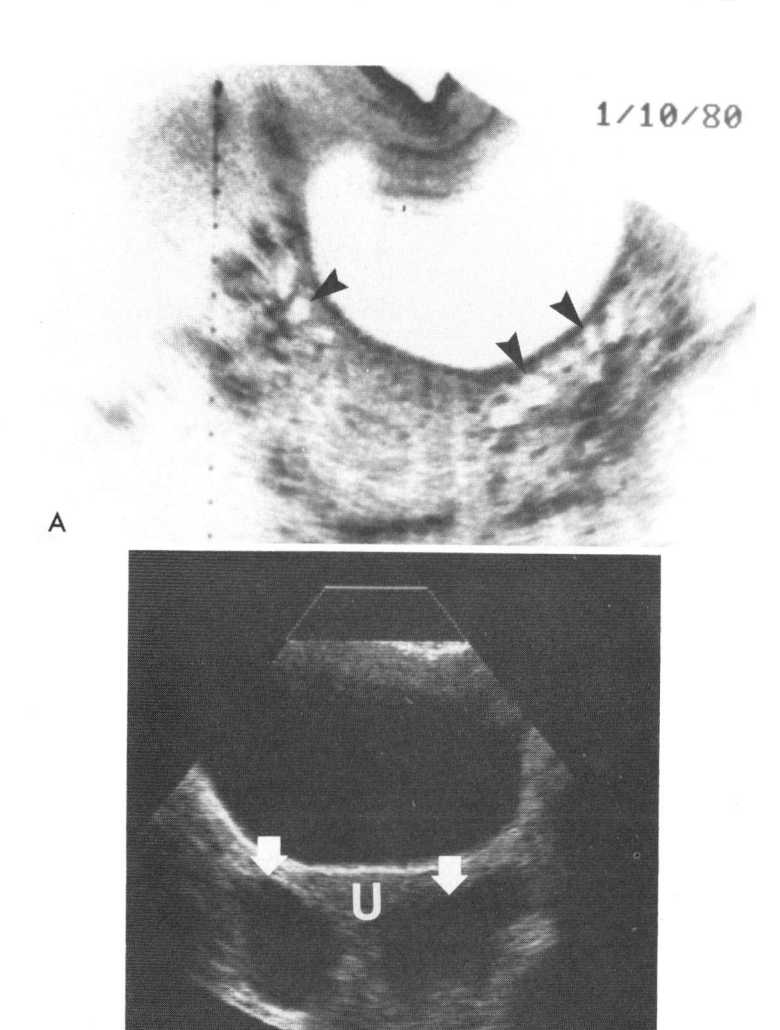

Figure 7. *A*, Transverse sonogram demonstrates beaded tubular adnexal structures (*arrowheads*) which were laparoscopically confirmed as bilateral hydrosalpinx. (Case courtesy of Dr. G. Leland Melson, St. Louis, Missouri.) *B*, Transverse sonogram in another patient with a more distended bilateral hydrosalpinx (*arrows*). The uterus (U) is seen in the midline. Despite their larger size, the tubes have retained their characteristic contours.

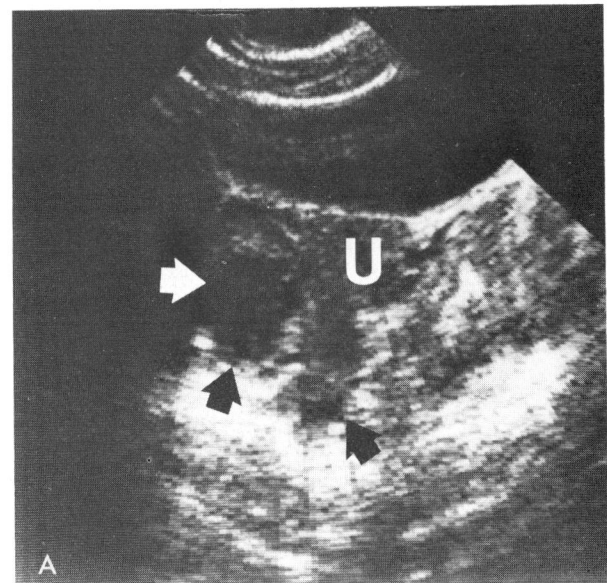

Figure 8. *A*, Transverse sonogram in a patient with an acute tubo-ovarian abscess (*arrows*). U, uterus. *B*, Several weeks later, the abscess (*arrows*) has decreased in size and has become more sharply defined. U, uterus.

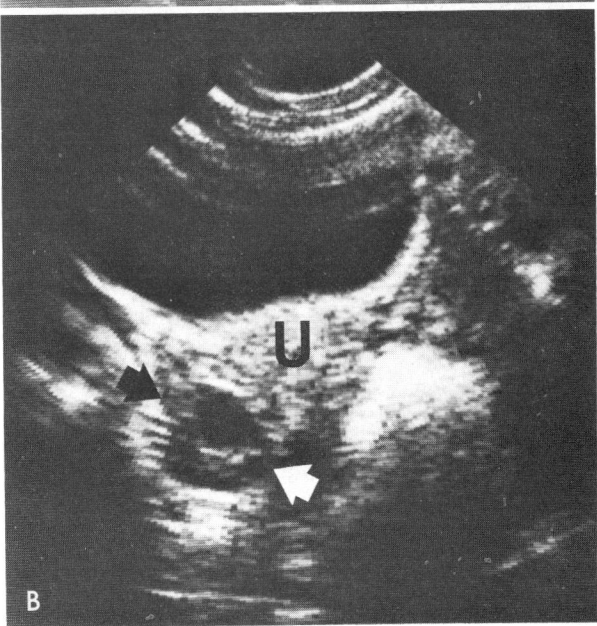

The limited role of sonography in chronic pelvic inflammatory disease is to document the appearance of sequelae, to gauge the effectiveness of therapy, and to help elucidate causes of infertility. However, clinical examination usually adequately serves these purposes. When further information is necessary, laparoscopy or hysterosalpingography is required for more specific diagnosis.[29, 31] As with acute pelvic inflammatory disease, radionuclide and computed tomographic studies are almost never necessary.

PELVIC INFECTIONS AND THE INTRAUTERINE DEVICE (IUD)

There is a significantly increased incidence of pelvic infection in patients with an intrauterine device (IUD),[22, 38] but the nature of such infection differs from pelvic inflammatory disease of venereal origin in both pathophysiology and bacteriology. Although most bacteria are cleared from the uterus after placement of an IUD,[38] the tail of the IUD provides a path for the introduction of bacteria from the vagina and

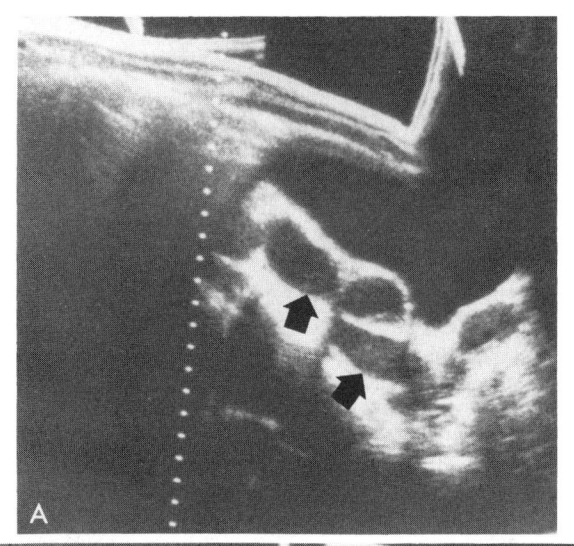

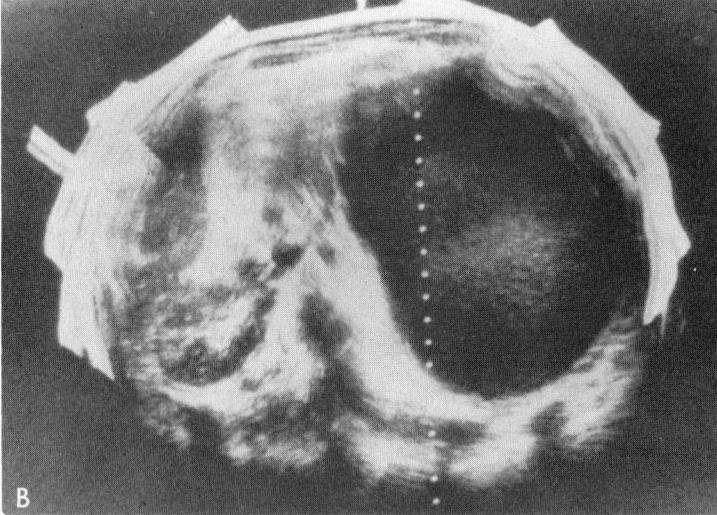

Figure 9. A, Longitudinal sonogram in a patient with left flank pain who had an echo-free tubular left adnexal mass compatible with a hydrosalpinx (arrows). B, However, a more cephalad transverse sonogram in this patient revealed a massive pyohydronephrosis of a left upper pole duplicated collecting system. (Case courtesy of Dr. G. Leland Melson, St. Louis, Missouri.)

cervix[35] into the uterus. Multifilament tails have been implicated as the most serious offenders because bacteria thrive in the microscopic spaces between filaments,[35] and thus such IUDs are no longer marketed; however, monofilament tails may also lead to bacterial infection.[35]

Once within the endometrial cavity, bacteria invade the uterine wall at the site of contact with the IUD and travel through lymphatics and veins to the salpinges, causing unilateral tubo-ovarian abscesses or pelvic abscesses.[35] The infecting organisms are often anaerobes, as with pelvic inflammatory disease, but actinomyces may be the causative agent in a minority of patients.[35, 42] The IUD may also migrate through the uterine wall into the peritoneal space, but may not cause an abscess in such cases.[12] A prodromal syndrome of vague lower abdominal pain, dyspareunia, and pelvic tenderness commonly heralds pelvic infection from an IUD. Although pelvic infections in women with IUDs have been associated with increased sexual activity, these infections are not true venereal pelvic inflammatory disease and the gonococcus is usually not isolated.[22]

Sonography

Adnexal sonographic findings in patients with infections from IUDs are similar to findings in acute pelvic inflammatory disease, except that tubo-ovarian abscesses associated with IUDs are more often unilateral. However, finding only a unilateral adnexal mass does not necessarily indicate that the infection is caused by an IUD. Unilateral or bilateral disease may occur with or without an IUD, and only unilateral disease may be sonographically detected even when bilateral disease is present, because one tubo-ovarian abscess may be much larger than the other. An intrauterine device is usually visible as an intensely echoing structure in the central uterine cavity but may occasionally be difficult to identify.[34] Metallic IUDs produce bright echoes, with a posterior acoustic shadow, but may also cause intense posterior echo enhancement. A similar effect has been recently observed with other metallic foreign bodies and is caused by sound reverberations within the metal.[1, 43] Nonmetallic devices may not produce strong central uterine echoes, but the loop-type IUD may be identified by the regularly spaced shadow caused by looping within the plane of section (Fig. 11). An IUD that has perforated the uterine wall may be impossible to see even if it remains within the pelvis.

The simultaneous identification of an IUD and a pelvic mass may suggest infection from IUD, but the differential diagnosis is broad and similar to that of acute pelvic inflammatory disease. Sonographi-

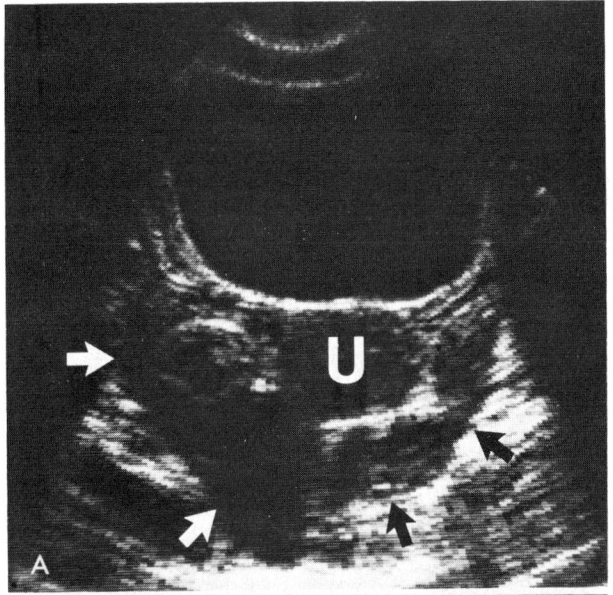

Figure 10. *A*, Transverse sonogram in a patient with a large, bilateral pelvic abscess (*arrows*). U, uterus. *B*, Transverse sonogram in a different patient with bilateral adnexal collections (*arrows*). However, these collections were simply fluid-filled loops of bowel as confirmed by real-time sonography. U, uterus.

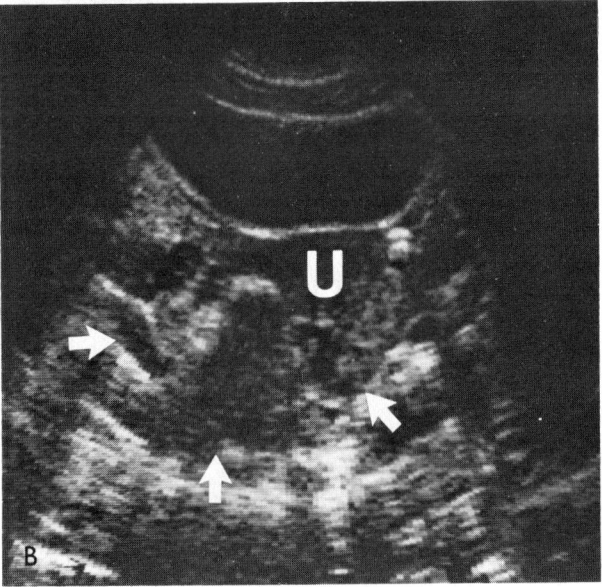

nostically in patients with the prodromal symptom complex. Plain film radiography may detect an IUD, but ultrasonography localizes the device more specifically.

NONVENEREAL PELVIC INFECTIONS

Pathology

Because the pelvis is the most dependent point of the peritoneal space in the supine person, the pelvis is a common site of an intraperitoneal abscess.[24] Abscesses may develop in postsurgical and posttraumatic patients even when the site of original infection is distant, and blood and ascites in these patients provide fertile media for bacterial growth. Most tubo-ovarian abscesses occur through ascending infection, but hematogenous seeding from distant sites may occasionally occur.[26] Uncommonly, a fistulous communication between a tubo-ovarian abscess and the sigmoid colon develops as occurred in 3 of 45 patients in a radiologic review of tubo-ovarian abscesses.[27] Such fistulas are usually simply a late consequence of abscess formation. Causative organisms depend upon the source of the abscess but anaerobes predominate and multiple organisms may coexist.[38] Multiple intraperitoneal abscesses commonly occur simultaneously and tend to form in other dependent areas such as Morison's pouch between the right hepatic

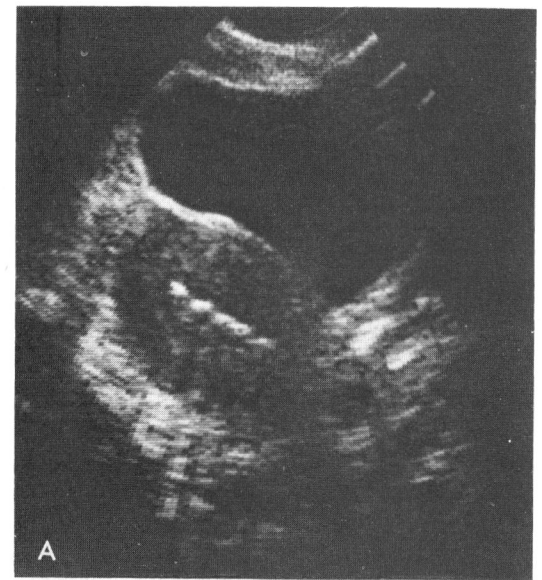

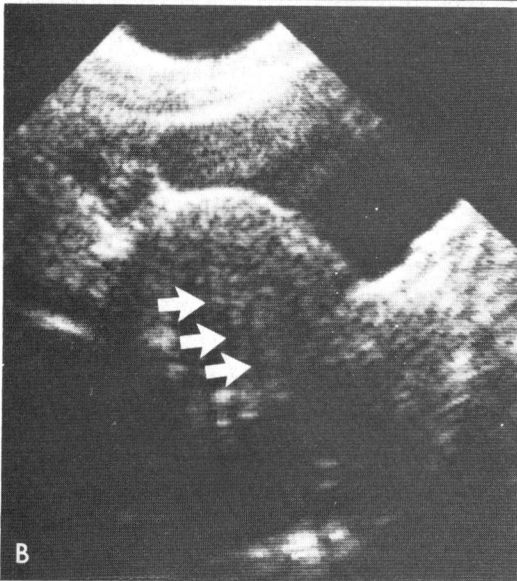

Figure 11. *A,* Longitudinal sonogram through a nonmetallic intrauterine device. High amplitude reflections and posterior acoustic shadows are seen as the device loops within the plane of section. *B,* Longitudinal sonogram through a similar intrauterine device in a different patient. Although the periodic shadows are present (*arrows*), there are no high amplitude echoes from the device itself, indicating that such devices may occasionally be difficult to identify.

cally localizing an IUD when a tail is not seen on physical examination may contribute significantly to managing patients with pelvic infections because the IUD provides a nidus for infection and must be removed.[35] Also, a patient may be unaware of the presence of an IUD, and thus its sonographic recognition is important diag-

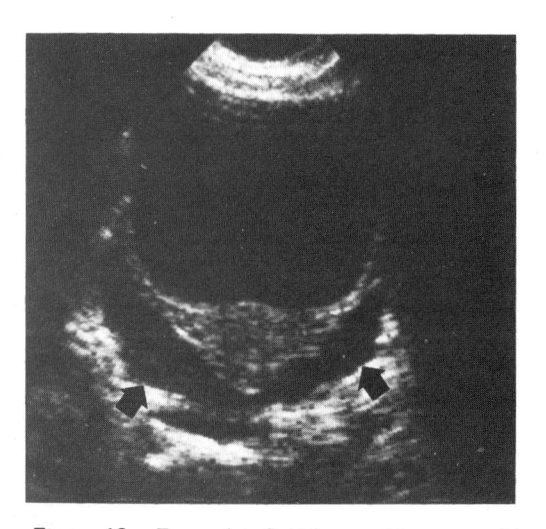

Figure 12. Free pelvic fluid (*arrows*) is seen on this transverse scan. This patient had a periappendiceal abscess which ruptured, causing the contents of the abscess to flow into the more dependent pouch of Douglas.

lobe and right kidney, the subphrenic spaces, and the paracolic gutters.[24] Abscesses originating in the pelvis may also rupture, leading to more widespread involvement, or infected ascites may loculate within the peritoneal cavity. Pelvic malignant disease and the effects of its treatment by surgery, radiation therapy, and chemotherapy predispose to both systemic and localized infections. At times, the tumor itself becomes infected. Periappendiceal and diverticular abscesses may occur within or rupture into the pelvis (Fig. 12), and inflammatory masses and abscesses of Crohn's disease are common in this location. Conversely, abscesses originating from pelvic organs may first appear clinically outside the pelvis (Figs. 13 and 14).

Sonography

The sonographic appearance of posttraumatic or postsurgical pelvic abscess is identical to a pelvic abscess complicating pelvic inflammatory disease. It is impossible to distinguish an infected from an uninfected fluid collection, but irregularity of the wall,

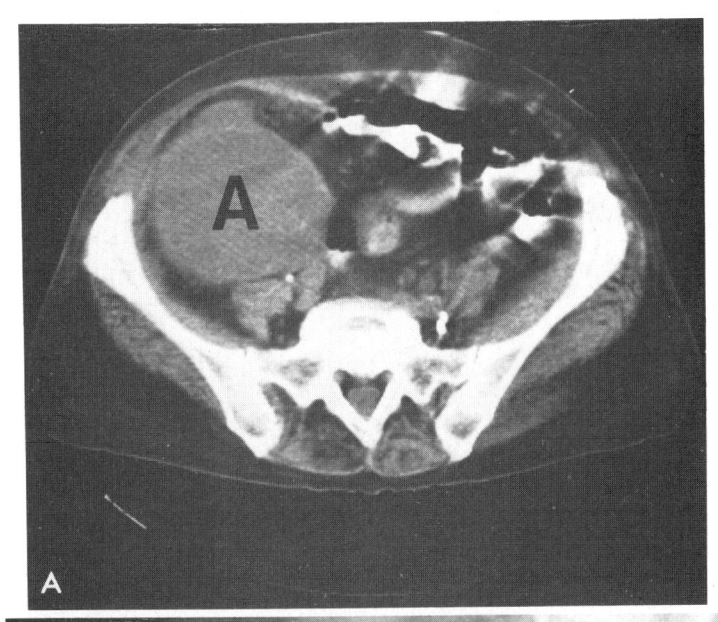

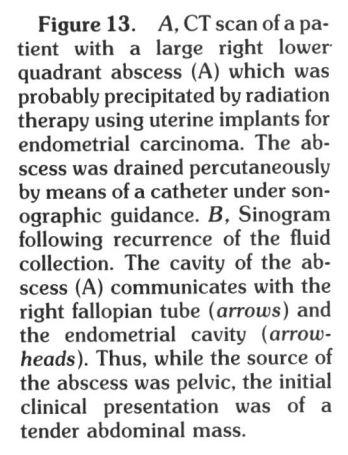

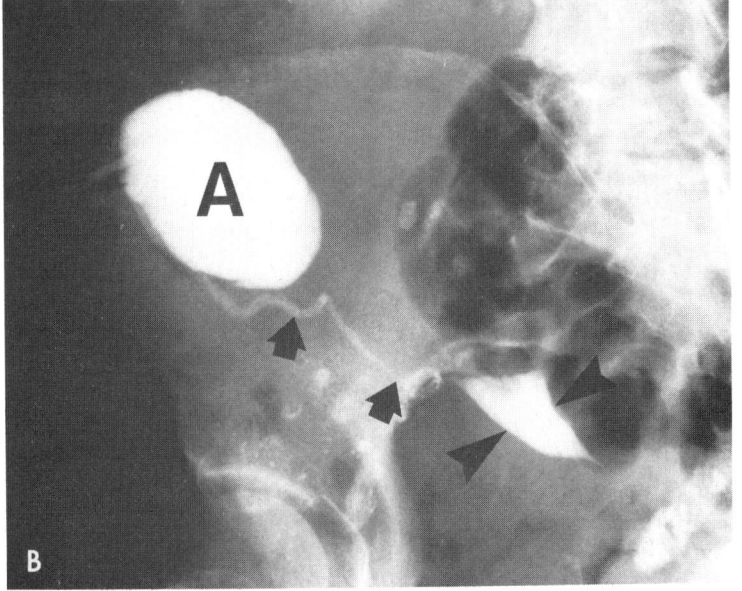

Figure 13. *A,* CT scan of a patient with a large right lower quadrant abscess (A) which was probably precipitated by radiation therapy using uterine implants for endometrial carcinoma. The abscess was drained percutaneously by means of a catheter under sonographic guidance. *B,* Sinogram following recurrence of the fluid collection. The cavity of the abscess (A) communicates with the right fallopian tube (*arrows*) and the endometrial cavity (*arrowheads*). Thus, while the source of the abscess was pelvic, the initial clinical presentation was of a tender abdominal mass.

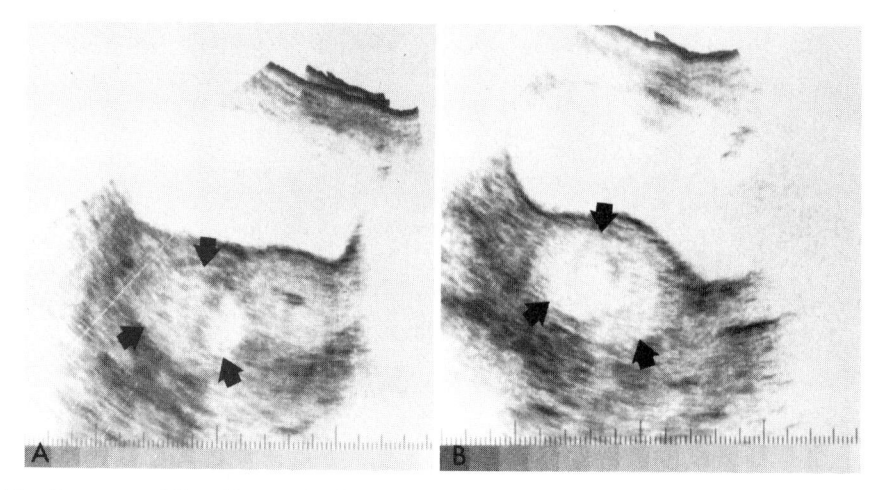

Figure 14. Transverse (A) and longitudinal (B) sonograms of a pelvic abscess (*arrows*). Prior to this study, this patient had surgery for presumed acute appendicitis. However, only the tip of the appendix was inflamed, and the abscess recurred. This abscess and the original "appendicitis" were probably from the patient's intrauterine device, which was removed before the sonogram was performed. (Case courtesy of Dr. G. Leland Melson, St. Louis, Missouri.)

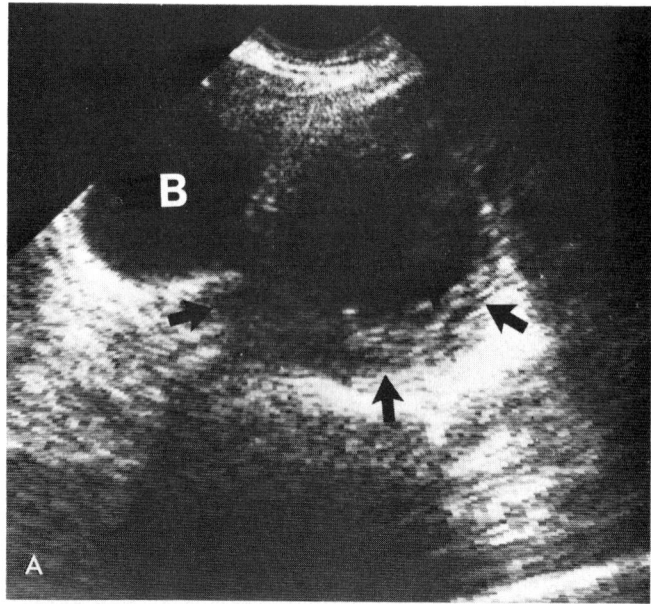

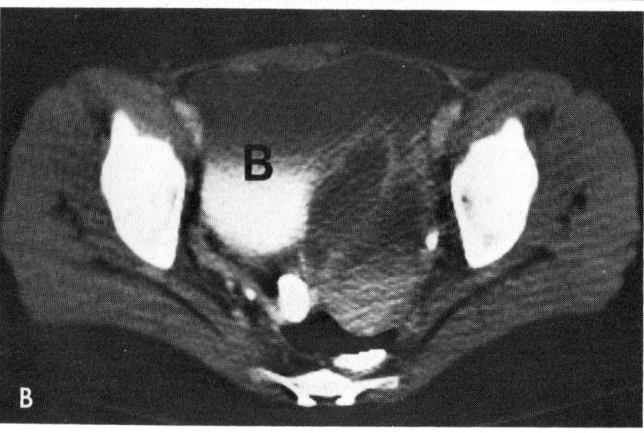

Figure 15. *A*, Transverse sonogram craniad to the uterus in a patient with an abscess (*arrows*) from gastrointestinal origin. The abscess has a thick irregular wall. B, bladder. *B*, CT scan of the same patient was originally misinterpreted as probable cystic ovarian tumor. There is some contrast material in the bladder (B). Thus the sonogram better demonstrated an appearance suggesting the proper diagnosis.

internal echoes, or the appearance of numerous bright echoes suggesting microbubbles increase the probability of infection (Fig. 15).

The diagnostic approach to pyogenic pelvic abscess often includes using several modalities. We prefer computed tomography as the first method of searching for abscess for several reasons. First, computed tomography provides a thorough assessment of the entire peritoneal cavity and may thus identify multiple abscesses (Fig. 16). Second, while a sonographic examination may produce difficulty in excluding an abscess especially in the presence of an ileus, a good quality computed tomographic examination may produce no difficulty in doing so.[15] Third, computed tomography may permit identification of gas or fresh hemorrhage within a fluid collection (Fig. 17), whereas sonography may not. Fourth, sonography is often limited by bandages, wounds, ileus, and the inability of some patients to fill the bladder.

Thus, as a nondirected survey examination of the pelvis, computed tomography is most likely to reveal a pelvic abscess. However, when computed tomography is inconclusive, sonography may be a helpful adjunct, especially when done as a directed study to ascertain the nature of an abnormality suspected by computed tomography.

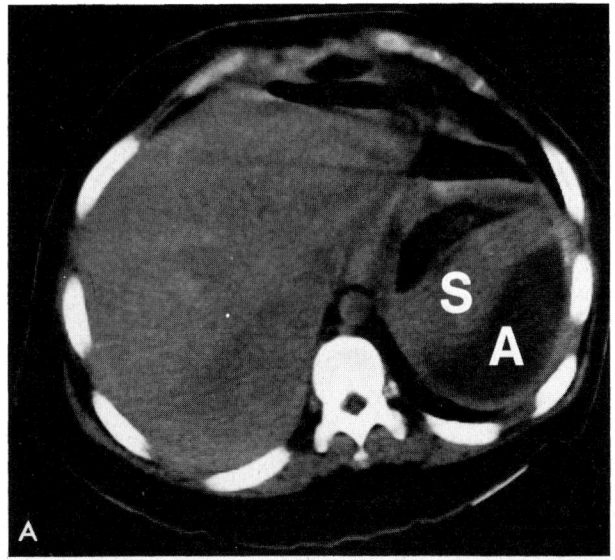

Figure 16. *A*, CT scan of the upper abdomen in a patient with a recent gastrectomy. An abscess collection (A) is lateral to the spleen (S). *B*, Pelvic CT scan in the same patient shows a second large abscess (A) which contains a small bubble of gas (*arrow*). The rectum (*open arrow*) is collapsed dorsal to the abscess. Computed tomography is preferred to sonography for the first evaluation of patients suspected of having abscesses because it can more easily detect multiple areas of involvement.

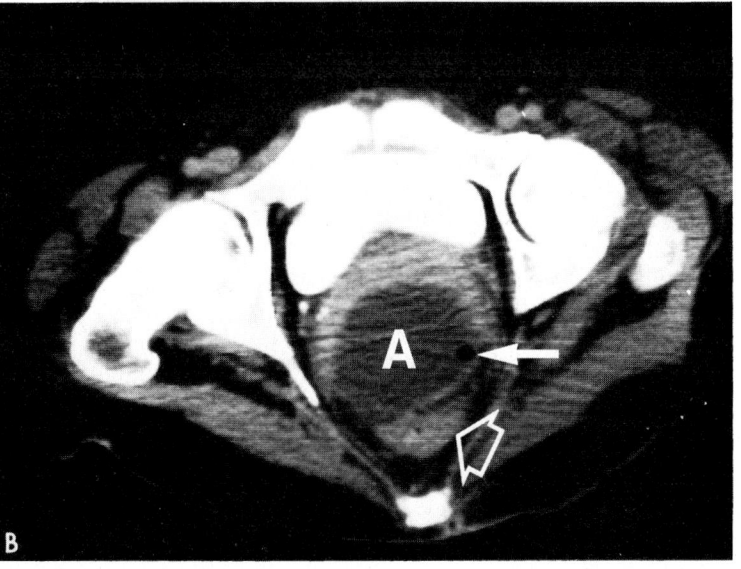

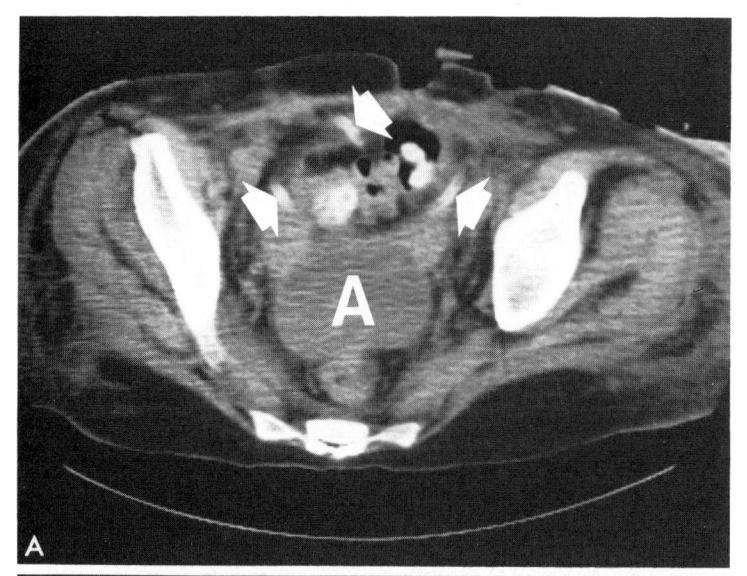

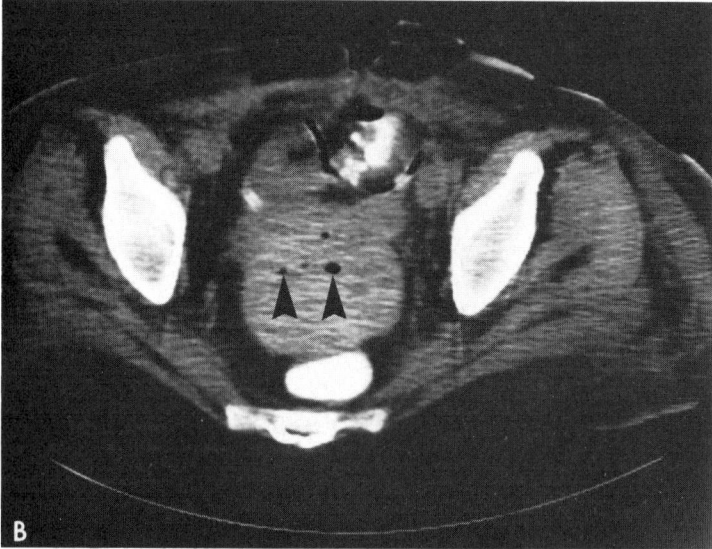

Figure 17. *A*, Pelvic CT scan of a patient with loculated, infected ascites. Despite a suprapubic drain (*arrows*), an abscess (A) was present within the deep pelvis. *B*, CT scan taken after vaginal drainage of the abscess shows a recurrence of the collection, but its high attenuation indicates that it is fresh hemorrhage rather than a recurrent abscess. Gas (*arrowheads*) is also seen within this collection because of the drainage procedure.

The identity of questionable fluid collections may be clarified with sonography by determining the anatomic relationship of a collection to surrounding structures or by identifying peristalsis. Also, abscesses recognized by computed tomography are often best localized for percutaneous aspiration using sonographic guidance,[10] particularly with real-time instruments.

Gallium-67 and indium-111 labeled white blood cell scans image the entire body and thus may detect systemic disease or disease outside areas scanned by sectional imaging techniques.[5, 23] These radionuclide studies also effectively highlight regions of suspected abnormality for further study with higher resolution imaging methods, but radionuclide scans produce many false normal and false abnormal results. Potentially life-threatening abdominal and pelvic abscesses require accurate diagnosis, and thus more than one type of imaging study is often necessary because of their complementary features.[4, 14, 15, 23]

PELVIC ABSCESS IN RENAL TRANSPLANT AND IMMUNOSUPPRESSED PATIENTS

Renal transplant and immunosuppressed patients present special problems in diagnosis and treatment of pelvic infections. Renal transplants are usually placed in an extraperitoneal location within the pelvis and are associated with several types of fluid collections, including seromas, hematomas, lymphangiomas, and urinomas (Fig. 18). Postoperative seromas are most often seen as echo-free collections and usually resolve slowly, as do the less common peritransplant hematomas. However, hematomas often show a sonographically changing character of internal echoes from an echogenic mass to an echo-free mass as clot liquifies and resorbs. In contrast to seromas and hematomas, lymphangiomas are often multiseptated and may slowly grow to remarkable size rather than disappear.

Urinomas are difficult to discriminate from seromas or echo-free hematomas, and all three can become infected without demonstrating any specific sonographic signs of infection. However, such peritransplant fluid collections are usually superficial and accessible to percutaneous needle aspiration for diagnosis or for drainage using sonographic guidance. While ultrasonography is the first choice for evaluating renal transplants, some patients may be difficult to examine, or bladder filling may be contraindicated, and thus computed tomography will detect collections located deep within the pelvis which cannot be seen by sonography.

Transplant patients also commonly have ascites which may become infected, occasionally from peritoneal dialysis. Ascitic fluid containing septations and internal echoes is probably complicated by infection or hemorrhage, but a definitive diagnosis is obtained by paracentesis. Diagnosing infections in transplant patients is difficult because of the variety of other problems that may occur and mimic abscess, and because such immunosuppressed patients with marginal renal function often do not manifest the classic physical signs of infection. Indeed, the most typical findings of an abscess are fever and tenderness, which usually imply allograft rejection in the transplant patient.

Similar problems in diagnosis occur in other immunosuppressed patients. Women with gynecologic malignant disease may develop ascites, and in the presence of a preexisting pelvic mass, diagnostic studies may be difficult to interpret. A necrotic tumor may mimic an abscess, or the tumor may become infected through surgical manipulation or fistula formation. The uncertainty in sonographic and clinical diagnosis emphasizes the importance of obtaining tissue or fluid, which can often be accomplished with sonographic or computed tomographic guidance.

TUBERCULOSIS AND PARASITES

These infections differ from acute pelvic inflammatory disease because with tuberculosis, the fallopian tubes tend to remain patent, despite the bilateral involvement always found.[13] Also, the ovary, which is relatively resistant to pyogenic infection, may develop deep infection when affected by tuberculosis. With progression of dis-

Figure 18. Oblique sonogram of a renal transplant. There is massive ascites, mild hydronephrosis, and several peritransplant fluid collections. One collection (*arrowheads*) is echo-free. Another, containing internal echoes (*arrows*), probably represents a hematoma. Sonography cannot specifically identify the presence of infection in the several types of fluid collections occurring in transplant patients.

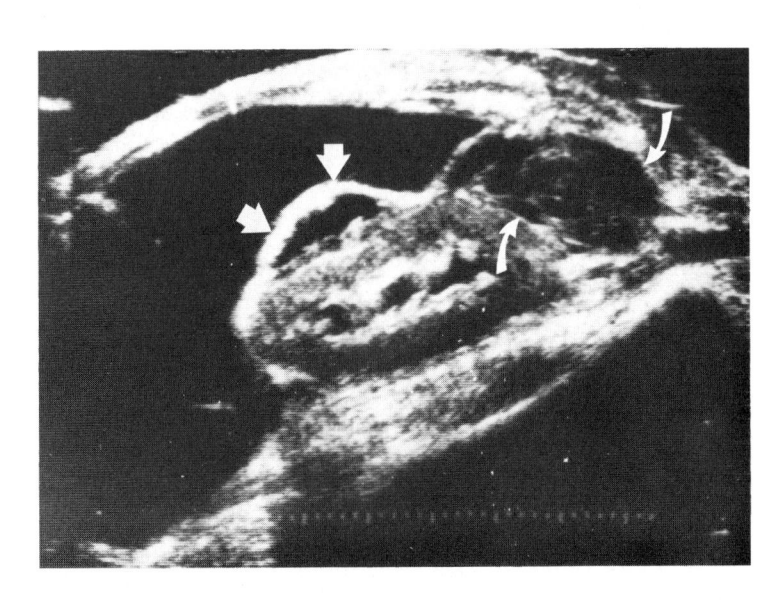

ease, dense, extensive adhesions form and thus tubercular pelvic infections commonly lead to infertility.

Tuberculosis of the pelvis is very uncommon in the United States, and there are probably no specific sonographic signs. The severe form might clinically and sonographically simulate an indolent chronic pelvic inflammatory disease.

Parasitic infestations, including schistosomiasis, involving the female genital tract are rare within the United States.[13] However, such diseases might be encountered among immigrants or those who have traveled abroad.

INFECTION RELATED TO PREGNANCY

Typical acute pelvic inflammatory disease is rare in pregnancy, probably because the gestation blocks the ascent of bacteria;[38] however, other causes of infection may be catastrophic to the mother and fetus. Puerperal sepsis usually begins as an ascending infection involving amnionitis and endometritis which may progress to salpingitis and peritonitis.[25] Intrauterine fetal monitoring may cause amniotic fluid contamination and subsequent postpartum infection.[38] Other risk factors for infection are prolonged labor with ruptured membranes, pregnancy with an intrauterine device, and cesarean section (Fig. 19).[38] Post-abortal sepsis may be caused by Clostridium or anaerobes, but this is much less common with the legalization of abortion.[12,38] Pelvic abscess may also occur in post-abortal sepsis and be indistinguishable from other types of abscesses. Promptly recognizing the clinical signs of infection is the key to successful therapy, and therefore ultrasound is usually of limited value. However, sonography may localize and follow the progress of fluid collections in patients responding poorly to antibiotic treatment.

TECHNICAL CONSIDERATIONS

Numerous technical variables including the experience and diligence of the sonographer influence the adequacy of the pelvic sonogram, but the impact of recent changes in ultrasound technology has not yet been thoroughly clarified. We now use high resolution real-time sector scanning without articulated arm imaging for sonographically evaluating the abdomen and pelvis in most patients. In the pelvis, this method decreases scanning time while improving the examination of adnexal structures because an organ or lesion is easily viewed in numerous planes. This capability of real-time scanning also helps to identify the three-dimensional shape of structures and, for example, may permit demonstration of the typical tubular shape of a hydrosalpinx. Using real-time scanning, a sonographer easily perceives peristalsis and fluid flow and thus masses are better differentiated from fluid-filled or matted bowel loops. Also, the technique of administering a water enema for differentiating adnexal cysts from fluid-filled distal colon[30] is improved with real-time imaging for the same reason.

With rapid frame rates and high frequencies of 3 to 5 MHz, which require higher gain settings, increased electronic noise may interfere with accurate assessment of whether a structure is fluid or solid. However, differentiating solid from cystic lesions may be difficult even if there is an accurate determination of whether a mass is echogenic or echo-free.[39] Clear fluid-

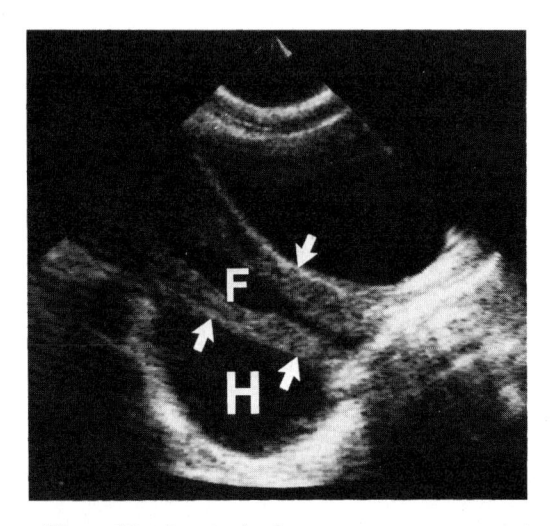

Figure 19. Longitudinal sonogram in a woman with postpartum pelvic pain. A hematoma (H) is present posterior to the lower uterine segment (*arrows*) Fluid (F) is present within the normally involuting uterus. Either the fluid or the hematoma might be accessible to percutaneous fine-needle aspiration if infection was suspected.

filled structures less than 2 cm in diameter may be difficult to identify as echo-free because of ultrasonic partial volume effects.[3] Fluid containing abscesses may contain numerous echoes because of purulent and/or hemorrhagic exudate, or because of sound scatter through overlying tissues, particularly in obese patients. Posterior echo enhancement may be impossible to identify because echogenic bowel contents may lie immediately deep to adnexal masses.

Previously described ultrasonic signs must be reevaluated in light of present technology. For example, several authors have described a loss of uterine borders in acute pelvic inflammatory disease,[2, 6, 9, 18] but recent changes in pre- and post-processing methods allow the operator the ability to vary the relative amplification of signals from strong specular reflectors and weak parenchymal reflectors.[11] Therefore, restoring or obliterating borders may be possible by modifying pre- or post-processing curves. Furthermore, this "indefinite uterus" sign has never been adequately explained. Is this loss of borders caused by inflammatory edema, or is it an ultrasonic "masking sign"[17] caused by contiguity of the uterus with purulent fluid of equivalent echogenicity? Might the higher resolution offered by newer scanners affect the ability to elicit this sign?

Another sign of uterine infection is decreased myometrial echogenicity. In our experience, the evaluation of this sign and other signs mentioned above is difficult, and the inability to consistently recognize such subtle sonographic findings further decreases diagnostic specificity.

FUTURE OF PELVIC SONOGRAPHY IN DIAGNOSING INFLAMMATORY DISEASE

Because of the technical limitations of pelvic sonography, we probably cannot improve substantially on present accuracy and sensitivity rates. Thus, when used in its present manner, the sonogram will continue to hold a secondary place in diagnosis. However, one method for possible investigation is the simultaneous pelvic examination and real-time ultrasound study as described by Platt et al.[28] This technique offers the potential for better detecting and better appreciating the location, shape, consistency, and fixation of mass lesions by real-time observation during manual manipulation of the pelvic organs. However, such procedures require close cooperation between the gynecologist and the sonographer, and thus would also require solving major logistic and political problems in many ultrasound laboratories.

A second area for further exploration is ultrasonic guidance for percutaneous aspiration of the adnexa and endometrium for bacterial culture. Blind endometrial percutaneous aspiration has been attempted by one author who achieved modest results,[19] and the success of ultrasonic guidance for biopsy of abdominal mass lesions and for amniocentesis suggests that such aspiration procedures may be a valuable technique. Infectious diseases of the pelvis are caused by a variety of organisms including aerobes,[38] anaerobes,[38] chylamydia,[26] mycoplasma,[37] actinomycosis,[21, 42] and tuberculosis,[26] and bacteriologic diagnosis can be crucial to selecting the proper antibiotic therapy.[21]

SUMMARY

Sonography is used infrequently for diagnosing acute pelvic inflammatory disease because the physical examination is highly sensitive, because the sonogram lacks specificity, and because the patient is often scheduled for surgery or laparoscopy or treated medically based on clinical findings, obviating the need for diagnostic studies.[33] Sonography is usually reserved for identifying, localizing, and following pelvic abscesses complicating pelvic inflammatory disease. The sonogram is valuable in identifying the location of intrauterine devices because of the increased incidence of inflammatory pelvic disease in these patients. Postoperative and posttraumatic abscesses and abscesses of gastrointestinal origin may require the concomitant use of computed tomography and radionuclide studies, with ultrasonography performing a complementary function. The ultrasound examination may be valuable both in improving diagnostic confidence and providing guidance for aspiration. Because of the limited spectrum of appearances of numerous pelvic diseases, the most accurate diagnoses are obtained when the sonogram is interpreted in light of the detailed clinical information.

REFERENCES

1. Amazeen, P. G., Whitehead, F., and Questo, W.: Ultrasonic appearance of metallic foreign bodies (letter). J. Clin. Ultrasound, 9:A–31, 1981.
2. Bowie, J. D.: Ultrasound of gynecologic pelvic masses: The indefinite uterus and other patterns associated with diagnostic error. J. Clin. Ultrasound, 5:323, 1977.
3. Bree, R. L., and Silver, T. M.: Differential diagnosis of hypoechoic and anechoic masses with gray scale sonography: New observations. J. Clin. Ultrasound, 7:249, 1979.
4. Callen, P. W.: Computed tomographic evaluation of abdominal and pelvic abscesses. Radiology, 131:171, 1979.
5. Carroll, B., Silverman, P. M., Goodwin, D. A., et al.: Ultrasonography and indium-111 white blood cell scanning for the detection of intraabdominal abscesses. Radiology, 140:155, 1981.
6. Cassoff, J., and Hanna, T.: Grey-scale ultrasonography for assessment of gynecologic pelvic masses. Can. Med. Assoc. J., 120:38, 1979.
7. Cochrane, W. J., and Thomas, M. A.: Ultrasound diagnosis of gynecologic pelvic masses. Radiology, 110:649, 1974.
8. Doust, B. D., and Doust, V. L.: Ultrasonic diagnosis of abdominal abscess. Dig. Dis., 21:569, 1976.
9. Fleischer, A. C., James, A. E., Millis, J. B., et al.: Differential diagnosis of pelvic masses by gray scale sonography. Am. J. Roentgenol., 131:469, 1978.
10. Gerzof, S. G., Robbins, A. H., Johnson, W. C., et al.: Percutaneous catheter drainage of abdominal abscesses: A five-year experience. N. Engl. J. Med., 305:653, 1981.
11. Jaffe, C. C., and Harris, D. J.: Physical factors influencing numerical echo-amplitude data extracted from B-scan ultrasound images. J. Clin. Ultrasound, 8:327, 1980.
12. Jones, H. W., and Jones, G. S.: Pelvic inflammatory disease. In Novak's Textbook of Gynecology. Edition 10. Baltimore, Williams and Wilkins Co., 1981.
13. King, T. M., and Burkman, R. T.: Pelvic inflammatory disease. In deAlvarez, R. R. (ed.): Textbook of Gynecology. Philadelphia, Lea and Febiger, 1977.
14. Knochel, J. Q., Koehler, P. R., Lee, T. G., et al.: Diagnosis of abdominal abscesses with computed tomography, ultrasound and in ^{111}In leukocyte scans. Radiology, 137:425, 1980.
15. Koehler, P. R., and Moss, A. A.: Diagnosis of intraabdominal and pelvic abscesses by computerized tomography. J.A.M.A., 244:49, 1980.
16. Kressel, H. Y., and Filly, R. A.: Ultrasonographic appearance of gas-containing abscesses in the abdomen. Am. J. Roentgenol., 130:71, 1978.
17. Kurtz, A. B., Dubbins, P. A., Rubin, C. S., et al.: Echogenicity: Analysis, significance, and masking. Am. J. Roentgenol., 137:471, 1981.
18. Lawson, T. L., and Albarelli, J. N.: Diagnosis of gynecologic pelvic masses by gray scale ultrasonography: Analysis of specificity and accuracy. Am. J. Roentgenol., 128:1003, 1977.
19. Ledger, W. J., Gee, C. L., Pollin, P. A., et al.: A new approach to patients with suspected anaerobic postpartum pelvic infections. Transabdominal uterine aspiration for culture and metronidazole for treatment. Am. J. Obstet. Gynecol., 126:1, 1976.
20. Lees, R. F., Feldman, P. S., Brenbridge, A. N. A. G., et al.: Inflammatory cysts of the pelvic peritoneum. Am. J. Roentgenol., 131:633, 1978.
21. Louria, D. B., and Sen, P.: Anaerobic infections of the pelvis. Obstet. Gynecol., 55:114S, 1980.
22. Luukkainen, T., Nielsen, N. C., Nygren, K. G., et al.: Nulliparous women, IUD and pelvic infection. Ann. Clin. Res., 11:121, 1979.
23. McNeil, B. J., Sanders, R., Alderson, P. O., et al.: A prospective study of computed tomography, ultrasound, and gallium imaging in patients with fever. Radiology, 139:647, 1981.
24. Meyers, M. A.: Dynamic Radiology of the Abdomen: Normal and Pathologic Anatomy. New York, Springer-Verlag, 1976.
25. Monif, G. R. G.: Significance of polymicrobial bacterial superinfection in the therapy of gonococcal endometritis-salpingitis-peritonitis. Obstet. Gynecol., 55:154S, 1980.
26. Novak, E. R., and Woodruff, J. D.: Salpingitis and inflammatory diseases of the ovary. In Gynecologic and Obstetric Pathology. Edition 8. Philadelphia, W. B. Saunders Co., 1979.
27. Phillips, J. C.: A spectrum of radiologic abnormalities due to tubo-ovarian abscess. Radiology, 110:307, 1974.
28. Platt, L. D., Manning, F. A., and Hill, L. M.: Simultaneous real-time ultrasound scanning and pelvic examination in assessment of pelvic disease. Am. J. Obstet. Gynecol., 136:693, 1980.
29. Reeves, R. D., Drake, T. S., and O'Brien, W. F.: Ultrasonographic versus clinical evaluation of a pelvic mass. Obstet. Gynecol., 55:551, 1980.
30. Rubin, C., Kurtz, A. B., and Goldberg, B. B.: Water enema: A new ultrasound technique in defining pelvic anatomy. J. Clin. Ultrasound, 6:28, 1978.
31. Scaling, S. T., Levinson, C. J., Plavidal, F., et al.: The correlation of pelvic ultrasound and laparoscopy in the diagnosis and management of gynecologic disorders. J. Reprod. Med., 21:53, 1978.
32. Schlensker, K. H., and Beckers, H.: The use of ultrasound in the diagnosis of pelvic pathology. Arch. Gynecol., 229:91, 1980.
33. Schwartz, P. E., and Weiner, M.: Ultrasound in gynecology: A clinician's viewpoint. Clin. Diag. Ultrasound, 2:183, 1979.
34. Spiegel, R. M., and Ben-Ora, A.: Ultrasound of inflammatory disease in the pelvis. Semin. Ultrasound, 1:41, 1980.
35. Taylor, E. S., McMillan, J. H., Greer, B. E., et al.: The intrauterine device and tubo-ovarian abscess. Am. J. Obstet, Gynecol., 123:338, 1975.
36. Taylor, K., Graaf, C., Wasson, J., et al.: Accuracy of grey-scale ultrasound diagnosis of abdominal and pelvic abscesses in 220 patients. Lancet, 1:83, 1978.

37. Taylor-Robinson, D., and McCormack, W. M.: The genital mycoplasmas. N. Engl. J. Med., *302*:1003, 1980.
38. Thadepalli, H.: Anaerobic infections of the female genital tract. Scand. J. Infect. Dis. Suppl. *19*:80, 1979.
39. Thurber, L. A., Cooperberg, P. L., Clement, J. G., et al.: Echogenic fluid: A pitfall in the ultrasonographic diagnosis of cystic lesions. J. Clin. Ultrasound, *7*:273, 1979.
40. Uhrich, P. C., and Sanders, R. C.: Ultrasonic characteristics of pelvic inflammatory masses. J. Clin. Ultrasound, *4*:199, 1976.
41. Walsh, J. W., Taylor, K. J. W., Wasson, J. M., et al.: Gray-scale ultrasound in 204 proved gynecologic masses: Accuracy and specific diagnostic criteria. Radiology, *130*:391, 1979.
42. Wagner, M., Kiselow, M. C., Goodman, J. J., et al.: The relationship of intrauterine device, actinomycosis infection, and bowel abscesses. Wisconsin Med. J., *78*:23, 1979.
43. Wendell, B. A., and Athey, P. A.: Ultrasonic appearance of metallic foreign bodies in parenchymal organs. J. Clin. Ultrasound, *9*:133, 1981.

18

Ultrasound Evaluation of Ectopic Pregnancy

Faye C. Laing, M.D., and R. Brooke Jeffrey, M.D.

The diagnosis of ectopic pregnancy must constantly be kept in mind as a potential threat to any woman in her reproductive years. Despite this maxim, this diagnosis is missed by the initial examining physician in up to 70 per cent of cases.[5, 10, 13–16] Although ectopic pregnancy is a life-threatening condition, responsible for up to 26 per cent of maternal deaths,[38] the correct diagnosis is delayed for a period of up to three weeks in 14.4 per cent of cases.[15] Compounding these disturbing statistics is the fact that the incidence of ectopic pregnancy appears to be increasing.[16, 17] The early detection of ectopic pregnancy has been hampered because the clinical signs and symptoms are nonspecific, and because until recently, no single test was particularly helpful for suggesting the correct diagnosis.

The purpose of this chapter is to reevaluate ectopic pregnancy, particularly in light of recent laboratory and ultrasonographic developments. This updated approach should enable an earlier and more accurate diagnosis to be made, with a concomitant diminution of associated morbidity and mortality.

HISTORY AND PREDISPOSING FACTORS

Ectopic pregnancy was first described in the Eleventh Century. It was an almost uniformly fatal condition until approximately 100 years ago when Lawson Tait developed a surgical treatment wherein success was equated to early surgical intervention.[37] Throughout history it has been estimated that no less than 3 per cent of women of childbearing age have died from ectopic pregnancy.[18]

Although modern medicine has been successful in conquering and limiting the ravages of many diseases, one of the consequences of its therapeutic and surgical triumphs has been an increase in the incidence of ectopic pregnancy. For example, it is a well known fact that underlying tubal damage promotes an environment which is receptive to tubal implantation. Indeed, at the time of laparotomy for ectopic pregnancy, up to 50 per cent of patients have a history of or pathologic evidence for pelvic inflammatory disease.[5, 10] Modern antibiotic therapy has contributed to the development of these partially obstructed and scarred fallopian tubes, in contrast to total tubal obstruction and sterility which occurred before the antibiotic era. Prior tubal surgery for reconstructive purposes or for antecedent ectopic gestation also promotes scarring which in turn increases the risk of ectopic pregnancy. The availability and popularity of therapeutic abortion and widespread use of intrauterine contraceptive devices have also contributed to a relatively higher incidence of ectopic pregnancy. These latter two predisposing factors, however, may bias the statistics in that they prevent intrauterine fetal development without affecting extrauterine fetal implantation.

The overall incidence of ectopic pregnancy varies dramatically throughout the world and appears to be closely related to socioeconomic status and the prevalence of salpingitis. In Kingston, Jamaica, there is a reported incidence of 1 ectopic pregnancy per 28 deliveries,[30] while in parts of the United States, the incidence is 1 per 280 deliveries.[14] The most frequently reported incidence is between 0.5 and 1 per cent of all pregnancies.[10]

SIGNS AND SYMPTOMS

The overwhelming majority (greater than 95 per cent) of ectopic implantations occur within the fallopian tubes, particularly within the isthmic and ampullary portions.[14, 16–18] In up to one third of cases, the ovum appears to migrate from one ovary to the opposite tube where implantation occurs.[5, 10, 17] This can result in a contralateral corpus luteum cyst.

The most frequent clinical symptom is pain, which ranges in severity from a mild ache to a severe localized or generalized pain. Because of the relatively high incidence of a contralateral corpus luteum cyst, it is not uncommon for this symptom to occur on the side opposite the ectopic pregnancy. Pain, which occurs in virtually every patient, most often develops within three to five weeks after a missed menstrual period.[5] Because the pain is so varied in intensity, duration, and location, it is frequently attributed to other organ systems, including the gastrointestinal, biliary, and urinary tracts. Tubal rupture, which occurs in 80 to 90 per cent of cases, is heralded by a sudden and dramatic exacerbation of pain.[5, 17, 38] Although associated bleeding may result in hypovolemic shock, signs and symptoms of advanced intraabdominal hemorrhage are evident in fewer than 15 per cent of cases.[17, 38]

Another presenting symptom is amenorrhea, which occurs in 50 to 75 per cent of patients.[5, 10, 15–17, 38] Abnormal vaginal bleeding due to hormonal withdrawal commonly accompanies the amenorrhea, and may be misinterpreted by the physician and patient as a normal menstrual cycle.[5, 10, 16–18, 38]

Common physical findings include abdominal tenderness, the presence of an adnexal mass, and cervical motion tenderness. The classic presenting triad for ectopic pregnancy, therefore, is pain, abnormal vaginal bleeding, and an abnormal mass. Unfortunately, these findings are nonspecific and are frequently misleading. Schwartz et al. recently reported an interesting analysis of a group of 234 patients who were clinically suspected of having ectopic pregnancies.[35] The classic presentation occurred most commonly in patients with "pelvic pain of undetermined etiology," and ectopic pregnancy was found to be the fourth most common cause for these signs and symptoms. Of the patients with ectopic pregnancy, the classic triad was present only 45 per cent of the time. Most large clinical series stress the fact that pelvic inflammatory disease is most commonly confused with ectopic pregnancy. Indeed, as many as one half of the patients with an ectopic pregnancy will receive an initial diagnosis and treatment for pelvic inflammatory disease.[10, 16] This is not surprising in light of the common association of pelvic inflammatory disease in patients with ectopic pregnancy, and their identical presenting signs and symptoms. In patients with intrauterine devices the problem of diagnosis is compounded by the fact that in up to 85 per cent of patients, the symptoms of ectopic pregnancy are initially attributed to the intrauterine device.[14]

The net effect of the nonspecific clinical presentation and poorly localized physical findings in ectopic pregnancies is that the correct diagnosis is delayed an average of 10 days.[15] This delay occurs despite the fact that most patients are seen, examined, and are frequently treated medically and even surgically by a physician during the time when they are symptomatic. In most instances the correct diagnosis is not made until the dramatic events accompanying tubal rupture occur.

AVAILABLE DIAGNOSTIC MODALITIES

It is obvious that increased emphasis must be placed on earlier and more accurate diagnosis of ectopic pregnancy if the morbidity and mortality attending tubal rupture are to be diminished. Despite the fact that clinicians frequently ask themselves, "Does this patient have an ectopic pregnancy?", until recently false-positive and false-negative results from available diagnostic tests and procedures have contributed to frequent misdiagnosis and, hence, mismanagement. Traditional diagnostic tools have included the results of a urine pregnancy test and/or culdocentesis. Recently, more accurate pregnancy tests, ultrasound, and laparoscopy have been added to the diagnostic armamentarium.

Table 1. *Historical Development of Pregnancy Tests**

TEST	END POINT	POSITIVE TEST (DAYS AFTER OVULATION)	TEST TIME	SENSITIVITY (IU OF HCG/ML)
Biologic	Rabbit—ovulation	25	2 days	10
	Frog—sperm ejection		2 hours	
Immunologic	HI (tube test)	18–20	1.5 hours	1–3
	LPI (slide test)	25	2 minutes	4–15
Radioassay	^{125}I competition for AB/receptors	6–12	1–24 hours	<.5

* Data adapted from Derman, R., et al.: Int. J. Gynaecol. Obstet., *17*:190, 1979.

Pregnancy Tests

The basis of almost all pregnancy tests is the detection of human chorionic gonadotrophin (HCG) in urine or plasma. This glycoprotein is elaborated by placental trophoblastic cells beginning the eighth day following conception.[8] Under normal circumstances the measurable amount of HCG doubles approximately every two days until it peaks at a level of approximately 100 IU per ml during the sixth week after conception.[9,32]

Historically, biologic pregnancy tests were the first available type (Table 1). Because these tests lack sensitivity, they were not able to detect the presence of a normal pregnancy until approximately three to four weeks after ovulation. In addition, they were time consuming and depended upon a qualitative biologic response such as ovulation or sperm ejection.

A great advancement occurred in 1960 when a commercially available immunologic pregnancy test was introduced.[41] This type of test, which is performed on a urine specimen, is still the most readily available and easiest pregnancy test to perform. It utilizes the principle of indirect agglutination and can be carried out in a test tube or on a slide. The 2 minute slide test is somewhat less sensitive than the 1½ to 2 hour test tube modification. Because these tests are sensitive enough to detect HCG concentrations greater than 1 IU of HCG per ml, they normally become positive at about seven days after the missed menstrual period.[9] Despite the obvious advantages of being rapidly performed and readily available, immunologic pregnancy tests are not without problems. The major limitations of this type of pregnancy test are frequent false-positive and false-negative results (Table 2).

Because of a structural similarity between the HCG molecule and other hormones, cross-reactivity is possible. This most often occurs in patients with levels of luteinizing hormone which become elevated in the preovulatory phase of the midmenstrual cycle, or in perimenopausal and postmenopausal women.[32] In practice, however, the threshold sensitivity of immunologic pregnancy tests is adjusted so that this type of cross-reactivity does not usually occur. Various other conditions may be associated with false-positive immunologic pregnancy tests. These include the presence of proteinuria in excess of 1 gm per 24 hours,[9] hematuria,[9] and the administration of pharmaceuticals, particularly aspirin,[19] major tranquilizers,[19] and methadone.[8] A 21 per cent false-positive rate has been reported with tubo-ovarian abscess.[19] This is particularly troublesome in light of the fact that pelvic inflammatory disease and ectopic pregnancy are often clinically confused. A variety of nongynecologic neoplasms, such as anterior pituitary tumors and bronchogenic carcinoma, have also been associated with false-positive pregnancy tests. In addition, several

Table 2. *Causes of False-Positive Pregnancy Tests*

Proteinuria
Hematuria
Luteinizing hormone
  Ovulation
  Menopause
Pharmaceuticals
  Aspirin
  Major tranquilizers
  Methadone
Tubo-ovarian abscess
Neoplasm
  Gynecologic
  Pituitary
  Lung

gynecologic neoplasms, including teratoma, leiomyoma, gestational and nongestational choriocarcinoma, and uterine and cervical malignant lesions may result in false-positive pregnancy tests.[19] In general, the less sensitive 2 minute slide test has been responsible for the majority of false-positive results. In order to minimize false-positive results, the widely used immunologic pregnancy tests have been made insensitive to low levels of HCG.[31]

Unfortunately, HCG titers in ectopic pregnancy are frequently lower than in patients with normal intrauterine pregnancies. The evidence suggests that during the first four weeks of pregnancy, HCG levels may approximate normal values, but in extrauterine gestations of five or more weeks, the HCG level is usually significantly lower than in a normal pregnancy of the same duration.[10, 31, 32] This may be due to defective trophoblastic function or lack of placental mass.[31] The net result is that 20 to 50 per cent of patients with ectopic pregnancy have a false-negative immunologic pregnancy test.[10, 16–18, 31, 38] This lack of sensitivity and specificity has led to a general sense of frustration among clinicians asked to clinically differentiate pelvic inflammatory disease (often associated with a false-positive pregnancy test) and ectopic pregnancy (often associated with a false-negative pregnancy test). Frequently, the immunologic pregnancy test is omitted altogether because it proves to be more harmful than helpful in directing management.

A significant breakthrough occurred in 1972 with the introduction of a radioimmunoassay able to detect plasma HCG levels of 0.5 IU of HCG per ml or less.[40] This test is specific for the beta chain of HCG, and therefore does not cross-react with other hormones or medications. It is positive only if a gestational event has occurred, whether intrauterine (normal or abnormal) or extrauterine. It will also be markedly positive in patients with trophoblastic disease processes, that is, hydatidiform mole and choriocarcinoma associated with production of HCG.

This test has several distinct advantages over the more readily available immunologic pregnancy tests: (1) it is specific for HCG; (2) it is capable of detecting the low levels of HCG which are commonly present in women with ectopic pregnancy; (3) a negative radioimmunoassay excludes a gestational event in 100 per cent of cases;[26, 32] and (4) the quantitative levels have specific clinical implications. Serial HCG determinations can be performed to help determine whether or not a pregnancy is progressing normally. The limitation of the radioimmunoassay test is that it requires specialized laboratory equipment and personnel. Initially, the test required 24 hours to perform, but more recent modifications allow it to be completed in approximately three hours.[32] Continued efforts are being made to shorten the length of time required for completion of this and related tests, and to make them technically easier to perform.[3, 36] To date, these modifications have not been as sensitive[36] or specific[3] in their ability to aid in the diagnosis of ectopic pregnancy.

In summary, a variety of pregnancy tests are currently available. Those which are easier to perform, the immunologic tests, are much less sensitive and specific for the diagnosis of pregnancy. These tests pose a particular problem in patients in whom the pregnancy is not progressing normally in that they are frequently false-negative. More recently, however, the highly sensitive and specific radioimmunoassay test has been introduced. Although it is becoming more readily available, it is still limited by the fact that it is a technically difficult and lengthy process.

Ultrasonography

Because it allows direct imaging of the uterus and adnexa, ultrasonography has assumed a leading role in the evaluation of patients with obstetric and gynecologic problems. Early publications of results obtained with bistable equipment demonstrated the remarkable accuracy of ultrasound in the diagnosis of ectopic pregnancy. The classic appearance consisted of uterine enlargement which did not contain a gestational sac associated with an irregular adnexal mass, "ectopic fetal head" or fluid in the cul-de-sac.[11, 21, 42] An initial description utilizing gray scale ultrasound was similarly gratifying with an accuracy greater than 90 per cent for the diagnosis of ectopic pregnancy.[27] As more reports appeared in the literature, however, it soon became apparent that the ultrasonographic findings in patients with ectopic pregnancy frequently lacked the classic findings.[6, 24, 34]

Current opinion is that visualization of an extrauterine gestational sac is unusual, and visualization of a viable extrauterine fetus is rare. Furthermore, it is not at all unusual to see an intrauterine fluid collection that mimics a gestational sac in patients with ectopic pregnancy.[28]

Because ultrasonographic findings may be difficult to interpret in patients with ectopic gestations, how should patients who are at risk be evaluated? Ideally, this group should initially undergo a serum radioimmunoassay pregnancy test. If the result of this test is negative, then pregnancy, either intrauterine or extrauterine, is excluded. If the test result is positive, an ultrasound examination should be performed in an effort to establish whether the pregnancy is intrauterine or extrauterine. Because radioimmunoassay tests are time-consuming and are not usually available on an emergency basis, a more realistic approach is to obtain a urine immunologic pregnancy test in high risk patients. Based on the subsequent sonographic findings, selected individuals may then also undergo one or more serum pregnancy tests.

The ultrasonographic findings vary widely in patients suspected of having ectopic pregnancies. The most common observation is a normal intrauterine pregnancy.[6,24] This discovery virtually excludes an ectopic pregnancy because concurrent intrauterine and extrauterine pregnancies occur in only 1 of 30,000 pregnancies.[2]

Uterine Changes. Since ultrasound is often most helpful for excluding an ectopic pregnancy by identifying a normal intrauterine gestation, great effort and care should be exercised in evaluating the uterus and its contents. Real-time equipment is essential to search for a small fetal pole and to assess whether or not cardiac activity or movement is present. Fetal movements are invariably detected after eights weeks of fetal life,[25] and with currently available high-resolution real-time equipment, fetal life may sometimes be confirmed 1 to 2 weeks earlier. Detection of embryonic echoes at approximately 5 to 6 weeks after conception also permits a fairly reliable and specific diagnosis of intrauterine pregnancy, although occasionally blood or other particulate material may be present within an intrauterine fluid collection and mimic a fetal pole.

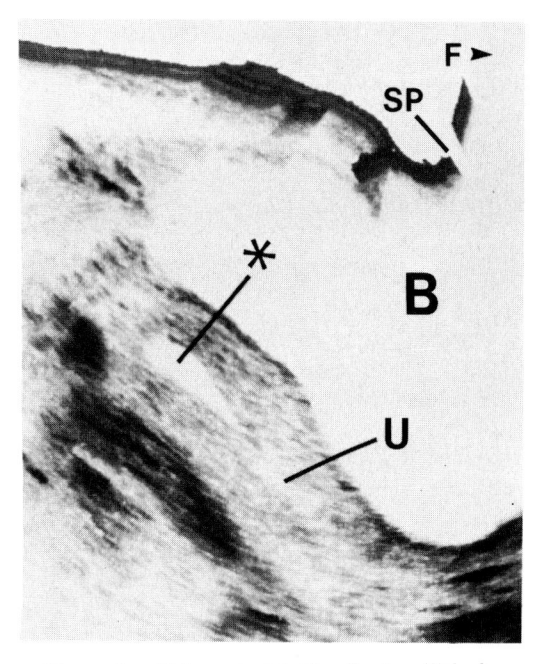

Figure 1. This central fluid collection (*) lacks a surrounding ring of high amplitude echoes. This appearance excludes a normal intrauterine pregnancy. An ectopic pregnancy was found at surgery. U, uterus; B, bladder; SP, symphysis pubis; F, feet.

Unfortunately, many pregnant patients who are clinically at risk for an ectopic gestation present early in pregnancy, at a time when fetal motion and fetal echoes may be lacking. The ultrasonographer, confronted with a scan demonstrating an intrauterine fluid collection, has to decide if this finding is due to an early intrauterine pregnancy (normal or abnormal) or to a pseudogestational sac of ectopic pregnancy.[28]

Close scrutiny of the fluid collection may reveal that it is not surrounded by a prominent ring of high amplitude echoes (Fig. 1), in which case the differential diagnosis is limited to either: (1) an abnormal intrauterine pregnancy (a blighted ovum or incomplete abortion); or (2) an ectopic pregnancy with an associated decidual cast. Uterine dilatation and curettage can often resolve this dilemma by revealing the presence or absence of chorionic villi. If chorionic villi are discovered, then an intrauterine gestational event can be confirmed. If chorionic villi are lacking, however, an ectopic pregnancy cannot be excluded.

A more difficult diagnostic problem occurs if a symptomatic patient with a positive pregnancy test has an intrauterine fluid collection surrounded by a rim of high amplitude echoes (Fig. 2). This appearance could be due to an early normal intrauterine pregnancy (prior to visualization of a fetal pole) or could be due to a decidual cast associated with an ectopic gestation. Marks and associates demonstrated pseudogestational sacs in 20 per cent of patients with ectopic pregnancies.[28] They are probably caused by decidual changes within endometrial tissues which result in enlarged and

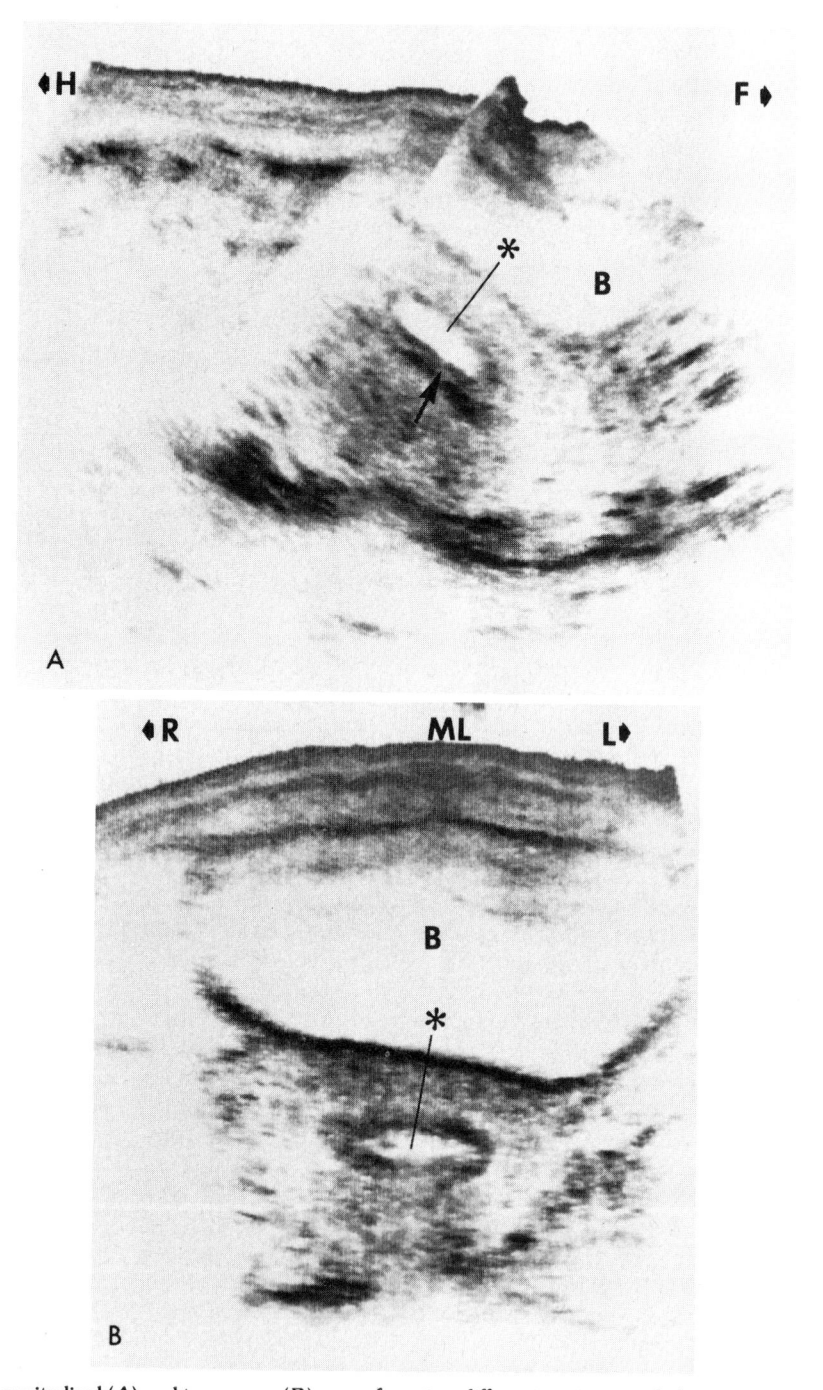

Figure 2. Longitudinal (*A*) and transverse (*B*) scans from two different patients each demonstrate an intrauterine fluid collection (*) surrounded by a rim of high amplitude echoes. The longitudinal scan, however, was obtained in a patient with a normal early intrauterine pregnancy and demonstrates double decidual sac findings (*arrow*). The transverse scan (*B*) lacks a double decidual sac and represents a prominent decidual reaction associated with an ectopic pregnancy. B, bladder; ML, midline; R, right; L, left; H, head; F, feet.

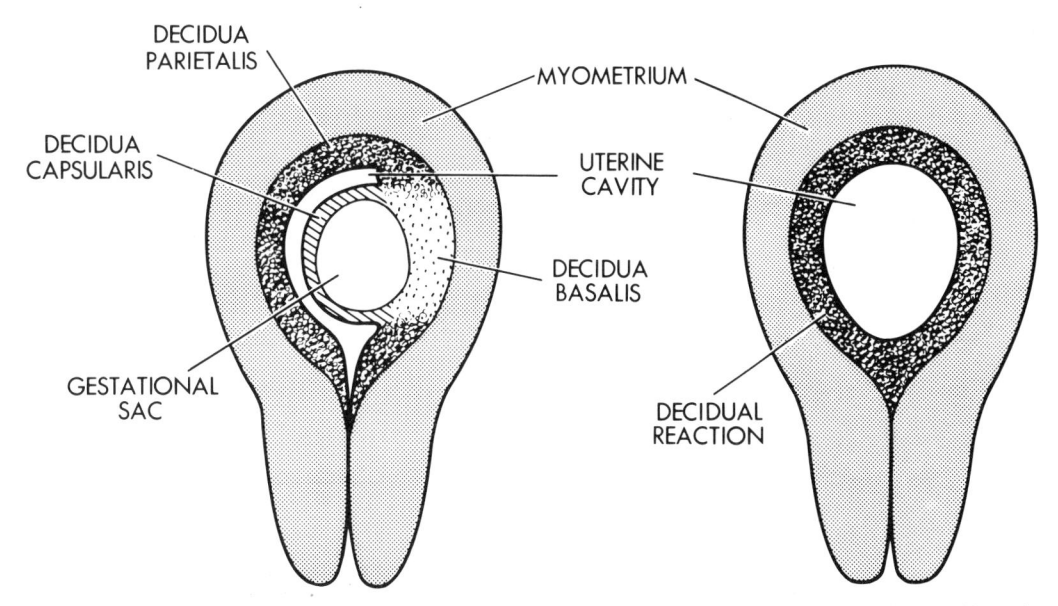

Figure 3. This diagram shows the uterine appearance in an early intrauterine pregnancy (left side of figure) with close apposition of the decidua capsularis and decidua parietalis. This accounts for the double decidual sac sign and allows a diagnosis of an intrauterine pregnancy to be made, despite nonvisualization of fetal echoes. On the right side of the figure, wide separation of the uterine walls is present. This appearance can be seen in patients with pseudogestational sacs of ectopic pregnancy. High amplitude echoes surrounding the uterine cavity are due to a prominent decidual reaction. (*From* Nyberg, D.A., et al.: Ultrasonographic differentiation of the gestational sac of early intrauterine pregnancy from the pseudogestational sac of ectopic pregnancy. Radiology, in press, with permission.)

edematous stromal cells. Pathologically, decidual changes are present in approximately 50 per cent of patients with ectopic pregnancy.

Recent evidence suggests that it is possible to differentiate the pseudogestational sac of ectopic pregnancy from an early intrauterine pregnancy with a high degree of confidence by observing two closely spaced concentric lines around a portion of the gestational sac in patients with early intrauterine pregnancies.[4, 29] This finding is absent in patients with intrauterine fluid collections associated with ectopic pregnancy. Although precise pathoanatomic correlation is not possible, gestational morphology suggests that the double lines detected by ultrasound represent the decidua parietalis (decidua vera) and adjacent decidua capsularis (Fig. 3). A recent retrospective analysis of 131 consecutively scanned pregnant patients revealed that this double decidual sac appearance correlated 98.4 per cent of the time with an intrauterine pregnancy (both normal and abnormal).[29] Patients whose uteri lacked a double decidual sac had either ectopic pregnancies or abnormal intrauterine pregnancies. The sonographic demonstration of a double decidual sac, even in the absence of a fetal pole, strongly suggests an intrauterine pregnancy and puts the patient at low risk for an ectopic pregnancy.

It is extremely important to use meticulous scanning technique, and utilize both static and real-time equipment in assessing intrauterine morphology. Occasionally, a patient may have an apparent double decidual sac on one view which cannot be confirmed on multiple other views (Fig. 4). If a definite intrauterine pregnancy cannot be confirmed ultrasonographically, the patient should still be considered at risk for an ectopic pregnancy. From the point of view of patient management, patients with indeterminant ultrasound studies pose a definite problem. If the patient is not acutely ill, serum HCG determinations should be obtained at two day intervals in order to look for the normal doubling pattern. Serial sonography may also be extremely helpful for further evaluation. If the patient is acutely ill, most clinicians would favor a laparoscopic examination.

A final appearance which may be observed in a symptomatic patient with a pos-

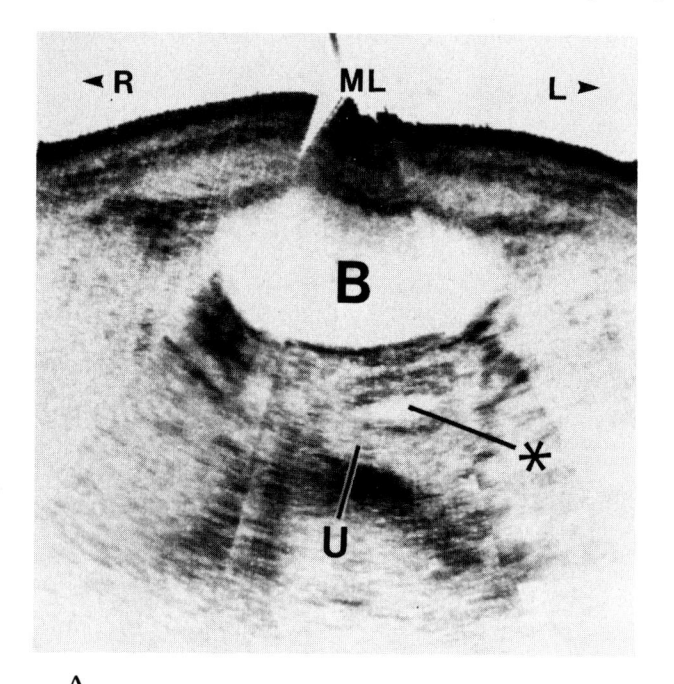

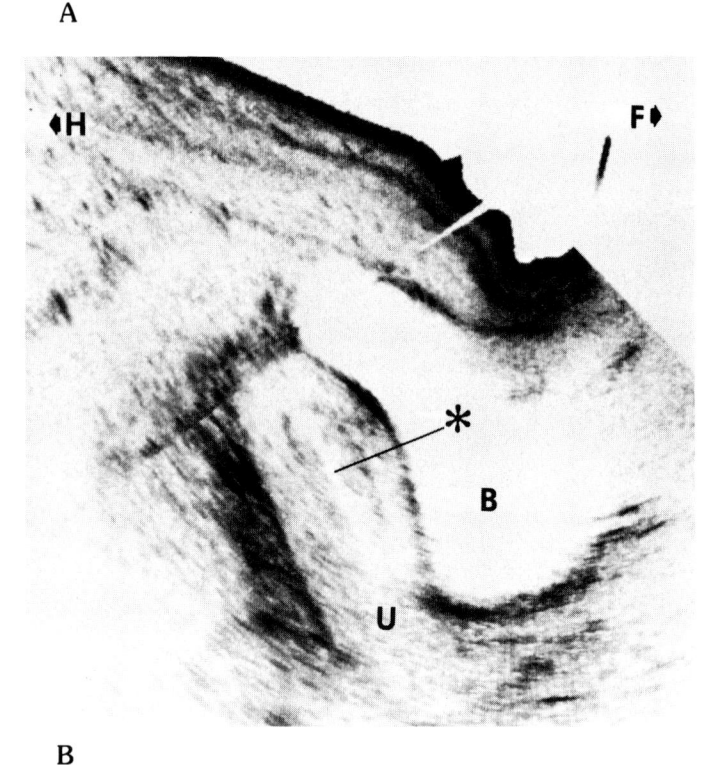

Figure 4. This transverse scan (A) reveals an intrauterine fluid collection (*) surrounded by an apparent double decidual sac. The longitudinal scan (B), however, fails to confirm the double decidual sac. Surgery revealed an ectopic pregnancy with an intrauterine decidual cast. U, uterus; B, bladder; ML, midline; R, right; L, left; H, head; F, feet.

itive pregnancy test is a slightly enlarged uterus with a normal central cavity echo (Fig. 5). If the pregnancy test is truly positive (see discussion on false-positive immunologic pregnancy tests), the differential diagnosis is limited to: (1) an early intrauterine pregnancy; (2) a recent abortion which accounts for the positive pregnancy test; or (3) an ectopic pregnancy. Uterine evacuation is usually performed under these circumstances to look for chorionic villi, which, if present, confirm that an intrauterine gestational event has occurred. If chorionic villi are absent, but the

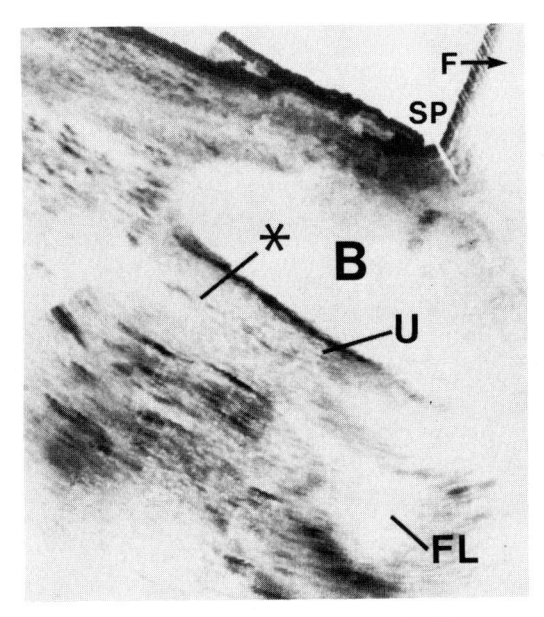

Figure 5. A normal central cavity echo (*) is seen within this patient's uterus (U). This appearance, in conjunction with a positive pregnancy test, strongly suggests an ectopic pregnancy. Fl, blood in the cul-de-sac; B, bladder; SP, symphysis pubis; F, feet.

patient is not acutely ill, serial serum HCG determinations may be effective for distinguishing between an ectopic pregnancy or a recent abortion.

Adnexal Changes. The clinical significance of an adnexal mass is very difficult to assess in patients suspected of having an ectopic pregnancy. Only in the rare situation in which a living ectopic pregnancy is discovered (Fig. 6) can one be certain that the visualized adnexal mass represents an ectopic pregnancy. In many cases interpretation of the adnexal finding without consideration of the uterine findings will lead to misdiagnosis. For example, a hemorrhagic corpus luteum cyst of pregnancy can closely mimic an ectopic pregnancy. Also, noteworthy is the fact that corpus luteum cysts, which are frequently contralaterally positioned, may be more prominent to the ultrasonographer than the actual ectopic pregnancy.[6] Because of the high association of pelvic inflammatory disease in patients with ectopic pregnancy, it is frequently impossible to state whether a visualized mass is an ectopic pregnancy or an inflammatory process (Fig. 7). Even a ring-like structure which may have the appearance of a gestational sac is not diagnostic.[6] Furthermore, adnexal masses of a variety of etiologies, including endometrioma and dermoid, can ultrasonographically mimic an ectopic pregnancy.

Because of the varied appearance of adnexal masses, it should be apparent that frequently the diagnosis of ectopic pregnancy cannot be established by ultrasound alone. In a patient with a negative serum pregnancy test, an ectopic pregnancy is effectively excluded regardless of the appearance of an adnexal mass. On the other

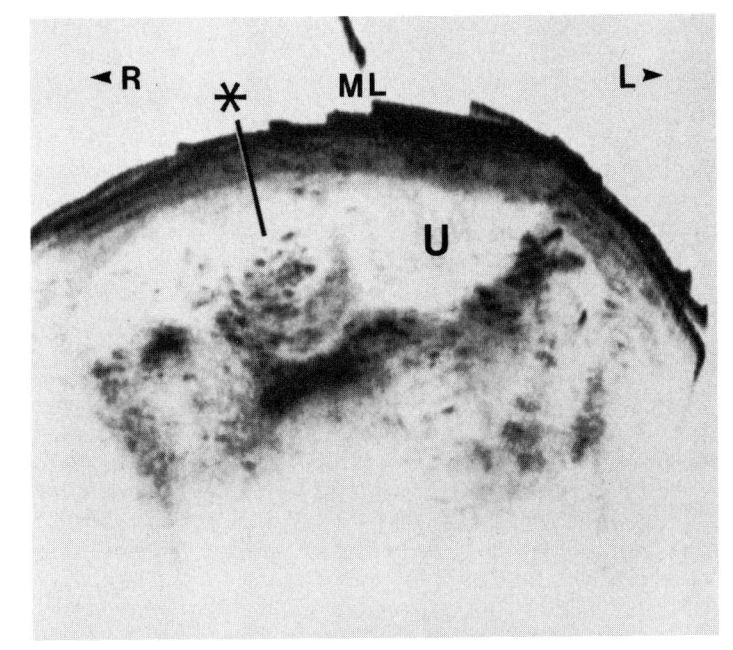

Figure 6. Transverse sonogram reveals an extrauterine gestational sac which contained a living fetus (*). The uterus (U) is situated to the left of the ectopic pregnancy. ML, midline; R, right; L, left.

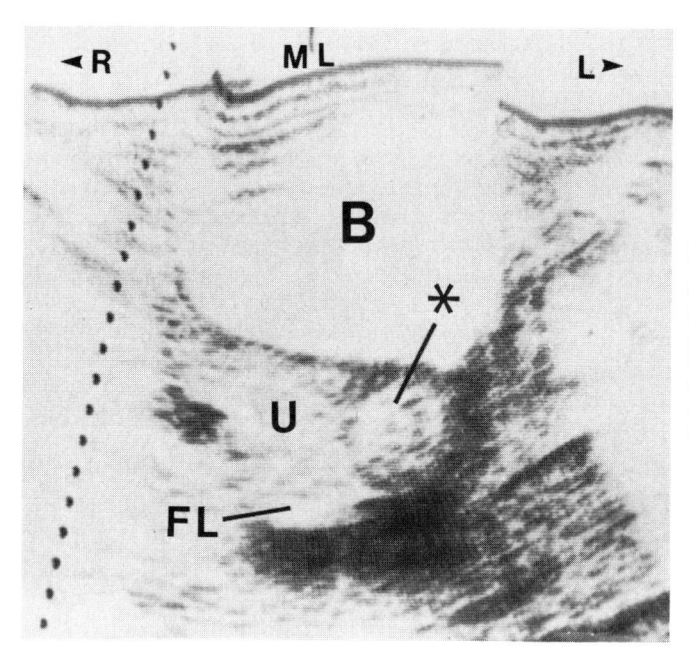

Figure 7. This sonogram demonstrates changes that mimic an ectopic pregnancy. The left adnexa contains a ring-like structure surrounded by high amplitude echoes. The multiple internal echoes (*) simulate a fetal pole. In addition, there is fluid (FL) posterior to the uterus (U). These changes were secondary to a tubo-ovarian abscess with associated pus in the pelvis. B, bladder; ML, midline; R, right; L, left.

hand, if a patient has a positive pregnancy test, empty uterus, and adnexal mass, the probability for an ectopic pregnancy is very high.

Changes in the Cul-de-Sac. Although fluid in the cul-de-sac increases the probability that a pregnant patient has an ectopic gestation, occasionally it may be due to a ruptured or hemorrhagic corpus luteum cyst, or may be secondary to a concurrent inflammatory process. If cul-de-sac fluid is visualized shortly after a culdocentesis has been performed, it may have been iatrogenically produced.

Like adnexal masses, cul-de-sac fluid should be interpreted in light of the intrauterine findings and the result of a pregnancy test. Visualizing a living intrauterine pregnancy makes it much less likely that cul-de-sac fluid is due to a concurrent ectopic pregnancy.

In a pregnant patient whose uterus fails to reveal products of conception, the presence of fluid in the cul-de-sac not only suggests an ectopic pregnancy, but also intimates that rupture may be occurring. At the time of surgery 80 to 90 per cent of tubal pregnancies will have ruptured.[15, 17, 38] More often than not, however, this is a subacute process because attendant signs of hypovolemic shock are present in fewer than 15 per cent of cases.[17, 38] Clot, in association with hemorrhage, may cause the cul-de-sac fluid to become echogenic. This appearance can deceive the unwary because the fluid may be misconstrued as a solid mass (Fig. 8). On the other hand, experienced sonographers recognize that this appearance is highly suggestive of hemoperitoneum. In the appropriate clinical setting, the diagnosis of ruptured ectopic pregnancy can be suggested solely on the basis of this finding. Jeffrey et al., in a recent review of 34 patients with hemoperitoneum, observed echogenic material in the cul-de-sac 26 per cent of the time.[20] The echo intensity of clotted blood is often dramatic in that it is of the same or greater intensity than uterine myometrial echoes in the majority of patients (Fig. 8).[20]

In addition to examining the cul-de-sac for fluid and/or clot, specific attention should also be given to the paracolic gutters and subhepatic space (Morison's pouch) in an effort to discover whether or not free intra-abdominal fluid is present. Occasionally, if the urinary bladder is overdistended, or if a patient has pelvic adhesions, fluid may be visible only in extrapelvic locations.

Unusual Types of Ectopic Pregnancy. Although greater than 80 per cent of ectopic pregnancies occur within the isthmic or ampullary portions of the fallopian tubes, they occasionally are found in other sites.[18] Because of the rarity of these implantations, however, there are few descriptions of their ultrasonographic appearances.

An interstitial ectopic pregnancy is a

particularly hazardous entity because of its propensity to cause fatal exsanguination.[12] Implantation occurs in the medial one third of the salpinx where the fallopian tube traverses the wall of the uterus (Fig. 9). Because the myometrium can expand and accommodate the gestational products, this form of ectopic pregnancy frequently ruptures at a later date when the surrounding vasculature is more prominently developed. Ultrasonographically, an interstitial ectopic pregnancy may look either intra- or extrauterine.[12] If the sac and its contents are clearly extrauterine, the diagnosis is readily apparent. If the sac is in close proximity to the uterus, the diagnosis of an in-

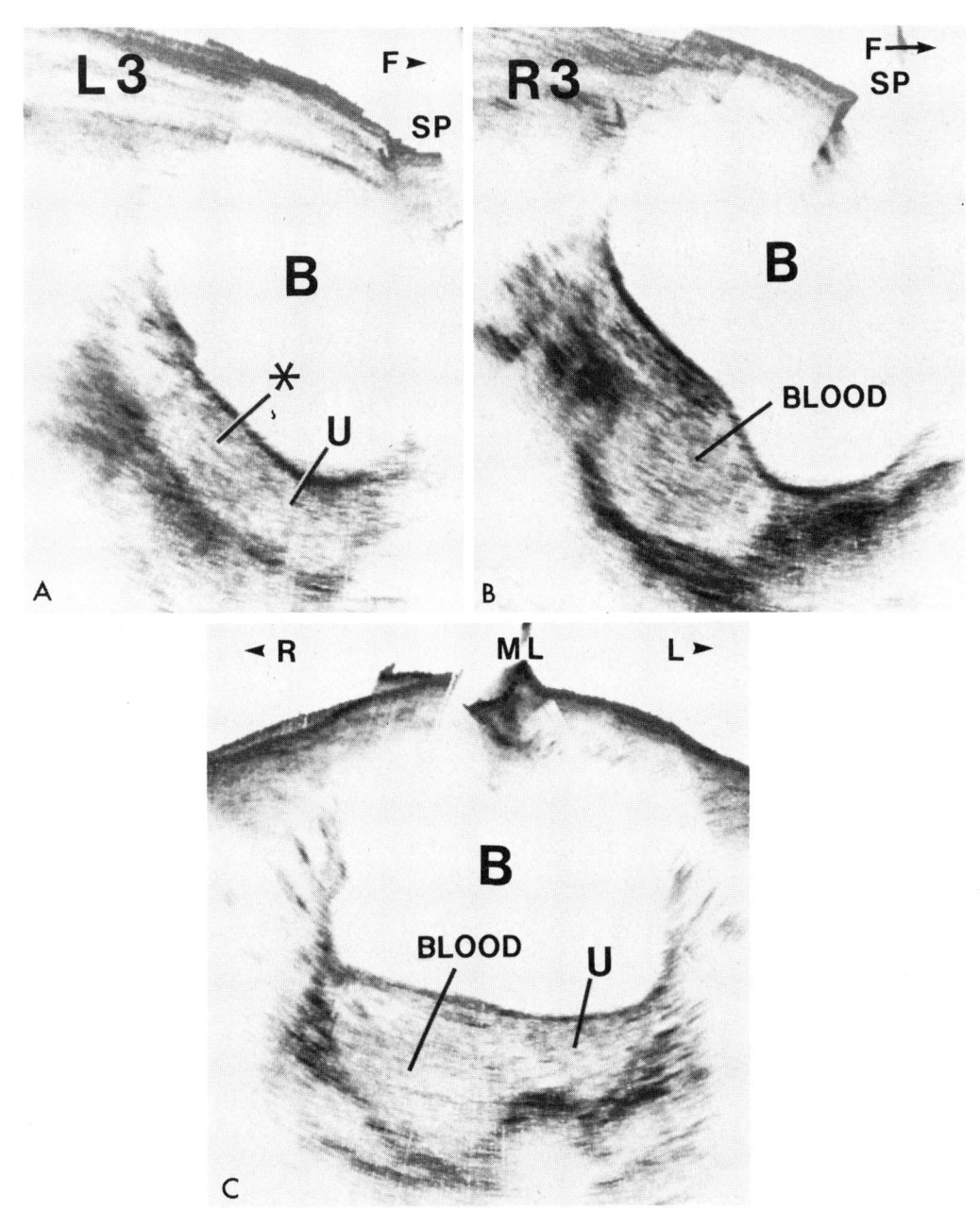

Figure 8. An echogenic clot should not be construed as a solid mass. In this patient, the uterus (U) is displaced toward the left (A). Its position is most readily defined by visualizing a normal central cavity echo (*). A large echogenic mass evident on the right (B and C) was caused by clotted blood which occurred following rupture of a right tubal pregnancy. Free fluid was visible sonographically in Morrison's pouch. B, bladder; SP, symphysis pubis; ML, midline; R, right; L, left; F, feet.

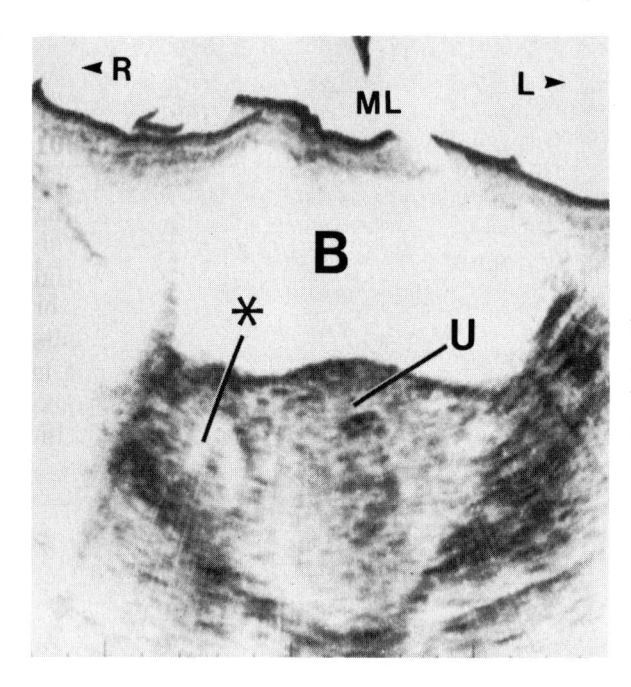

Figure 9. An unusual ectopic pregnancy is one that implants in the interstitial portion of the fallopian tube (*). A prominent decidual reaction within the uterus (U) is also seen. This type of ectopic pregnancy can be difficult to diagnose because it may occasionally look intrauterine. B, bladder; ML, midline; R, right; L, left.

terstitial ectopic pregnancy can be suggested. Two additional findings which suggest that an interstitial ectopic pregnancy is present have been described.[12] These include the lack of a complete myometrial mantle around the gestational sac as well as an eccentric location of the sac in relation to the remainder of the uterus. The latter appearance may occasionally be seen, however, as a result of a gestation in one horn of a bicornuate uterus or if a myoma is in one wall of the uterus.[12] Furthermore, compression and elongation of the lower uterine segment due to overdistention of the urinary bladder may cause the gestational sac to "migrate" cephalically, thereby mimicking this form of ectopic pregnancy.[22] Performing the ultrasound examination without overly distending the bladder combined with recognition of these pitfalls should allow the correct diagnosis to be made.

An ectopic cervical pregnancy, which has a reported incidence of 0.1 per cent of ectopic gestations,[18] is suggested if a gestational sac appears to be lodged within the region of the cervical canal. An aborting fetus, however, could have a similar ultrasonographic appearance.

An abdominal pregnancy occurs as a result of a tubal pregnancy that has either aborted or ruptured into the peritoneal cavity.[1] Very rarely, an intrauterine fetus can pass through a preexisting uterine wall defect into the abdominal cavity.[33] Because these fetuses may survive, they are frequently not diagnosed until relatively late in pregnancy. Sonographic features which suggest an intra-abdominal pregnancy include:[1] (1) visualization of the uterus as separate from the fetus; (2) failure to visualize the uterine wall between the fetus and the urinary bladder; (3) close approximation of fetal parts to the maternal abdominal wall; (4) eccentric position and/or abnormal attitude of the fetus; and (5) visualization of extrauterine placental tissue. These findings, which may be subtle, require close attention to detail and, ultimately, a high level of suspicion. Other entities that may mimic an intra-abdominal pregnancy include fetal development within a persistently retroverted uterus,[23] as well as the presence of fetal or uterine anomalies that cause the fetus to assume an unusual position.

Culdocentesis and Laparoscopy

Because they are more invasive procedures, it is desirable to perform culdocentesis and/or laparoscopy only in selected cases or under certain clinical conditions.

Prior to the advent of high resolution ultrasonography and sensitive pregnancy tests, culdocentesis was frequently performed as part of the initial evaluation of any patient clinically suspected of having an ectopic pregnancy. Because this technique, which consists of needle aspiration through the posterior vagina into the region of the cul-de-sac, will detect the presence of free intra-abdominal blood, it has been considered the most useful diagnostic procedure for ectopic pregnancy.[18] A positive test consists of obtaining blood which fails to clot within 10 to 15 minutes. Aspirated blood that clots indicates that a vessel has been entered. It is a nonspecific test, however, in that bleeding from any abdominal or pelvic source will similarly fail to clot. In addition, the procedure will not detect an ectopic pregnancy if bleeding is not present or if the needle fails to penetrate the peritoneal cavity. In a negative tap clear yellow fluid is obtained, whereas the absence of fluid (dry tap) is nondiagnostic.[10] Despite its limitations, culdocentesis has been reported positive for nonclotting blood in 75 to 97 per cent of patients with ectopic pregnancy.[5, 10, 16, 17, 38]

Ultrasonographers should urge their clinical colleagues not to perform a culdocentesis if they are contemplating an ultrasound examination shortly thereafter, because the iatrogenic introduction of blood into the cul-de-sac could be misinterpreted as a hemoperitoneum secondary to an ectopic pregnancy. Of course, if the patient is acutely ill, the clinician may favor an immediate culdocentesis which, if positive, would necessitate urgent laparotomy.

Laparoscopy is generally reserved for patients with a suspicious history, an equivocal sonogram, or a negative culdocentesis. It is a useful technique for directly visualizing the uterus, tubes, ovaries, and free intrapelvic blood. It should not be used indiscriminately, however, since general anesthesia is required. In addition, complications including bowel perforation and vessel laceration can occur. This technique is contraindicated in patients who have undergone prior laparotomy since adhesions will increase the risk of bowel perforation. Nondiagnostic laparoscopic examinations may also occur in patients with extensive pelvic adhesions which frequently accompany pelvic inflammatory disease. Finally, laparoscopy is also not indicated in acutely ill patients who have a positive culdocentesis, since it will delay definitive therapy.

SUMMARY

The combined use of a serum radioimmunoassay pregnancy test and high resolution ultrasonography allows a more direct approach to be made in the diagnosis of ectopic pregnancy. It is important for ultrasonographers to understand the limitations of the more readily available immunologic pregnancy tests in order to avoid misinterpreting ultrasonograms in the event that a pregnancy test is either falsely positive or falsely negative.

Clinical suspicion is mandatory if the early diagnosis of ectopic pregnancy is to be made. The referring physician should take advantage of the highly accurate information resulting from the combined findings of a positive serum HCG and the ultrasonographic images. If the statistics regarding diagnostic delay and tubal rupture are to be improved, these tests should be obtained when a patient is initially evaluated.

It is important to recognize that the ultrasonographic interpretation rests primarily upon the uterine findings. A normal living intrauterine pregnancy essentially excludes the diagnosis of ectopic pregnancy. Other uterine appearances may result from an early intrauterine pregnancy, an abnormal intrauterine gestational event, or, as in approximately 1 per cent of pregnancies, an ectopic gestation. Subsequent evaluation in suspicious cases may require a variety of tests including serial HCG determinations, repeat ultrasound examination, uterine dilatation and curettage, culdocentesis, or laparoscopy. It is impossible to recommend a specific schematic approach for any given patient. In part, the pattern of management depends upon availability of tests, the presence or absence of adnexal or cul-de-sac findings, and, of course, the clinical status of the patient.

REFERENCES

1. Allibone, G. W., Fagan, C. J., and Porter, S. C.: The sonographic features of intra-abdominal pregnancy. J. Clin. Ultrasound, 9:383, 1981.
2. Berger, M. J., and Taymor, M. L.: Simultaneous intrauterine and tubal pregnancies following ovulation induction. Am. J. Obstet. Gynecol., 113:812, 1972.
3. Berry, C. M., Thompson, J. D., and Hatcher, R.:

The radioreceptor assay for HCG in ectopic pregnancy. Obstet. Gynecol., *54*:43, 1979.
4. Bradley, W. B., Fiske, C. E., and Filly, R. A.: The double sac sign of early intrauterine pregnancy: Use in exclusion of ectopic pregnancy. Radiology, *143*:223, 1982.
5. Breen, J. L.: A 21 year survey of 654 ectopic pregnancies. Am. J. Obstet. Gynecol., *106*:1004, 1970.
6. Brown, T. W., Filly, R. A., Laing, F. C., et al.: Analysis of ultrasonographic criteria in the evaluation for ectopic pregnancy. Am. J. Roentgenol., *131*:967, 1978.
7. Chow, T. T. S., and Lindahl, S.: Ectopic cervical pregnancy. J. Clin. Ultrasound, *7*:217, 1979.
8. Derman, R.: Early diagnosis of pregnancy. A symposium. J. Reprod. Med., *26*:149, 1981.
9. Derman, R., Edelman, D. A., and Berger, G. S.: Current status of immunologic pregnancy tests. Int. J. Gynaecol. Obstet., *17*:190, 1979.
10. Dodson, M. G: Bleeding in pregnancy. *In* Aladjem, S. (ed.): Obstetrical Practice. St. Louis, C. V. Mosby Co., 1980, pp. 451–472.
11. Donald, J.: Diagnostic uses of sonar (ultrasonic echo sounding) in obstetrics and gynecology. *In* Marcus, S. L., and Marcus, G. (eds.): Advances in Obstetrics and Gynecology. Baltimore, Williams and Wilkins Co., 1967, pp. 314–329.
12. Graham, M., and Cooperberg, P. L.: Ultrasound diagnosis of interstitial pregnancy: Findings and pitfalls. J. Clin. Ultrasound, *7*:433, 1979.
13. Hallatt, J. G.: Repeat ectopic pregnancy: A study of 123 consecutive cases. Am. J. Obstet. Gynecol., *122*:520, 1975.
14. Hallatt, J. G.: Ectopic pregnancy associated with the intrauterine device: A study of seventy cases. Am. J. Obstet. Gynecol., *125*:754, 1976.
15. Hazekamp, J. T.: Ectopic pregnancy: Diagnostic dilemma and delay. Int. J. Gynaecol. Obstet., *17*:598, 1980.
16. Helvacioglu, A., Long, E. M., Jr., and Yang, S.-L.: Ectopic pregnancy. An eight-year review. J. Reprod. Med., *22*:87, 1979.
17. Hlavin, G. E., Ladocsi, L. T., and Breen, J. L.: Ectopic pregnancy: An analysis of 153 patients. Int. J. Gynaecol. Obstet., *16*:42, 1978–1979.
18. Iffy, L.: Ectopic pregnancy. *In* Iffy, L., and Kaminetzky, H. A. (eds.): Principles and Practice of Obstetrics and Perinatology. New York, John Wiley and Sons, 1981, pp. 609–633.
19. Jacobson, E., and Rothe, D.: False-positive hemagglutination inhibition tests for pregnancy with tubo-ovarian abscess. Int. J. Gynaecol. Obstet., *17*:307, 1980.
20. Jeffrey, R. B., and Laing, F. C.: Echogenic clot: A useful sign of pelvic hemoperitoneum. Radiology (in press).
21. Kobayashi, M., Hellman, L., and Fillisti, L.: Ultrasound: An aid in the diagnosis of ectopic pregnancy. Am. J. Obstet. Gynecol., *103*:1131, 1969.
22. Laing, F. C.: Letter to the editor. J. Clin. Ultrasound, *8*:287, 1980.
23. Laing, F. C.: Sonography of a persistently retroverted gravid uterus. Am. J. Roentgenol., *136*:413, 1981.
24. Lawson, T. L.: Ectopic pregnancy: Criteria and accuracy of ultrasonic diagnosis. Am. J. Roentgenol., *131*:153, 1978.
25. Levine, S. C., and Filly, R. A.: Accuracy of real time sonography in the determination of fetal viability. Obstet. Gynecol., *49*:475, 1977.
26. Lundstrom, V., Bremme, K., Eneroth, P., et al.: Serum beta-human chorionic gonadotropin levels in the early diagnosis of ectopic pregnancy. Acta Obstet. Gynecol. Scand., *58*:231, 1979.
27. Maklad, N. F., and Wright, C. H.: Grey scale ultrasonography in the diagnosis of ectopic pregnancy. Radiology, *126*:221, 1978.
28. Marks, W. M., Filly, R. A., Callen, P. W., et al.: The decidual cast of ectopic pregnancy. A confusing ultrasonographic appearance. Radiology, *133*:451, 1979.
29. Nyberg D. A., Laing, F. C., Filly, R. A., et al.: Ultrasonographic differentiation of the gestational sac of early intrauterine pregnancy from the pseudo-gestational sac of ectopic pregnancy. Radiology, in press.
30. Pathak, V. N., and Stewart, D. B.: Autotransfusion in ectopic pregnancy. Lancet, *1*:961, 1970.
31. Pelosi, M. A.: Use of the radioreceptor assay for human chorionic gonadotropin in the diagnosis of ectopic pregnancy. Surg. Gynecol. Obstet., *152*:149, 1981.
32. Rasor, J. L., and Braunstein, G. D.: A rapid modification of the beta-hCG radioimmunoassay. Use as an aid in the diagnosis of ectopic pregnancy. Obstet. Gynecol., *50*:553, 1977.
33. Sauerbrei, E., Toi, A., Effer, S. B., et al.: Intrauterine to intraabdominal pregnancy: Ultrasound demonstration. Am. J. Roentgenol., *133*:132, 1979.
34. Schoenbaum, S., Rosendorf, L., and Kappelman, N.: Gray-scale ultrasound in tubal pregnancy. Radiology, *127*:757, 1978.
35. Schwartz, R. O., and Di Pietro, D. L.: β-hCG as a diagnostic aid for suspected ectopic pregnancy. Obstet. Gynecol., *56*:197, 1980.
36. Seppala, M., Tontiti, K., Ranta, T., et al.: Use of a rapid hCG-beta-subunit radioimmunoassay in acute gynaecological emergencies. The Lancet, *1*:165, 1980.
37. Tait, L.: Five cases of extra-uterine pregnancy operated upon at the time of rupture. Br. Med. J., *1*:1250, 1884.
38. Tancer, M. L., Delke, I., and Veridiano, N. P.: A fifteen year experience with ectopic pregnancy. Surg. Gynecol. Obstet., *152*:179, 1981.
39. Unanswered questions on ectopic pregnancy. (Unsigned editorial.) Br. Med. J., *280*:1127, 1980.
40. Vaitukaitis, J. L., Braunstein, G. D., and Ross, G. T.: Radioimmunoassay which specifically measures human chorionic gonadotropin in the presence of luteinizing hormone. Am. J. Obstet. Gynecol., *113*:751, 1972.
41. Wide, L., and Gemzell, C. A.: An immunological pregnancy test. Acta Endocrinol., *35*:261, 1960.
42. Zacutti, A., and Brugnoli, C. A.: The usefulness of ultrasonic scanning in the diagnosis of ectopic pregnancy. Acta Eur. Fertil., *2*:445, 1970.

19
Pelvimetry

Michael P. Federle, M.D.

The process of labor involves a series of accommodations of the fetus to the bony passage through which it must pass. Accordingly, the size and shape of the pelvis and the size and position of the fetus are of vital importance in obstetrics.

PELVIC ANATOMY

The adult pelvis is a bony ring composed of four bones: the sacrum, the coccyx, and the two innominate bones. Each innominate bone is formed by the fusion of the ilium, the ischium, and the pubis. The innominate bones are joined to the sacrum at the sacroiliac synchondrosis and to each other anteriorly at the symphysis pubis. The female pelvis differs rather markedly from the usual male pelvis, being wider and rounded in adaptation to childbearing. In addition, the ligamentous structures constituting part of the wall of the pelvis and the fibrocartilaginous joints between the pelvic bones possess a degree of mobility, softening, and stretching that increases during pregnancy under hormonal stimulation.

The linea terminalis (iliopectineal line) demarcates the false pelvis from the true pelvis (Fig. 1), with the true pelvis lying below this boundary. Although the false pelvis may vary considerably among women, it is of no particular obstetric significance. The true pelvis is the portion important in childbearing, and it is bounded above by the promontory and alae of the sacrum, the linea terminalis, and the upper margins of the pubic bones, and below by the pelvic outlet (tip of sacrum, ischial tuberosities, pubic arch, and sacrosciatic ligaments).

Planes and Diameters of the Pelvis

The pelvis has been described as having several planes through which the fetus must pass; those of clinical importance will be discussed.

Pelvic Inlet. In most women, the pelvic inlet or superior strait is nearly round. Various diameters have been described and measured, although the anteroposterior diameter is most important obstetrically. The shortest distance between the sacral promontory and the posterior surface of the symphysis pubis is called the obstetric conjugate (Fig. 1). Normally, the obstetric conjugate measures 10 cm or more (average, 11 cm), but it may be considerably shortened in abnormal pelves. The distance between the promontory and the top of the symphysis has been designated the true conjugate, although it does not represent the shortest diameter of the inlet.

Neither the obstetric nor true conjugate can be measured directly with the obstetrician's examining fingers. Instead, one can palpate the distance between the lower margin of the symphysis to the sacral promontory; this is designated the diagonal conjugate. The length of the obstetric conjugate is estimated by subtracting 1.5 to 2 cm from the diagonal conjugate, depending upon the height and inclination of the symphysis pubis.[20] The transverse diameter represents the greatest distance between the linea terminalis on either side, averaging about 13.5 cm (see Fig. 1).

Midpelvis. The midpelvis is at the level of the ischial spines and is often called the plane of least pelvic dimensions. The interspinous diameter, normally greater than 10 cm (average, 10.5 cm), is usually the smallest diameter of the pelvis. The anteroposterior diameter of the midpelvis,

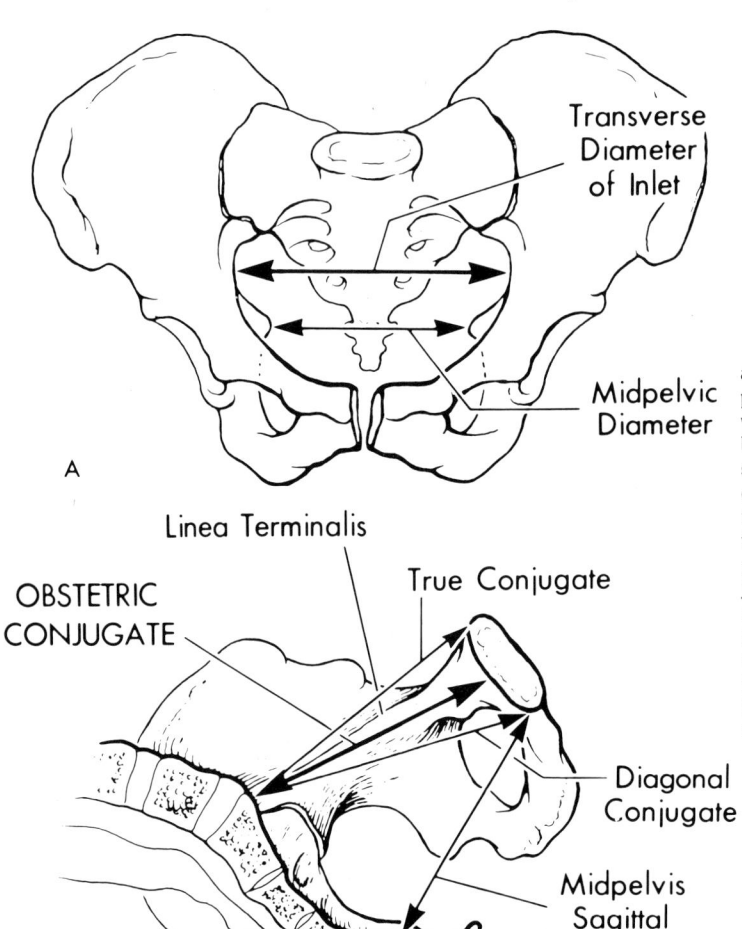

Figure 1. Important pelvic diameters. *A*, Anteroposterior view of pelvis. Transverse diameter of pelvic inlet is the maximum distance between the linia terminalis on either side. The midpelvic diameter is the distance between the ischial spines, usually the smallest pelvic diameter. *B*, Lateral view showing sagittal pelvic diameters. The obstetric conjugate (sacral promontory to back of symphysis pubis) is the most useful measurement. The diagonal conjugate is palpated by the obstetrician as the distance between the bottom of the symphysis pubis and the sacral promontory.

from sacrum to symphysis at the level of the ischial spines, measures an average of 11.5 cm (see Fig. 1).

Pelvic Outlet. The important dimension of the pelvic outlet, the diameter between the ischial tuberosities, is accessible for clinical measurement and is normally greater than 8 cm. Although more refined techniques for measurement, including x-ray pelvimetry, have been employed, the pelvic outlet is rarely the cause of obstructed labor. If the pelvic inlet and midpelvis are adequate, such techniques are usually unwarranted.[21]

Clinical Estimation of Pelvic Size. Clinical evaluation of pelvic adequacy is a fundamental part of the obstetric examination. In most cases, adquate pelvic capacity is assured, and further evaluation is therefore obviated. Inadequate pelves because of congenital, metabolic, or traumatic abnormalities are also frequently evident.[8]

The diagonal conjugate provides an estimate of the obstetric conjugate, and the transverse diameter of the outlet (between the ischial tuberosities) is directly accessible. Clinical assessment of midpelvic capacity is more limited. One's suspicion of pelvic contraction should be raised by unusual prominence of the ischial spines, convergence of pelvic side walls ("funnel pelvis"), or shallow concavity of the sacrum.[20]

X-RAY PELVIMETRY

The value of x-ray pelvimetry remains a highly controversial topic; opinions range from enthusiastic support for its frequent use to the contention that it is a useless and potentially harmful procedure. The prevailing opinion of practicing obstetricians seems to be somewhere between these two extremes. A consensus can be reached on at least several points. The prognosis for successful labor in any given case cannot be established by x-ray pelvimetry alone, since pelvic capacity is only one of several factors that determine the outcome. Other important factors include the size of the fetal head, the force of uterine contractions, moldability of the fetal head and maternal pelvis, and presentation and position of the fetus.[16] X-ray pelvimetry does offer certain advantages over manual estimation of pelvic size, including more accurate measurements of the pelvic inlet and midpelvis. Two important diameters can be measured on radiographs that are not otherwise obtainable: the transverse diameter of the inlet and the interischial spinous diameter. X-ray pelvimetry should be delayed until near term or, preferably, until early labor to minimize radiation hazards to the developing fetus.

Indications for X-ray Pelvimetry

Almost as many different lists of indications for pelvimetry exist as authors of journal articles or textbook chapters. Some lists are broad in their suggested indications, such as a history of difficult labor or traumatized fetus, presence of an unengaged head in a primiparous woman in active labor, or contemplated use of oxytocin for induction of labor in a nulliparous woman.[6,14] Many obstetricians do not consider the preceding indications to be adequate but would agree that a pelvis judged to be too small by clinical evaluation would warrant x-ray pelvimetry if demonstration of a contracted pelvis would indicate elective cesarean section without an attempt at labor.[20] Others suggest that all mothers without an obviously deformed or contracted pelvis be given a trial of labor if the fetus is in vertex presentation.[8,11] Some authors recommend pelvimetry in cases of arrested labor;[9,20] others claim that such cases require a more "aggressive" approach to labor management (oxytocin infusion, monitoring intrauterine pressure) and decide for or against cesarean section on clinical rather than pelvimetry data.[8,18]

Although no consensus is possible, it seems that the conduct of labor in fetal vertex presentation is rarely altered by findings with x-ray pelvimetry.[8,11,12] The study is, however, of value in breech presentation, since it may deter unwarranted attempts to deliver a relatively unmolded head through an inadequate maternal pelvis.[5,11,12,14,15] Films may also reveal a deflexed or hyperextended fetal head, which, because of the associated risk of

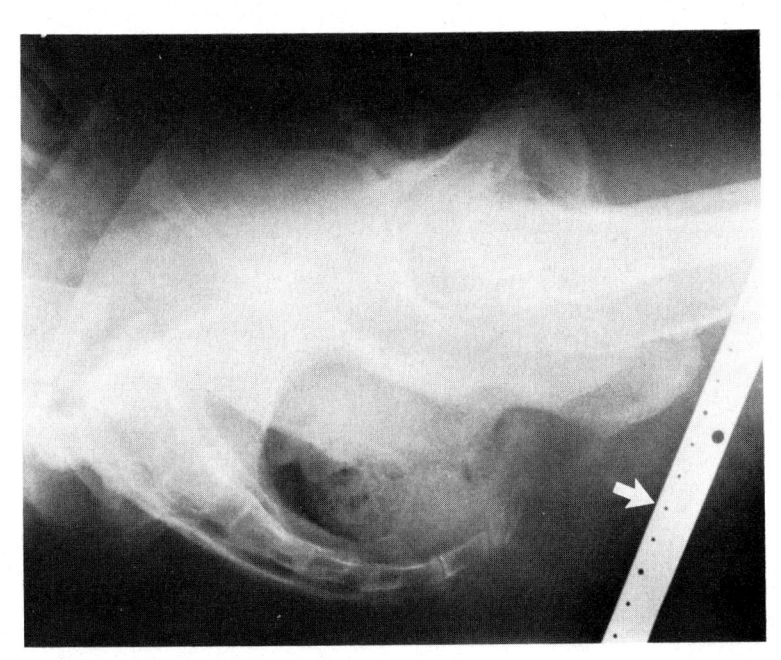

Figure 2. Conventional lateral pelvimetry radiograph. A metal ruler (*arrow*) with centimeter calibrations is placed between the thighs. Measurement of sagittal pelvic diameters is corrected for magnification by reference to this centimeter scale.

cervical cord damage, is a contraindication to vaginal delivery.[5]

Technique of X-ray Pelvimetry

Numerous methods of pelvimetry have been described, and all are reasonably accurate if used properly.[25] Sagittal (anteroposterior) diameters can be measured relatively easily since all lie in the same plane at the midline. A centimeter scale can be placed in the midline between the thighs and can be used in direct measure of the sagittal diameters (Fig. 2). Transverse pelvic diameters lie in different planes and are less simple to calculate. Some correction for radiographic magnification is necessary since those pelvic diameters lying farther from the radiographic film cassette will measure disproportionately larger than those that lie closer. Various attempts at correction include stereoscopic views and placement of metal rulers with calibrated distortion factors. These techniques are further described elsewhere.[3, 22]

A major concern with any pelvimetry technique is the amount of ionizing radiation to which the fetus and the maternal gonads are exposed. Radiation dose varies considerably with measurement technique, screen-film systems, and the number and types of views obtained.[1, 3] As a general indication, the mean fetal gonadal exposure from pelvimetry has been estimated as 885 ± 111 mrads by the British Committee on Radiological Hazards to Patients.[19] More recently, the 1977 report of the United Nations Scientific Committee on the Effects of Atomic Radiation estimated the mean fetal whole body dose at about 620 mrads.[23] In the United States, pelvimetry is the major single source of ionizing radiation to the fetus.[4]

Though estimates of the hazard of low-level diagnostic radiation remain controversial, fetal irradiation does appear to be associated with an increased risk of subsequent childhood malignant disease. Data from both England and the United States show an increased incidence of leukemia and other malignant diseases in children exposed in utero to diagnostic x-rays.[2, 15, 17] Besides the somatic carcinogenic effects, in utero irradiation may also be associated with genetic effects due to mutations induced by gonadal irradiation.

CT-DIGITAL PELVIMETRY

In consideration of the potential deleterious effects and technical problems associated with conventional x-ray pelvimetry, we have developed a new, low-dose technique based on digital radiographs generated on a computed tomographic (CT) scanner.[7] Most recently manufactured CT scanners contain a modification "package" that allows one to generate a digital radiograph, similar in appearance to a conventional radiograph, that is generally used for subsequent selection of levels for axial CT sections. The digital radiograph is produced by mechanically moving the patient

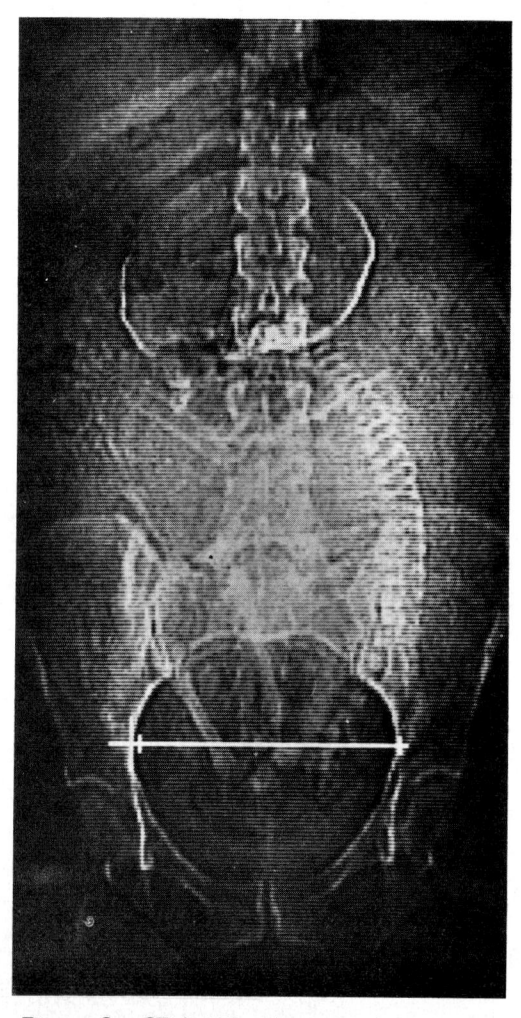

Figure 3. CT-digital pelvimetry. Anteroposterior view demonstrates single fetus in frank breech presentation with head flexed. Electronic cursors are used to measure transverse diameter of pelvic inlet (*white line*). Result is read on the television monitor with no need for magnification correction.

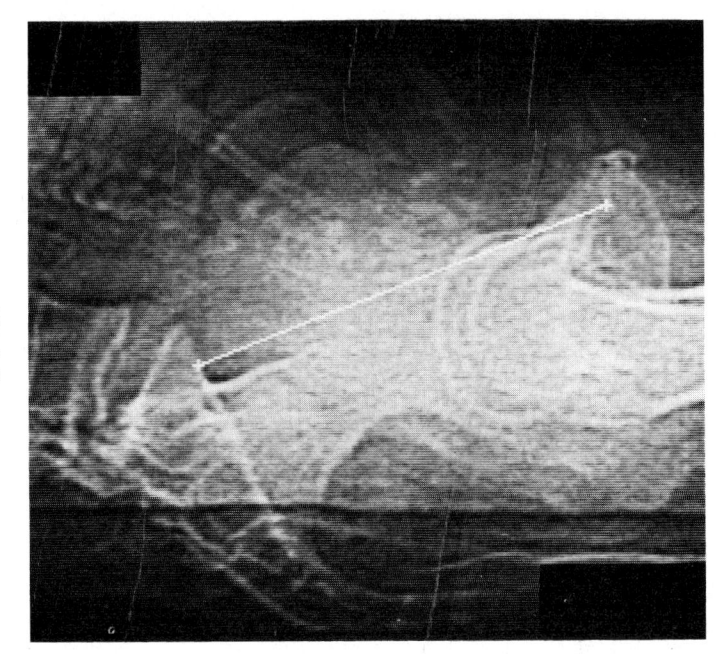

Figure 4. CT-digital pelvimetry. Electronic cursors measure shortest sagittal diameter from sacral promontory to back of symphysis, the obstetric conjugate.

through a rapidly pulsed, narrowly collimated x-ray beam. Multiple xenon detectors collect the x-rays transmitted through the patient and produce an electrical signal which is converted into a digital format. An anteroposterior view is obtained with the x-ray tube and detectors positioned above and below the patient, respectively; for a lateral view, the tube and detectors are placed to the sides of the patient.

Digital pelvimetry has several distinct advantages over conventional techniques. Digital images are generated by using a standard set of radiographic factors, not requiring adjustments for different patients that often result in suboptimal or even uninterpretable conventional studies. Digital images are stored electronically, allowing the viewer to manipulate the brightness, contrast, magnification, and other factors

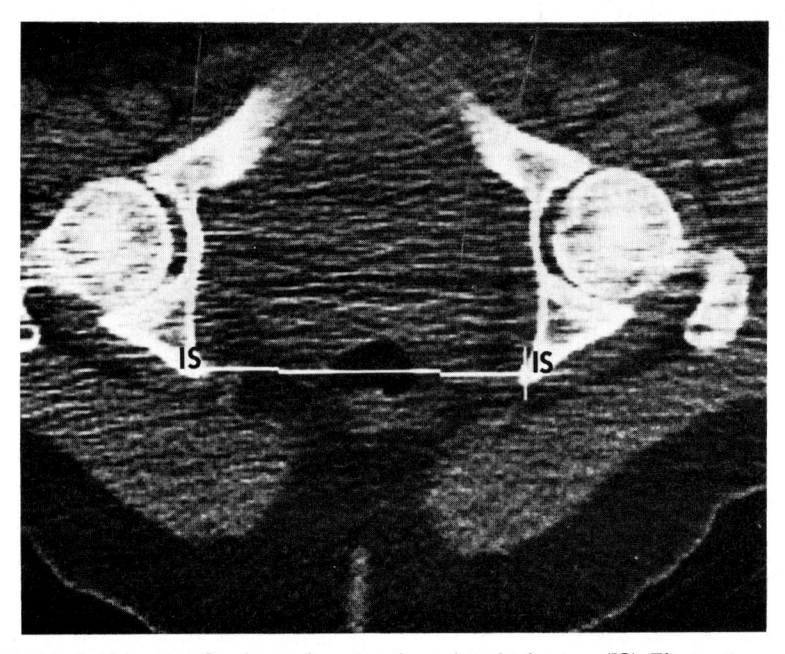

Figure 5. CT-digital pelvimetry. Single axial section through ischial spines (IS). Electronic cursor measures interspinous diameter or transverse midpelvic diameter.

after the study has been completed. Sagittal and transverse pelvic diameters are measured by electronic calipers on the television screen with no need to correct for magnification (Figs. 3 and 4). Most important, the absorbed dose for the fetus and maternal gonads is 20 mrads for each of the two digital exposures, only 5 per cent of the dose from conventional x-ray pelvimetry.

Because the important interischial spine diameter is difficult to identify on both conventional and digital pelvimetry, we perform a single axial CT section using very reduced factors (40 mA) through the level of the ischial spines. If the spines cannot be seen on the anteroposterior digital radiograph, a level is chosen through the fovea of the femoral head, which usually corresponds to the level of the ischial spines on supine positioning. This single axial CT section permits a highly accurate direct measurement of the interspinous diameter and midpelvic capacity (Fig. 5). The absorbed dose from this section is 380 mrads, but both the fetus and the maternal gonads are effectively shielded from this exposure because of the low position and the tight collimation of the CT section.

In breech presentation, the position of the fetal head should be noted since deflexion may be a contraindication to vaginal delivery. Although one can measure the fetal head on digital radiographs, this is of little value. Distance measurements are accurate only if the structures measured lie in the center of the CT gantry. The maternal pelvis is placed in the center, but the fetal head usually lies anteriorly. In addition, a true biparietal diameter is rarely visualized on the films. Ultrasonography more accurately measures the fetal head.

Since CT-digital pelvimetry is simple, accurate, and extremely low in ionizing radiation, it has completely replaced conventional pelvimetry at this institution.

SUMMARY

The indications for x-ray pelvimetry and its technique have changed greatly in recent years. Many former indications for its use (size and position of fetus, fetal anomalies or death, placental abnormalities) have been supplanted by ultrasonography. Decreased use in fetal vertex presentation has been a general trend, whereas pelvimetry remains of value in breech presentation and other individually selected cases. Any pelvimetry technique must properly shield the fetus and mother and must be exacting in radiographic technique to reduce radiation exposure. CT-digital pelvimetry, a promising new alternative, offers improved accuracy and a substantially lower radiation dose.

REFERENCES

1. Axelson, B., and Ohlsen, H.: Radiation doses in low-dose pelvimetry using rare-earth screens. Acta Radiol. Oncol. Radiat. Phys. Biol., *18*:470, 1979.
2. Bithell, J., and Stewart, A.: Prenatal irradiation and childhood malignancy: A review of the British data from the Oxford Survey. Br. J. Cancer, *31*:271, 1975.
3. Brown,, R. C.: A modification of the Colcher-Sussman technique of x-ray pelvimetry. Am. J. Roentgenol., *115*:623, 1972.
4. Campbell, J. A.: X-ray pelvimetry: Useful procedure or medical nonsense? J. Natl. Med. Assoc. *68*:524, 1976.
5. Collea, J. V., Chien, C., and Quilligan, E. J.: The randomized management of term frank breech presentation: A study of 208 cases. Am. J. Obstet. Gynecol. *137*:235, 1980.
6. Doust, B. D., and Doust, V. L.: Ultrasound, roentgenography, and radionuclide imaging in obstetric diagnosis. *In* Danforth, D. N. (ed.): Obstetrics and Gynecology. Edition 3. New York, Harper and Row, 1977, p. 493–579.
7. Federle, M. P., Cohen, H. A., Rosenwein, M. F., et al.: Pelvimetry by digital radiography: A low dose examination. Radiology, *143*:733–735, 1982.
8. Fine, E. A., Bracken, M., and Berkowitz, R. L.: An evaluation of the usefulness of x-ray pelvimetry: Comparison of the Thoms and modified Ball methods with manual pelvimetry. Am. J. Obstet. Gynecol. *137*:15, 1980.
9. Friedman, E. A.: The therapeutic dilemma of arrested labor. Contemp. Ob/Gyn, *11*:34, 1978.
10. Friedman, E. A., and Taylor, M. B.: A modified nomographic aid for x-ray cephalopelvimetry. Am. J. Obstet. Gynecol., *105*:1110, 1969.
11. Joyce, D. N., Giwa-Osagie, F., and Stevenson, G. W.: Role of pelvimetry in active management of labor. Br. Med. J., *4*:505, 1975.
12. Kelley, K. M., Madden, D. A., Arcarese, J. S., et al.: The utilization and efficacy of pelvimetry. Am. J. Roentgenol., *125*:66, 1975.
13. Klapholz, H.: A computerized aid to Ball pelvimetry. Am. J. Obstet. Gynecol., *121*:1067, 1975.
14. Langer, A., and Kennedy, K. W.: The normal pelvis. *In* Iffy, L., and Kaminetzky H. A. (eds.): Principles and Practice of Obstetrics and Perinatology. New York, John Wiley and Sons, 1981, pp. 733–745.
15. MacMahon, B.: Prenatal x-ray exposure and childhood cancer. J. Natl. Cancer Instit., *28*:1173, 1962.
16. Mengert, W. F.: Estimation of pelvic capacity. J.A.M.A., *138*:169, 1948.
17. Newcombe, H. B., and McGregor, J. F.: Childhood

cancer following obstetric radiography. Lancet, 2:1151, 1971.
18. O'Driscoll, P.: Active management of labor and CPD. J. Obstet. Gynecol. Br. Commonw., 77:385, 1970.
19. Osborne, S. B.: The implications of the reports of the Committee on Radiologic Hazards to Patients (Adrian Committee). I. Variations in the radiation dose received by the patient in diagnostic radiology. Br. J. Radiol., 36:229, 1963.
20. Pritchard, and MacDonald, P. C. (eds.): Williams Obstetrics, Edition 16. New York, Appleton-Century-Crofts, 1980, p. 275–292.
21. Steer, C. M.: X-ray pelvimetry and the outcome of labor. Am. J. Obstet. Gynecol., 76:118, 1958.
22. Thoms, H.: The clinical application of roentgen pelvimetry and a study of the results in 1,100 white women. Am. J. Obstet. Gynecol., 42:957, 1941.
23. United Nations Scientific Committee on the Effects of Atomic Radiation 1977 Report to the General Assembly. Sources and Effects of Ionizing Radiation. United Nations, New York, 1977.
24. Varner, M. W., Cruikshank, D. P., and Laube, D. W.: X-ray pelvimetry in clinical obstetrics. Obstet. Gynecol., 56:296, 1980.
25. Weinberg, A.: Radiological estimation of pelvic capacity. Obstet. Gynecol. Surv. 7:455, 1952.

20

Ultrasound Instrumentation: Physical Principles

Frederick W. Kremkau, Ph.D.

Ultrasound is useful for diagnosis in obstetrics and gynecology because it provides a way of visualizing internal female pelvic anatomy and the fetus in utero. This is accomplished by sending pulses of ultrasound into the patient (Fig. 1), receiving the reflected and scattered pulses (echoes) (Fig. 2), and processing them in the electronics of the instrumentation to produce a displayed image of the internal cross-sectional anatomy.

The principal components of the imaging system include the electronic instrumentation, the transducer, and the tissues (patient). The instrumentation produces electrical pulses that drive the transducer, receives and processes electrical voltages from the transducer corresponding to received echoes, and produces the cross-sectional image on a display. In some cases, the instrumentation also has the capability of storing the information corresponding to one cross-sectional image in a memory. The transducer is the interface between the instrumentation and the tissues. It produces ultrasound pulses when stimulated by electrical pulses from the instrumentation, and converts returning echoes back into electrical voltages which are sent to the instrumentation. The ultrasound pulses produced by the transducer interact with the tissues in several ways, imparting information that can then be used by the instrumentation to yield an image useful for evaluation and diagnosis.

ULTRASOUND

Ultrasound is like the ordinary sound that we hear except that its pitch is beyond the range of human hearing. The principles that govern its behavior are the same as those for audible sound.

The ultrasound used for medical imaging is delivered in the form of pulses rather than continuously (Fig. 3). About 1000 pulses are produced each second, each being about one microsecond long. Each pulse consists of two or three cycles (complete variations) in the acoustic variables associated with sound (pressure, density, temperature, and particle motion). These sound pulses travel through tissues with a speed that depends upon the particular type of tissue. For soft tissues, the average propagation speed is 1540 meters per second (m/sec), with fat being the only significantly different case (1450 m/sec). As we shall see later, reducing the length of the pulse improves resolution. The pulse length may be reduced by reducing the number of cycles in the pulse or by reducing the length of each cycle. The number of cycles in the pulse is determined by the transducer. The length of each cycle is determined by the propagation speed and the frequency. Frequency is the number of cycles occurring in one second (assuming that the sound is continuous, i.e., the quiet spaces between the pulses are assumed to have sound in them). As frequency is increased, the length of each cycle (wavelength) is decreased. Therefore as frequency increases, spatial pulse length decreases (Fig. 4 shows a pulse for a frequency higher than that for Fig. 3).

The strength of the pulses (which depends upon the magnitude of the variations of the acoustic variables illustrated in Figs. 3 and 4) is described by the intensity. Intensity is equal to the sound power divided by the area over which the sound is spread (cross-sectional area of the beam). Several intensities are defined because the sound power is not distributed uniformly over the cross-section of the beam and because the sound is not delivered uniformly in time

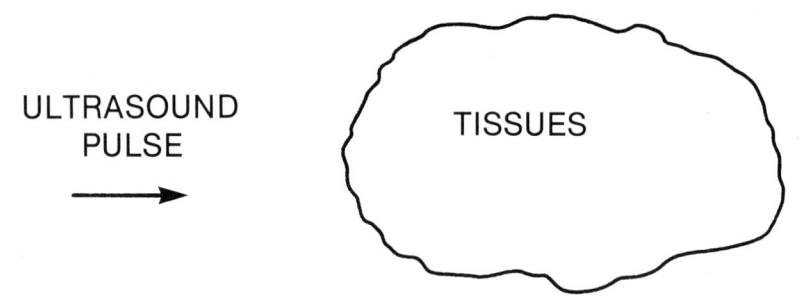

Figure 1. In diagnostic imaging, ultrasound pulses are sent into the tissues to interact with them obtaining information about them.

(pulsed rather than continuous). The use of spatial peak and average values and temporal peak and average values results in four possibilities for intensity: spatial and temporal average intensity; spatial peak, temporal average intensity; spatial average, temporal peak intensity; spatial and temporal peak intensity. The spatial and temporal average will yield the lowest value for a given pulsed sound beam, whereas the spatial and temporal peak value will be the highest. Spatial or temporal averaging yields intermediate values.

TISSUE INTERACTIONS

As sound pulses travel through tissues, various interactions occur. One aspect of this which has already been discussed and can be considered to be an interaction is the determination of the propagation speed by the medium through which the sound passes. Figure 5 shows a pulse in two positions during its travel. As the pulse travels from left to right, time is required (about 6.5 microseconds for each centimeter of travel). Figure 5 also shows that as the pulse travels it becomes weaker. This reduction in intensity with travel is called attenuation. Attenuation results from reflection and scattering of sound (discussed later) and absorption (conversion of sound to heat). Attenuation depends upon the type of tissue involved and the frequency used. In soft tissues, attenuation is approximately proportional to frequency such that attenuation in decibels per centimeter is approximately equal to the frequency in megahertz. The decibel unit is a description of intensity reduction as described in Table 1. For example, at 3.5 megahertz, attenuation will be approximately 3.5 dB/cm so that over a 2 cm distance, 7 dB of attenuation will occur. Table 1 shows that this corresponds to a reduction in intensity of 80 per cent; i.e., 20 per cent of the intensity at the beginning of the path remains at the end of the 2 cm path. At 10 MHz, the attenuation is approximately 10 dB/cm and a 2 cm path will result in 20 dB of attenuation corresponding to a 99 per cent intensity reduction. Increasing frequency results in increasing attenuation and thus decreased imaging depth. Therefore, as frequency is increased pulses are shortened for better resolution but imaging depth is reduced. In medical imaging, frequencies from about 1 to 10 MHz are used, the lower frequencies when greater depths of imaging are required and the higher frequencies for visualizing superficial structures.

As sound encounters boundaries between different tissues, it can be reflected and scattered. Partial reflection of the sound at

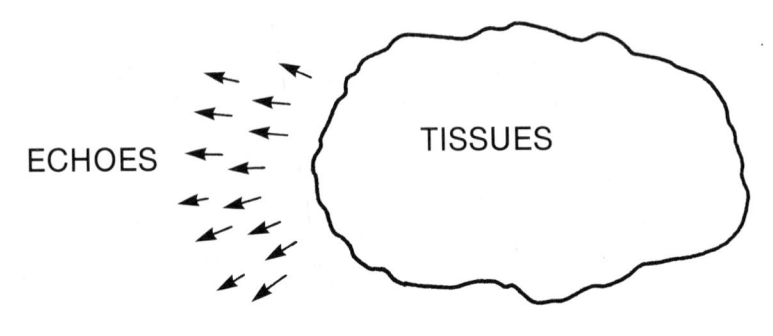

Figure 2. Reflected and scattered ultrasound pulses (echoes) return from the tissues to the sound source providing information useful for imaging and diagnosis.

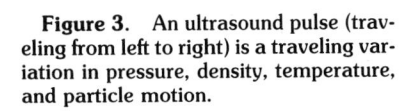

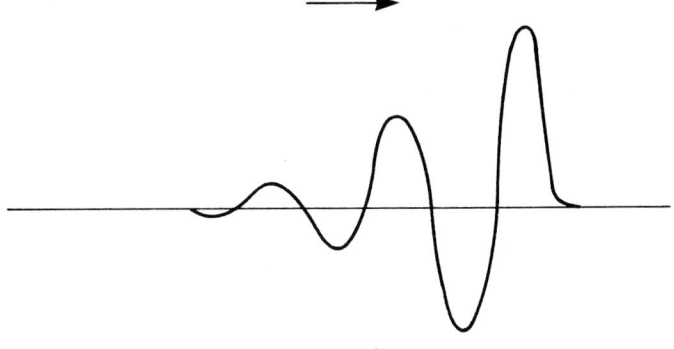

Figure 3. An ultrasound pulse (traveling from left to right) is a traveling variation in pressure, density, temperature, and particle motion.

a boundary occurs when the impedances (propagation speed times density) of the two tissues are different (Fig. 6). As the ratio of the impedances departs from one (when the ratio is one, the impedances are equal) the reflected intensity increases and the intensity of the sound transmitted into the second tissue decreases. The sum of the reflected and transmitted intensities (Fig. 6B) is equal to the incident intensity (Fig. 6A). Reflections from tissue boundaries allow ultrasonographic visualization of organs in the body.

If the tissues boundaries are not smooth (irregularities comparable to or greater than the wavelength), the sound, in addition to being reflected at the boundary, will be scattered (Fig. 7A). Scattering also occurs from within heterogeneous media like tissues (Fig. 7B) allowing tissue parenchyma to be visualized. In the frequency range of diagnostic ultrasound, the intensity of scattered sound generally increases as frequency increases.

TRANSDUCERS

A transducer is a device which converts energy from one form to another. An ultrasound transducer (Fig. 8) converts electrical voltages into ultrasound pulses and vice versa. The transducer element, which is made out of piezoelectric (Greek: pressure electricity) material, performs this function. Since the transducer element and the skin have different impedances, a reflection will occur at this boundary. The matching layer in front of the transducer element helps to reduce this reflection and improve sound transmission from the element into the tissues. Coupling gel or oil is used between the matching layer and skin to eliminate the air space which would produce a prohibitive reflection. The damping material behind the element reduces the number of cycles in each pulse to about two or three. Without the damping material the pulses would be much longer and resolution would be unacceptable.

The sound pulses produced by flat circular disk transducer elements have a width or diameter which decreases as the pulse travels away from the element in the near zone and then increases in the far zone (Fig. 9). The lateral extent of these pulses as they travel out from the transducer is described by the beam width or diameter. The lateral resolution of the imaging system depends upon the pulse diameter. Re-

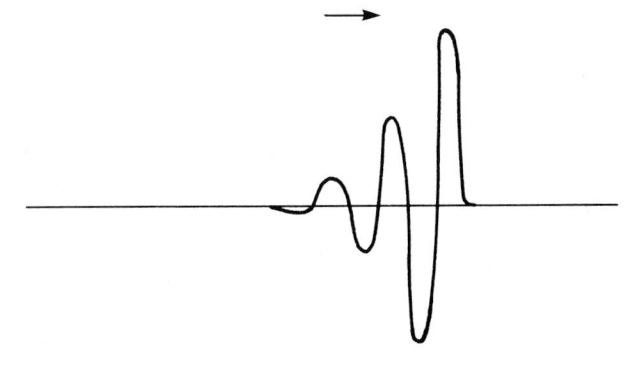

Figure 4. Increasing the frequency of the ultrasound shortens the pulse (assuming the same number of cycles—three in this case—in the pulse).

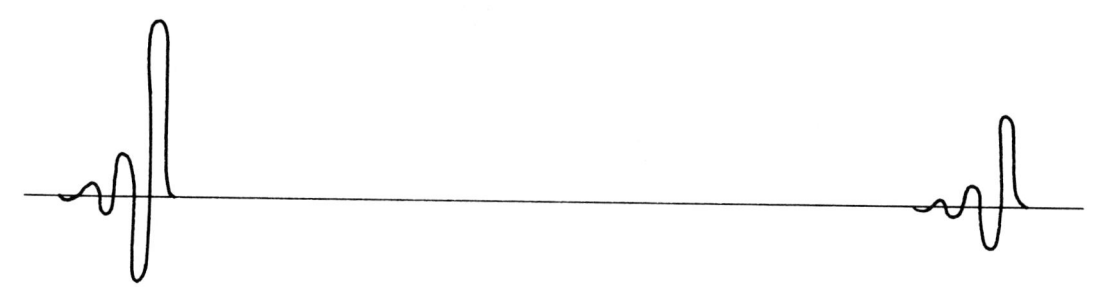

Figure 5. As a sound pulse travels from left to right, time is required (determined by the speed in the medium). Also the pulse intensity is reduced.

ducing the pulse diameter improves the lateral resolution. This can be accomplished by focusing (curving of the transducer element). Focusing can be accomplished only in the near zone for the comparable flat transducer element. In the far zone, focusing will result in increased beam diameter and degraded lateral resolution. In the focal region of a focused transducer, lateral resolution is optimum.

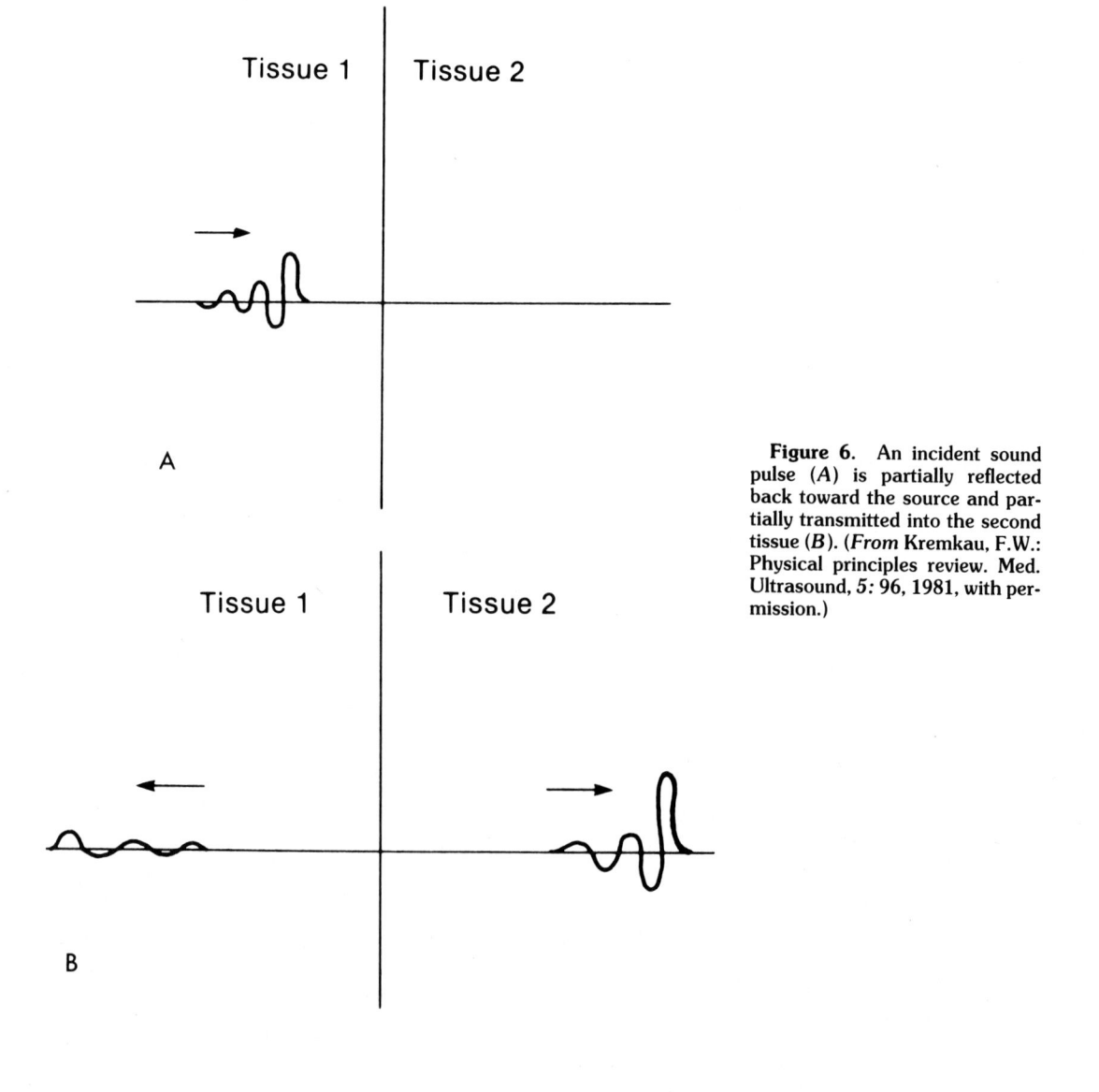

Figure 6. An incident sound pulse (A) is partially reflected back toward the source and partially transmitted into the second tissue (B). (*From* Kremkau, F.W.: Physical principles review. Med. Ultrasound, 5: 96, 1981, with permission.)

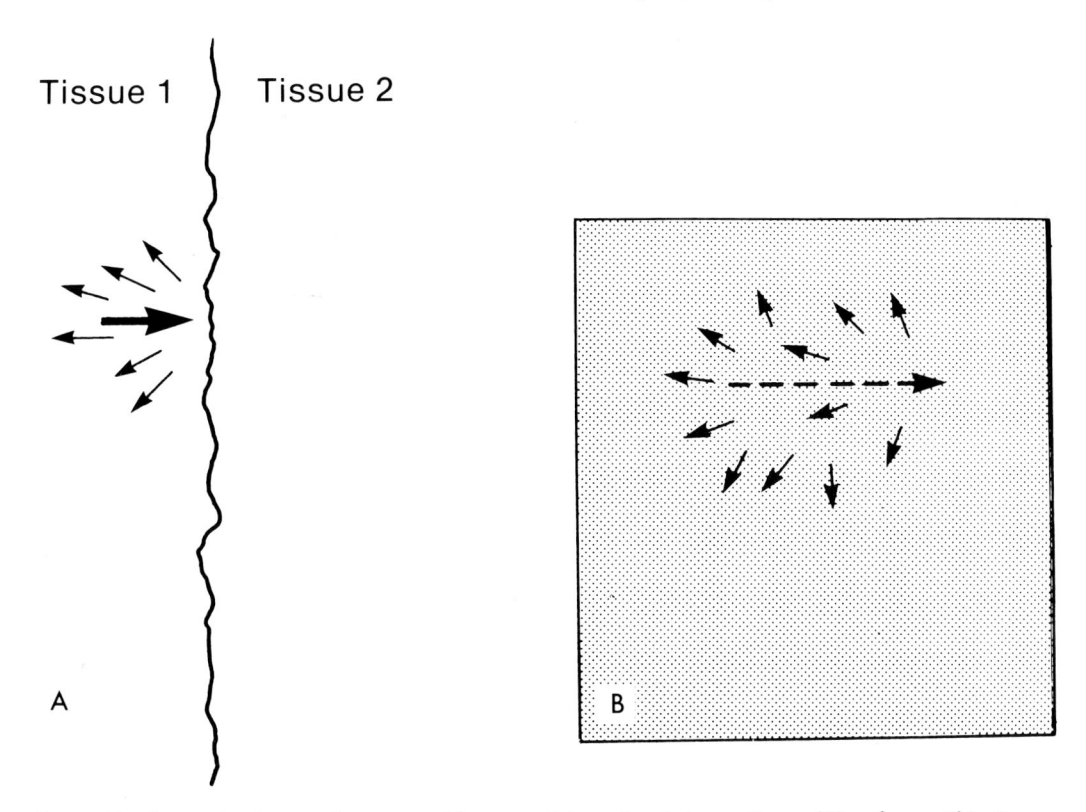

Figure 7. A sound pulse may be scattered by a rough boundary between tissues (A) or from within tissues owing to their heterogenous character (B). (*From* Kremkau, F.W.: Physical principles review. Med. Ultrasound, 6: 37–38, 1982, with permission.)

Real-Time Transducers

For real-time or dynamic imaging, means must be provided for rapidly and repeatedly scanning the ultrasound beam through the patient. This is done with mechanical real-time transducers (Fig. 10) or with electronic transducer arrays (Fig. 11). Mechanical real-time transducers may consist of an oscillating single element disk transducer (Fig. 10A) or a rotating assembly of several elements (Fig. 10B). Transducer arrays can be operated in two modes: the linear switched or sequenced array (Fig. 11A) applies each electrical pulse to a group of elements, with each subsequent pulse being applied to another group shifted by one. For example, if the first electrical pulse is applied to elements one through five, then the next electrical pulse will be applied to elements two through six, and so forth. This results in a lateral linear

Figure 8. The components of a transducer assembly. (*From* Kremkau, F.W.: Diagnostic Ultrasound: Physical Principles and Exercises. New York, Grune and Stratton, 1980, with permission.)

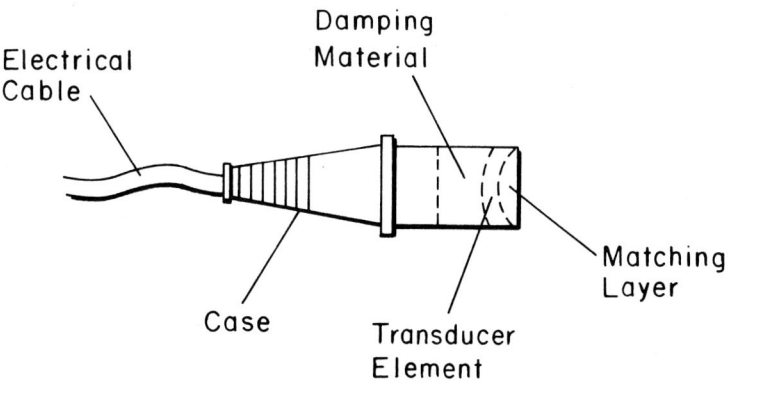

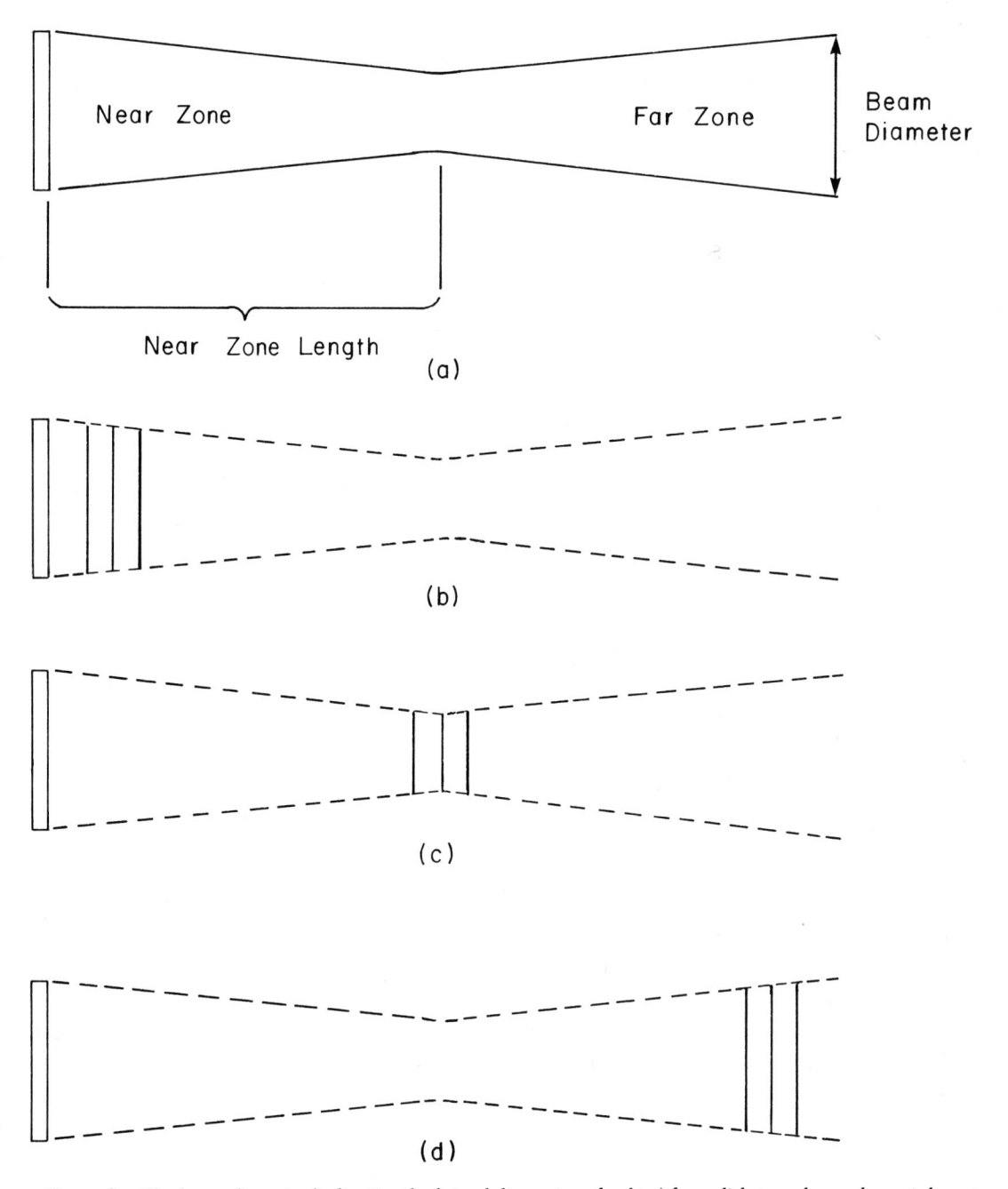

Figure 9. The beam diameter (indicating the lateral dimension of pulses) for a disk transducer element decreases in the near zone and increases in the far zone (a). A sound pulse narrows as it travels through the near zone (b) until it reaches the far zone (c) after which it widens (d). (*From* Kremkau, F.W.: Diagnostic Ultrasound: Physical Principles and Exercises. New York, Grune and Stratton, 1980, with permission.)

sweeping or scanning of the sound beam. The phased array (Fig. 11*B*) rotates the beam (each subsequent pulse goes out in a slightly different direction). Each electrical pulse is applied to all elements but the timing of the application of the pulse to the various elements (phasing) is adjusted for each pulse so that the corresponding ultrasound pulse goes out in a slightly different direction. Proper phasing can also produce electronic focusing of the beam for phased arrays (Fig. 12). Linear switched or se-

Table 1. *The Decibel Unit as a Decription of Intensity Reduction*

dB	INTENSITY REDUCTION (%)
1	21
2	37
3	50
4	60
5	68
6	75
7	80
8	84
9	87
10	90
20	99

quenced arrays have a linear scan format and result in a rectangular display format (Fig. 13A). Mechanical real-time transducers and phased arrays have a sector scan format and result in a pie-shaped or sector display format (Fig. 13B).

INSTRUMENTATION

A block diagram of the electronic instrumentation for diagnostic ultrasound imaging is shown in Figure 14. The pulser produces the electrical pulses which are applied to the transducer resulting in the production of ultrasound pulses. These electrical pulses are very short (much less than a microsecond) electrical pulses of several hundred volts. Voltages from the transducer, corresponding to received echoes, go to the receiver which performs several functions. The receiver must first amplify (increase in strength) these voltages to values usable for storage and display. This amplification is also called gain and it is measured in decibels (attenuation was measured in decibels also). Table 2 gives a list of examples of gain in dB with corresponding increases in electrical power. The strongest echo received by the transducer might be

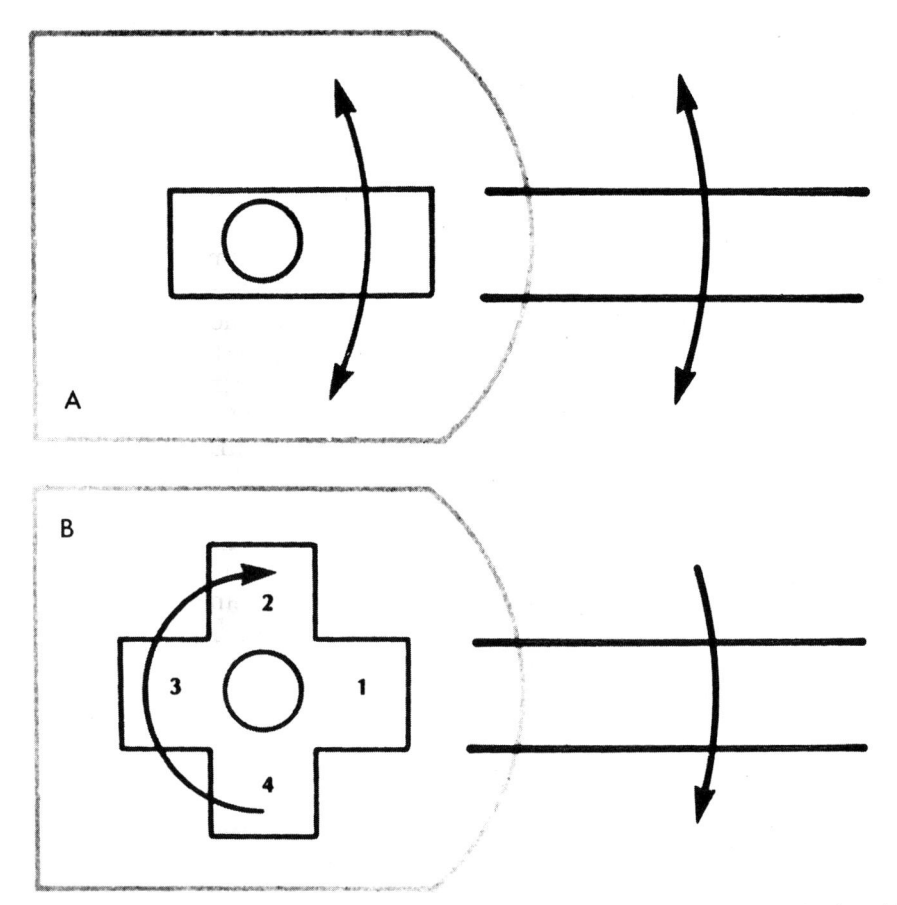

Figure 10. Mechanical real-time transducer assemblies have a single transducer angling back and forth (A) or a group of transducers rotating (B) to produce a sector scan. (*From* Nelson, L.H., and Kremkau, F.W.: Real-time diagnostic ultrasound in obstetrics. Am. Fam. Physician, *25:*149–156, with permission.)

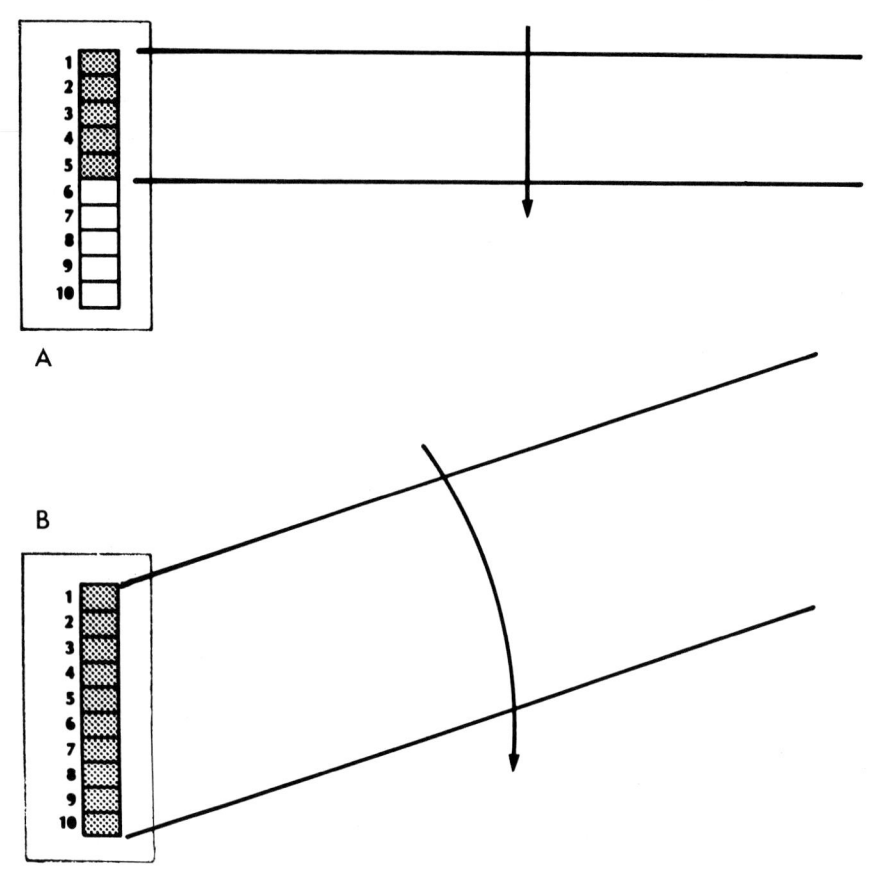

Figure 11. Real-time transducer arrays may be operated in the linear switched or sequenced mode (A) or in the phased mode (B). (*From* Nelson, L.H., and Kremkau, F.W.: Real-time diagnostic ultrasound in obstetrics. Am. Fam. Physician, 25:149–156, with permission.)

ten billion times the intensity of the weakest (a 100 dB relation). Much of this difference is caused by attenuation in tissues resulting in deeper structures returning weaker echoes to the transducer because of the longer path length. One of the jobs of the receiver is to compensate for tissue attenuation. This is done by increasing echoes from deeper structures with more amplification (higher gain). Echoes from deeper structures return later because of increased path length, therefore attenuation compensation is achieved by increasing gain with time after each pulse is sent out. This process is called time gain compensation or depth gain compensation. After this is performed the strongest voltage corresponding to the strongest echo might be 10,000 times the intensity of the weakest (a 40 dB relation).

After amplification and compensation the voltages corresponding to echoes are converted to numbers which are placed in storage positions corresponding to the location of the anatomic structures which produced them. The storage block is a dig-

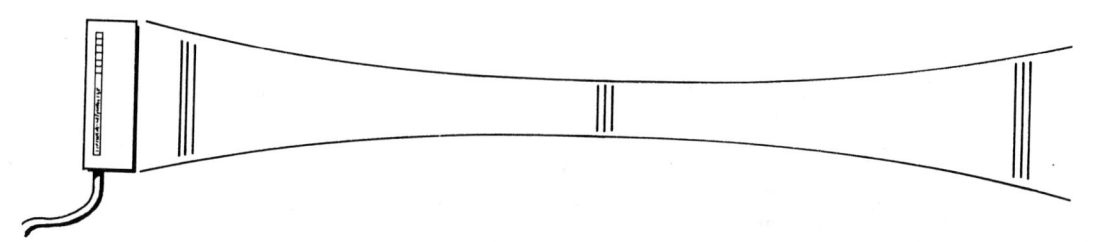

Figure 12. Focusing reduces pulse diameter (width) in the focal region.

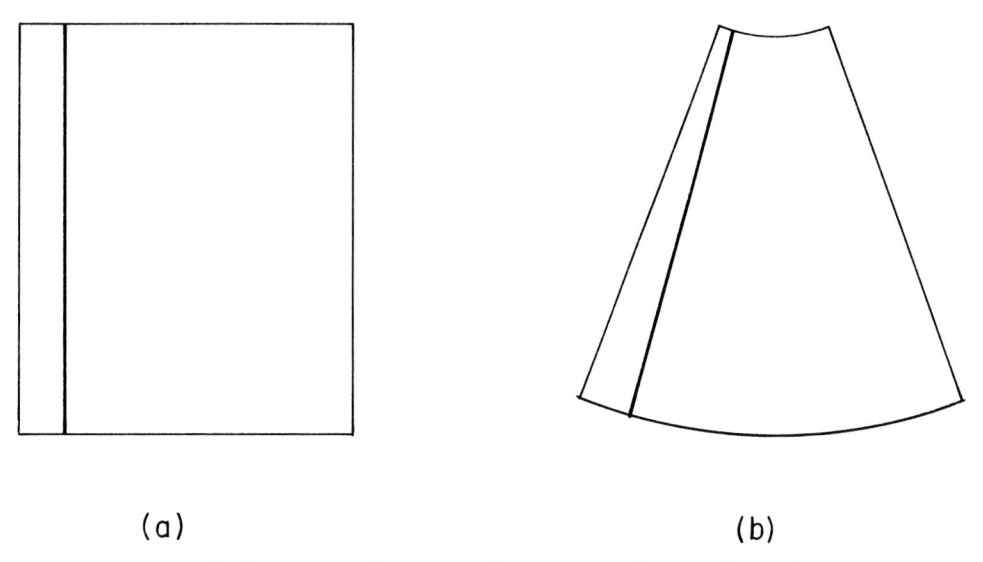

Figure 13. Linear switched or sequenced arrays produce a rectangular scan format (a) whereas mechanical real-time and phased array transducers produce a sector scan format (b).

ital computer memory. The numbers corresponding to echo strengths are placed in proper position in storage utilizing information from the transducer scanning arm concerning transducer location and orientation when each pulse is sent out. This is indicated by the dashed line in Figure 14. By knowing the location of the transducer and the direction in which it is pointing and by knowing the travel time for a pulse to a reflector and back, the proper location for each echo generating structure can be determined. Using this information, each number corresponding to the echo strength is placed in storage in the proper position. By scanning the transducer over the surface of the patient while many pulses are emitted and echoes returned, echo information is built up in storage yielding a complete cross sectional image information matrix in memory which may then be applied to a display to produce a two dimensional cross sectional image corresponding to the anatomy (Fig. 15).

Real-time or dynamic imaging instrumentation must produce several cross-sectional images per second. This requires the use of mechanical or array real-time transducers as discussed previously. Ten to 60 images are displayed per second, yielding what appears to be a continuously changing image. Real-time instruments may or

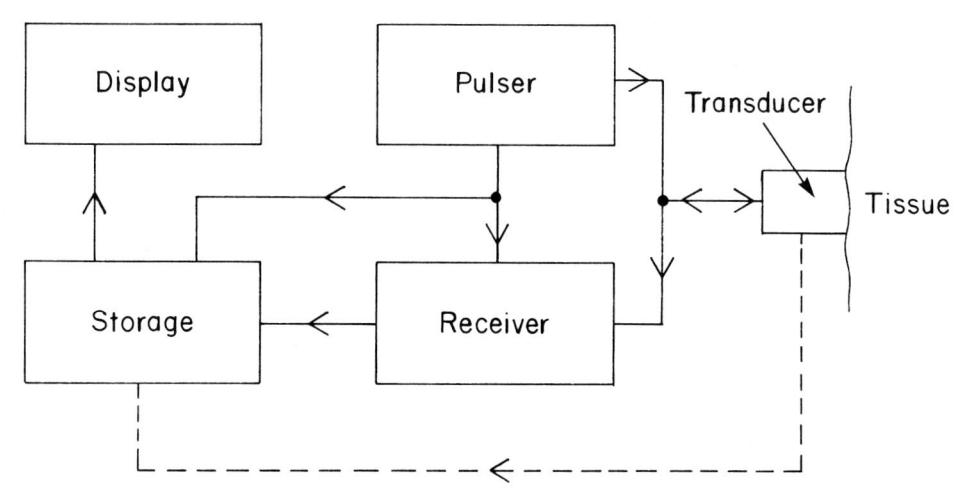

Figure 14. Block diagram of a diagnostic ultrasound imaging instrument.

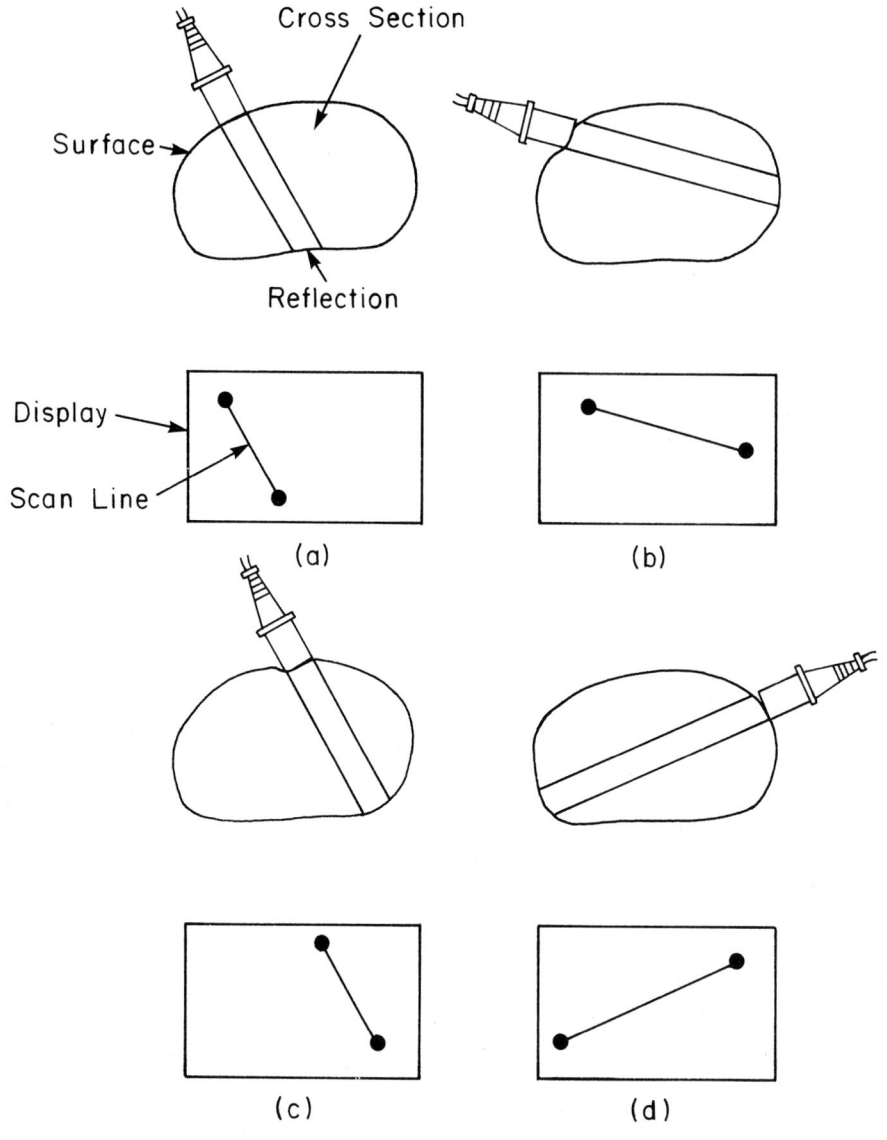

Figure 15. Pulse reflections produce corresponding bright spots on the display (a). Transducer orientation is different in (b) and (a). Transducer location is different in (c) and (a). Transducer orientation and location are different in (d) and (a). (*From* Kremkau, F.W.: Diagnostic Ultrasound: Physical Principles and Exercises. New York, Grune and Stratton, 1980, with permission.)

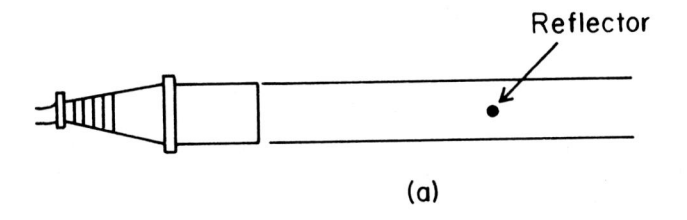

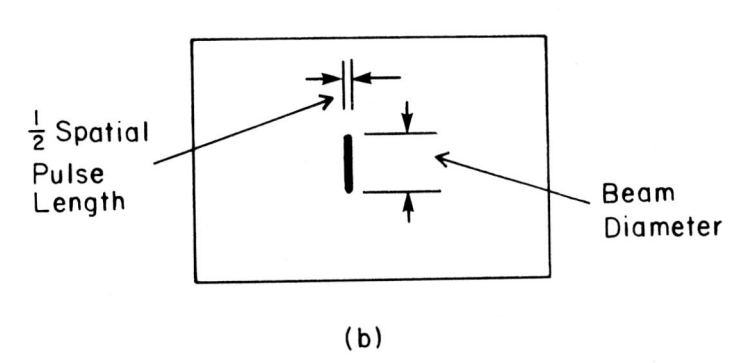

Figure 16. As the sound beam is scanned across a small reflector (a), the lateral resolution of the image produced depends on the beam diameter whereas the axial resolution depends on the pulse length. (*From* Kremkau, F.W.: Diagnostic Ultrasound: Physical Principles and Exercises. New York, Grune and Stratton, 1980, with permission.)

Table 2. *Gain in Decibels with Corresponding Increases in Electrical Power*

dB	POWER INCREASE
3	×2
6	×4
10	×10
20	×100
30	×1000
40	×10,000
50	×100,000

may not have a memory. Since the images are produced rapidly in sequence, memory is not required as it is in the manual scan which takes a second or two to produce and then is observed for several seconds. If a real-time instrument has static image or freeze frame capability, it must have a memory. Advantages and disadvantages of static and real-time systems are given in Table 3.

The imaging resolution of diagnostic ultrasound systems depends first on the acoustic resolution. This has an axial (in

Table 3. *Advantages and Disadvantages of Various Imaging Systems*

IMAGING SYSTEM	ADVANTAGES	DISADVANTAGES
Static scanner	flexible scanning technique—determined by operator high resolution frequency change easy, inexpensive large field of view	no dynamic information more training and skill required not portable
Real-time scanner	image quality less dependent on operator skill often portable	resolution and quality of individual scans not as good as real-time sequence or static scanners
Sector	better accessibility, smaller transducer assembly	limited lateral field of view close to transducer
Linear	lateral field of view constant with depth	limited accessibility, larger transducer assembly

the direction of sound propagation) and a lateral (perpendicular to propagation direction) aspect. The acoustic axial resolution is equal to one-half the spatial pulse length while the acoustic lateral resolution is equal to the beam diameter (Fig. 16). Axial resolution is improved by increasing frequency. Lateral resolution is improved by decreasing beam diameter (focusing). The imaging system resolution may be comparable to or worse than the acoustic resolution. Electronic signal processing and characteristics of the display may degrade the resolution from the value determined by the pulse geometry.

SUMMARY

By sending short pulses of ultrasound into the body and using reflections received from tissue interfaces to produce images of internal structures, ultrasound is used as a medical diagnostic tool. Pulsed ultrasound is used in medical imaging. It is described by frequency, propagation speed, intensity, attenuation, and pulse length. Reflections and scattering occur at organ boundaries and scattering from within tissues. The distance to refectors and scatterers is determined by travel time.

Transducers convert electrical voltages into ultrasound and vice versa by piezoelectricity. Acoustic axial resolution is equal to half the pulse length. It can be improved by increasing frequency. Acoustic lateral resolution is equal to beam diameter. It can be improved by focusing. Imaging system resolutions are usually worse than the acoustic resolutions. Disk transducers produce sound beams with near and far zones. Focusing reduces beam diameter in the near zone. Mechanical and array real-time transducers can scan, steer, and shape beams repeatedly, permitting real-time imaging.

Pulse-echo imaging systems use intensity, direction, and arrival time of echoes to produce cross-sectional images. Imaging systems consist of pulser, transducer, receiver, memory, and display. The pulser applies voltages to the transducer resulting in the production of ultrasound pulses. Received echoes are converted into voltages which are amplified in the receiver (where attenuation is compensated for also). Numbers corresponding to echo strengths are stored in the digital memory at locations corresponding to reflector and scatterer positions. After a cross-sectional number representation is built up in the memory, the stored numbers are converted to brightness dots on the display resulting in a cross-sectional anatomic image.

REFERENCES

1. Kremkau, F. W.: Diagnostic Ultrasound: Physical Principles and Exercises. New York, Grune and Stratton, 1980.
2. McDicken, W. N.: Diagnostic Ultrasonics: Principles and Use of Instruments. New York, John Wiley and Sons, 1981.
3. Wells, P. N. T.: Biomedical Ultrasonics. New York, Academic Press, 1977.
4. Wells, P. N. T., and Ziskin, M. C.: New techniques and instrumentation in ultrasonography. In Taylor, K. J. W. (ed.): Clinics in Diagnostic Ultrasound, Vol. 5. New York, Churchill Livingstone, 1980.

Appendix

Table 1. *Clinical Parameters in Estimation of Gestational Age**

PRIORITY FOR ESTIMATING GESTATIONAL AGE	"ESTIMATED" RANGE FOR 95% CASES
1. In vitro fertilization	less than 1 day
2. Ovulation induction	3–4 days
3. Recorded basal body temperature	4–5 days
4. Ultrasound crown-rump length (CRL)	± .7 weeks
5. First trimester physical examination (normal uterus)	± 1 week
6. Ultrasound BPD prior to 20 weeks	+ 1 week
7. Ultrasound gestational sac volume	± 1.5 weeks
8. Ultrasound BPD from 20 to 26 weeks	± 1.6 weeks
9. LNMP from recorded dates (good history)†	± 2–3 weeks
10. Ultrasound BPD 26 to 30 weeks	+ 2–3 weeks
11. LNMP from memory (good history)	3–4 weeks
12. Ultrasound BPD after 30 weeks	3–4 weeks
13. Fundal height measurement	4–6 weeks
14. LNMP from memory (not good history)	4–6 weeks
15. Fetal heart tones first heard	4–6 weeks
16. Quickening	4–6 weeks

* *Rule* is to always use a more reliable indicator in preference to a less reliable one.
† A "good" history requires knowledge of both LNMP and previous period with regular periods and no use of birth control pills for at least six months prior to the LNMP.

Table 2. *Fetal Crown-Rump Length Against Gestational Age**

CRL (mm)	−2 SD	MEAN WEEKS	+2 SD	CRL (mm)	−2 SD	MEAN WEEKS	+2 SD
7		6.25	7.15	39	10	10.65	11.35
8		6.45	7.3	40	10.1	10.75	11.45
9		6.7	7.55	41	10.2	10.8	11.55
10	6.25	6.9	7.7	42	10.3	10.9	11.65
11	6.5	7.1	7.9	43	10.4	11.05	11.7
12	6.6	7.25	8.1	44	10.45	11.1	11.8
13	6.85	7.45	8.25	45	10.55	11.2	11.9
14	7.00	7.60	8.45	46	10.66	11.3	12
15	7.15	7.75	8.60	47	10.7	11.35	12.05
16	7.3	7.9	8.70	48	10.8	11.45	12.15
17	7.45	8.1	8.9	49	10.9	11.55	12.25
18	7.60	8.2	9.0	50	10.95	11.6	12.3
19	7.75	8.4	9.15	51	11.1	11.7	12.4
20	7.9	8.5	9.3	52	11.15	11.8	12.5
21	8.05	8.6	9.4	53	11.2	11.85	12.55
22	8.15	8.8	9.55	54	11.3	11.95	12.65
23	8.3	8.9	9.65	55	11.4	12.05	12.75
24	8.4	9.05	9.8	56	11.5	12.1	12.8
25	8.55	9.15	9.9	57	11.55	12.2	12.9
26	8.7	9.3	10	58	11.65	12.3	12.95
27	8.8	9.4	10.1	59	11.7	12.35	13.05
28	8.9	9.5	10.25	60	11.8	12.45	13.15
29	9.05	9.65	10.35	61	11.85	12.5	13.2
30	9.15	9.7	10.45	62	11.9	12.6	13.3
31	9.25	9.85	10.55	63	12	12.65	13.4
32	9.35	9.95	10.65	64	12.05	12.75	13.45
33	9.45	10.05	10.75	65	12.1	12.85	13.55
34	9.55	10.15	10.85	66	12.2	12.9	13.6
35	9.6	10.2	10.95	67	12.3	12.95	13.7
36	9.7	10.35	11.05	68	12.35	13.05	13.75
37	9.8	10.4	11.15	69	12.45	13.1	13.8
38	9.9	10.55	11.25	70	12.5	13.15	13.9

* *From* Robinson, H. P., and Fleming, J. E. E.: A critical evaluation of sonar crown-rump length measurements. Br. J. Obstet. Gynecol., *82:*702, 1975, with permission.

Table 3. *Correlation of Predicted Menstrual Age Based upon Biparietal Diameters*

MENSTRUAL AGE (WEEKS)	BPD MEAN VALUES (mm)					
	Composite Sabbagha and Hughey[1]	Composite Kurtz et al.[2]	Kurtz et al.[2] < 1974	Kurtz et al.[2] > 1974	Hadlock et al.[3] 1982	Shepard and Filly[4] 1982
14	28	27	28	26	27	28
15	32	31	31	29	30	31
16	36	34	35	33	33	34
17	39	38	39	36	37	37
18	42	41	42	40	40	40
19	45	45	46	43	43	43
20	48	48	49	46	46	46
21	51	51	52	50	50	49
22	54	54	55	53	53	52
23	58	57	58	56	56	55
24	61	60	61	59	58	57
25	64	63	64	61	61	60
26	67	66	67	64	64	63
27	70	69	69	67	67	65
28	72	71	72	70	70	68
29	75	74	75	72	72	71
30	78	76	77	75	75	73
31	80	79	79	77	77	76
32	82	81	81	79	79	78
33	85	83	83	82	82	80
34	87	85	85	84	84	83
35	88	87	87	86	86	85
36	90	89	89	88	88	88
37	92	91	91	90	90	90
38	93	92	92	92	91	92
39	94	94	94	94	93	95
40	95	95	95	95	95	97

[1] Sabbagha, R. E., and Hughey, M.: Standardization of sonar cephalometry and gestational age. Obstet. Gynecol., *52:*402, 1978.

[2] Kurtz, A. B., Wapner, R. J., Kurtz, R. J., et al.: Analysis of biparietal diameter as an accurate indicator of gestational age. J. Clin. Ultrasound, *8:*319, 1980.

[3] Hadlock, F. P., Deter, R. L., Harrist, R. B., et al.: Fetal biparietal diameter: A critical re-evaluation of the relation to menstrual age by means of real-time ultrasound. J. Ultrasound Med., *1:*97–104, 1982.

[4] Shepard, M., and Filly, R. A.: A standardized plane for biparietal diameter measurement. J. Ultrasound Med., *1:*145–150, 1982.

Table 4. Comparison of Predicted Femur Lengths at Points in Gestation

MENSTRUAL AGE (WEEKS)	FEMUR LENGTH (mm)			
	Filly et al.[1] 1981	Jeanty et al.[2] 1981†	Hadlock et al.[3] 1982*	Hadlock et al.[3] 1982†
12		09	14	08
13		12	16	11
14	16	16	19	15
15	19	19	21	18
16	22	23	23	21
17	25	26	26	24
18	28	30	28	27
19	32	33	30	30
20	35	36	33	33
21	38	39	35	36
22	41	42	38	39
23	44	45	40	42
24	47	48	42	44
25	50	51	45	47
26	53	54	47	49
27	55	57	49	52
28	57	59	52	54
29	61	62	54	56
30	63	65	57	58
31		67	59	61
32		70	61	63
33		72	64	65
34		74	66	66
35		77	69	68
36		79	71	70
37		81	73	72
38		83	76	73
39		85	78	75
40		87	80	76

* Linear function
† Linear quadratic function

[1] Filly, R. A., Golbus, M. S., Carey, J. C., et al.: Short-limbed dwarfism: Ultrasonographic diagnosis by mensuration of fetal femoral length. Radiology, *138:*653–656, 1981.

[2] Fetal femur length as a predictor of menstrual age: Sonographically measured. Am. J. Roentgenol., *138:*875–878, 1982.

[3] Jeanty, P. Kirkpatrick, C., Dramaix-Wilmet, M., et al.: Ultrasonic evaluation of fetal limb growth. Radiology, *140:*165–168, 1981.

Table 5. *Head Circumference: Normal Values*

	DETER ET AL.[13]			HADLOCK ET AL.[30]		
MENSTRUAL AGE (WKS)	Lower Limit* (cm)	Predicted Value† (cm)	Upper Limit‡ (cm)	−2 S.D.‖ (cm)	Predicted Value§ (cm)	+2 S.D.‖ (cm)
12	5.8	7.3	8.8	5.1	7.0	8.9
13	7.2	8.7	10.2	6.5	8.9	10.3
14	8.6	10.1	11.6	7.9	9.8	11.7
15	9.9	11.4	12.9	9.2	11.1	13.0
16	11.3	12.8	14.3	10.5	12.4	14.3
17	12.6	14.1	15.6	11.8	13.7	15.6
18	13.9	15.4	16.9	13.1	15.0	16.9
19	15.2	16.7	18.2	14.4	16.3	18.2
20	16.4	17.9	19.4	15.6	17.5	19.4
21	17.7	19.2	20.7	16.8	18.7	20.6
22	18.9	20.4	21.9	18.0	19.9	21.8
23	20.0	21.5	23.0	19.1	21.0	22.9
24	21.2	22.7	24.2	20.2	22.1	24.0
25	22.3	23.8	25.3	21.3	23.2	25.1
26	23.4	24.9	26.4	22.3	24.2	26.1
27	24.4	25.9	27.4	23.3	25.2	27.1
28	24.4	26.9	29.4	24.3	26.2	28.1
29	25.4	27.9	30.4	25.2	27.1	29.0
30	26.3	28.8	31.3	26.1	28.0	29.9
31	27.2	29.7	32.2	27.0	28.9	30.8
32	28.1	30.6	33.1	27.8	29.7	31.6
33	28.9	31.4	33.9	28.5	30.4	32.3
34	29.7	32.2	34.7	29.3	31.2	33.1
35	30.4	32.9	35.4	29.9	31.8	33.7
36	31.1	33.6	36.1	30.6	32.5	34.4
37	31.7	34.2	36.7	31.1	33.0	34.9
38	32.3	34.8	37.3	31.9	33.6	35.5
39	32.9	35.4	37.9	32.2	34.1	36.0
40	33.4	35.9	38.4	32.6	34.5	36.4

* <28 weeks: predicted value −1.5 cm.
  >28 weeks: predicted value −2.5 cm.
† HC = −10.3676 + 1.5021 (MA) − .0002136 (MA)^3 [R^2 = 97.3%].
‡ <28 weeks: predicted value +1.5 cm.
  >28 weeks: predicted value +2.5 cm.
§ HC = −10.339 + 1.481 (MA) − .0002259 (MA)^3 [R^2 = 98.3%].
‖ 2 S.D. = 1.9 cm.

Table 6. *Head Circumference: Normal Growth Rates*

	DETER ET AL.[15]		
MENSTRUAL AGE INTERVAL (WKS)	−2 S.D.† (cm/wk)	Predicted Value* (cm/wk)	+2 S.D.† (cm/wk)
12–13	1.4	1.6	1.8
13–14	1.3	1.5	1.7
14–15	1.3	1.5	1.7
15–16	1.3	1.5	1.7
16–17	1.3	1.5	1.7
17–18	1.2	1.4	1.6
18–19	1.2	1.4	1.6
19–20	1.2	1.4	1.6
20–21	1.1	1.3	1.5
21–22	1.1	1.3	1.5
22–23	1.2	1.3	1.4
23–24	1.1	1.2	1.3
24–25	1.1	1.2	1.3
25–26	1.1	1.2	1.3
26–27	1.0	1.1	1.2
27–28	1.0	1.1	1.2
28–29	0.9	1.0	1.1
29–30	0.9	1.0	1.1
30–31	0.8	0.9	1.0
31–32	0.8	0.9	1.0
32–33	0.7	0.8	0.9
33–34	0.6	0.8	1.0
34–35	0.5	0.7	0.9
35–36	0.5	0.7	0.9
36–37	0.4	0.6	0.8
37–38	0.4	0.6	0.8
38–39	0.3	0.5	0.7
39–40	0.1	0.4	0.7

* Date represent first derivative values of the function

$$HC = -13.84 + 1.68 \times (MA) - 2.67 \times 10^{-4} (MA)^3$$

which describes the average longitudinal growth curve. These values are calculated as follows:

$$\frac{dHc}{dMA} = 1.68 + 3(-2.67 \times 10^{-4}) MA^2$$

The values given are mid-week values (i.e., 12–13 week interval: derivative value at 12.5 weeks).

† Values calculated as follows:

$$2\text{ S.D.} = \left(\frac{2}{9}\left[\sum_{i=1}^{19}(a_{1i} - 1.68)^2 + 9(MA)^4 \right.\right.$$
$$\times \sum_{i=1}^{19}(a_{3i} + 2.67 \times 10^{-4})^2 + 6(MA)^2$$
$$\left.\left.\times \sum_{i=1}^{19}(a_{1i} - 1.68)(a_{3i} + 2.67 \times 10^{-4})\right]\right)^{\frac{1}{2}}$$

where a_{1i} and a_{3i} are coefficients of the individual HC growth curves.[15]

Table 7. *Abdominal Circumference: Normal Values*

	DETER ET AL.[13]			HADLOCK ET AL.[31]		
MENSTRUAL AGE (WKS)	Lower Limit* (cm)	Predicted Value† (cm)	Upper Limit‡ (cm)	−2 S.D.‖ (cm)	Predicted Value§ (cm)	+2 S.D.‖ (cm)
12	5.4	6.3	7.1	3.1	5.6	8.1
13	6.4	7.4	8.3	4.4	6.9	9.4
14	7.4	8.4	9.5	5.6	8.1	10.6
15	8.3	9.5	10.8	6.8	9.3	11.8
16	9.3	10.6	12.0	8.0	10.5	13.0
17	10.2	11.7	13.3	9.2	11.7	14.2
18	11.2	12.8	14.5	10.4	12.9	15.4
19	12.1	13.9	15.7	11.6	14.1	16.6
20	13.1	15.0	17.0	12.7	15.2	17.7
21	14.0	16.1	18.2	13.9	16.4	18.9
22	15.0	17.2	19.5	15.0	17.5	20.0
23	16.0	18.3	20.7	16.1	18.6	21.1
24	16.9	19.4	22.0	17.2	19.7	22.2
25	17.9	20.5	23.2	18.3	20.8	23.3
26	18.8	21.6	24.4	19.4	21.9	24.4
27	19.8	22.7	25.7	20.4	22.9	25.4
28	20.7	23.8	26.9	21.5	24.0	26.5
29	21.7	24.9	28.2	22.5	25.0	27.5
30	22.6	26.0	29.4	23.5	26.0	28.5
31	23.6	27.1	30.6	24.5	27.0	29.5
32	24.6	28.2	31.9	25.5	28.0	30.5
33	25.5	29.3	33.1	26.5	29.0	31.5
34	26.5	30.4	34.4	27.5	30.0	32.5
35	27.4	31.5	35.6	28.4	30.9	33.4
36	28.4	32.6	36.9	29.3	31.8	34.3
37	29.3	33.7	38.1	30.2	32.7	35.2
38	30.3	34.8	39.3	31.1	33.6	36.1
39	31.2	35.9	40.6	32.0	34.5	37.0
40	32.2	37.0	41.8	32.9	35.4	37.9

* Predicted value − .13 (predicted value).
† AC = −6.9300 + 1.0985 (MA) [R^2 = 95.5%].
‡ Predicted value + .13 (predicted value).
§ AC = −10.4997 + 1.4256 (MA) − .00697 (MA)^2 [R^2 = 97.9%].
‖ 2 S.D. = 2.5 cm.

Table 8. *Ratio of Head Circumference to Abdominal Circumference: Normal Values*

	DETER ET AL.			HADLOCK ET AL.		
MENSTRUAL AGE (WKS)	−2 S.D.[†] (cm)	Predicted Value* (cm)	+2 S.D.[†] (cm)	−2 S.D.[§] (cm)	Predicted Value[‡] (cm)	+2 S.D.[§] (cm)
12	1.16	1.29	1.41	1.12	1.22	1.31
13	1.15	1.28	1.40	1.11	1.21	1.30
14	1.14	1.27	1.39	1.11	1.20	1.30
15	1.13	1.26	1.38	1.10	1.19	1.29
16	1.12	1.25	1.37	1.09	1.18	1.28
17	1.11	1.24	1.36	1.08	1.18	1.27
18	1.10	1.22	1.35	1.07	1.17	1.26
19	1.09	1.21	1.34	1.06	1.16	1.25
20	1.08	1.20	1.33	1.06	1.15	1.24
21	1.07	1.19	1.32	1.05	1.14	1.24
22	1.06	1.18	1.30	1.04	1.13	1.23
23	1.05	1.17	1.29	1.03	1.12	1.22
24	1.04	1.16	1.28	1.02	1.12	1.21
25	1.03	1.15	1.27	1.01	1.11	1.20
26	1.02	1.14	1.26	1.00	1.10	1.19
27	1.01	1.13	1.25	1.00	1.09	1.18
28	1.00	1.12	1.24	.99	1.08	1.18
29	.99	1.11	1.23	.98	1.07	1.17
30	.97	1.10	1.22	.97	1.07	1.16
31	.96	1.09	1.21	.96	1.06	1.15
32	.95	1.08	1.20	.95	1.05	1.14
33	.94	1.07	1.19	.95	1.04	1.13
34	.93	1.05	1.18	.94	1.03	1.13
35	.92	1.04	1.17	.93	1.02	1.12
36	.91	1.03	1.16	.92	1.01	1.11
37	.90	1.02	1.15	.91	1.01	1.10
38	.89	1.01	1.13	.90	1.00	1.09
39	.88	1.00	1.12	.89	.99	1.08
40	.87	.99	1.11	.89	.98	1.08

* HC/AC = 1.42104 − .0106229(MA) [R^2 = 58.9%].
[†] 2 S.D. = 0.12.
[‡] HC/AC = 1.32293 − .0084471(MA) [R^2 = 67.2%].
[§] 2 S.D. = 0.10.

Table 9. *Mean Values for TIUV as a Quadratic Function of Weeks of Gestation with Upper and Lower 2.5 and 10% Tolerance Limits**

MENSTRUAL WEEKS	LOWER 2.5%	LOWER 10%	MEAN	UPPPER 10%	UPPPER 2.5%
21	502	789	912	1036	1322
22	507	801	1020	1238	1533
23	536	836	1134	1432	1732
24	589	895	1256	1616	1922
25	667	981	1384	1788	2101
26	771	1091	1520	1949	2269
27	895	1221	1663	2105	2431
28	1033	1364	1813	2262	2593
29	1179	1516	1970	2425	2762
30	1329	1672	2134	2597	2940
31	1483	1832	2306	2780	3129
32	1642	1996	2485	2973	3327
33	1806	2165	2670	3175	3535
34	1980	2345	2863	3381	3746
35	2171	2541	3062	3585	3955
36	2384	2759	3270	3781	4156
37	2623	3004	3484	3965	4346
38	2887	3273	3705	4138	4524
39	3175	3566	3934	4302	4693
40	3484	3880	4170	4459	4855

* *From* Filly, R. A.: J. Clin. Ultrasound, 7:24, 1979, with permission.

Table 10. *Estimated Fetal Weights**

Biparietal diameter	\multicolumn{12}{c}{Abdominal circumference}
	15.5	16.0	16.5	17.0	17.5	18.0	18.5	19.0	19.5	20.0	20.5	21.0
3.1	212	219	227	236	244	253	262	272	282	292	303	314
3.2	218	226	234	243	252	261	270	280	290	301	312	323
3.3	225	233	242	250	260	269	279	289	299	310	321	333
3.4	232	241	249	258	268	277	287	298	308	319	331	343
3.5	239	248	257	266	276	286	296	307	318	329	341	353
3.6	247	256	265	274	284	294	305	316	327	339	351	364
3.7	254	263	273	283	293	303	314	325	337	349	361	374
3.8	262	271	281	291	302	312	324	335	347	359	372	385
3.9	270	280	290	300	311	322	333	345	357	370	383	397
4.0	278	288	299	309	320	331	343	355	368	381	394	408
4.1	287	297	308	318	330	341	353	366	379	392	406	420
4.2	296	306	317	328	340	352	364	377	390	404	418	433
4.3	305	315	326	338	350	362	375	388	401	416	430	445
4.4	314	325	336	348	360	373	386	399	413	428	443	458
4.5	323	334	346	358	371	384	397	411	425	440	455	471
4.6	333	344	356	369	382	395	409	423	438	453	469	485
4.7	343	355	367	380	393	407	421	435	450	466	482	499
4.8	353	365	378	391	404	418	433	448	463	479	496	513
4.9	364	376	389	402	416	431	445	461	477	493	510	527
5.0	374	387	401	414	428	443	458	474	490	507	524	542
5.1	386	399	412	426	441	456	472	488	504	521	539	558
5.2	397	410	424	439	454	469	485	502	519	536	554	573
5.3	409	422	437	452	467	483	499	516	533	551	570	589
5.4	421	435	449	465	480	496	513	531	548	567	586	606
5.5	433	447	463	478	494	511	528	546	564	583	602	622
5.6	446	461	476	492	508	525	543	561	580	599	619	640
5.7	459	474	490	506	523	540	558	577	596	616	636	657
5.8	472	488	504	520	538	555	574	593	612	633	654	675
5.9	486	502	518	535	553	571	590	609	629	650	672	694
6.0	500	516	533	550	568	587	606	626	647	668	690	712
6.1	514	531	548	566	584	604	623	644	665	686	709	732
6.2	529	546	564	582	601	620	641	661	683	705	728	751
6.3	544	561	580	598	618	638	658	679	701	724	747	772
6.4	559	577	596	615	635	655	676	698	721	744	768	792
6.5	575	594	613	632	653	673	695	717	740	764	788	813
6.6	592	610	630	650	671	692	714	737	760	784	809	835
6.7	608	628	648	668	689	711	733	757	780	805	831	857
6.8	626	645	666	686	708	730	753	777	801	827	853	879
6.9	643	663	684	705	727	750	774	798	823	848	875	902
7.0	661	682	703	725	747	771	795	819	845	871	898	926
7.1	680	701	722	745	768	791	816	841	867	894	921	950
7.2	699	720	742	765	789	813	838	863	890	917	945	974
7.3	718	740	763	786	810	835	860	886	913	941	970	999
7.4	738	760	783	807	832	857	883	910	937	966	995	1,025
7.5	758	781	805	829	854	880	906	934	962	991	1,020	1,051
7.6	779	803	827	851	877	903	930	958	987	1,016	1,047	1,078
7.7	801	825	849	874	900	927	955	983	1,012	1,042	1,073	1,105
7.8	823	847	872	898	924	952	980	1,008	1,038	1,069	1,100	1,133
7.9	845	870	895	922	949	977	1,005	1,035	1,065	1,096	1,128	1,161
8.0	868	893	919	946	974	1,002	1,031	1,061	1,092	1,124	1,157	1,190
8.1	892	918	944	971	999	1,028	1,058	1,088	1,120	1,152	1,186	1,220
8.2	916	942	969	997	1,026	1,055	1,085	1,116	1,148	1,181	1,215	1,250
8.3	941	967	995	1,023	1,052	1,082	1,113	1,145	1,177	1,211	1,245	1,281
8.4	966	993	1,021	1,050	1,080	1,110	1,142	1,174	1,207	1,241	1,276	1,312
8.5	992	1,020	1,048	1,078	1,108	1,139	1,171	1,203	1,237	1,272	1,307	1,344
8.6	1,018	1,047	1,076	1,106	1,136	1,168	1,200	1,234	1,268	1,303	1,339	1,377
8.7	1,046	1,074	1,104	1,134	1,166	1,198	1,231	1,265	1,300	1,335	1,372	1,410
8.8	1,073	1,103	1,133	1,164	1,196	1,228	1,262	1,296	1,332	1,368	1,405	1,444
8.9	1,102	1,132	1,162	1,194	1,226	1,259	1,294	1,329	1,365	1,402	1,439	1,478
9.0	1,131	1,161	1,193	1,225	1,257	1,291	1,326	1,361	1,398	1,436	1,474	1,514
9.1	1,161	1,192	1,223	1,256	1,289	1,324	1,359	1,395	1,432	1,470	1,509	1,550
9.2	1,191	1,223	1,255	1,288	1,322	1,357	1,393	1,429	1,467	1,506	1,545	1,586
9.3	1,222	1,254	1,287	1,321	1,355	1,391	1,427	1,464	1,503	1,542	1,582	1,624

*Log(BW) = −1.599 + 0.144(BPD) + 0.032(AC) − 0.111(BPD$_2$ × AC)/1,000. S. D. = + OR − 106.0 Gm. per kilogram of body weight.
From Warsof, S. T., Gohari, P., Berkowitz, R. L., et al.: The estimation of fetal weight by computer assisted analysis. Am. J. Obstet. Gynecol., *128*:881, 1977.

Table 10. *Estimated Fetal Weights* (Continued)

\multicolumn{13}{c	}{Abdominal circumference}
21.5	*22.0*	*22.5*	*23.0*	*23.5*	*24.0*	*24.5*	*25.0*	*25.5*	*26.0*	*26.5*	*27.0*	*27.5*
325	337	349	362	375	388	402	417	432	448	464	481	498
335	347	359	372	386	400	414	429	445	461	478	495	513
345	357	370	384	397	412	427	442	458	475	492	509	528
355	368	381	395	409	424	439	455	471	488	506	524	543
366	379	393	407	421	436	452	468	485	503	521	539	559
377	390	404	419	434	449	465	482	499	517	536	555	575
388	402	416	431	446	462	479	496	514	532	551	571	591
399	413	428	443	459	476	493	510	528	547	567	587	608
411	426	441	456	473	489	507	525	543	563	583	603	625
423	438	453	470	486	503	521	540	559	579	599	620	642
435	451	467	483	500	518	536	555	575	595	616	638	660
448	464	480	497	514	533	551	571	591	612	633	656	679
461	477	494	511	529	548	567	587	607	629	651	674	697
474	491	508	526	544	563	583	603	624	646	669	692	716
488	505	522	541	559	579	599	620	642	664	687	711	736
502	519	537	556	575	595	616	637	659	682	706	731	756
516	534	552	572	591	612	633	655	678	701	725	750	776
531	549	568	588	608	629	650	673	696	720	745	771	797
546	564	584	604	625	646	668	691	715	740	765	791	819
561	580	600	621	642	664	687	710	734	760	786	812	840
577	596	617	638	660	682	705	729	754	780	807	834	862
593	613	634	655	678	701	724	749	774	801	828	856	885
609	630	651	673	696	720	744	769	795	822	850	879	908
626	647	669	692	715	739	764	790	816	844	872	901	932
643	665	687	710	734	759	784	811	838	866	895	925	956
661	683	706	730	754	779	805	832	860	888	918	949	981
679	702	725	749	774	800	826	854	882	912	942	973	1,006
698	721	745	769	795	821	848	876	905	935	966	998	1,031
717	740	764	790	816	843	870	899	929	959	991	1,023	1,057
736	760	785	811	837	865	893	922	953	984	1,016	1,049	1,084
756	780	806	832	859	887	916	946	977	1,009	1,042	1,076	1,111
776	801	827	854	882	910	940	970	1,002	1,034	1,068	1,103	1,138
797	822	849	876	905	934	964	995	1,027	1,060	1,095	1,130	1,166
818	844	871	899	928	958	989	1,020	1,053	1,087	1,122	1,158	1,195
839	866	894	922	952	982	1,014	1,046	1,079	1,114	1,150	1,186	1,224
861	889	917	946	976	1,007	1,039	1,072	1,106	1,142	1,178	1,215	1,254
884	912	941	970	1,001	1,033	1,065	1,099	1,134	1,170	1,207	1,245	1,284
907	936	965	995	1,027	1,059	1,092	1,126	1,162	1,198	1,236	1,275	1,315
931	960	990	1,021	1,052	1,085	1,119	1,154	1,190	1,227	1,266	1,305	1,346
955	984	1,015	1,046	1,079	1,112	1,147	1,183	1,219	1,257	1,296	1,337	1,378
979	1,009	1,041	1,073	1,106	1,140	1,175	1,212	1,249	1,287	1,327	1,368	1,410
1,004	1,035	1,067	1,100	1,133	1,168	1,204	1,241	1,279	1,318	1,359	1,400	1,443
1,030	1,061	1,094	1,127	1,161	1,197	1,233	1,271	1,310	1,350	1,391	1,433	1,477
1,056	1,088	1,121	1,155	1,190	1,226	1,263	1,302	1,341	1,382	1,424	1,467	1,511
1,083	1,115	1,149	1,184	1,219	1,256	1,294	1,333	1,373	1,414	1,457	1,501	1,546
1,110	1,143	1,177	1,213	1,249	1,286	1,325	1,364	1,405	1,447	1,491	1,535	1,581
1,138	1,172	1,207	1,242	1,279	1,317	1,356	1,397	1,438	1,481	1,525	1,570	1,617
1,166	1,201	1,236	1,273	1,310	1,349	1,389	1,430	1,472	1,515	1,560	1,606	1,653
1,195	1,230	1,266	1,303	1,342	1,381	1,421	1,463	1,506	1,550	1,595	1,642	1,690
1,225	1,260	1,297	1,335	1,374	1,414	1,455	1,497	1,541	1,585	1,632	1,679	1,728
1,255	1,291	1,329	1,367	1,406	1,447	1,489	1,532	1,576	1,621	1,668	1,716	1,766
1,286	1,323	1,361	1,400	1,440	1,481	1,523	1,567	1,612	1,658	1,706	1,755	1,805
1,317	1,355	1,393	1,433	1,473	1,515	1,559	1,603	1,648	1,695	1,744	1,793	1,844
1,349	1,387	1,426	1,467	1,508	1,551	1,594	1,639	1,686	1,733	1,782	1,832	1,884
1,382	1,420	1,460	1,501	1,543	1,586	1,631	1,676	1,723	1,772	1,821	1,872	1,925
1,415	1,454	1,495	1,536	1,579	1,623	1,668	1,714	1,762	1,811	1,861	1,913	1,966
1,449	1,489	1,530	1,572	1,615	1,660	1,705	1,752	1,801	1,850	1,901	1,954	2,007
1,483	1,524	1,565	1,608	1,652	1,697	1,744	1,791	1,840	1,891	1,942	1,995	2,050
1,519	1,560	1,602	1,645	1,690	1,736	1,783	1,831	1,881	1,931	1,984	2,037	2,093
1,554	1,596	1,639	1,683	1,728	1,775	1,822	1,871	1,921	1,973	2,026	2,080	2,136
1,591	1,633	1,677	1,721	1,767	1,814	1,862	1,912	1,963	2,015	2,069	2,124	2,180
1,628	1,671	1,715	1,760	1,807	1,854	1,903	1,953	2,005	2,058	2,112	2,168	2,225
1,666	1,709	1,754	1,800	1,847	1,895	1,945	1,996	2,048	2,101	2,156	2,213	2,270

Table 10. *Estimated Fetal Weights* (Continued)

Biparietal diameter	\multicolumn{12}{c}{Abdominal circumference}
	15.5	16.0	16.5	17.0	17.5	18.0	18.5	19.0	19.5	20.0	20.5	21.0
9.4	1,254	1,287	1,320	1,354	1,389	1,425	1,462	1,500	1,539	1,579	1,620	1,661
9.5	1,287	1,320	1,354	1,388	1,424	1,461	1,498	1,536	1,576	1,616	1,658	1,700
9.6	1,320	1,354	1,388	1,423	1,460	1,497	1,535	1,574	1,614	1,655	1,697	1,740
9.7	1,354	1,388	1,423	1,459	1,496	1,533	1,572	1,611	1,652	1,694	1,736	1,780
9.8	1,389	1,424	1,459	1,496	1,533	1,571	1,610	1,650	1,691	1,733	1,776	1,821
9.9	1,425	1,460	1,496	1,533	1,571	1,609	1,649	1,690	1,731	1,774	1,817	1,862
10.0	1,461	1,497	1,534	1,571	1,609	1,648	1,689	1,730	1,772	1,815	1,859	1,905

Biparietal diameter	\multicolumn{12}{c}{Abdominal circumference}
	28.0	28.5	29.0	29.5	30.0	30.5	31.0	31.5	32.0	32.5	33.0	33.5
3.1	517	535	555	575	596	617	640	663	687	712	738	765
3.2	532	551	571	591	613	635	658	682	707	732	759	786
3.3	547	567	587	608	630	653	677	701	726	753	780	808
3.4	563	583	604	626	648	672	696	721	747	774	802	831
3.5	579	600	621	644	667	691	715	741	768	795	824	853
3.6	595	617	639	662	685	710	735	762	789	817	847	877
3.7	612	634	657	680	705	730	756	783	811	840	870	901
3.8	629	652	675	699	724	750	777	804	833	863	893	925
3.9	647	670	694	719	744	771	798	826	856	886	918	950
4.0	665	689	713	738	765	792	820	849	879	910	942	976
4.1	684	708	733	759	786	813	842	872	903	934	967	1,002
4.2	703	727	753	779	807	835	865	895	927	959	993	1,028
4.3	722	747	773	801	829	858	888	919	951	985	1,019	1,055
4.4	742	767	794	822	851	881	911	943	976	1,011	1,046	1,082
4.5	762	788	816	844	874	904	936	968	1,002	1,037	1,073	1,110
4.6	782	809	838	867	897	928	960	994	1,028	1,064	1,101	1,139
4.7	803	831	860	890	920	952	985	1,019	1,055	1,091	1,129	1,168
4.8	825	853	883	913	945	977	1,011	1,046	1,082	1,119	1,158	1,198
4.9	847	876	906	937	969	1,003	1,037	1,073	1,109	1,148	1,187	1,228
5.0	869	899	930	961	994	1,028	1,064	1,100	1,138	1,177	1,217	1,259
5.1	892	922	954	986	1,020	1,055	1,091	1,128	1,166	1,206	1,247	1,290
5.2	915	946	978	1,012	1,046	1,082	1,118	1,156	1,196	1,236	1,278	1,322
5.3	939	971	1,004	1,038	1,073	1,109	1,146	1,185	1,225	1,267	1,310	1,354
5.4	963	996	1,029	1,064	1,100	1,137	1,175	1,215	1,256	1,298	1,342	1,387
5.5	988	1,021	1,055	1,091	1,127	1,165	1,204	1,245	1,286	1,330	1,374	1,420
5.6	1,013	1,047	1,082	1,118	1,156	1,194	1,234	1,275	1,318	1,362	1,407	1,454
5.7	1,039	1,074	1,109	1,146	1,184	1,224	1,264	1,306	1,350	1,395	1,441	1,489
5.8	1,065	1,100	1,137	1,175	1,213	1,254	1,295	1,338	1,382	1,428	1,475	1,524
5.9	1,092	1,128	1,165	1,203	1,243	1,284	1,326	1,370	1,415	1,462	1,510	1,560
6.0	1,119	1,156	1,194	1,233	1,273	1,315	1,358	1,403	1,449	1,496	1,545	1,596
6.1	1,147	1,184	1,223	1,263	1,304	1,347	1,391	1,436	1,483	1,531	1,581	1,633
6.2	1,175	1,213	1,253	1,293	1,335	1,379	1,424	1,470	1,517	1,567	1,618	1,670
6.3	1,204	1,243	1,283	1,325	1,367	1,411	1,457	1,504	1,553	1,603	1,655	1,708
6.4	1,233	1,273	1,314	1,356	1,400	1,445	1,491	1,539	1,588	1,639	1,692	1,746
6.5	1,263	1,304	1,345	1,388	1,433	1,478	1,526	1,574	1,625	1,677	1,730	1,786
6.6	1,294	1,335	1,377	1,421	1,466	1,513	1,561	1,610	1,662	1,714	1,769	1,825
6.7	1,325	1,367	1,410	1,454	1,500	1,548	1,597	1,647	1,699	1,753	1,808	1,865
6.8	1,356	1,399	1,443	1,488	1,535	1,583	1,633	1,684	1,737	1,792	1,848	1,906
6.9	1,388	1,432	1,476	1,522	1,570	1,619	1,670	1,722	1,776	1,831	1,888	1,947
7.0	1,421	1,465	1,511	1,557	1,606	1,656	1,707	1,760	1,815	1,871	1,929	1,989
7.1	1,454	1,499	1,545	1,593	1,642	1,693	1,745	1,799	1,854	1,912	1,971	2,032
7.2	1,488	1,533	1,580	1,629	1,679	1,730	1,784	1,838	1,895	1,953	2,013	2,075
7.3	1,522	1,568	1,616	1,666	1,716	1,769	1,823	1,878	1,936	1,995	2,055	2,118
7.4	1,557	1,604	1,653	1,703	1,754	1,808	1,862	1,919	1,977	2,037	2,098	2,162
7.5	1,592	1,640	1,690	1,741	1,793	1,847	1,903	1,960	2,019	2,080	2,142	2,207
7.6	1,628	1,677	1,727	1,779	1,832	1,887	1,943	2,001	2,061	2,123	2,186	2,252
7.7	1,665	1,714	1,765	1,818	1,872	1,927	1,985	2,044	2,104	2,167	2,231	2,297
7.8	1,702	1,752	1,804	1,857	1,912	1,968	2,026	2,086	2,148	2,211	2,276	2,344
7.9	1,740	1,791	1,843	1,897	1,953	2,010	2,069	2,130	2,192	2,256	2,322	2,390
8.0	1,778	1,830	1,883	1,938	1,994	2,052	2,112	2,173	2,237	2,302	2,368	2,437
8.1	1,817	1,869	1,923	1,979	2,036	2,095	2,155	2,218	2,282	2,348	2,415	2,485
8.2	1,857	1,910	1,964	2,021	2,079	2,138	2,200	2,263	2,327	2,394	2,463	2,533

Appendix

Table 10. *Estimated Fetal Weights* (Continued)

					Abdominal circumference							
21.5	22.0	22.5	23.0	23.5	24.0	24.5	25.0	25.5	26.0	26.5	27.0	27.5
1,705	1,749	1,794	1,840	1,888	1,937	1,987	2,038	2,091	2,145	2,201	2,258	2,316
1,744	1,788	1,834	1,881	1,930	1,979	2,030	2,082	2,135	2,190	2,246	2,304	2,363
1,784	1,829	1,875	1,923	1,972	2,022	2,073	2,126	2,180	2,235	2,292	2,350	2,410
1,824	1,870	1,917	1,966	2,015	2,066	2,117	2,171	2,225	2,281	2,339	2,397	2,458
1,866	1,912	1,960	2,009	2,059	2,110	2,162	2,216	2,271	2,328	2,386	2,445	2,506
1,908	1,955	2,003	2,052	2,103	2,155	2,208	2,262	2,318	2,375	2,433	2,493	2,555
1,951	1,998	2,047	2,097	2,148	2,200	2,254	2,309	2,365	2,423	2,482	2,542	2,604

					Abdominal circumference							
34.0	34.5	35.0	35.5	36.0	36.5	37.0	37.5	38.0	38.5	39.0	39.5	40.0
792	821	851	882	914	947	981	1,017	1,054	1,092	1,131	1,172	1,215
814	844	875	906	939	973	1,008	1,045	1,082	1,122	1,162	1,204	1,248
837	867	899	931	965	1,000	1,036	1,073	1,112	1,152	1,194	1,237	1,281
860	891	924	957	991	1,027	1,064	1,102	1,142	1,183	1,226	1,270	1,316
884	916	949	983	1,018	1,055	1,093	1,132	1,173	1,215	1,258	1,304	1,350
908	941	975	1,010	1,046	1,083	1,122	1,162	1,204	1,247	1,292	1,338	1,386
933	966	1,001	1,037	1,074	1,112	1,152	1,193	1,236	1,280	1,325	1,373	1,422
958	992	1,028	1,064	1,102	1,142	1,182	1,224	1,268	1,313	1,360	1,408	1,459
984	1,019	1,055	1,093	1,131	1,172	1,213	1,256	1,301	1,347	1,395	1,445	1,496
1,010	1,046	1,083	1,121	1,161	1,202	1,245	1,289	1,335	1,382	1,431	1,481	1,534
1,037	1,074	1,111	1,151	1,191	1,233	1,277	1,322	1,369	1,417	1,467	1,519	1,573
1,064	1,102	1,140	1,181	1,222	1,265	1,310	1,356	1,404	1,453	1,504	1,557	1,612
1,092	1,130	1,170	1,211	1,254	1,298	1,343	1,390	1,439	1,489	1,542	1,596	1,652
1,120	1,160	1,200	1,242	1,285	1,330	1,377	1,425	1,475	1,527	1,580	1,635	1,692
1,149	1,189	1,231	1,274	1,318	1,364	1,411	1,461	1,512	1,564	1,619	1,675	1,734
1,179	1,220	1,262	1,306	1,351	1,398	1,447	1,497	1,549	1,603	1,658	1,716	1,776
1,209	1,250	1,294	1,338	1,385	1,433	1,482	1,534	1,587	1,642	1,698	1,757	1,818
1,239	1,282	1,326	1,372	1,419	1,468	1,519	1,571	1,625	1,681	1,739	1,799	1,861
1,270	1,314	1,359	1,406	1,454	1,504	1,555	1,609	1,664	1,721	1,780	1,842	1,905
1,302	1,346	1,392	1,440	1,489	1,540	1,593	1,647	1,704	1,762	1,822	1,885	1,949
1,334	1,379	1,426	1,475	1,525	1,577	1,631	1,687	1,744	1,804	1,865	1,929	1,994
1,366	1,413	1,461	1,510	1,562	1,615	1,670	1,726	1,785	1,846	1,908	1,973	2,040
1,400	1,447	1,496	1,547	1,599	1,653	1,709	1,767	1,826	1,888	1,952	2,018	2,086
1,433	1,482	1,532	1,583	1,637	1,692	1,749	1,808	1,868	1,931	1,996	2,064	2,133
1,468	1,517	1,568	1,621	1,675	1,731	1,789	1,849	1,911	1,975	2,041	2,110	2,181
1,503	1,553	1,605	1,658	1,714	1,771	1,830	1,891	1,954	2,020	2,087	2,157	2,229
1,538	1,589	1,642	1,697	1,753	1,812	1,872	1,934	1,998	2,065	2,133	2,204	2,277
1,574	1,626	1,680	1,736	1,793	1,853	1,914	1,977	2,043	2,110	2,180	2,252	2,327
1,611	1,664	1,719	1,775	1,834	1,894	1,957	2,021	2,088	2,156	2,227	2,301	2,377
1,648	1,702	1,758	1,816	1,875	1,937	2,000	2,066	2,133	2,203	2,275	2,350	2,427
1,686	1,741	1,798	1,856	1,917	1,979	2,044	2,111	2,179	2,251	2,324	2,400	2,478
1,724	1,780	1,838	1,898	1,959	2,023	2,088	2,156	2,226	2,298	2,373	2,450	2,530
1,763	1,820	1,879	1,939	2,002	2,067	2,133	2,202	2,273	2,347	2,423	2,501	2,582
1,803	1,860	1,920	1,982	2,046	2,111	2,179	2,249	2,321	2,396	2,473	2,552	2,634
1,843	1,901	1,962	2,025	2,090	2,156	2,225	2,296	2,370	2,445	2,524	2,604	2,687
1,883	1,943	2,005	2,068	2,134	2,202	2,272	2,344	2,419	2,495	2,575	2,657	2,741
1,924	1,985	2,048	2,113	2,179	2,248	2,319	2,393	2,468	2,546	2,627	2,710	2,795
1,966	2,028	2,091	2,157	2,225	2,295	2,367	2,441	2,518	2,597	2,679	2,763	2,850
2,008	2,071	2,136	2,202	2,271	2,342	2,415	2,491	2,569	2,649	2,732	2,817	2,905
2,051	2,115	2,180	2,248	2,318	2,390	2,464	2,541	2,620	2,701	2,785	2,871	2,960
2,094	2,159	2,226	2,294	2,365	2,438	2,513	2,591	2,671	2,754	2,839	2,926	3,017
2,138	2,204	2,271	2,341	2,413	2,487	2,563	2,642	2,723	2,807	2,893	2,981	3,073
2,183	2,249	2,318	2,388	2,461	2,536	2,614	2,693	2,776	2,860	2,947	3,037	3,130
2,228	2,295	2,365	2,436	2,510	2,586	2,665	2,745	2,828	2,914	3,002	3,093	3,187
2,273	2,342	2,412	2,485	2,559	2,636	2,716	2,798	2,882	2,969	3,058	3,150	3,245
2,319	2,388	2,460	2,533	2,609	2,687	2,768	2,850	2,936	3,023	3,114	3,207	3,303
2,366	2,436	2,508	2,583	2,659	2,738	2,820	2,904	2,990	3,079	3,170	3,264	3,361
2,413	2,484	2,557	2,633	2,710	2,790	2,872	2,957	3,044	3,134	3,227	3,322	3,420
2,460	2,532	2,606	2,683	2,761	2,842	2,926	3,011	3,099	3,190	3,284	3,380	3,479
2,508	2,581	2,656	2,734	2,813	2,895	2,979	3,066	3,155	3,247	3,341	3,438	3,538
2,557	2,631	2,707	2,785	2,865	2,948	3,033	3,121	3,211	3,303	3,399	3,497	3,598
2,606	2,681	2,757	2,836	2,918	3,001	3,087	3,176	3,267	3,360	3,457	3,556	3,658

Table 10. *Estimated Fetal Weights* (Continued)

Biparietal diameter	\multicolumn{12}{c}{Abdominal circumference}
	28.0	28.5	29.0	29.5	30.0	30.5	31.0	31.5	32.0	32.5	33.0	33.5
8.3	1,897	1,951	2,006	2,063	2,122	2,182	2,244	2,308	2,374	2,441	2,511	2,582
8.4	1,937	1,992	2,048	2,106	2,165	2,226	2,289	2,354	2,420	2,489	2,559	2,631
8.5	1,978	2,034	2,091	2,149	2,210	2,271	2,335	2,400	2,468	2,537	2,608	2,681
8.6	2,020	2,076	2,134	2,193	2,254	2,317	2,381	2,447	2,515	2,585	2,657	2,731
8.7	2,063	2,120	2,178	2,238	2,300	2,363	2,428	2,495	2,564	2,634	2,707	2,781
8.8	2,106	2,163	2,222	2,283	2,345	2,410	2,475	2,543	2,612	2,684	2,757	2,832
8.9	2,149	2,208	2,267	2,329	2,392	2,457	2,523	2,592	2,662	2,734	2,808	2,884
9.0	2,194	2,252	2,313	2,375	2,439	2,504	2,572	2,641	2,711	2,784	2,859	2,936
9.1	2,238	2,298	2,359	2,422	2,486	2,552	2,620	2,690	2,762	2,835	2,911	2,988
9.2	2,284	2,344	2,406	2,469	2,534	2,601	2,670	2,740	2,812	2,887	2,963	3,041
9.3	2,330	2,391	2,453	2,517	2,583	2,650	2,720	2,791	2,864	2,938	3,015	3,094
9.4	2,376	2,438	2,501	2,566	2,632	2,700	2,770	2,842	2,915	2,991	3,068	3,147
9.5	2,423	2,485	2,549	2,615	2,682	2,750	2,821	2,893	2,967	3,043	3,121	3,201
9.6	2,471	2,534	2,598	2,664	2,732	2,801	2,872	2,945	3,020	3,096	3,175	3,256
9.7	2,519	2,583	2,648	2,714	2,782	2,852	2,924	2,997	3,073	3,150	3,229	3,310
9.8	2,568	2,632	2,698	2,765	2,833	2,904	2,976	3,050	3,126	3,204	3,283	3,365
9.9	2,618	2,682	2,748	2,816	2,885	2,956	3,029	3,103	3,180	3,258	3,338	3,420
10.0	2,668	2,733	2,799	2,867	2,937	3,009	3,082	3,157	3,234	3,313	3,393	3,476

\multicolumn{13}{c}{Abdominal circumference}
34.0	34.5	35.0	35.5	36.0	36.5	37.0	37.5	38.0	38.5	39.0	39.5	40.0
2,655	2,731	2,809	2,888	2,971	3,055	3,142	3,231	3,323	3,418	3,515	3,615	3,718
2,705	2,782	2,860	2,941	3,024	3,109	3,197	3,287	3,380	3,475	3,573	3,674	3,778
2,756	2,833	2,912	2,994	3,078	3,164	3,252	3,343	3,437	3,533	3,632	3,734	3,838
2,807	2,885	2,965	3,047	3,132	3,219	3,308	3,400	3,494	3,591	3,691	3,794	3,899
2,858	2,937	3,018	3,101	3,186	3,274	3,364	3,457	3,552	3,650	3,750	3,854	3,960
2,910	2,989	3,071	3,155	3,241	3,330	3,420	3,514	3,610	3,708	3,810	3,914	4,021
2,962	3,042	3,125	3,209	3,296	3,385	3,477	3,571	3,668	3,767	3,869	3,974	4,082
3,015	3,096	3,179	3,264	3,352	3,442	3,534	3,629	3,726	3,826	3,929	4,035	4,143
3,068	3,149	3,233	3,319	3,407	3,498	3,591	3,687	3,785	3,886	3,989	4,095	4,204
3,121	3,203	3,288	3,374	3,463	3,555	3,649	3,745	3,844	3,945	4,049	4,156	4,265
3,175	3,258	3,343	3,430	3,520	3,612	3,706	3,803	3,902	4,004	4,109	4,216	4,326
3,229	3,313	3,398	3,486	3,576	3,669	3,764	3,861	3,961	4,064	4,169	4,277	4,388
3,283	3,368	3,454	3,542	3,633	3,726	3,822	3,920	4,020	4,123	4,229	4,338	4,449
3,338	3,423	3,510	3,599	3,690	3,784	3,880	3,979	4,080	4,183	4,289	4,398	4,510
3,393	3,479	3,566	3,656	3,748	3,842	3,938	4,037	4,139	4,243	4,349	4,459	4,571
3,449	3,535	3,623	3,713	3,805	3,900	3,997	4,096	4,198	4,302	4,410	4,519	4,632
3,505	3,591	3,679	3,770	3,863	3,958	4,055	4,155	4,257	4,362	4,470	4,580	4,692
3,561	3,647	3,736	3,827	3,920	4,016	4,114	4,214	4,317	4,422	4,529	4,640	4,753

Index

Page numbers in italics refer to illustrations; (t) indicates tables.

Abdomen, anterior wall defects of, 71–72, *71–72*
  circumference of, as index of fetal growth, 124–128, *125, 126,* 127(t), *128,* 331(t). See also *Circumference, abdominal.*
  fetal, 46–54, *48–57*
    normal values, 127(t), 330(t)
    abnormalities of, 67–78
Abnormalities. See also *Malformations.*
  fetal, anterior wall, 71–72, *71–72*
    cervical region, 61–64, *62–64, 111*
    gastrointestinal tract, 67–72
    genitourinary tract, 72–77, *180*
    heart, 65, *65–69*
    limb reduction, 92–94, 93(t)
    multiple congenital, 77, *78*
    of meninges, 108–112
    of thorax and abdomen, 61–78
  ovarian, 211, *212*
Abortion, selective, malformations best treated by, 177, 178(t)
Abruptio placentae, 152–153, *153*
Abscess, pelvic. See also *Infections, pelvic; Pelvic inflammatory disease.*
  periappendiceal, *280,* 281
  tubo-ovarian, *218,* 272, *272, 273, 277*
Acheiria, 93(t)
Achondroplasia, dwarfism and, 88, *89*
Acoustic shadowing, in identifying intrauterine contraceptive device, 250–251, *252–253*
Acrania, *102*
Adactyly, 93(t)
Adenocarcinoma, of ovary, *221*
Adenomatoid malformation, cystic, 65, *65*
Adenomyosis, of uterus, 242–243, *243*
Adnexa, uterine, *205,* 206
  changes in ectopic pregnancy, 299–300, *299, 300*
  cystic masses of, 216–217, 216(t), *217*
Adrenal gland, fetal, *49, 51–54, 56, 57*
Age, gestational, assigning of in utero, 34, 34(t)
  biochemical estimation of, 22–24
  biparietal diameter and, 24, 25–33. See also *Biparietal diameter.*
  clinical estimation of, 22
  clinical parameters for, 34, 34(t), 325(t)
  crown-rump length and, 24–25, *25, 26,* 26(t), 325(t)
  estimation of in newborn infant, 37
  estimation of in utero, 21–37
  femur length and, 24, 34, *35,* 36(t), 327(t)
  gestational sac measurements and, 24–26, *25*
  placental grading and, 147
  radiologic and ultrasonic estimation of, 24–37
  menstrual, correlation of biparietal diameter with, 33(t)
  in assessing fetal growth, 120
Agenesis, renal, 72–73, *73*
Alpha-fetoprotein, 108–109
Amelia, in amniotic band syndrome, 92, *92*

Amniocentesis, 169–173
  in twin pregnancies, 171–172, 172(t)
  technique of, 169, *171*
  ultrasound guidance of, 171, 172(t)
Amnion. See *Chorioamniotic elevation; Chorioamniotic separation; Membranes, fetal.*
Amniotic band syndrome, amelia in, 92, *92*
Amniotic sac, prolapse of, 245, *245*
Anembryonic gestation, of blighted ovum, 15–16, *16*
Anencephaly, 101–102, *102, 103*
Anomalies, See also *Abnormalities; Malformation.*
  congenital, of uterus, 17, *17*
Aorta, fetal *47*
Area, surface, of placenta, 148–149
Artery, umbilical, 57, *58*
Ascites, fetal, 77–78
  urinary, 74–75, *75*
Atresia, esophageal, 67
  intestinal, 67–71, *69, 70,* 77
Axis, neural, of fetus, normal and abnormal, 97–112

Beam diameter, in ultrasound, 315, *318*
Biparietal diameter. See also *Circumference, fetal head.*
  and fetal weight versus abdominal circumference, 134(t)–135(t)
  and standard growth curves, 115–117, *116, 117*
  "coronal" views in, 27, *28*
  correlation of with predicted menstrual age, 33(t), 326(t)
  in estimating gestational age, 24, 25–33
  interpretation of, 29–32, 33(t)
  in twin pregnancies, 33
  points of measurement for, 27, *27*
  steps in obtaining, 29, *30–31*
  versus femoral length, 86, 87(t), *89*
Birth weight, in identifying intrauterine well nourished versus malnourished infants, *119*
Bladder, urinary, fetal, 50–51, *56*
  normal female, *194–196, 201–204, 203*
Blastocyst, development of, 1, *2*
  implanted, 1, *2*
Blighted ovum, anembryonic gestation and, sonogram of, 15–16, *16*
Bone(s), dysplasias of, short-limbed, 87–91
  fetal, fractures of, 94–96, *95*
  hypomineralization of, 94–96, *95*
Bowel, See also *Gastrointestinal tract.*
  obstruction of, 67–71, *69, 70,* 77
Brain, fetal, normal sonogram of, *99–101*
  normal development of, 97–101, *98–101*
  pathologic lesions of, 101–108
Breathing movements, by fetus, 162–163, *164*

337

Calvarium, fetal, pathologic lesions of, 108–112
Carcinoma, ovarian, *219*, *221*
  endometrial, 239–241, *240*
  of uterus, cervical, 241, *241*
Catheters, indwelling, fetal, *182*, 183, *183*, *184*
Cerclage suture, in incompetent cervix, *243*, 245
Cervix, uterine, incompetent, 243, *244*, 245
  normal length of, *244*, 245
Cesarean section, malformations requiring, 178–179, 178(t)
  uterus following, 228, *231*, *232*
Chest, fetal, 44–46, *45–48*
Chondroectodermal dysplasia, 88
Chorioadenoma destruens, 259. See also *Gestational trophoblastic disease; Invasive mole.*
Chorioamniotic elevation, 10–13, *12–14*
Chorioamniotic separation, 10, *11*
Choriocarcinoma, 259, 266–269, *267*, *268*
  pathology of, 267–269, *267*
Chorion, in fetus of 10 weeks, *4*
Choroid plexus, *98*, 99–101, *99*, *100*
Circulatory system, fetal, 44–50, *48–54*
Circumference, abdominal, of fetus, and fetal weight versus biparietal diameter, 134(t)–135(t)
    as index of fetal growth, 124–128, *125*, *126*, 127(t), *128*
    data evaluation in, 126–128, 127(t)
    measurement procedure for, 125–126, *126*, *128*
    normal values of, 127(t), 330(t)
    ratio of to head circumference, 137(t), 331(t)
  fetal head, as index of fetal growth, 115, *116*, *117*, 120–124, *121*, *122*, 123(t), 124(t), 328(t), 329(t)
    data evaluation and, 122–124, 123(t), 124(t)
    measurement procedure for, 121–122, *121*, *122*
    normal growth rates of, 123(t)
    ratio of to abdominal circumference, 137(t)
  fetal thigh, as index of fetal growth, 128–131, *129*, *130*, 131(t)
    data evaluation in, 131, 131(t)
    measurement procedure for, 129, *129*, *130*
    normal values of, 131(t)
Clot, extramembranous, in abruptio placentae, 152, *153*
  retroplacental, in abruptio placentae, 152, *153*
Club hand deformity, 93, *94*
Colon, See also *Gastrointestinal tract.*
  rectosigmoid, 206–207, *207*
Computed tomography, digital radiographs and, in pelvimetry, 308–310, *308*, *309*
Congestive heart failure, 159–160, *160*
Conjugate, obstetric, 306, *306*
Contraception, failed, 13–15, 256–257, *257*
Contraceptive devices, intrauterine. See *Intrauterine contraceptive devices.*
Cord, umbilical, 54–57, *58*
  hernia of, 71
  insertion of into placenta, *148*, 149–150, *149*
Corpus luteum cyst, 13, *15*

Counseling, genetic, for prenatal diagnosis of genetic defects, 169, *170*
Crown-rump length, of fetus, 7, *8*, *44*
  for determining gestational age, 24–25, *25*, *26*, 26(t), 325(t)
CT-digital pelvimetry, 308–310, *308*, *309*
Cul-de-sac, changes in ectopic pregnancy, 300, *301*
Culdocentesis, in ectopic pregnancy, 302–303
Cyst(s), corpus luteum, 13, *15*
  dermoid, of ovary, 217, *219*, 220, *221*
  nabothian, 229, *233*
  ovarian, 216–223. See also *Ovary, masses in.*
  para-ovarian, *222*, 223
  theca lutein, in gestational trophoblastic disease, 262–263, *262*
Cystadenocarcinoma, mucinous, 219
Cystadenoma, mucinous, 217, *218*
  papillary serous, *219*
Cystic adenomatoid malformation, 65, *65*
Cystic hygroma, differentiation of from meningomyelocele, 64, *64*, 111
  fetal, 63–64, *63*, *64*, 111

Dandy-Walker syndrome, 107, *108*
Decibel, as description of intensity reduction, 314, 319(t)
  gain in, with increasing electric power, 319, 322(t)
Decidua, in fetus of 10 weeks, 3, *4*
Defects, developmental, See also *Abnormalities; Malformation.*
  of anterior wall of fetus, 71–72, *71–72*
  perinatal management of, 177–192
Deficiency states, fetal, requiring treatment in utero, 179, 179(t)
Deformity. See also *Abnormalities; Malformation.*
  club hand, 93, *94*
Delivery, cesarean, malformations requiring, 178–179, 178(t)
  preterm, malformations requiring, 177, 178(t)
Dermoid cyst, 217, *219*, 220, *221*
Diagnosis, prenatal, impact of fetal therapy on, 185–186
  of genetic defects, genetic counseling for, 169, *170*
  ultrasound in, 169–175
Diameter, biparietal. See *Biparietal diameter.*
Diaphragm, congenital hernia of, treatment of in utero, 183–184, *187*, *188*
  inversion of, 66, *68–69*
Double bubble sign, in intestinal atresia, 68, *69*, *77*
Duodenum, atresia of, 68, *69*, *77*
Ductus venosus, 47–50, *50*, *51*, *53*
Dwarfism, thanatophoric, 88, *90*, *91*
Dysplasia(s), bone, short-limbed, 87–91
  chondroectodermal, 88
  thanatophoric, 88, *90*, *91*

Echocardiography, 174–175, *174*, *175*
  M-mode, of fetal heart, 46, *46*
Ectopic pregnancy, See *Pregnancy, ectopic.*

Index

Edema, fetal, 63, *63*
Elevation, chorioamniotic, 10–13, *12–14*
Ellis-van Creveld syndrome, 88
Embryo, normal sonographic appearance of, 3–10, *4–7*
Encephalocele, mediastinal, 65, *65*
Encephalomeningocele, 109, *110–111*
Endometrial cavity, persistence of, *6*
Endometrial hyperplasia, 242
  adenomatous, 231, *235*
Endometriomas, multiple, 223, *223*
Endometritis, 231, *234*
  with pelvic inflammatory disease, 231, *234*, *235*
Endometrium, polyps of, 239
Entrance-exit reflections, of intrauterine contraceptive devices, 251, *254*
Epiphysis, distal femoral, fetal, 83, *85*
Erythroblastosis fetalis, 159–160, *160*
Esophagus, atresia of, 67
Expulsion, of intrauterine contraceptive device, 252–253, *255*
Extremities, fetal, measuring of, 85–87. See also *Femur*.
  limb reduction abnormalities of, 92–94, 93(t)
  short-limbed bone dysplasias of, 87–91
Eyes, movements of by fetus, 163–164, *164–166*

Failure, contraceptive, 13–15, 256–257, *257*
  heart, congestive, 159–160, *160*
Fallopian tube, abscess of. See *Tubo-ovarian abscess*.
  ectopic pregnancy in, 301, *302*
Femur, fetal, abnormalities of, 87
  bowing of in osteogenesis imperfecta, *95*
  distal epiphysis of, 83, *85*
  fracture of, *95*
  in thanatophoric dwarfism, *91*
  length of, as index of fetal growth, 131–132, *132*, 133(t)
    data evaluation of, 132, 133(t)
    in estimating gestational age, 24, 34, *35*, 36(t), 327(t)
    measurement of, *83*, 131–132, *132*
    versus biparietal diameter, 86, 87(t), *89*
  normal growth rates of, 133(t)
  normal length of, 133(t)
Fetal pole, on sonogram, 6–7
Fetoscopy, conditions diagnosed by, 173–174, 173(t)
  technique for blood drawing in, 149, *150*
Fetus, abdomen of, 46–54, *48–57*
  abnormalities of thorax and abdomen in, 61–78
  and fetal membranes, 2, *3*
  anterior wall defects of, 71–72, *71–72*
  ascites in, 77–78
    urinary, 74–75, *75*
  behavior and condition of, 159–175
  body proportionality of, as index of fetal growth, 136–137, 137(t)
  bone fractures of, 94–96, *95*
  bone hypomineralization in, 94–96, *95*
  breathing activity of, on sonogram, 36–37
  breathing movements by, 162–163, *164*
  chest of, 44–46, *45–48*

Fetus (*Continued*)
  circulatory system of, in abdomen, 47, *48–54*
  congestive heart failure in, 159–160, *160*
  crown-rump length of, 7, *8*
  cystic hygroma of, 63–64, *63*, *64*, *111*
  early development of, 44, *44*, *45*
  extremities of, measuring, 85–87
  eye movements of, 163–164, *164–166*
  femur of. See *Femur*.
  general body movements of, 161–162, *163*
  genitalia of, 54–56, *57*
  growth retardation of. See *Intrauterine growth retardation*.
  head size of, as index of growth, *115*, *116*, *117*, 120–124, *121*, *122*, 123(t), 124(t), 328(t), 329(t)
  hearing and habituation by, 165–166
  heart of, 45–46, *45–48*
    M-mode echocardiography of, 46, *46*
  heart rate of, 160–161
  hydropic, 63, *63*
  indwelling catheter for, *182*, 183, *183*, *184*
  length of, as index of fetal growth, 131–132, *132*, 133(t). See also *Femur, fetal, length of*.
  lie of, 41, *43*
  limb reduction abnormalities of, 92–94, 93(t)
  lung maturity of, lecithin/sphingomyelin ratio and, 23, 150
    placental grading and, 150, 150(t)
  multiple congenital abnormalities in, 77, *78*
  neck abnormalities of, 61–64, *62–64*, *111*
  neural axis of, normal and abnormal, 97–112
  normal anatomy of, 41–58
  normal growth of, 113–119
  osteogenesis imperfecta in, 94, *95*
  pathologic lesions of brain of, 101–108
  pathologic lesions of calvarium, spine, and meninges of, 108–112
  short-limbed bone dysplasias of, 87–91
  skeleton of, ultrasonography of, 81–96
  soft tissue mass of, as index of fetal growth, 128–131, *129*, *130*, 131(t)
  sonographic examination of, technique of, 41–44, *42*, *48*
  spine of, 84–85, *86*
  surgery on in utero, technique of, 179–183, *181*
  therapy of, in utero, 179–192
    assessing risk and benefit, 186–187
    future of, 187–192
  trunk size of, as index of fetal growth, 124–128, *125*, *126*, 127(t), *128*
  weight of, as index of fetal growth, 132–136, 134(t)–135(t)
    estimated, 332–336(t)
  with correctable defect, perinatal management of, 177–192
  yawning by, *162*
Fibroid, of uterine fundus, 18, *18*
Fibula, fetal, *82*, *84*
Fingers, fetal, *83*
Follicle, ovarian, normal dimensions of, 213, 213(t)
  sonographic monitoring of maturation of, 211–215, *214*
Foot, fetal, *82*
Foramen ovale, *45*
Fractures, of fetal bones, 94–96, *95*

Gallbladder, fetal, *49–51, 53, 54*
Gas, intrauterine, 231, *235*
Gastrointestinal tract, abnormalities of, 67–72
Gastroschisis, 71–72, *71–72*
Genetic counseling, for prenatal diagnosis of genetic defects, 169, *170*
Genitalia, fetal, 54–56, *57*
Genitourinary tract, abnormalities of, 72–77, *180*
Gestation, anembryonic, 15–16, *16*
   multiple, biparietal diameter in, 33
      genetic amniocentesis in, 171–172, 172(t)
      placenta in, 153–156, *155, 156*
      sonogram of, 8–10, *9, 10*
Gestational age. See *Age, gestational.*
Gestational sac, growth of, 4–6, *5–7*
   measurements of, in estimating gestational age, 24–25, *25*
   sonogram of, 10–13, *11–15*
Gestational trophoblastic disease, 259–270. See also *Choriocarcinoma; Hydatidiform mole; Invasive mole.*
   classification of, 259
   complications of, 261–263
   diagnosis of, 259
   hemorrhage in, 261, *262*
   progression of, *268*, 269. *269*
   sonogram in, 16, *17, 262, 268, 269*
   theca lutein cysts in, 262–263, *262*
   treatment of, 264
Grading, placental, 141–144, *142–146*, 143(t)
   and fetal lung maturity, 150, 150(t)
   and gestational age, 147
   and obstetric or medical complications, 150, 150(t)
Growth, fetal, 113–119. See also *Intrauterine growth retardation.*
   normal versus abnormal, boundary between, 117–119, *118*
   parameters for evaluating, 113–115
   retardation of, and fetal stress, 160
   standard growth curves and, 115–117, *116, 117*
Growth curves, standard, 115–117, *116, 117*
Growth profile, fetal, use of, 137–138
   for intrauterine growth retardation, 120–138

Hand, fetal, 82–83, *83*
   club hand deformity of, *93*, 94
Head, fetal, circumference of, as index of fetal growth, 115, *116, 117*, 120–124, *121, 122,* 123(t), 124(t), 328(t), 329(t). See also *Biparietal diameter.*
      normal growth rates of, 123(t), 328(t)
Hearing, by fetus, 165–166
Heart, fetal, 45–46, *45–48*
   abnormalities of, 65, *65–69*
   M-mode echocardiography of, 46, *46*
Heart failure, congestive, 159–160, *160*
Heart rate, fetal, 160–161
Hematoma, following cesarean section, 228, *232*
Hematometra, 243–245
Hemimelia, 93(t)
Hemorrhage, as complication of gestational trophoblastic disease, 261, *262*
Hepatic veins, fetal, *52*
Hepatobiliary system, fetal, 47–50, *48–54*

Hernia, diaphragmatic, congenital, treatment of in utero, 183–184, *187, 188*
   umbilical cord, 71
Holoprosencephaly, 107, *108*
Hourglass membranes, 245, *245*
Humerus, fetal, 82, *83*
Hydatidiform mole 259–264, *260–263*. See also *Choriocarcinoma; Invasive mole; Pregnancy, molar.*
   complications of, 261–263
   diseases simulating, 263, *263*
   sonogram of, 16, *17, 262, 268, 269*
   ultrasonographic appearance of, 260–261, *261*
   with coexistent normal fetus, 264, *264*
Hydranencephaly, 77, 107, *107*
Hydrocele, *76*, 77
Hydrocephalus, 103–106, *104–106*
   congenital obstructive, treatment of in utero, 184–185
Hydrometra, 243–245
Hydronephrosis, congenital, 73–75, *74–76*
   "expectant management" of, 188–192, *189–191*
      treatment of in utero, 179–183, *180, 183*
   ureterostomy in, *186*
Hydrops, fetal, 63, *63*
   and placental thickness, 148, *148*
Hydrosalpinx, in chronic pelvic inflammatory disease, 275–276, *276, 278*
Hygroma, cystic, fetal, 63–64, *63, 64, 111*
   differentiation of from meningomyelocele, 64, *64, 111*
Hyperplasia, endometrial, 242
   adenomatous, 231, *235*
Hyperstimulation syndrome, ovarian, 215, *215*
Hypomineralization, of fetal bones, 94–96, *95*

Implantation, cornual, 3, *5*
   sonographic appearance, 3, *4*
Infant(s), newborn, estimation of gestational age in, 37
   normal versus growth-retarded, *114*
   small-for-dates, 119. See also *Intrauterine growth retardation.*
Infantile polycystic kidney, 76–77
Infections, pelvic, 271–288. See also *Pelvic inflammatory disease.*
   and intrauterine contraceptive device, 277–280, *280*
   in renal transplant and immunosuppressed patients, 284–285, *285*
   nonvenereal, 280–284, *280–284*
   parasites and, 285–286
   related to pregnancy, 286
   technical considerations for sonography, 286–287
   tuberculosis and, 285–286
   venereal, 271–280
Instrumentation, for ultrasound, 319–324, *321–323*
   physical principles of, 313–324
Intensity reduction, decibel unit and, 314, 319(t)
Intestine, obstruction of, 67–71, *69, 70,* 77

Index

Intrauterine contraceptive devices, acoustic beam and, 250–251, *252–253*
 and pelvic infections, 277–280, *280*
 complications of use, 252–256
 contraceptive failure and, 13–15, 256–257, *257*
 detection of by ultrasound, 249–257
 entrance-exit reflections of, 251, *254*
 explusion of, 252–253, *255*
 identification of, 249–252, *251–254*
 localization of, 252, *255*
 pelvic inflammatory disease and, 254–255, *256*
 perforation by, 253–254, *256*
 pregnancy and, 13–15, 256–257, *257*
 type-specific morphology of, on sonography, 250, *251, 253*
 types of, 249, *250*
Intrauterine growth retardation, and fetal "stress," 160
 growth profile for, 120–138
 indices of, body proportionality and, 136–137, 137(t)
 fetal head size and, 120–124, *121, 122,* 123(t), 124(t)
 fetal length and, 131–132, *132,* 133(t)
 fetal weight and, 132–136, 134(t)–135(t)
 fetal thigh circumference and, 128–131, *129, 130,* 131(t)
 fetal trunk size and, 124–128, *125, 126,* 127(t), *128*
 types of, 119–120
 ultrasound assessment of, 120–137
Invasive mole, 259, 264–265, *265*

Jejunum. See also *Gastrointestinal tract.*
 atresia of, 69, *70*

Kidney, agenesis of, 72–73, *73*
 fetal, *49,* 50, *54, 55*
 hydronephrotic, 73–75, *74–76*
 multicystic, 75–76, *75, 76*
 polycystic, infantile, 76–77
 rupture of collecting system of, 74, *75*
 transplant of, pelvic infections and, 284–285, *285*

Laparoscopy, in ectopic pregnancy, 302–303
Last normal menstrual period (LNMP), for dating duration of pregnancy, 21–22
Lecithin/sphingomyelin ratio, for assessing fetal lung maturity, 23, 150
Leg, fetal, bones of, 81, *82, 84.* See also *Femur.*
Leiomyoma, in pregnancy, sonogram of, 17–19, *18*
 uterine, *231, 233,* 236–239, *238–240*
Leiomyosarcoma, uterine, 241
Length, femoral, as index of fetal growth, 131–132, *132,* 133(t)
Limb, reduction abnormalities of, 92–94, 93(t). See also *Extremities.*
Lippes Loop. See *Intrauterine contraceptive devices.*

Liver, fetal, *48, 49*
LNMP. See *Last normal menstrual period.*
L/S ratio, 83, 150, 150(t)
Lung, cystic adenomatoid malformation of, 65, *65*
 fetal, *48*
 maturity of, L/S ratio and, 23, 150
 placental grading and, 150, 150(t)
 sequestration of, 65, *66–67*
 underdevelopment of, 66, *68–69*
Lymphoma, ovarian, *221*

Malformation. See also *Abnormalities.*
 adenomatoid, cystic, 65, *65*
 fetal, best treated after term delivery, 177, 178(t)
 best treated by selective abortion, 177, 178(t)
 requiring early delivery, 177, 178(t)
 requiring treatment in utero, 179–185, 179(t)
 urinary tract, treatment plan, *180*
Masses, ovarian. See *Ovary, masses in; Tumors, ovarian.*
Mediastinal encephalocele, 65, *65*
Membranes, fetal, 2, *3*
 sonogram of, 10–13, *11, 14*
 hourglass, 245, *245*
Meninges, fetal, pathologic lesions of, 108–112
Meningomyelocele, differentiation of from cystic hygroma, 64, *64, 111*
Menstrual age, in assessing fetal growth, 120
Menstrual period, last normal, for dating duration of pregnancy, 21–22
Microcephaly, 106–107, *106*
Molar pregnancy. See *Pregnancy, molar.*
Mole, hydatidiform. See *Hydatidiform mole.*
 incomplete or partial, 264, *265*
 invasive. See *Invasive mole.*
Morula, *2*
Mucinous cystadenocarcinoma, *219*
Mucinous cystadenoma, 217, *218*
Multicystic kidneys, 75–76, *75, 76*
Multiple gestation, biparietal diameter in, 33
 genetic amniocentesis in, 171–172, 172(t)
 placenta in, 153–156, *155, 156*
 sonogram in, 8–10, *9, 10*
Musculature, pelvic, normal female, 193–196, *194–200*
Myelomeningocele, 109–112, *111*
Myoma, uterine, 236–239, *238–240*
 with pregnancy, *237*

Nabothian cyst, 229, *232*
Neck, fetal, abnormalities of, 61–64, *62–64, 111*
Neoplasm. See also *Carcinoma; Choriocarcinoma; Gestational trophoblastic disease; Tumor.*
 ovarian, 215–223
 uterine, 236–242
Neural axis, fetal, normal and abnormal, 97–112

Obstetric conjugate, 306, *306*
Obstruction, intestinal, 67–71, *69, 70,* 77
   urethral, 74, *75*
      in fetus, developmental consequences of, *180,* 182
Oligohydramnios, 72, *73,* 74, *75*
   in congenital hydronephrosis, *180,* 181
Omphalocele, 71, *71–72*
Osteogenesis imperfecta, in fetus, 94, *95*
Ovary, anatomic abnormalities of, 211, *212*
   carcinoma of, *219,* 221
   follicles of, normal dimensions of, 213, 213(t)
      sonographic monitoring of maturity of, 211–215, *214*
   hyperstimulation syndrome of, 215, *215*
   masses in, 215–223
      completely cystic, 216–217, 216(t), *217*
      complex, predominantly cystic, 216(t), 217–219, *218*
         predominantly solid, 216(t), 219–222, *219–220*
      sonographic appearance of, 216(t)
      sonographic mimics of, 222–223, *222–223*
      monitoring follicular maturation of, 211–215, *214*
   normal, *205, 206, 210*
   normal anatomy and scanning techniques, 209–211, *210*
   normal volume of, 209, 210(t), *211*
   polycystic, 211, *212*
   sonography of, 209–224
   tumors of, cystic, 215–222
      solid, 222, *222*
Ovum, blighted, sonogram of, 15–16, *16*

Pancreas, fetal, 50, *53, 54*
Papillary serous cystadenoma, *219*
Para-ovarian cyst, *222,* 223
Parasites, pelvic infections and, 285–286
Pelvic inflammatory disease, 228, *232, 234*
   acute, 271–275
      differential diagnosis of, 274–275, *274*
      sonographic appearance of, 272–274, *272, 273*
   chronic, 275–277
      sonographic appearance of, 275–277, *275–279*
   future of sonography in, 287
   in patients with intrauterine contraceptive devices, 254–255, *256*
   with endometritis, 231, *234, 235*
Pelvic inlet, 305, *306*
Pelvimetry, 305–310
Pelvic outlet, 306
   computed tomographic-digital, 308–310, *308, 309*
   x-ray, 306–308, *307*
      indications for, 307
      technique of, 308
Pelvis, female, infections of. See *Infections, pelvic; Pelvic inflammatory disease.*
   blood vessels of, 196–199, *194–202*
   inlet of, 305, *306*

Pelvis, female, infections of (*Continued*)
   midpelvis measurements, 305, *306*
   musculature of, 193–196, *194–200*
   normal anatomy of, 193–207, 305–306, *306*
   obstetric conjugate of, 306, *306*
   outlet of, 306
   pelvimetry of, 305–310
   planes and diameters of, 305–306, *306*
   size of, clinical estimation of, 306
   fetal, 85
Penis, fetal, *57*
Perforation, by intrauterine contraceptive device, 253–254, *256*
Periappendiceal abscess, *280,* 281
Peritoneum, reflections of, 207
Phalanges, of hand, fetal, 82, *83*
Phocomelia, 93(t)
PID. See *Pelvic inflammatory disease.*
Placenta, 10, 141–156
   grading system of, 141–144, *142–146,* 143(t)
   and fetal lung maturity, 150, 150(t)
   and gestational age, 147
   and obstetric or medical complications, 150, 150(t)
   in multiple gestation, 153–156, *155, 156*
   insertion of umbilical cord into, *148,* 149–150, *149*
   scanning techniques for, 144–147, *146, 147*
   surface area of, 148–149
   thickness of, 147–148, *148*
Pole, fetal, on sonogram, 6–7, *45*
Placenta previa, *13,* 151, *151, 152*
Polycystic kidney, infantile, 76–77
Polycystic ovaries, 211, *212*
Polydactyly, 94, *94*
Polyhydramnios, 67–71, *69,* 77
Polyps, endometrial, 239
Potter's syndrome, 72–73, *73*
Pregnancy, anembryonic, 15–16, *16*
   duration of, last normal menstrual period and, 21–22
   ectopic, adnexal changes in, 299–300, *299, 300*
      cul-de-sac changes in, 300, *301*
      culdocentesis in, 302–303
      diagnostic modalities for, 292
      evaluation of, 291–303
      history and predisposing factors of, 291
      laparoscopy in, 302–303
      signs and symptoms of, 292
      sonogram of, 16–17, *295, 296, 298–302*
      ultrasonography for, 294–302
      unusual types of, 300–302, *302*
      uterine changes in, 295–299, *295–299*
   first trimester of, normal sonographic appearance, 3–13
   ultrasound in, 1–19
   from failed contraception, 13–15, 256–257, *257*
   leiomyomata in, 17–19, *18*
   molar, variations of, 264, *264.* See also *Hydatidiform mole.*
   multiple, biparietal diameter in, 33
      genetic amniocentesis in, 171–172, 172(t)
      placenta in, 153–156, *155, 156*
      sonogram in, 8–10, *9, 10*
   normal uterine changes in, *297*
   pelvic infections and, 286

Pregnancy (*Continued*)
    tests for, 293–294, 293(t)
        causes of false-positive results in, 293(t)
    with coexistent mole and fetus, 264, *264*
    with intrauterine contraceptive device, 256–257, *257*
Profile, growth, for intrauterine growth retardation, 120–138
Proportionality, body, of fetus, as index of growth, 136–137, 137(t)
Pseudosac, on sonogram, *6*
Pulses, sonographic, 313–324, *314–318, 320, 322*
    physical principles of, 313–318
Pyometra, 243–245

Radiography, in estimation of gestational age, 24–37
Radius, fetal, 82, *83*
Rapid eye movements, by fetus, 164, 166
Real-time transducers, for ultrasound, 317–319, *319–321*
REM. See *Rapid eye movements.*
Renal agenesis, 72–73, *73*. See also *Kidney.*
Respiratory system, fetal, 64–67, *65–68*
Rh-sensitization, placental thickness in, 148, *148*
Ribs, fetal, 82

Sac, amniotic, prolapse of, 245, *245*
    gestational. See *Gestational sac.*
    yolk, *2, 3*
        sonogram of, 7–8, *9*
Sacrum, fetal, *85*
Scapula, fetal, 82, *82*
Scrotum, hydrocele of, 76, *77*
Separation, chorioamniotic, 10, *11*
Sequestration, pulmonary, 65, *66–67*
Short-limbed bone dysplasias, 87–91
Skeleton, fetal, and short-limbed bone dysplasias, 87–91
    normal, 81–85
    ultrasonography of, 81–96
Small-for-dates infants, 119. See also *Intrauterine growth retardation.*
Soft tissue, fetal, mass of as index of fetal growth, 128–131, *129, 130,* 131(t)
    thickening of, in thanatophoric dwarfism, 91
Sonogram. See also *Ultrasound.*
    crown-rump length measurements on, 7, *8*
    for measuring fetal femoral length, *83*
    in abruptio placentae, *153*
    in adenomyosis, 243
    in differentiating benign from malignant uterine masses, 242
    in erythroblastosis fetalis, 160
    in first trimester of pregnancy, abnormalities in, 13–19
        normal, 3–13
    in gestational trophoblastic disease, 16, 17, *262, 268, 269*
    in monitoring ovarian follicular maturation, *214*

Sonogram (*Continued*)
    in pelvic inflammatory disease, 232, 234
        acute, 272, *273*
        chronic 275–279
        in patient with IUD, *256*
    in Potter's syndrome, 72–73, *73*
    in renal agenesis, 73
    in severe Rh sensitization, 148
    in thanatophoric dysplasia, 90, *91*
    of abnormal femur in fetus with multiple anomalies, *87*
    of amelia in amniotic band syndrome, 92, *92*
    of anembryonic gestation with blighted ovum, 15–16, *16*
    of anencephaly, *102, 103*
    of bicornuate uterus with pregnancy, *237*
    of brain, normal developing, *99–101*
    of cerclage suture in incompetent cervix, 243
    of cervical teratoma, *62*
    of cervical uterine carcinoma, 241
    of choriocarcinoma, 268
    of club hand deformity, 93, *94*
    of coexistent hydatidiform mole and normal fetus, *264*
    of congenital uterine anomalies, 17, *17*
    of cornual implantation, 5
    of corpus luteum cyst, 13, *15*
    of cystic adenomatoid malformation of lung, *65*
    of cystic hygroma, *63, 64,* 111
    of dermoid cyst, *219, 221*
    of distal femoral epiphysis, *85*
    of distal fetal leg and foot, 82, *84*
    of duodenal atresia, 69, *77*
    of ectopic pregnancy, 16–17, 295, 296, 298–302
    of encephalomeningocele, 110, *111*
    of endometrial adenomatous hyperplasia, *235*
    of endometrial carcinoma, 240
    of extraembryonic structures, 10–13, *11–15*
    of fetal abdomen, 48–48
        circumference of, *125,* 128
    of fetal breathing movements, *164*
    of fetal eye movements, 163–164, *164–166*
    of fetal femur profile, *132*
    of fetal hand, *83*
    of fetal head circumference, *121, 122*
    of fetal heart, 45, *47*
    of fetal hepatobiliary system, 47–50, *48–54*
    of fetal humerus, *83*
    of fetal pole, 6–7, *45*
    of fetal spine, *86*
    of fetal thigh circumference, *129, 130*
    of fetal urinary ascites, *75*
    of fetus in early development, 44, *45*
    of gastroschisis, *71*
    of gestational sac growth, 4–6, *5–7*
    of hemorrhage in gestational trophoblastic disease, 261, *262*
    of holoprosencephaly, *108*
    of hydranencephaly, 77, 107, *107*
    of hydatidiform mole, 16, *17,* 261
    of hydrocele, 76, *77*
    of hydrocephalus, *104–106*
    of hydronephrotic kidney, 73–75, *74–76*
    of hydropic fetus, *63*
    of hydrosalpinx, *276, 278*
    of implantation site, 3, *4*

Sonogram (*Continued*)
 of intrauterine contraceptive device, *252–257*
  and infections from, 278–280, *280*
  and pregnancy, 13–15
 of intrauterine gas, 231, *235*
 of invasive mole, *265*
 of inverted diaphragm, 68–69
 of jejunal atresia, *70*
 of jet effect of urine entering bladder, *203*
 of leiomyomata in pregnancy, 17–19, *18*
 of malignant ovarian teratoma, *218*
 of mediastinal encephalocele, *65*
 of meningomyelocele, *64*, 77
 of microcephaly, *106*
 of mucinous cystadenocarcinoma, *219*
 of mucinous cystadenoma, *218*
 of multicystic kidneys, 75, *76*
 of multiple congenital abnormalities, 77
 of multiple endometriomas, 223, *223*
 of multiple gestation, 8–10, *9, 10, 155, 156*
 of nabothian cyst, *232*
 of omphalocele, *71–72*
 of osteogenesis imperfecta, *95*
 of ovarian adenocarcinoma, *221*
 of ovarian carcinoma, *219*
 of ovarian hyperstimulation syndrome, 215, *215*
 of ovarian lymphoma, *221*
 of ovarian masses, completely cystic, *217*
  complex, predominantly cystic, *218*
  complex, predominantly solid, *219–220*
  structures mimicking, 222–223
 of ovarian tumors, solid, *222*
 of ovaries, *205, 206, 210*
 of papillary serous cystadenoma, *219*
 of para-ovarian cyst, *222*
 of partial mole, *265*
 of pelvic blood vessels, *202*
 of pelvis, normal female, *197–200, 202*
 of periappendiceal abscess, 280, *281*
 of placenta and endocervical canal, normal, *142*
 of placenta previa, 151, *152*
 of polycystic ovaries, 211, *212*
 of polydactyly, *94*
 of postpartum involuting uterus, *286*
 of pregnancy in fallopian tube, *302*
 of pregnancy with intrauterine contraceptive device, *257*
 of prolapsed amniotic sac, *245*
 of pulmonary sequestration, *66–67*
 of renal transplant with pelvic infection, *285*
 of rectosigmoid colon, *207*
 of skeleton, normal fetal, *82–86*
 of soft tissue thickening thanatophoric dwarfism, *91*
 of spina bifida, *111*
 of structures mimicking ovarian masses, 222–223
 of tubo-ovarian abscess, *218, 272, 273, 277*
 of ureter, 202, *203*
 of uterine fibroids, 17–19, *18*
 of uterine leiomyomata, 231, *233*
 of uterine leiomyomata, *238–240*
 of uterine myoma with pregnancy, *237*
 of uterine retroposition, *230*
 of uterus and vagina, normal *204, 228–230*
 of uterus following cesarean section, 228, *231, 232*

Sonogram (*Continued*)
 of yawning by fetus, *162*
 of yolk sac, 7–8, *9*, 45
Spina bifida, 109–112, *111*
Spine, fetal, *48, 54, 84–85, 86*
 open defect of, *111*
 pathologic lesions of, 108–112
Spleen, fetal, *49*
Startle reaction, 165
Stomach, fetal, *48, 49, 53, 54*
Stress, to fetus and growth retardation, 160
Surgery, fetal, technique of, 179–183, *181*

Teratoma, cervical, in fetus, 61, *62*
 malignant, of ovary, *218*
Tests, pregnancy, 293–294, 293(t)
 causes of false-positive results, 293(t)
Testes, fetal, 57
Thanatophoric dysplasia, 88, *90, 91*
Thigh, fetal, circumference of, as index of fetal growth, 128–131, *129, 130,* 131(t)
 normal circumference of, 131(t)
Thorax, fetal abnormalities of, 61–67
 small, in thanatophoric dwarfism, *91*
Theca lutein cysts, in gestational trophoblastic disease, 262–263, *262*
Thumb, fetal, *83*
Tibia, fetal, *82, 84*
Tissues, reactions of to ultrasound, 314–315, *316, 317*
Toes, polydactyly of, *94*
Tomography, computed, digital radiographs and, in pelvimetry, 308–310, *308, 309*
Transducers, for ultrasound, 315–319, *317–322*
 real-time, 317–319, *319–321*
Transplant, renal, pelvic infections and, 284–285, *285*
Trimester, of pregnancy, first, ultrasound in, 1–19
Trophoblastic disease, gestational, 259–270. See also *Gestational trophoblastic disease.*
Trunk, fetal, size of as index of intrauterine growth retardation, 124–128. See also *Circumference, abdominal.*
Tube, fallopian. See *Fallopian tube; Tubo-ovarian abscess.*
Tuberculosis, pelvic infections and, 285–286
Tubo-ovarian abscess, *218, 272, 272, 273, 277*
Tumors. See also *Carcinoma; Choriocarcinoma; Gestational trophoblastic disease; Neoplasm.*
 ovarian, cystic, 215–222
  solid, 222, *222*
Twins. See Gestation, multiple.

Ulna, fetal, 82, *83*
Ultrasonography. See also *Sonogram; Ultrasound.*
Ultrasound. See also *Sonogram.*
Ultrasound, acoustic shadowing in, and intrauterine contraceptive devices, 250–251, *252–253*
 advantages and disadvantages of various imaging systems in, 323, 323(t)
 amniocentesis and 169–175, 172(t)

Ultrasound (*Continued*)
  beam diameter for, 315, *318*
  biparietal diameter measurements in, 24, 25–33. See also *Biparietal diameter.*
  characterization of trophoblastic disease by, 269–270
  crown-rump length determinations by, 24–25, *25, 26,* 26(t)
  echocardiography and, 174–175, *174, 175*
  entrance-exit reflections of intrauterine contraceptive devices and, 251, *254*
  femur length determinations in, 24, 34, *35,* 36(t)
  fetal breathing activity and, 36–37
  fetoscopy and, 173–174, 173(t)
  focusing in, 318, *320*
  for measuring fetal extremities, 85–87
  gestational sac measurements and, 24–25, *25*
  in assessing fetal growth profile, 120–137
  in detecting intrauterine contraceptive devices, 249–257
  in detecting intrauterine growth retardation, 119–138
  in diagnosing pelvic inflammatory disease, future of, 287
  in estimation of gestational age, 24–37
  in evaluating ectopic pregnancy, 291–303
  in evaluating fetal behavior and condition, 159–175
  in evaluating gestational trophoblastic disease, 259–270
  in evaluating normal and abnormal fetal neural axis, 97–112
  in evaluating normal fetal growth, 113–119
  in evaluating pelvic infections, 271–288
    technical considerations, 286–287
  in evaluating placenta, 141–156
  in limb reduction abnormalities, 92–94
  in perinatal management of correctable defects, 177–192
  in pregnancy, in first trimester, 1–19
    abnormal findings, 13–19
    normal findings, 3–13
  in short-limbed bone dysplasias, 87–91
  instrumentation for, 319–324, *321–323*
    physical principles of, 313–324
  modes of, 317–319, *320*
  normal fetal anatomy on, 41–58
  of fetal abnormalities involving thorax and abdomen, 61–78
  of fetal bone fractures of hypomineralization, 94–96, *95*
  of fetal heart and respiratory system, 64–67, *65–68*
  of fetal skeleton, 81–96
    normal and pathologic 81–96
  of fetus, technique of, 41–44, *42, 43*
  of gastrointestinal tract abnormalities, 67–72
  of genitourinary tract abnormalities, 72–77
  of normal female pelvis, 193–207
  of ovary, 209–224
  of uterus, 227–246
  reflection and scattering of pulses in, 313–314, *314*
  role of in prenatal diagnostic procedures, 169–175
  tissue interactions in, 314–315, *316, 317*
  transducers for, 315–319, *317–322*
    real-time, 317–319, *319–321*

Umbilical artery, 57, *58*
Umbilical cord, 54–57, *58*
  hernia of, 71
  insertion of into placenta, *148,* 149–150, *149*
Umbilical vein, 47–50, *48–54*
  size of, as index of fetal growth, 124–125, *125, 126*
Ureter, normal female, *194,* 199–201, *201–203*
Urethra, obstruction of, 74, *75*
  in fetus, developmental consequences of, *180,* 182
Ureterostomy, in fetus with hydronephrosis, *186*
Urinary ascites, fetal, 74–75, *75*
Urinary bladder, fetal, 50–51, *56*
  normal female, *194–196,* 201–204, *203*
Urinary tract, fetal, malformation of, treatment plan, *180*
Uterus, acquired disorders of, 236–245
  adenomyosis of, 242–243, *243*
  bicornuate, with pregnancy, *237*
  carcinoma of, cervical, 241, *241*
    endometrial, 239–241, *240*
  cervix of, incompetent, *243, 244,* 245
    normal length of, *244,* 245
  changes in, in ectopic pregnancy, 295–299, *295–299*
  changes in size and shape of, 13
  congenital anomalies of, sonogram of, 17, *17*
  contour of, 228–229, *231, 232*
  developmental variants of, 232–236, *236, 237*
  double, 17, *17*
  echo of central cavity of, 229–232, *229, 232, 235*
  endometrial hyperplasia of, 242
  endometrial adenomatous hyperplasia of, 231, *235*
  fibroids of, 18, *18*
  following cesarean section, 228, *231, 232*
  gas in, 231, *235*
  hydrometra of, 243–245
  indistinct contours of, 228, *232*
  involuting, *286*
  leiomyomata of, 228, *231, 233,* 236–239, *238–240*
  leiomyosarcoma of, 241
  nabothian cyst of, 229, *232*
  neoplastic diseases of, 236–242
    differentiation between benign and malignant, 241–242, *242*
  nonneoplastic disorders of, 242–245
  normal, 204–205, *204*
  normal sonographic appearance of, 227, *228–230*
  position of, 227, *228*
  retroposition of, 228, *230*
  shape of, 227–228, *228, 229, 230*
  size of, 227, *228*
  sonography of, 227–246, *228–230*
  texture of, 228–229

Vagina, normal, 204–205, *204*
Vein, hepatic, fetal, *52*
  of abdomen, fetal, 47, *48–54*
  portal, fetal, *52*

Vein, hepatic, fetal (*Continued*)
  umbilical, 47–50, *48–54*
    as index of fetal growth, 124–125, *125*, *126*
  uterine, differentiation of from abruptio placentae, 152, *154*

Weight, fetal, as index of fetal growth, 132–136, 134(t)–135(t)
  data evaluation of, 133–136, 134(t)–135(t)
  estimated, 332–336(t)
  versus biparietal diameter and abdominal circumference, 134(t)–135(t)
  infant, in intrauterine well nourished versus malnourished conditions, *119*

X-ray pelvimetry, 306–308, *307*
  indications for, 307
  technique of, 308

Yawning, by fetus, *162*
Yolk sac, *2*, *3*, 45
  sonogram of, 7–8, *9*

Zygote, development of, 1, *2*